Contents

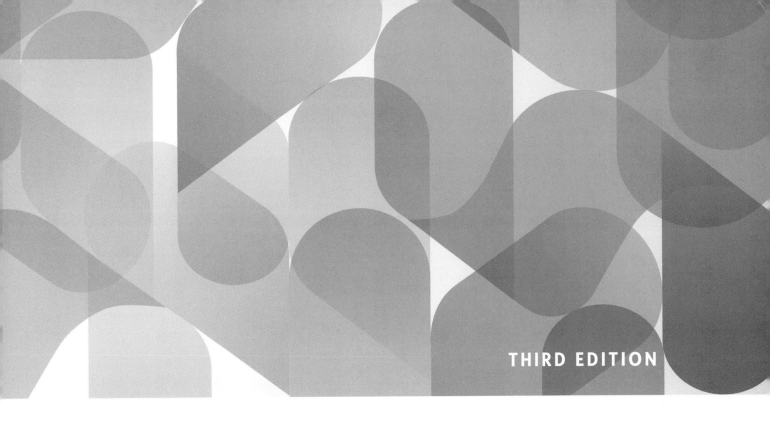

THIRD EDITION

FAMILY NURSE PRACTITIONER
CERTIFICATION REVIEW

JoAnn Zerwekh, EdD, RN
President/CEO
Nursing Education Consultants, Inc.
Chandler, Arizona;
Director of Nursing Education
Picmonic, Inc.
Tempe, Arizona;
Faculty
University of Phoenix Online
Phoenix, Arizona

ELSEVIER

ELSEVIER

3251 Riverport Lane
St. Louis, Missouri 63043

FAMILY NURSE PRACTITIONER CERTIFICATION REVIEW,
THIRD EDITION

ISBN: 978-0-323-42819-4

Notices

Knowledge and best practice in this field are constantly changing. As new research and experience broaden our understanding, changes in research methods, professional practices, or medical treatments may become necessary.

Practitioners and researchers must always rely on their own experience and knowledge in evaluating and using any information, methods, compounds, or experiments described herein. In using such information or methods, they should be mindful of their own safety and the safety of others, including parties for whom they have a professional responsibility.

With respect to any drug or pharmaceutical products identified, readers are advised to check the most current information provided (i) on procedures featured or (ii) by the manufacturer of each product to be administered, to verify the recommended dose or formula, the method and duration of administration, and contraindications. It is the responsibility of practitioners, relying on their own experience and knowledge of their patients, to make diagnoses, to determine dosages and the best treatment for each individual patient, and to take all appropriate safety precautions.

To the fullest extent of the law, neither the Publisher nor the authors, contributors, or editors, assume any liability for any injury and/or damage to persons or property as a matter of products liability, negligence or otherwise, or from any use or operation of any methods, products, instructions, or ideas contained in the material herein.

Library of Congress Cataloging-in-Publication Data

Names: Zerwekh, JoAnn Graham, author.
Title: Family nurse practitioner certification review / JoAnn Zerwekh.
Description: Third edition. | St. Louis, Missouri : Elsevier Inc., [2017] |
    Includes bibliographical references.
Identifiers: LCCN 2016030999 (print) | LCCN 2016031841 (ebook) | ISBN
    9780323428194 (pbk. : alk. paper) | ISBN 9780323428132 (Ebook)
Subjects: | MESH: Family Nurse Practitioners--education | Nursing Process |
    Certification | United States | Examination Questions
Classification: LCC RT120.F34 (print) | LCC RT120.F34 (ebook) | NLM WY 18.2 |
    DDC 610.73076--dc23
LC record available at https://lccn.loc.gov/2016030999

Executive Content Strategist: Lee Henderson
Content Development Manager: Laurie Gower
Associate Content Development Specialist: Elizabeth Fifer
Publishing Services Manager: Hemamalini Rajendrababu
Project Manager: Manchu Mohan
Designer: Brian Salisbury

Printed in United States of America.

Last digit is the print number: 9 8 7 6 5 4 3 2 1

Working together
to grow libraries in
developing countries

www.elsevier.com • www.bookaid.org

About the Author

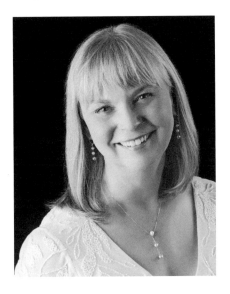

JoAnn Zerwekh has worked as a family nurse practitioner at Carondelet Health Care primary health care clinics in southern Arizona. She taught FNP students at the University of Phoenix and worked for a brief period of time as the advance practice consultant for the Arizona Board of Nursing. She is the author of numerous publications, including *Nursing Today: Transition & Trends*, NCLEX® RN and PN review books, and the popular Memory NoteCards of Nursing and Memory Notebooks of Nursing. She is the President/CEO of Nursing Education Consultants and is the Director of Nursing Education for Picmonic, the visual learning community for nursing and medical students.

KAREN ABATE, PhD, APRN-BC, FNAP
Family Nurse Practitioner
Simmons College
Boston, Massachusetts

CAROL BAFALOUKOS, DNP, WHNP-BC, MSN
Program Manager MSN/FNP
University of Phoenix
Tempe, Arizona

COURTNEY BETTS, ANP-BC
Adult Nurse Practitioner
New England Community Medical Services
North Andover, Massachusetts

WENDY BIDDLE, PhD, RN, MSN, FNP-BC
Program Director MSN-FNP Program
College of Nursing and Public Health
South University
Virginia Beach, Virginia

LYNN BLACKBURN, DNP, APRN, WHNP-BC
Clinical Assistant Professor
University of Tennessee, College of Nursing
Knoxville, Tennessee

JANEEN DAHN, PhD, RN, FNP-C
Faculty
School of Nursing
University of Phoenix
Phoenix, Arizona

SHARON K. DAVIS, DNP, APRN, WHNP-BC
Clinical Assistant Professor
Interim Chair Doctor of Nursing Practice Program
College of Nursing
University of Tennessee
Knoxville, Tennessee

JOHN DISTLER, DPA, MBA, MS, FNP-C, FAANP
Dean Nurse Practitioner Tracks
Chamberlain College of Nursing
Downers Grove, Illinois

THERESA J. FRIMEL, FNP-C
Provider
Arthritis Health Limited; Rheumatology
Scottsdale, Arizona

ASHLEY GARNEAU, PhD, RN
Nursing Faculty
GateWay Community College
Phoenix, Arizona

MELLISA HALL, DNP, AGPCNP-BC, FNP-BC
Chair
Graduate Nursing Department
University of Southern Indiana
Evansville, Indiana

ELAINE KAUSCHINGER, PhD, MS, ARNP, FNP-BC
Family Nurse Practitioner/Assistant Professor
School of Nursing
Duke University
Durham, North Carolina

PETER MELENOVICH, PhD, RN, CCRN, CNE
Nursing Faculty
GateWay Community College
Phoenix, Arizona

CATHERINE (KATIE) O'KEEFE, DNP, APRN-NP, CPNP-PC
Associate Professor and NP Curriculum Coordinator
College of Nursing
Creighton University
Omaha, Nebraska

COL. RICHARD M. PRIOR, DNP, FNP-BC, FAANP
Chief Nursing Officer
Ireland Army Community Hospital
Fort Knox, Kentucky

MARYLOU V. ROBINSON, PhD, FNP-C
Associate Professor
College of Nursing
University of Colorado
Aurora, Colorado

RUTH K. ROSENBLUM, DNP, RN, PNP-BC
Assistant Professor
School of Nursing
San José State University;
Pediatric Nurse Practitioner, Child Neurology
Department of Pediatrics
Santa Clara Valley Medical Center
San Jose, California

ERICH WIDEMARK, PhD, RN, FNP-BC
Director of Simulation Education
College of Health Professions, School of Nursing
University of Phoenix
Tempe, Arizona

Reviewers

ROBIN WEBB CORBETT, PhD, RNC, FNP-BC
Associate Professor
Interim Chair – Graduate Nursing Science
College of Nursing
East Carolina University
Greenville, North Carolina

DIANE DADDARIO, MSN, ANP-C, ACNS-BC, RN-BC, CMSRN
Adjunct Faculty, RN to BSN Program
Pennsylvania State University
University Park, Pennsylvania

KARI GALI, DNP, CNP
Pediatric Nurse Practitioner
Cleveland Clinic
Department of Clinical Transformation
Cleveland, Ohio;
Quality Improvement Scholar and Patient Safety
Leadership Program Instructor
College of Medicine
University of Illinois-Chicago
Chicago, Illinois

SHELLEY Y. HAWKINS, PhD, FNP-BC, GNP, FAANP
Associate Professor and Director
DNP & MSN Nurse Practitioner Programs
Hahn School of Nursing & Health Science
University of San Diego
San Diego, California

KATHLEEN S. JORDAN, DNP, MS, RN, FNP-BC, ENP-BC, SANE-P
Clinical Assistant Professor
UNC Charlotte School of Nursing;
Nurse Practitioner
Mid-Atlantic Emergency Medicine Associates
Charlotte, North Carolina

SARAH E. MANNLE, DNP, FNP-C
Assistant Professor
DNP Program Director
School of Nursing
Western Carolina University
Asheville, North Carolina

LUCY MAYS, DNP, APRN, FNP-BC, CNE
Coordinator of Online Nursing Programs
Morehead State University
Morehead, Kentucky

PAULA D. RUEDEBUSCH, DNP, ARNP, FNP-BC, MSN, BSN, RN
Clinical Assistant Professor
Psychosocial and Community Health
University of Washington
Seattle, Washington

VIRGINIA B. SCHNEIDER, MSN, Ed, FNP-BC
Academic Chair – Nursing IV
Associate Professor of Nursing
St. Petersburg College of Nursing
St. Petersburg, Florida

MICHELE WALTERS, DNP, APRN, FNP-BC, CNE
Associate Professor of Nursing
Morehead State University
St. Claire Regional Medical Center
Morehead, Kentucky

Preface

With the proliferation of new DNP programs, there is an increasing need for additional reference information and study materials for the certification examinations. Nurse practitioners are playing a vital role in the health care delivery system in the United States. With the assistance of certified nurse practitioners and my editorial expertise in test item writing, *Family Nurse Practitioner Certification Review*, Third Edition, has been developed to assist the advanced practice nurse to prepare for the FNP certification exam. Extensive efforts have been made to include current information that is representative of the content, based on the blueprints for the certification exams. This book of questions is not intended to be an exhaustive review of the content but an adjunct to the review process.

Test-taking strategies are included in Chapter 1. As a candidate prepares for the exam, it is vitally important to be familiar with and to practice good testing strategies. Testing strategies can prevent the candidate from making mistakes and selecting the wrong answer. As the review process begins, a review of the test-taking strategies chapter and the practice of good testing strategies is critical. With many years' experience in the field of testing, I consistently have identified the importance that practice testing plays in the review process. Practice questions give the candidate an opportunity to review questions written from different perspectives. To enhance the review process, answers with complete rationales are provided at the end of each chapter, along with a reference list. Not only does the candidate increase his/her knowledge of the subject area, but also, with more practice, testing skills become fine-tuned. Good testing skills make the candidate more comfortable and help decrease the stress associated with certification exams.

This book also includes chapters reviewing important concepts related to Growth & Development and Health Promotion & Maintenance. These chapters provide questions that test information related to growth and development, general health supervision, and health maintenance. The clinical chapters are developed using a systems approach (i.e., cardiovascular, respiratory, endocrine, etc.). In each of these chapters, the test questions are divided into three areas: Physical Examination & Diagnostic Tests, Disorders, and Pharmacology. This format assists the candidate to easily locate specific questions. Separate content chapters on mental health, pediatrics, and maternity are included. The last two chapters in the text are on Research & Theory and Professional Issues. The test questions in these chapters focus on professional competencies inherent in the role and function of the FNP.

My thanks to the many nurse practitioners across the country who provided questions and insight into the role of the nurse practitioner. I wish to thank Elizabeth Fifer, our Content Development Specialist at Elsevier, for her support and suggestions in the preparation of the manuscript. Thank you also goes to the nurse practitioners who took time from their busy schedules to review the questions for content correctness and clarity.

Acknowledgments

I want to express my appreciation to Lee Henderson at Elsevier and his "can-do" attitude that made the realization of this third edition possible.

I am especially grateful to the many people at Elsevier who assisted with this major revision effort, including the folks who have assisted with the online practice exams and the alternate item formats. In particular, I want to thank Elizabeth Fifer and Laurie Gower in Content, Manchu Mohan in Production, Kate Odem in Marketing, and Brian Salisbury in Design.

I want to thank the contributors and reviewers for their assistance in the revision process. Your current practice and clinical expertise is surely noted in your contribution to updating this edition.

I am particularly appreciative to the many nurse practitioners who used the previous editions to pass their certification exams and faculty who have requested a new edition of this test question review book.

And last, I want to thank my husband, John Masog, for his tolerance and sense of humor as I continued to work on a revision of another book! Thank you so much for the awesome meals you prepare for us and snatching me away from the computer for a round of golf—I appreciate the balance you bring to my life.

A special note to my amazing grandchildren (Maddie and Harper Zerwekh; Ben Garneau; Brooklyn and Alexis Parks; Owen and Emmet Masog) who have such bright futures; you always put a smile on Grandma's face and make her proud.

JoAnn Zerwekh

Contents

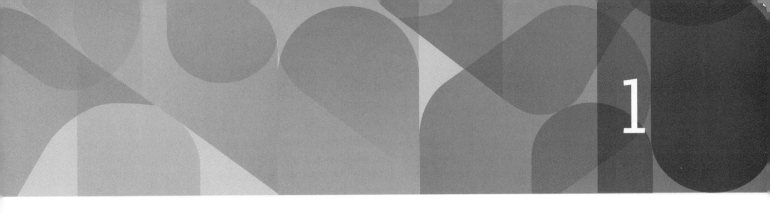

Test-Taking Strategies

Certification Exam Information

For the family nurse practitioner certification exam, there are two credentialing bodies, the American Nurses Credentialing Center (ANCC) and the American Academy of Nurse Practitioners Certification Board (AANPCP). Both groups provide detailed information in handbooks available for download at their respective websites. This information includes the application process, testing procedure, test content outline, bibliography of references, and other relevant information for the exam candidate. Certification from both agencies is recognized by the U.S. Department of Veterans Affairs, Centers for Medicare & Medicaid (CMS), health insurance companies, the National Council State Boards of Nursing (NCSBN), and state boards of nursing. Both exams are computer based, and the candidate will schedule the exam at a designated testing center.

ANCC

The ANCC certification exam consists of multiple-choice test questions, drag and drop (ordered response or a proper sequence), hot spot (click on a particular feature or area of a graphic image), and multiple responses (asked to select a specific number of correct responses). There are a total of 200 questions on the family nurse practitioner exam with 175 items scored and 25 pilot test items that do not count toward the final score. The passing score is a scale score of 350 or higher. The raw score (number of test items answered correctly, e.g., 122 out of 175) is converted to a scale score using a conversion formula before the results are given to the exam candidate at the testing site. Candidates who successfully complete the ANCC certification exam may use the credential Family Nurse Practitioner-Board Certified (FNP-BC).

AANPCP

Each AANPCP exam consists of 150 multiple-choice questions (135 test items are scored and 15 pretest items are not counted in the final score). A "preliminary" exam score is provided to the candidate at the completion of the exam. The scaled score ranges from 200 to 800 points with a minimum passing score of 500. Candidates who successfully complete the AANPCP certification exam may use the credential Nurse Practitioner-Certified (NP-C).

Testing Strategies

Knowing how to take an exam is a skill that is developed through practice and experience. Being able to take an exam effectively is almost as important as the basic knowledge required to answer the question. Everyone has taken an exam only to find in the review of the exam that questions were missed because of inadequate testing skills.

Nurse practitioner programs provide the graduate student with a comprehensive base of knowledge; how you utilize this knowledge will determine your success on a certification exam. The certification exam is an objective test that covers knowledge, understanding, and application of professional nursing theory and practice.

Read the information in this chapter carefully to make sure you understand the strategies discussed. This chapter is designed to help you identify problem areas in testing skills and learn how to use strategy and judgment in selecting correct answers. It is important for you to practice testing skills if you are going to be able to utilize these skills on the certification exam.

1. Do not read extra meaning into the question. The question is asking for specific information; if it appears to be simple "common sense," then assume it is simple. Do not look for a hidden meaning in what appears to be an easy question.

> **EXAMPLE**
>
> The family nurse practitioner understands that the most common form of facial paralysis in the adult patient is:
>
> 1. Facial nerve fasciitis.
> 2. Trigeminal neuralgia.
> 3. Bell's palsy.
> 4. Herpes zoster.

The correct answer is Option #3. Be careful not to "read into" the question and add pain to the facial paralysis symptom. Instead, concentrate on the question's key words, "the most common form of facial paralysis," which is Bell's palsy, a disorder that affects the facial nerve and is characterized by muscle flaccidity of the affected side of the face. Trigeminal neuralgia is a disorder of cranial nerve V that is characterized by an abrupt onset of pain in the lower and upper jaw, cheek, and lips. Herpes zoster affects the dermatomes and does not cause a paralysis but rather pain, herpetic grouped skin vesicles, and possibly postherpetic neuralgia.

2. Read the stem correctly. Make sure you understand exactly what information the question is asking. It is important to understand the question before reviewing the options for the correct answer.

EXAMPLE

The family nurse practitioner would refer a child with the following findings to a pediatric cardiologist for workup and evaluation in 1–2 weeks:

1. Signs of exercise intolerance, dyspnea, and elevated pulse.
2. Poor feeding, increased cyanosis with crying, and dizziness.
3. Nonfunctional heart murmur, respiratory crackles, and retarded growth and development.
4. Systolic ejection murmur, grade II, which disappears on sitting.

The question asks you to determine which child's symptoms would require a referral to a pediatric cardiologist in the next 1–2 weeks. Options #1, #2, and #3 are considered unstable and acute and should be immediately referred to a pediatric cardiologist. Option #4 is not considered an emergency, as long as the child who has the murmur is asymptomatic, has normal activity and exercise, and is growing normally.

3. Before considering the options, think about the characteristics of the condition and the critical concepts to consider. Begin by assessing each option with regard to the concepts of the condition.

EXAMPLE

A mother who is 3 days' postpartum has been complaining of soreness and fullness in her breasts and that she wants to stop breast-feeding her infant until her breasts feel better. The family nurse practitioner:

1. Shows the patient how to apply a breast binder to decrease the discomfort and the production of milk.
2. Tells the patient that breast fullness may be a sign of infection and to stop breast-feeding.
3. Suggests to the patient that she decrease her fluid intake for the next 24 hours to suppress lactation temporarily.
4. Explains to the patient that the breast discomfort is normal and that the infant's sucking will promote the flow of milk.

Formulate in your mind critical information for the care of this patient. Think to yourself, "Is it normal to have fullness and soreness in the breasts during the first 3 days of lactation?" If you are unsure, go back and reassess the question. In this instance Option #4 is

correct. Initially, breast soreness may occur for about 2–3 minutes during each feeding until the let-down reflex is established.

4. Identify what type of response the question is asking. A positive stem requires identification of three false items and one correct answer.

EXAMPLE

How soon after exposure should patients who believe they have been exposed to human immunodeficiency virus (HIV) have an HIV antibody test?

1. The next day and 2 months later.
2. 6 months after exposure and again at 12 months.
3. 6–12 weeks after exposure and again at 6 months.
4. 4 weeks and 12 weeks later.

The correct answer is Option #3. This question requires you to identify three incorrect responses and one correct response. The HIV antibody develops between 6 and 12 weeks after exposure. Because of the variability of antibody development, it is recommended that the test be repeated in 6 months to confirm the findings.

5. Identify questions that require identification of something the family nurse practitioner should not or would not do (i.e., an unsafe action, contraindication, or inappropriate action).

EXAMPLE

An older adult patient is diagnosed with chronic open-angle glaucoma. The patient has a past history of bradycardia and first-degree atrioventricular block. In consideration of her treatment, what medication is to be avoided?

1. Pilocarpine (Isopto Carpine).
2. Timolol (Timoptic).
3. Hydrochlorothiazide (HydroDiuril).
4. Acetazolamide (Diamox).

The correct answer is Option #2. Topical beta blockers, such as timolol, lower intraocular pressure but can be absorbed systemically. The major side effects are similar to those associated with systemic beta-blocker therapy, which can include a worsening of heart failure, bradycardia, and heart block. Topical beta blockers are contraindicated in some patients who have cardiac or pulmonary disease.

6. Questions may also be analytical. These questions may ask the nurse practitioner to identify findings and statements that are consistent or inconsistent with the patient's presenting problem and/or differentiate between them.

EXAMPLE

A child is being evaluated for attention deficit hyperactivity disorder (ADHD). Which test is helpful in evaluating the difference between ADHD and a learning disability?

1. Standardized IQ achievement test.
2. Denver Developmental Screening Test.
3. Audiologic and visual testing.
4. Complete neurologic exam.

Before you examine the options in this question, it is important to think about the differences between ADHD and learning disabilities. The correct answer is Option #1. Children who have learning disabilities and ADHD are often impulsive, inattentive, and overactive. Usually, children with ADHD do not have lower IQ achievement scores; however, children with a learning disability usually demonstrate a level of educational achievement substantially below that of the IQ.

7. Identify key words that affect your understanding of the question. Make sure you understand exactly what information the question is asking. Be aware of questions in the stem such as *except, contraindicated, avoid, least, not applicable,* and *does not occur.* These words change the direction of the question. It may help to rephrase the question in your own words to better understand what information is being requested.

EXAMPLE

A patient complains of intolerable itching in the pubic hair. On exam, the family nurse practitioner notes erythematous papules and tiny white specks in the pubic hair. The differential diagnosis includes all except:

1. Pediculosis pubis.
2. Scabies.
3. Impetigo.
4. Atopic dermatitis.

Rephrase the question and look for the three conditions associated with itching, "What are the three differential diagnoses for pruritus or itching in the pubic hair?" Intense itching is characteristic of pediculosis pubis, scabies, and atopic dermatitis. Impetigo starts out as a tender erythematous papule and progresses through a vesicular to a honey-crusted stage with no itching. The correct answer is Option #3, because impetigo is not in the differential diagnosis with conditions that are characterized by itching.

8. As you read the options, eliminate the options you know are not correct. This will help narrow the field of choice. When you select an answer or eliminate a distracter, you should have a specific reason for doing so. Do not try to predict a correct answer; it is distressing if the answer you want is not a selection.

EXAMPLE

A 45-year-old female patient complains of knee pain while kneeling and a "clicking" noise when walking up steps. On exam, there is a slight knee effusion and tenderness when palpating the patella against the condyles. The diagnosis for this patient is:

1. Anterior cruciate tear. (No, the patient generally cannot bear weight on the extremity without its buckling or giving way.)
2. Dislocated patella. (No, there would be considerable effusion and locking of the knee in flexion.)
3. Chondromalacia patella. (Yes, there is clicking and anterior knee pain around or under the kneecap, aggravated by knee extensor stress.)
4. Patellar tendonitis. (No, there would be no clicking sound with movement.)

After systematically evaluating the options, Option #3 is the correct answer.

9. Identify similarities in the distracters. Frequently, three distracters will contain similar information, and one will be different. The different one may be the correct answer.

EXAMPLE

An older adult patient is encouraged to increase protein intake. The addition of which of these foods to 100 mL of milk will provide the greatest amount of protein?

1. 50 mL of light cream and 2 tbsp of corn syrup.
2. 30 g of powdered skim milk and 1 egg.
3. 1 small scoop (90 g) of ice cream and 1 tbsp of chocolate syrup.
4. 2 egg yolks and 1 tbsp of sugar.

Options #1, #3, and #4 all contain a simple sugar. The correct answer, Option #2, has the greatest amount of protein. Notice that three of the options are similar and the one that is different is the correct answer. This strategy is not a substitute for basic knowledge but may help you figure out the answer.

10. Select the most comprehensive answer. All options may be correct, but one will include the other three options or will need to be considered first.

EXAMPLE

A new mother tells the family nurse practitioner that her infant was born HIV positive. She asks the family nurse practitioner how long her baby has to live. The family nurse practitioner's response would be based on the knowledge that:

1. The antibodies present in the baby's blood may reflect the antibodies received from the mother at birth.
2. If antibodies are present at birth, the baby has AIDS in an active form.
3. Although the baby is HIV positive, the child will develop AIDS within 3 years.
4. The antibodies detected at birth indicate the presence of the HIV; the test does not indicate whether the child will develop AIDS.

The correct answer is Option #4. It is important to give the mother as much hope as possible but still be realistic about the condition. There is no way to tell whether the child will develop active AIDS, and many infants seroconvert to HIV-negative status.

11. Select the best answer that is most specific to what the question asks. All options may be correct, but one is more specific or essential to the question being asked.

EXAMPLE

When a child visits a health maintenance clinic, what is essential for the family nurse practitioner to do?

1. Order routine laboratory tests.
2. Perform vision and auditory screening.
3. Plot height and weight on charts.
4. Review immunization record.

The correct answer is Option #4. The other alternatives may be correct but should be prioritized. It is absolutely essential that the immunization record be reviewed. The other options are important but are not essential for a health maintenance visit. Recognize key words that identify the question that is asking for a priority of care—first, initial, essential, best, and most.

12. Watch questions in which the options contain several items to consider. After you are sure you understand what information the question is requesting, evaluate each part of the option. Is it appropriate to what the question is asking? If an option contains one incorrect item, the entire option is incorrect. All items listed in the selection must be correct if the option is to be the answer to the question.

EXAMPLE

Which diagnostic tests are typically abnormal when ruling in systemic lupus erythematosus (SLE) as a differential diagnosis?

1. Complete blood count (CBC), electrolyte panel, and erythrocyte sedimentation rate (ESR).
2. Chest x-ray and coagulation profile.
3. Antinuclear antibodies (ANA), ESR, and C-reactive protein.
4. CBC, urinalysis (UA), and chest x-ray.

The correct answer is Option #3. In a methodical evaluation of the diagnostic tests in the options, you can eliminate Options #1, #2, and #4. Although all tests included in the answer may be included in a complete physical exam, the laboratory test specific to the diagnosis of SLE includes the ANA, ESR, and C-reactive protein. During flares, ESR and C-reactive protein are elevated. The ANA titer in a patient with SLE is positive at a 1:80 ratio.

13. Be alert to relevant information contained in previous questions. Sometimes as you are answering questions, you will find information similar to the question being tested. Previous questions may assist you in identifying relevant information in the current question. This strategy is particularly helpful when you are answering paper-and-pencil tests.

EXAMPLE

The Advisory Committee of Immunization Practices (ACIP) recommends that healthy older adults receive the Tdap vaccination:

1. Every 5 years.
2. At age 75.
3. At age 65.
4. Every 10 years.

The correct answer to this question is Option #3. On February 22, 2012, ACIP approved the use of Tdap (tetanus toxoid, reduced diphtheria toxoid, and acellular pertussis) for all adults aged 65 years and older. Boostrix should be used for adults aged 65 years and older; however, ACIP concluded that either vaccine (Boostrix or Adacel) administered to a person 65 years or older is immunogenic and would provide protection. In another question involving immunizations, you read the question in the next example.

EXAMPLE

In taking the history of an alert older adult, the family nurse practitioner determines the patient is an avid gardener and spends much time outside. The patient had a pneumococcal vaccination last year but cannot remember whether a tetanus vaccination was ever administered. A health maintenance recommendation for this patient would be to obtain:

1. Pneumococcal vaccine.
2. Tdap/Td vaccine.
3. Hepatitis B vaccine.
4. No recommendation.

The correct answer is Option #2. A clue to the correct answer may be found in the previous question. Older adults who enjoy gardening and outdoor activities should have a Tdap/Td booster once, as recommended by the ACIP. As part of standard wound management care to prevent tetanus, a tetanus toxoid–containing vaccine might be recommended for wound management in adults aged 19 years and older if 5 years or more have elapsed since last receiving the vaccine. If a tetanus booster is indicated, Tdap is preferred over Td for wound management in adults aged 19 years and older who have not received Tdap previously.

When you are taking the test on a computer, it is more difficult to remember previous questions because you may not be able to go back and change answers or review previous questions; therefore, this strategy is often most helpful for when you are taking paper-and-pencil tests.

14. Multiple-choice mathematic computations may be included in the exam. Mathematic computations may include calculations of IM, PO, and IV dosages; calculations of pediatric dosage; determining creatinine clearance; and conversion of units of measurement.

EXAMPLE

The family nurse practitioner is ordering amoxicillin (Amoxil) for a 15-month-old child who has otitis media. The child weighs 22 lb. How would the order be written?

1. Amoxicillin 250 mg/5 mL Sig: 5 mL PO tid × 10 days.
2. Amoxicillin 500 mg Sig: 1 tab PO tid × 3 days.
3. Amoxicillin 350 mg/5 mL Sig: 5 mL PO bid × 14 days.
4. Amoxicillin 125 mg/5 mL Sig: 5 mL PO tid × 10 days.

The correct answer is Option #4. First, you must convert pounds (lb) to kilograms (kg). By using the formula 2.2 lb = 1 kg, the child who weighs 22 lb is 10 kg (22 lb ÷ 2.2 = 10 kg). The dose for amoxicillin is 20–40 mg/kg/day given every 8 hours for a child older than 3 months and less than 40 kg. 10 kg × 40 mg/kg/day = 400 mg/day. Dosing 3 times a day would be approximately 133 mL for each dose. Amoxicillin is supplied in 125 mg/5 mL. The easiest to administer for the parent and closest correct dose for this child would be the 5 mL PO every 8 hours.

15. Evaluate priority questions carefully. Frequently, all answers are appropriate to the situation. You need to decide which actions you should do first.

While attending a rural public school, a 7-year-old child was bitten on the hand by a raccoon. At the rural clinic, the family nurse practitioner cleansed the wound. The next action is:

1. Administer tetanus antitoxin.
2. Contact local animal control authorities.
3. Administer rabies immune globulin (RIG) and human diploid cell vaccine (HDCV).
4. Teach the family how to do hourly soaks to the hand using normal saline and peroxide.

The correct answer is Option #3. Any type of animal bite that might be associated with an animal that may harbor rabies (skunks, bats, raccoons, foxes, coyotes, rats) should be treated with both active and passive rabies immunization. The priority action is to prevent rabies. Tetanus antitoxin would be indicated if the child was not current on the immunization. Animal authorities would be called after the initial treatment to locate the animal and sacrifice it so that the brain can be examined for rabies.

Techniques to Increase Critical Thinking Skills

Memory aids and Mindmapping™ are tools that assist in drawing associations from other ideas with the use of visual images. **Mnemonics** are words, phrases, or other techniques that help you remember information. **Imagery** is a tool that helps you identify a problem and visualize a mental picture. Learning content that uses these techniques will assist you to recall information more effectively.

Mindmapping™ is a method of organizing important information that is in sharp contrast to the traditional outline format. A thought or concept is written in the center of the page, and images and color are added to information as ideas begin to flow from the center focus (see Figure 1-1).

Acronyms help you recall specific information through word associations or letter arrangements. Examples of these are the "6-Ps" of dyspnea (see Figure 1-2), the "6-Ps" of circulatory assessment (see Figure 1-3), and the "ABCDE" of malignant melanoma (see Figure 1-4).

Acrostics are catchy phrases in which the first letter of each word stands for something to recall. For example, in

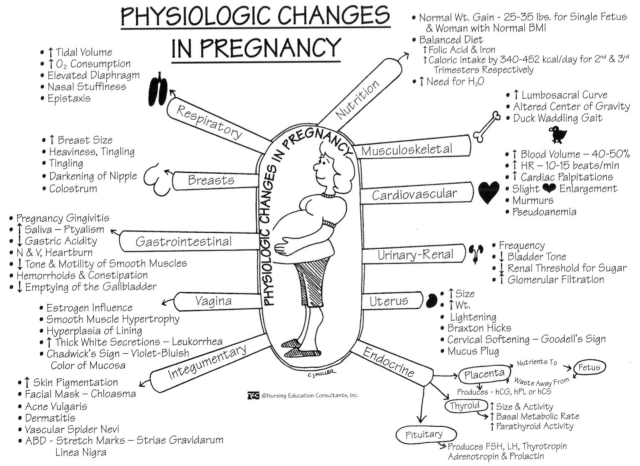

FIGURE 1-1 Example of Mindmapping™: Physiologic Changes in Pregnancy. From: Zerwekh J, Garneau A, Miller CJ: *Memory Notebook of Nursing, CD*. Chandler, AZ: Nursing Education Consultants Publishing, 2016.

remembering the use of canes and walkers, think of "Wandering Wilma's Always Late" (**W**alker **W**ith **A**ffected **L**eg) (see Figure 1-5). Everyone remembers the cranial nerve mnemonic (see Figure 1-6).

Memory aids/images are pictures or caricatures that help you recall information more effectively (see Figure 1-7).

Rhymes are phrases or words spoken in a rhythmic or musical manner that increase recall, such as the rhyme

for hypoglycemia versus hyperglycemia (see Figure 1-8). Another rhyme, "fingers, nose, penis, toes," identifies the areas where lidocaine with epinephrine is contraindicated as a local anesthetic. "Two is too much" may help you remember toxic levels of lithium, digoxin, and theophylline, which have a narrow margin of safety (see Figure 1-9). Books and electronic resources are available on these helpful aids (see References at the end of the book).

Testing Skills for Paper-and-Pencil Tests

Because your certification exams are available on computer, the following skills are applicable for **paper-and-pencil tests**, which you may encounter as a student in your program.

1. Go through the exam and mark all answers that you know are correct. This ensures you have adequate time to answer the questions you know. Then go back and evaluate those questions for which you did not readily recognize the answer.
2. Do not indiscriminately change answers. If you go back and change an answer, you should have a specific reason for doing so. You may remember information and realize you answered the question incorrectly. Frequently, test takers "talk themselves out of" the correct answer and change it to an incorrect one.
3. After you have completed the exam, go back and check your booklet to make sure all questions are answered. Be sure to answer all questions, even if you must guess at some.

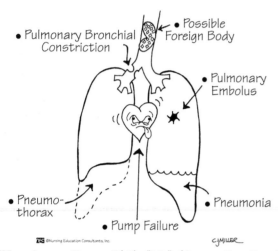

FIGURE 1-2 Acronym Memory Aid: The "6-Ps" of Dyspnea. From: Zerwekh J, Garneau A, Miller CJ: *Memory Notebook of Nursing, CD.* Chandler, AZ: Nursing Education Consultants Publishing, 2016.

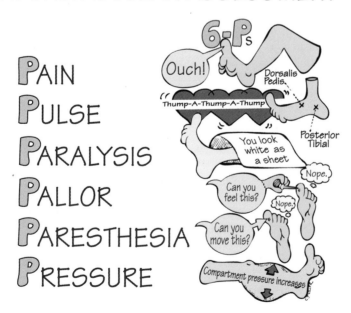

FIGURE 1-3 Circulation Assessment: The "6-Ps." From: Zerwekh J, Garneau A, Miller CJ: *Memory Notebook of Nursing, CD.* Chandler, AZ: Nursing Education Consultants Publishing, 2016.

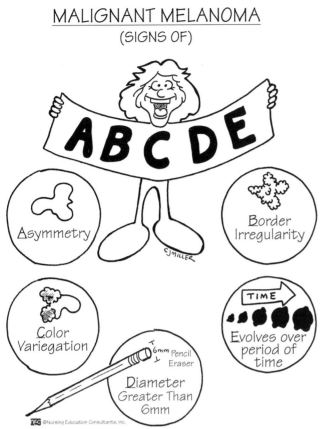

FIGURE 1-4 Indications of Possible Malignant Melanoma: "ABCDE." From: Zerwekh J, Garneau A, Miller CJ: *Memory Notebook of Nursing, CD.* Chandler, AZ: Nursing Education Consultants Publishing, 2016.

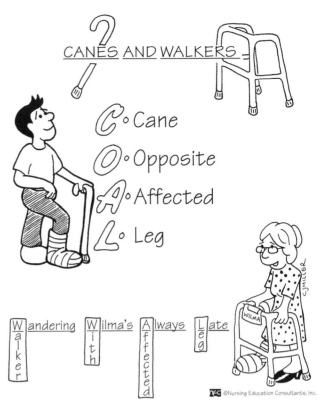

FIGURE 1-5 Mnemonics for Canes ("COAL") and Walkers ("WWAL"). From: Zerwekh J, Garneau A, Miller CJ: *Memory Notebook of Nursing, CD.* Chandler, AZ: Nursing Education Consultants Publishing, 2016.

Successful Test Taking

1. Listen carefully to the instructions given at the beginning of the exam. Make sure you understand all information given and exactly how to mark your answers and/or how to use the keyboard and mouse. Adjust the computer screen for optimum viewing.
2. Watch your timing. Do not spend too much time on one question. It is very important that you practice your timing on the sample exams. You may not be able to review your questions and answers on completion of the computerized test; therefore, watch your timing on the computerized tests, and make use of a computer clock if it is available.
3. Be aware of your "first hunch" because it is frequently the correct answer. Sometimes information is processed by the brain without your awareness. If something about an answer "feels right" or if you have a "gut feeling" about an answer, pay attention to it.
4. Eliminate options that assume the patient "would not understand" or "is ignorant of" the situation or those that "protect them from worry." For example, "The patient should not be told she has cancer because it would upset her too much."
5. Be aware of options that contain the words *always* and *never*.
6. There is no pattern of correct answers. Both computerized and paper-and-pencil exams are compiled by a computer, and the position of the correct answers is selected at random.
7. Watch the length of the options to consider. The number of words required to adequately state the correct answer is sometimes longer than the other options.

Decrease Anxiety

Your activities on the day of the exam strongly influence your level of anxiety. By carefully planning ahead, you will be able to eliminate some anxiety-provoking situations. If you are a diabetic or have special needs, contact the certification agency ahead of time to make arrangements to have accommodations that you may require.

1. Visit the exam site before the day of the exam. Evaluate travel time, parking, and time to reach the designated area. Be sure to get an early start to allow for extra time.
2. If you have to travel some distance to the exam site, try to spend the night in the immediate vicinity.
3. Do something pleasant the evening before the exam. This is not the time to "crash study."

CRANIAL NERVE MNEMONIC

S = Sensory	M = Motor	B = Both

O	Olfactory	O	On	S	Some
O	Optic	O	Old	S	Say
O	Oculomotor	O	Olympus	M	Marry
T	Trochlear	T	Towering	M	Money
T	Trigeminal	T	Tops	B	But
A	Abducens	A	A	M	My
F	Facial	F	Finn	B	Brother
A	Acoustic	A	And	S	Says
G	Glossopharyngeal	G	German	B	Bad
V	Vagus Nerve	V	Viewed	B	Business
S	Spinal	S	Some	M	Marry
H	Hypoglossal	H	Hops	M	Money

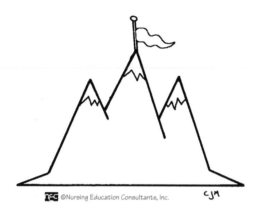
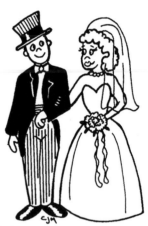

@Nursing Education Consultants, Inc.   CJM

FIGURE 1-6 Cranial Nerve Mnemonic. From: Zerwekh J, Garneau A, Miller CJ: *Memory Notebook of Nursing, CD*. Chandler, AZ: Nursing Education Consultants Publishing, 2016.

4. Anxiety is contagious. If those around you are extremely anxious, avoid contact with them before the exam.

5. Make your meal before the test a light, healthy one.

6. Avoid eating highly spiced or different foods. This is not the time for a gastrointestinal upset.

7. Wear comfortable clothes. This is not a good time to wear tight clothing or new shoes.

8. Wear clothing of moderate weight. It is difficult to control the temperature to keep everyone comfortable. Take a sweater or wear layered clothes. You may not be allowed to remove any garments once you are seated for the exam.

9. Wear soft soled shoes; this decreases the noise in the testing area.

10. Make sure you have the papers and proper identification that are required to gain admission to the exam site. If you wear reading glasses, do not forget to bring them with you.

11. Do not take study materials to the exam site. You will not be able to take such materials with you into the exam area.

12. Do not panic when you encounter content with which you are unfamiliar in a question. Use good test-taking strategies, select an answer, and continue. Remember, you are not going to know all of the correct answers.

13. Reaffirm to yourself that you know the material. It is not time for any self-defeating behavior or negative self-talk. You will pass! Build your confidence by visualizing yourself in 6 months working in the area you desire. Create that mental picture of where you want to be and who you want to be—a certified family nurse practitioner. Use your past successes to bring positive energy and "vibes" to your certification. You can do it!

HYPERTHYROIDISM

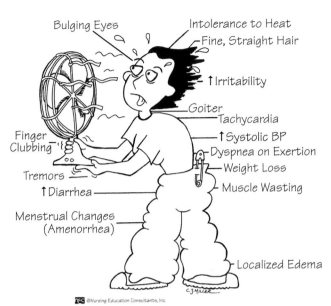

FIGURE 1-7 Image as Memory Aid for the Signs/Symptoms of Hyperthyroidism. From: Zerwekh J, Garneau A, Miller CJ: *Memory Notebook of Nursing, CD.* Chandler, AZ: Nursing Education Consultants Publishing, 2016.

BLOOD SUGAR MNEMONIC

HOT & DRY = SUGAR HIGH

COLD & CLAMMY = NEED SOME CANDY

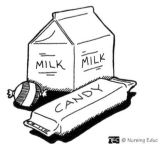

FIGURE 1-8 Blood Sugar Rhyme. From: Zerwekh J, Garneau A, Miller CJ: *Memory Notebook of Nursing, CD.* Chandler, AZ: Nursing Education Consultants Publishing, 2016.

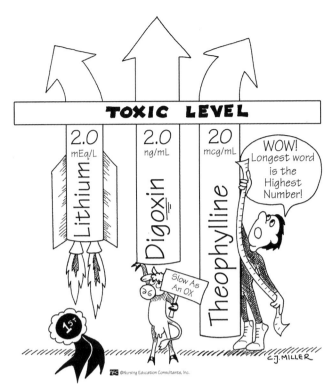

FIGURE 1-9 "Two Is Too Much": Toxic Levels of Lithium, Digoxin, and Theophylline. From: Zerwekh J, Garneau A, Miller CJ: *Memory Notebook of Nursing, CD.* Chandler, AZ: Nursing Education Consultants Publishing, 2016.

Study Habits

Enhancing Study Skills

- Decide on a realistic study schedule; write it down and stick with it.
- Divide the review material into segments—pediatrics, well woman, cardiac, and so forth.
- Prioritize the segments; review first the areas in which you seem deficient or weak.
- Identify areas that will require additional review.
- Establish a realistic schedule; study in short segments or "bursts." Avoid marathon sessions.
- Plan on achieving your study goal several days before the exam.
- Do not study when you are tired or when there are frequent distractions or interruptions.
- Review general concepts of practice from a variety of resources.

Group Study

- Keep the group limited to three to five people.
- Group members should be mature and serious about studying.
- The group should agree on the planned study schedule.
- If the group makes you anxious, or if you do not think the group meets your study needs, do not continue to participate.

Testing Practice

- Include testing practice in your schedule.
- Select about 50 questions for a practice testing session of 1 hour. This will allow you to evaluate the pace of the exam (i.e., approximately 1 question per minute).
- Try to answer the questions as if you were taking the real exam. Do not look up the correct answer immediately after answering the question. Complete all questions you have selected, and then go back and grade the questions.
- Utilize the testing strategies described in this chapter.
- Evaluate the practice exam for problem areas: testing skills and knowledge base.
- Evaluate the questions you answer incorrectly. Review the rationale for the right answer, and understand why you missed it.
- Utilize the questions at a later point to review the information again.

Growth & Development

Physical Assessment

1. The following sequence is recommended for well-child examinations up to the age of 5 years:

   1. 2 weeks, 2 months, 4 months, 6 months, 1 year, 15 months, 18 months, and every year from ages 2–5.

   2. 2 months, 4 months, 6 months, 9 months, and annually from years 1–5.

   3. 2 weeks, 2 months, 4 months, 6 months, 9 months, 12 months, 15 months, 18 months, and annually years 2–5.

   4. The same intervals recommended for immunizations.

2. An appropriate treatment for overweight children under 8 years of age would be to:

   1. Administer an appetite suppressant.

   2. Eliminate all carbohydrates in the diet.

   3. Plan a program of activity, balanced diet, and exercise.

   4. Use vitamin therapy and herbal teas.

3. The family nurse practitioner examines a 2-week-old newborn during a first clinic visit. The family nurse practitioner notes dysmorphic facial features. The family nurse practitioner's evaluation includes:

   1. Ordering a chromosome analysis.

   2. Completing a postnatal history.

   3. Writing a detailed physical exam and perinatal history.

   4. Avoiding discussion with parents until diagnostic studies are completed.

4. An 18-month-old's feet turn inward. The mother is concerned, although the child is unaware of the problem. The differential diagnosis includes all except:

   1. Femoral anteversion.

   2. Metatarsus adductus.

   3. Legg-Calvé-Perthes disease.

   4. Adducted great toe.

5. The characteristics of an innocent heart murmur in children include:

   1. Asymptomatic, loud diastolic rumble, grades I to V.

   2. Midsystolic, no thrill, and asymptomatic.

   3. Asymptomatic with an S_4 heard at lower left sternal border.

   4. May disappear on sitting and following any type of physical activity.

6. The family nurse practitioner is examining a 6-month-old infant. What would be the anticipated findings on examining the infant's fontanels?

   1. Both anterior and posterior should be open.

   2. The anterior should be open, the posterior closed.

   3. Both anterior and posterior should be closed.

   4. The anterior should be closed, the posterior open.

7. Genu varum up to 20 degrees is normal until age:

   1. 18 years.

   2. 5 years.

   3. 18 months.

   4. 6 months.

8. When approaching a toddler to complete a cardiac assessment, the family nurse practitioner would:

   1. Allow the toddler to handle the stethoscope while the history is being taken.

   2. Explain in detail what procedures will take place and get the toddler involved.

   3. Keep the child warm and covered to minimize discomfort.

   4. Approach the child by cheerfully calling out his name.

9. In performing a physical exam, the family nurse practitioner allows the child to touch the medical equipment first, and then begins by examining the extremities. This sequence would be most appropriate for a patient in what age group?

   1. Infant.

   2. Toddler.

   3. School-age child.

   4. Adolescent.

10. An appropriate test to check for color perception in a preschooler would be:

    1. Ishihara's test.

    2. Bruchner's test.

    3. Hirschberg's test.

    4. Jaeger's test.

11. When assessing the cranial nerves in a young child, the family nurse practitioner should:

    1. Obtain help from the parents to enlist the child's cooperation.

    2. Defer assessing the cranial nerve until the child is older.

    3. Modify the physical exam technique based on the child's developmental level.

    4. Expect minimal variations among age groups.

12. Genu valgum is considered normal from:

    1. 1–2 years old.

    2. 2–6 years old.

    3. 8–10 years old.

    4. 12–16 years old.

13. An African American mother and her newborn are seen by the family nurse practitioner for a well-baby visit. The mother is responsive to the baby's cries, and the baby comforts easily and makes frequent eye contact with the mother. On exam, the family nurse practitioner notes the following: height and weight are at the 75th percentile on growth charts, there is a strong sucking reflex, and there is a large blue-black macular area over the lumbosacral area. The family nurse practitioner should:

    1. Contact a social worker and report the mother to Child Protective Services immediately.

    2. Refer the mother and infant to a dermatologist.

    3. Recognize that the blue-black spot is a congenital skin spot, and counsel the mother that no treatment is necessary.

    4. Prescribe clotrimazole cream 1% (Mycelex) bid for 4 weeks.

14. The plantar fat pad, which makes a young child appear to have pes planus, is normal until:

    1. 6 months–1 year old.

    2. 1–2 years old.

    3. 2–5 years old.

    4. 6–8 years old.

15. Growth hormone secretion tests, along with a history and physical exam, have indicated a positive diagnosis for delayed puberty. The next step for the family nurse practitioner is to:

    1. Treat with hormone replacement.

    2. Refer to a pediatric endocrinologist.

    3. Treat with hormone stimulation therapy.

    4. Refer for possible pituitary tumor.

16. The family nurse practitioner is performing a physical exam on a 13-year-old female. It is important for the family nurse practitioner to incorporate developmental principles such as:

    1. Maintain a comfortable silence.

    2. Verbally affirm normalcy of physical findings.

    3. Discuss only the major areas of abnormality.

    4. Verbally address problems of sexually transmitted diseases.

17. At a school clinic, a 14-year-old girl comes in complaining of dizziness midmorning and then later that morning. The practitioner should question the adolescent regarding diet/nutrition, drug use, and:

    1. Asthma.

    2. Pregnancy.

    3. Heart disease.

    4. Stress.

18. **QSEN** The family nurse practitioner understands that sulfonamide medications are not recommended for children under which age?

    1. 18 months.

    2. 12 months.

    3. 6 months.

    4. 2 months.

Growth & Development

19. The major influence on the timing of puberty is:

    1. Exposure to light.

    2. Genetics.

    3. General health.

    4. Nutrition.

20. A 14-year-old girl is seen in the clinic by the family nurse practitioner because she has not achieved menarche. Physical exam reveals axillary and pubic hair and breast buds with increased size of areola. Based on these findings, the most appropriate intervention would be:

    1. Bone age studies.

    2. Labs for luteinizing hormone (LH) and follicle-stimulating hormone (FSH) levels.

    3. Chromosome analysis to rule out Turner's syndrome.

    4. Reassurance that she is developing normally.

21. A 13-year-old male is seen by the family nurse practitioner for a sports physical. The genital exam reveals straight dark pubic hair at the base of the penis and testicular enlargement. Using the Tanner scale, the family nurse practitioner would record these findings as:

    1. Tanner stage I.

    2. Tanner stage II.

    3. Tanner stage III.

    4. Tanner stage IV.

22. An 11-year-old girl who has just begun to show signs of breast development asks the family nurse practitioner when she will start having periods like her friends. The family nurse practitioner's response is based on the knowledge that:

    1. The average age of menarche is 12.8 years.

    2. Most girls will have a growth spurt following the onset of menarche.

    3. Menarche usually occurs about 3–6 months after the onset of breast development.

    4. Menarche usually occurs about 18–24 months after the onset of breast development.

23. A teenage girl with curly pubic hair on the mons pubis and breast enlargement without secondary contour would be classified on the Tanner scale (stages) as:

    1. Tanner stage I.

    2. Tanner stage II.

    3. Tanner stage III.

    4. Tanner stage IV.

24. A mother of a 2-year-old brings her child to see the family nurse practitioner because the child has been irritable and has a small "knot" under the left ear. The child has no history of fever, upper respiratory infection, or pulling at the ears. What condition is the most likely reason for these symptoms?

    1. Otitis media.

    2. Teething.

    3. Tonsillitis.

    4. Otitis externa.

25. A routine well-child visit for a healthy full-term infant should include a hemoglobin and hematocrit test at:

    1. 1 month of age.

    2. 4 months of age.

    3. 6–9 months of age.

    4. 1 year of age.

26. The mother of a 3-month-old infant is concerned because her baby seems to sleep most of the time. The family nurse practitioner's response is based on the knowledge that a 3-month-old infant usually spends:

    1. 10 hours daily sleeping.
    2. 15–16 hours daily sleeping.
    3. 18–19 hours daily sleeping.
    4. Most hours of the day sleeping, waking only to eat.

27. During a routine well-child exam, a mother reports that her 5-month-old who weighs 15 lb and was sleeping all night at 3 months of age is now waking up hungry in the middle of the night? A diet history reveals that the infant is taking six 6-oz bottles of formula in a 24-hour period and has 2 tbsp of rice cereal in the morning. What teaching should the family nurse practitioner give the mother?

    1. Increase the amount of formula at each feeding to 8 oz.
    2. Take the child off formula and switch to homogenized milk.
    3. Decrease the amount of formula to 32 oz in 24 hours and add fruits, cereals, and juices.
    4. Continue the same amount of formula and introduce a variety of baby foods.

28. The father of a 12-year-old male tells the family nurse practitioner that he is afraid that his son is "getting fat." The child is at the 50th percentile for height and the 75th percentile for weight on the growth chart. The most appropriate response would be:

    1. Reassure the father that the son is not "fat."
    2. Assess family for the presence of obesity and genetic factors.
    3. Suggest a low-calorie, low-fat diet.
    4. Explain that this is typical of the growth pattern of boys at this age, and encourage exercise and a healthy diet.

29. **QSEN** A mother asks the family nurse practitioner if an infant walker will help her 6-month-old learn to walk faster. The family nurse practitioner's response is based on the knowledge that:

    1. Infant walkers help strengthen the infant's extremities and prepare them to walk.
    2. Infants who are placed in walkers usually walk about 1 month earlier than other infants.

    3. Infant walkers are dangerous and should not be recommended for use.
    4. There have been very few injuries related to the use of infant mobile walkers.

30. **QSEN** The mother of a 6-month-old infant tells the family nurse practitioner that the baby was spitting up his formula so she put him on goat milk. The family nurse practitioner is concerned because goat milk places the infant at risk of developing:

    1. Rickets.
    2. Scurvy.
    3. Megaloblastic anemia secondary to folic acid deficiency.
    4. Botulism.

31. A 1-year-old reaches for the family nurse practitioner's stethoscope with his left hand and the father says, "It looks like he's going to be a lefty, just like his old man!" The nurse's response is based on the knowledge that:

    1. Male infants usually have the same hand preference as their fathers.
    2. Hand preference is well established by 9 months of age.
    3. Children will not demonstrate a hand preference until about age 6.
    4. Children usually develop handedness by 18–24 months of age.

32. A mother is concerned that her 7-month-old breast-fed infant is not getting enough to eat. The infant weighed 7 lb, 8 oz at birth and was 19 inches long. At 6 months of age, he weighed 15 lb and was 25 inches long. He now weighs 15 lb and is 25½ inches long. The family nurse practitioner's response is based on the knowledge that:

    1. Infants should gain 2–4 oz per week and ½ inch in height per month during the first 6 months of life.
    2. Infants should triple their birth weight by 6 months of age.
    3. Infants should gain 3–4 oz per week and ½ inch in height per month from 6–12 months of age.
    4. Infants should gain 1–2 oz per week and 1 inch in height per month from 6–12 months of age.

33. A child will be able to do which of the following fine motor skills first?

    1. Imitate a circle.

    2. Imitate a square.

    3. Copy a triangle.

    4. Copy a diamond.

34. The family nurse practitioner would expect a child to follow a one-step command that is given without a gesture and with only four to six individual words at what age?

    1. 7 months.

    2. 9 months.

    3. 14 months.

    4. 20 months.

35. The family nurse practitioner knows that language is the best single measure of normal cognitive development in early childhood. At what age do children begin to combine two words together?

    1. 8–10 months.

    2. 10–12 months.

    3. 12–15 months.

    4. 14–23 months.

36. A mother of 2-year-old twins is concerned that the twins do not talk very much and seem to have their own "private" language. The family nurse practitioner should:

    1. Tell the mother to spend some individual time with the twins so that they learn language skills.

    2. Perform a pure-tone audiometry.

    3. Tell the mother that this is normal for twins or siblings that are close in age.

    4. Refer to a speech pathologist for further testing.

37. The family nurse practitioner notices that a 9-month-old infant who was born 2 months prematurely only reaches for an object with his left hand. The nurse would:

    1. Record these findings as normal for a premature infant.

    2. Refer the infant for further evaluation.

    3. Order a muscle biopsy to rule out muscular dystrophy.

    4. Make a note on the chart that the child will probably be left-handed.

38. The mother of a 6-month-old infant tells the family nurse practitioner that her infant is now taking homogenized milk instead of an iron-fortified infant formula. The family nurse practitioner's response would be based on the knowledge that:

    1. Homogenized milk has the same solute load as formula and is a safe alternative to iron-fortified formula if vitamin supplements are given.

    2. There is an increased incidence of occult gastrointestinal bleeding and the development of iron-deficiency anemia in infants fed homogenized milk before 1 year of age.

    3. Once the infant is taking solid foods regularly, there is no need to continue offering iron-fortified formula.

    4. Homogenized milk has too high of a fat content and needs to be diluted 2:1 with water.

39. The development of the male sexual characteristics in utero is dependent on:

    1. Estrogen.

    2. Progesterone.

    3. Prolactin.

    4. Testosterone.

40. The production of sperm usually begins during the:

    1. Eighth week of gestation.

    2. Beginning of puberty.

    3. End of puberty.

    4. Eighth month of gestation.

41. What is true about the developmental process of sperm or spermatozoa?

    1. Each mature sperm contains 23 chromosomes.

    2. Sperm become motile immediately at maturation.

    3. Spermatogenesis takes place in the prostate.

    4. Higher than normal body temperature contributes to sperm production.

42. What is produced by the testes?

    1. Alkaline phosphate.

    2. Gonadotropin.

    3. Testosterone.

    4. Acid phosphate.

43. Which statement is correct concerning healthy sexual developmental tasks?

    1. At 9 years of age, children are less self-conscious and readily expose themselves to younger children or parents of the opposite sex.

    2. At 16 years of age, adolescents are significantly influenced by the media in terms of sexual content and conduct.

    3. At 4 years of age, children distinguish organs associated with each sex and demonstrate increased sexual curiosity.

    4. At 5 years of age, children begin to have concerns about body image and begin to investigate their own sexual organs.

44. The family nurse practitioner understands the following about birth defects and growth and developmental problems in mothers who have prenatal alcohol exposure:

    1. If alcohol is ingested late in the pregnancy, there is a higher incidence of postmaturity syndrome.

    2. The practice of drinking alcohol while eating a meal significantly reduces the risk of fully expressed fetal alcohol syndrome.

    3. If alcohol is ingested in large amounts early in the pregnancy, there is an increased incidence of fully expressed clinical features of fetal alcohol syndrome.

    4. Growth retardation is associated with early trimester alcohol consumption and postmaturity syndrome.

45. In response to a young adult male's question concerning the production of sperm, the family nurse practitioner knows that sperm is produced in the:

    1. Epididymis.

    2. Vas deferens.

    3. Prostate.

    4. Seminiferous tubules.

46. An adolescent female with breast budding and sparse, straight, lightly pigmented pubic hair along the medial border of the labia is at which Tanner stage of sexual maturity?

    1. Stage I.

    2. Stage II.

    3. Stage III.

    4. Stage IV.

47. Precocious puberty is defined as:

    1. Onset of puberty before age 8 in females and 9 in males.

    2. Onset of puberty before age 5 in females and 7 in males.

    3. Onset of puberty before age 10 in females and 12 in males.

    4. Onset of puberty for either gender before older siblings enter into puberty.

48. The mother of a 5-month-old infant brings her child to the clinic because the infant awakens frequently at night and cries. The family nurse practitioner understands that the most common cause of night awakening in healthy infants is:

    1. Night terrors and nightmares.

    2. Separation anxiety.

    3. Trained night crying.

    4. Hunger pain and wet diaper.

49. A 10-day-old breast-fed infant is brought to the clinic because the mother is concerned about the infant's "yellow-orange" color. History and findings are as follows: mother's blood type is AB-positive; infant's blood type is B-negative and total bilirubin 15 mg/dL. The family nurse practitioner understands that this is most likely caused by:

    1. Hemolytic jaundice.

    2. Breast-fed jaundice.

    3. Obstructive jaundice.

    4. Physiologic jaundice.

50. A new mother presents to the clinic inquiring about when she should start feeding her 2-month-old infant solid foods. The family nurse practitioner should recommend that the mother:

    1. Start the infant on meat and eggs now.

    2. Wait until the infant is 1 year old before introducing solid foods.

    3. Start the infant on cereals now.

    4. Introduce one new food at a time when the infant is 4–6 months old.

Aging

51. As an individual ages, which physiologic change would affect responses to pharmacologic agents?

    1. Increased gastric emptying.

    2. Increased glomerular filtration rate.

    3. Decreased percentage of body fat.

    4. Decreased albumin concentration.

52. **QSEN** The number one cause of accidental death in patients older than 65 years of age is:

    1. Motor vehicle accidents.

    2. Poisoning.

    3. Falls.

    4. Drowning.

53. **QSEN** The family nurse practitioner selects which assessment tool to evaluate balance and gait problems in older adult patients?

    1. Lawton & Brody Balance and Coordination Scale.

    2. Tinetti Balance and Gait Evaluation.

    3. Instrumental Activities of Daily Living Scale.

    4. Index of Independence of Activities of Daily Living.

54. In assessing the nutritional status of an older adult patient, the family nurse practitioner identifies the common physiologic change in the gastrointestinal system to be:

    1. Increased peristalsis.

    2. Decreased absorption of iron.

    3. Maintenance of normal fat metabolism.

    4. Increased drug metabolism.

55. What are the normal physiologic changes in the thyroid gland that occur with aging?

    1. Hypertrophy with a decrease in triiodothyronine (T_3) and thyroxine (T_4).

    2. Normal size with increase in thyroid-stimulating hormone (TSH) and decrease in T_4.

    3. Atrophy of the gland with a decrease in TSH, T_3, and T_4.

    4. Increase in nodularity with normal TSH and T_4.

56. The aging process causes what normal physiologic changes in the heart?

    1. Heart size stays the same, and the valves thicken and become rigid secondary to fibrosis and sclerosis.

    2. Cardiomegaly occurs along with the prolapse of the mitral valve and regurgitation.

    3. Dilation of the right ventricle with sclerosis of pulmonic and tricuspid valves.

    4. Hypertrophy of the right ventricle with decreasing capacity and compromised efficiency of the coronary arteries.

57. Which pulmonary physiologic change is commonly associated with the aging process?

    1. Increased cough response.

    2. Decrease in vital capacity.

    3. Decreased AP diameter of the thorax.

    4. Increase in residual pCO_2.

58. **QSEN** Which of these clinical findings would indicate a deviation from the normal age-related changes in the neurologic system that may have some diagnostic significance for the older patient?

    1. Decreased sense of touch.

    2. Increased tolerance to pain.

    3. Decreased short-term memory.

    4. Decreased ability to maintain balance.

59. During a teaching session, the family nurse practitioner instructs the patient regarding normal skin lesions in the older population. These would include:

    1. Seborrheic dermatitis.

    2. Senile keratosis.

    3. Senile lentigo.

    4. Squamous cell.

60. Which assessment is a normal physiologic change of the respiratory system that occurs with aging?

    1. Decreased residual lung volume.

    2. Hyperresonance.

    3. Increased forced vital capacity.

    4. Increased tactile fremitus.

61. The family nurse practitioner indicates an understanding of the normal aging process with which documentation of the gastrointestinal (GI) system in the physical examination?

    1. Increase in the size of the liver (16 cm).

    2. Absent bowel sounds.

    3. Femoral bruit.

    4. Increased adipose tissue.

62. **QSEN** During the physical exam of an older patient, the family nurse practitioner indicates an understanding of deviations in the neurologic system from the normal aging processs with which clinical finding?

    1. Decrease in short-term memory.

    2. Decrease in deep tendon and superficial reflexes.

    3. Decreased sense of touch.

    4. Positive Romberg's sign.

63. **QSEN** Which functional assessment tool should the family nurse practitioner use to evaluate the safety of a patient who had a stroke and is planning to return to a home environment?

    1. OARS ADL Scale.

    2. Bennet Social Isolation Scale.

    3. Mini Mental State Examination.

    4. Norton Scale.

64. **QSEN** The family nurse practitioner understands which factor is most influential in the driving ability of an older adult?

    1. Ability to coordinate a clutch transmission.

    2. Acuity of vision.

    3. Comprehension of the details of road rules.

    4. Reaction times.

65. As an individual ages, which physiologic change would affect sleep?

    1. Decreased REM sleep.

    2. Increased delta or stage IV sleep.

    3. Decreased nocturnal awakenings.

    4. Decreased sleep latency.

66. When treating an infection in the older adult, the family nurse practitioner must consider that:

    1. Thymus-derived immunity is increased.

    2. Immune function declines with age.

    3. Immune function increases with age.

    4. Antibody production increases.

67. The diminished immunity of the older adult can be attributed to a decline in:

    1. B-cell function.

    2. T-cell production.

    3. B-cell production.

    4. T-cell function.

68. Which physiologic factor of aging contributes to incontinence in older adults?

    1. Decreased vascularity of the bladder mucosa.

    2. Increased urethral closing pressure.

    3. Increased ability to concentrate urine.

    4. Decreased bladder capacity.

69. The family nurse practitioner understands that as the patient ages changes occur in the cells of the immune system. Which statement reflects these changes?

    1. The cells are able to proliferate as they would in the younger patient.

    2. The total number of T cells is decreased.

    3. There is an increased ability to respond to infections with previously produced "remembered" antibodies.

    4. The immune system is able to respond to antigenic stimulation as in the younger patient.

70. **QSEN** The parents of a newborn state, "We will probably not have our baby immunized because we are concerned about the risk of our child being injured." Which is the best response for the family nurse practitioner to make?

    1. "It is your decision, and I think it is wrong."

    2. "Have you talked with your parents about this? They can probably help you think about this decision."

    3. "The risks of not immunizing your baby are greater than the risks from the immunizations, not only to your child but to others around him."

    4. "You are making a mistake, but we don't need any permission to administer it anyway."

71. **QSEN** A nurse practitioner is assessing a 47-year-old patient who has come to the office for an annual physical examination. One of the first physical signs of aging is:

    1. Having more frequent aches and pains.

    2. Diminished eyesight, especially close vision.

    3. Increasing loss of muscle tone.

    4. Diminished hearing or taste.

72. The nurse who volunteers at a senior citizens center is planning activities for the members who attend the center. Which activity would best promote health and maintenance for these senior citizens?

    1. Gardening every day for an hour.

    2. Cycling 3 times a week for 20 minutes.

    3. Sculpting once a week for 40 minutes.

    4. Walking 3 to 5 times a week for 30 minutes.

73. Which of the following is NOT a developmental screening tool used for children?

    1. Modified Checklist for Autism in Toddlers (M-CHAT).

    2. Ages and Stages Questionnaire (ASQ).

    3. Denver Developmental Screening Test (DDST).

    4. Activities-specific Balance Confidence (ABC) Scale.

2 Growth & Development Answers & Rationales

Physical Assessment

1. Answer: 3

Rationale: These are the recommended health evaluation intervals for children to obtain regular assessment information regarding growth and development and to administer recommended immunizations.

2. Answer: 3

Rationale: An approach with a well-balanced diet, activity, and exercise is necessary for weight reduction. This allows for a slow approach to weight loss that incorporates healthy behavior habits.

3. Answer: 3

Rationale: The first and most important part of all data gathering starts with a detailed history and physical exam. A detailed, objective description of the dysmorphic features is essential for comparison to textbook descriptions and other data. Although chromosome analysis will probably be ordered, it is not done initially. Parents should be included in the discussion of the findings and kept informed of the progress throughout the evaluation process.

4. Answer: 3

Rationale: In-toeing is a common problem in children and can result from femoral anteversion, adduction of the great toe, medial tibial torsion, and metatarsus adductus. Legg-Calvé-Perthes disease is commonly seen in older children (ages 4 to 8 years) who have loss of hip medial rotation.

5. Answer: 2

Rationale: Characteristics of innocent murmurs include midsystolic; asymptomatic; less than a grade III; loudest in pulmonic area (2–3 left intercostal space at the left sternal border); no radiation to other areas; may disappear on sitting; and may intensify with fever, activity, anemia, and stress. Any S_4 sound is considered pathologic in children as well as in adults.

6. Answer: 2

Rationale: The posterior fontanel is usually closed by 2 months of age; the anterior fontanel closes at about 24 months of age.

7. Answer: 3

Rationale: Genu varum (bowleg) of up to 20 degrees is a normal finding in children until the age of 18 months.

8. Answer: 1

Rationale: Toddlers like to make the first move (i.e., let them move closer and initiate eye contact first; do not call out their name because this might frighten them). Allowing them to handle the stethoscope will decrease their fear. Detailed explanations and involvement are more appropriate when assessing a school-age child.

9. Answer: 2

Rationale: Allow a toddler to explore the instruments and start with the extremities. Save the most invasive exam (of the head) for last. In infants, auscultate the heart and lungs while the infant is quiet, then proceed to do a head-to-toe assessment. In school-age and adolescent children, a head-to-toe sequence is preferred.

10. Answer: 1

Rationale: Ishihara's test checks for color perception; Bruchner's test checks for the red reflex; Hirschberg's test checks for corneal light reflex; and Jaeger's test checks for near vision.

11. Answer: 3

Rationale: Because assessing cranial nerves can be a challenging task, the family nurse practitioner should employ techniques that consider the child's developmental level.

12. Answer: 2

Rationale: Genu valgum (knock knee) is considered normal from age 2 to 6 years.

13. Answer: 3

Rationale: Congenital dermal melanocytosis, also known as Mongolian spots, are often found in infants of African American, Hispanic, Native American, and Asian descent. These spots are benign and tend to fade and disappear by age 3, requiring no intervention or treatment. Abuse is not suspected because signs of a healthy mother-infant relationship are noted (e.g., mother and infant respond positively to each other, and the baby is thriving).

14. Answer: 3

Rationale: Most children are flat-footed (pes planus) up to 2–5 years of age due to the plantar fat pad under the medial longitudinal arch, which protects it while the arch develops.

15. Answer: 2

Rationale: Once the tentative diagnosis is made, the family nurse practitioner should refer to a pediatric endocrinologist for further workup. It is beyond the scope of the family nurse practitioner's practice to treat the patient at this point.

16. Answer: 2

Rationale: Early adolescence is a time when the child undergoing great physical changes continually wonders if these changes are normal. Verbal affirmation of areas of normalcy during the physical exam can decrease anxiety.

17. Answer: 2

Rationale: Although all areas would be assessed, pregnancy is a common reason for midmorning syncope in adolescents associated with altered nutrition.

18. Answer: 4

Rationale: Newborns and infants up to 2 months of age may develop kernicterus because sulfonamides displace bilirubin from the plasma proteins.

Growth & Development

19. Answer: 2

Rationale: Genetics is the primary determinant of the timing of puberty. Factors such as geographic location, exposure to light, nutritional status, and health status play a role, but genetics is the major influence.

20. Answer: 4

Rationale: Menarche usually occurs about 18–24 months after the onset of breast development. Bone age and laboratory studies are not necessary because development is within normal limits. Findings do not indicate a chromosomal abnormality, so chromosome analysis is unnecessary.

21. Answer: 2

Rationale:

Tanner Stage	Pubic Hair
I	None
II	Countable; straight; increased pigmentation and length
III	Darker; begins to curl; increased quantity
IV	Increased quantity; coarser texture; covers most of pubic area
V	Adult distribution; spread to medial thighs and lower abdomen
	Genital Development
I	Prepubertal
II	Testicular enlargement; slight rugation of scrotum
III	Further testicular enlargement; penile lengthening begins
IV	Testicular enlargement continues; increased rugation of scrotum; increased penile length
V	Adult genitalia

22. Answer: 4

Rationale: Menarche usually occurs about 18–24 months after the onset of breast development. Although the average age of menarche is 12.8 years, this should not be the basis for the family nurse practitioner's response. Most girls have a growth spurt at Tanner stage IV.

23. Answer: 3

Rationale:

Tanner Stage	Pubic Hair
I	None
II	Countable; straight; increased pigmentation and length
III	Darker; begins to curl; increased quantity on mons pubis
IV	Increased quantity; coarser texture; labia and mons well covered
V	Adult distribution; with feminine triangle and spread to medial thighs
	Breast Development
I	None
II	Breast bud present; increased areolar size
III	Further enlargement of breast; no secondary contour
IV	Areolar area forms secondary mound on breast contour
V	Mature; areolar area is part of breast contour; nipples project

24. Answer: 2

Rationale: At approximately 20 months of age, the lower second molars erupt and, at 24 months, the upper second molars erupt. With a history of irritability and lymph node enlargement without fever or other symptoms, teething is the most likely cause of discomfort. With otitis media and tonsilitis, the family nurse practitioner would not observe a temperature elevation. The child with otitis externa would have pain (around the tragus) and more than likely would not be pulling at the ears.

25. Answer: 4

Rationale: It is important in a healthy infant to check the hemoglobin and hematocrit levels at 1 year, as per current American Academy of Pediatrics (AAP) recommendations. For the first 4–6 months infants can rely on their body's own storage supply of iron.

26. Answer: 2

Rationale: Normally, 3-month-old infants sleep 15–16 hours in a 24-hour period.

27. Answer: 3

Rationale: Consumption of 32 oz of formula per day is usually an indicator of the need for solids. Formula is recommended for the first year of life. Nutritional requirements are 110–120 cal/kg/day. Introduction of solids usually occurs between 4 and 6 months of age.

28. Answer: 4

Rationale: It is normal for boys at this age to appear heavier before they have their "growth spurt." Reassuring the father, although appropriate, is not the best response. Although the findings are within normal limits, it would not be necessary to assess the family for the presence of obesity. Low-calorie, low-fat diets are contraindicated for the growing child. Encouraging exercise and a healthy diet would be important to prevent obesity.

29. Answer: 3

Rationale: The American Academy of Pediatrics (AAP) Committee on Injury and Poison Control issued a policy statement on the use of infant walkers (*Pediatrics* 108: 790–792). Because data indicate a considerable risk of major and minor injury and even death from the use of infant walkers, and because there is no clear benefit from their use, AAP recommends a ban on the manufacture and sale of mobile infant walkers. If a parent insists on using a mobile infant walker, it is vital that they choose a walker that meets the performance standards of ASTM F977-96 to prevent falls down stairs. Stationary activity centers should be promoted as a safer alternative to mobile infant walkers.

30. Answer: 3

Rationale: Goat milk can cause folic acid deficiency, which can lead to megaloblastic anemia. Rickets is caused by the lack of vitamin D. Scurvy is caused by a lack of ascorbic acid (vitamin C) in the diet. Botulism is food poisoning caused by an endotoxin produced by the bacillus *Clostridium botulinum*. Most botulism cases occur after eating improperly canned or cooked foods. Infants have been known to develop botulism from raw honey that is placed on their pacifiers.

31. Answer: 4

Rationale: Children usually develop handedness by 18–24 months of age. The hand preference is usually fixed after 5 years of age.

32. Answer: 3

Rationale: Infants should gain 3–4 oz per week and ½ inch in height per month from 6–12 months of age. This child also doubled his birth weight by 6 months of age, as expected.

Age	Weight	Length/Height
0–6 months	6–8 oz/week (doubles birth weight by 5–7 months)	1 in/month
6–12 months	3–4 oz/week (triples birth weight by 1 year)	½ in/month

33. Answer: 1

Rationale: A child should be able to imitate a circle at 2½ years, copy a square at 4 years, copy a triangle at 5 years, and copy a diamond at 6 years. The ability to draw a shape after watching someone else draw it first is called imitation. Children are always able to imitate a shape or form before being able to copy it.

34. Answer: 3

Rationale: A child should be expected to follow a one-step command (using no gestures and only four to six individual words) between 10½ and 16½ months of age.

35. Answer: 4

Rationale: Two-word combinations are expected at 14–23 months of age.

36. Answer: 3

Rationale: It is normal for twins or siblings close in age to develop a "private" language understood only by them. Although it is important for the mother to spend individual time with each child, this is not what the question is asking. Pure-tone audiometry is done after age 3. There is no need for a referral to a speech pathologist at this time.

37. Answer: 2

Rationale: The infant should be referred for further evaluation. Handedness before 1 year of age may be an early sign of cerebral palsy. The history of prematurity could be an indication of anoxia at birth and would warrant further investigation. The earlier a child is diagnosed; the earlier intervention can be started.

38. Answer: 2

Rationale: There is an increased incidence of occult gastrointestinal bleeding and iron-deficiency anemia in infants fed homogenized milk before 1 year of age. Homogenized milk does not have the same solute load as formula and is not a safe alternative to iron-fortified formula, even if vitamin supplements are given. The solute load of whole milk is too much for the infant's immature kidneys. The infant needs to continue taking iron-fortified formula for the first year of life, if possible.

39. Answer: 4

Rationale: The most important sex hormone during embryonic development is the primary male sex hormone, testosterone. Testosterone is produced by the gonads of the genetic male embryo, causing the male gonads to develop into two testes, which produce sperm. The other hormones are female hormones. Estrogen, the major female hormone, is produced by the ovaries (ovarian follicle and corpus luteum) and cortices of the adrenal glands and placenta during pregnancy. Progesterone, the second major female hormone, is produced by the corpus luteum. Prolactin is an anterior pituitary hormone and one of the somatotropic hormones that are secreted by lactotropic cells. Prolactin is also responsible for milk production in the female.

40. Answer: 3

Rationale: Between the ages of 9 and 12 years, the gonads produce more of the sex hormones, which trigger sexual maturation or puberty. Puberty in males begins at approximately age 11 and lasts for 2–3 years, ending with the first ejaculation that contains mature sperm.

41. Answer: 1

Rationale: Each mature sperm develops from mitotic division of diploid (46-chromosome) germ cells (spermatogonium) found on the basement membrane of each seminiferous tubule and becomes primary spermatocytes with 23 chromosomes each. Each of these two cells further divides into two more cells (spermatids), each of which has 23 chromosomes. Motility depends on the biochemicals in semen and in the female reproductive tract. Sperm production needs a temperature that is less than normal body temperature by at least 1°–2°F.

42. Answer: 3

Rationale: The testes have two functions: production of gonadotropin (androgens and testosterone) and production of gametes (sperm). The sperm are produced in the seminiferous tubules of the testes. The androgens and testosterone are produced mainly by Leydig cells of the testes (androgens and testosterone are also produced by the adrenal glands). Gonadotropin hormone is produced and secreted by the anterior pituitary gland.

43. Answer: 2

Rationale: Adolescents are greatly influenced by the media and tend to identify with their parents as sexually functioning people. At age 9, children are more interested in their own body and are quite self-conscious. Distinguishing organs and sexual curiosity is true for 6-year-olds, not 4-year-olds. Having concerns about body image and own sexual organs is true for 10-year-olds not 5-year-olds.

44. Answer: 3

Rationale: Large amounts of alcohol early in the pregnancy have the most devastating effects on the maturing fetus. There is no safe, established dose for alcohol in pregnancy. Food consumption along with alcohol intake does not reduce the risk of defects. Ingesting alcohol in the later months of pregnancy is associated with an increased incidence of premature and small-for-gestational-age neonates.

45. Answer: 4

Rationale: Sperm is produced in the seminiferous tubules of the testes.

46. Answer: 2

Rationale: Tanner has five stages of sexual maturity for both males and females. Stage I for both is preadolescent, and stage V for both is mature or adult development. Stages II, III, and IV chronicle development of breasts, pubic hair distribution, penis, and testes. This young female is demonstrating characteristics of Tanner stage II.

Tanner Stage	Pubic Hair
I	None
II	Countable; straight; increased pigmentation and length
III	Darker; begins to curl; increased quantity on mons pubis
IV	Increased quantity; coarser texture; labia and mons well covered
V	Adult distribution; with feminine triangle and spread to medial thighs
	Breast Development
I	None
II	Breast bud present; increased areolar size
III	Further enlargement of breast; no secondary contour
IV	Areolar area forms secondary mound on breast contour
V	Mature; areolar area is part of breast contour; nipples project

47. Answer: 1

Rationale: Precocious puberty is defined as beginning at age 8 for females and at age 9 for males.

48. Answer: 3

Rationale: Trained night crying can become a problem in infants who are not allowed to learn to "self-quiet." Activities such as rocking to sleep, exciting play activities before bedtime, and picking up the infant as soon as he cries can lead to trained night crying. Separation anxiety occurs in infants after 6 months of age. The majority of infants after 4 months of age are able to sleep throughout the night. Nightmares and night terrors occur at a later age.

49. Answer: 2

Rationale: This is a type of exaggerated physiologic jaundice that occurs frequently in breast-fed babies because of the infant's inadequate caloric intake before the mother's milk comes in. It typically occurs between 7 and 15 days of life, whereas physiologic jaundice occurs most often between the second and fourth day of life. Hemolytic jaundice occurs in an Rh-negative mother who has an Rh-positive infant who becomes isoimmunized.

50. Answer: 4

Rationale: Solid foods are not recommended until the infant is 4–6 months old. Cereals should be introduced first, followed by fruits, vegetables, meats, and eggs. All foods should be introduced based on the readiness of the child.

Aging

51. Answer: 4

Rationale: Medications are often protein bound (not fat bound); albumin decreases with age. A low albumin level decreases the number of protein-binding sites, causing an increase in the amount of free drug in the plasma. Drug overdose may occur in elderly patients. Gastric emptying and glomerular filtration rate *decrease* with the aging process.

52. Answer: 3

Rationale: Falls are the major cause of morbidity and mortality in the elderly. A fall is often the precipitating event for a cascade of problems leading to death. Complications from falls include fractures, pneumonia, pressure ulcers, pain, and immobility.

53. Answer: 2

Rationale: The Tinetti Balance and Gait Evaluation is an activity-based test that asks the patient to perform tasks, such as sitting and rising from a chair, turning, and bending. It requires no more than 15 to 20 minutes to perform. Another appropriate test for the assessment of falls is the timed "Up and Go" test, which assesses balance and gait speed. The Instrumental Activities of Daily Living Scale assesses complex tasks such as shopping, laundry, and food preparation. The Index of Independence of Activities of Daily Living helps identify daily activities with which the patient needs assistance.

54. Answer: 2

Rationale: Decreased hydrochloric acid, which occurs with aging, leads to decreased absorption of iron and vitamin B_{12}. Fat absorption would decrease, as would peristalsis and drug metabolism.

55. Answer: 4

Rationale: There is usually adequate secretion of thyroid-stimulating hormone (TSH) and a normal serum concentration of thyroxine (T_4). Aging may produce fibrosis and increased nodularity, but overall the thyroid function remains within normal limits.

56. Answer: 1

Rationale: The heart does not increase in size with normal aging. An enlarged heart is a result of cardiac dysfunction. Dilation of the left ventricle occurs with myocardial infarction and altered cardiac functioning secondary to cardiac disease, not from normal aging. The aging process does cause fibrosis and sclerosis of the cardiac valves; all valves are equally affected.

57. Answer: 2

Rationale: A decrease in the vital capacity, along with a 50% increase in residual volume, occurs during the aging process. Other aging changes include a less effective cough, impaired ciliary action, and weaker respiratory muscles. Increased AP diameter is associated with aging and in COPD patients. pCO_2 usually decreases, but pCO_2 usually remains unchanged.

58. Answer: 4

Rationale: Decreased ability to maintain balance may indicate a cerebellar complication. The first three findings are normal age-related changes.

59. Answer: 3

Rationale: The senile lentigo is a gray-brown, irregular, macular lesion on sun-exposed areas of the face, arms, and hands that are normal skin lesions. The other lesions are common abnormal skin lesions in the older adult.

60. Answer: 2

Rationale: A normal age-related change is an increase in the anteroposterior diameter that results in hyperresonance. Age-related changes result in an increase in the residual lung volume (RV) and decrease in the forced vital capacity (FVC). An increased tactile fremitus is a deviation that is of diagnostic significance.

61. Answer: 4

Rationale: Common age-related changes in the gastrointestinal (GI) system include increased adipose tissue, decreased liver size, reduced motility and peristalsis, decreased acid secretions and motor activity of the stomach, and decreased glomerular filtration rate. Absence of bowel sounds after five full minutes and bruits are deviations of clinical significance.

62. Answer: 4

Rationale: Romberg's sign indicates the inability to maintain balance, which indicates a need for further evaluation. A decrease in short-term memory, deep tendon and superficial reflexes, and sense of touch are normal age-related changes. If it affects the patient's functional ability, a decrease in short-term memory would

be considered a deviation. Also, the testing strategy of looking for similarities in the options applies here, as the three incorrect responses all relate to a *decrease* in a body change with age.

63. Answer: 1

Rationale: The OARS ADL Scale is the more appropriate screening tool for identifying at-risk populations. The Bennet Social Isolation Scale would be appropriate to evaluate social interactions and resources. The Mini Mental State Examination is used to evaluate memory, orientation, and attention. The Norton Scale is used to evaluate pressure ulcer risk.

64. Answer: 2

Rationale: The most age-dependent factor is sensory change. The older adult patient being assessed for driving capacity should use any prescribed corrective devices for optimal performance. Poor hearing by itself is generally not a limiting factor for motor vehicle operation, and vision assessment has received the greatest emphasis in assessing older drivers. Documenting the best-corrected binocular visual acuity, color perception, and dark vision is basic in assessing driving visual acuity. Laboratory performance studies have not clearly demonstrated that the other factors are highly applicable to the on-the-road skills of the older adult driver.

65. Answer: 1

Rationale: REM sleep begins approximately 120 minutes from sleep onset and recurs in three or four regularly spaced, 10- to 15-minute cycles. REM sleep, associated with skeletal muscle atonia and dreaming, decreases with aging. Delta sleep, or stage IV, is deep sleep and also decreases with age. Nocturnal wakening and sleep latency increase. Sleep is generally less efficient in older patients, who spend more time in bed and less time sleeping.

66. Answer: 2

Rationale: Immune function declines with age, making the older adult more susceptible to infection. The older adult has less thymus-derived immunity because of the shrinking of the thymus gland, thus making it more difficult for the older adult to produce antibodies.

67. Answer: 4

Rationale: The older adult has diminished cell-mediated immunity because of a decline in T-cell function. The T cells have a decreased ability to produce cytokines, which are needed to facilitate B-cell growth and maturation, and have a decreased ability to proliferate in response to an antigen.

68. Answer: 4

Rationale: Decreased bladder capacity, decreased ability to concentrate urine, and decreased urethral closing pressure after menopause lead to incontinence. Other factors are depression, decreased mobility, decreased vision, and lack of attention to bladder cues of feelings of fullness.

69. Answer: 3

Rationale: Older adult patients are able to respond to infections with previously produced "remembered" antibodies, but they are less able to respond to antigenic stimulation (new antigens) than younger patients. In the older adult patient, the cells of the immune system also are less likely to proliferate. The total number of T cells remains the same with age, but T-cell function decreases and cells have decreased cytotoxicity.

70. Answer: 3

Rationale: The benefits provided by most vaccines extend beyond benefit to the individual who is immunized. There is also a significant public health benefit. Parents who choose not to immunize their own children increase the potential for harm to other persons in four important ways. First, should an unimmunized child contract disease, that child poses a potential threat to other unimmunized children. Second, even in a fully immunized population, a small percentage of immunized individuals will either remain or become susceptible to disease. These individuals have done everything they can to protect themselves through immunization, yet they remain at risk. Third, some children cannot be immunized because of underlying medical conditions. These individuals derive important benefit from herd immunity and may be harmed by contract-ing disease from those who remain unimmunized. Finally, immunized individuals are harmed by the cost of medical care for those who choose not to immunize their children and whose children then contract vaccine-preventable diseases.

71. Answer: 2

Rationale: Refractive errors are the most frequent eye problems in the United States. Blurred vision results from an inappropriate length of the eye and/or shape of the eye or cornea, and almost all errors—myopia (nearsightedness), hyperopia (farsightedness), astigmatism (distorted vision at all distances), and presbyopia (a form of farsightedness that usually occurs between 40 and 45 years of age)—can be corrected by eyeglasses, contact lenses, or, in some cases, surgery. Recent studies conducted by the National Eye Institute showed that proper refractive correction could improve vision among 11 million Americans who are 12 years and older.

72. Answer: 4

Rationale: Exercise and activity are essential for health promotion and maintenance in the older adult and to achieve an optimal level of functioning. About half of the physical deterioration of the older patient is caused by disuse rather than by the aging process or disease. One of the best exercises for an older adult is walking, progressing to 30-minute sessions, 3 to 5 times each week. Swimming and dancing are also beneficial.

73. Answer: 4

Rationale: The Activities-specific Balance Confidence Scale (ABC) is used in older adults to assess for fall risk. All other scales and tests are pediatric related.

Health Promotion & Maintenance

1. What are the current American Cancer Society (ACS) dietary recommendations for cancer prevention?

   1. Maintaining a desirable body weight and eating a variety of foods, including fruits and vegetables, and foods that are high in fiber.

   2. Increasing the amount of protein in the diet.

   3. Alcohol use in small to moderate amounts.

   4. Increase in fresh fruits, fish, and dairy products.

2. In the presence of dyslipidemia and diabetes, the National Cholesterol Education Program guidelines set the goal for lipid levels as:

   1. LDL <100 mg/dL and triglyceride levels <200 mg/dL.

   2. LDL <160 mg/dL and triglyceride levels <240 mg/dL.

   3. LDL <100 mg/dL and triglyceride levels <180 mg/dL.

   4. LDL <150 mg/dL and triglyceride levels <220 mg/dL.

3. The American Diabetes Association recommends screening adults starting at age 45 with a fasting plasma glucose (FPG) test every:

   1. 1 year.

   2. 3 years.

   3. 5 years.

   4. 10 years.

4. What are tertiary prevention activities for an older adult woman who has had a stroke?

   1. Annual influenza vaccination.

   2. Physical therapy program.

   3. Annual mammogram.

   4. Annual ophthalmologic examination to evaluate for glaucoma.

5. A patient is continuing his recovery at home after an extensive surgery. The family nurse practitioner would instruct the patient to increase intake of what foods to promote healing?

   1. Tomatoes, rice, and whole-bran cereal.

   2. Milk, poultry, and yellow vegetables.

   3. Red meat, oranges, and green beans.

   4. Liver, corn, and eggs.

6. When an older adult patient has an alteration in the sensory-perceptual function of hearing, which plan would be most appropriate for the family nurse practitioner to implement during a health promotion session?

   1. Increase the pitch of the voice.

   2. Stand behind the patient when speaking.

   3. Speak in a tone that does not include shouting.

   4. Use typical complex sentences to prevent insulting the patient.

7. **QSEN** Which of the following management plans demonstrates an understanding of primary prevention of falls among older adults?

   1. Evaluate the need for assistive devices for ambulation after the patient has been injured in a fall.

   2. Provide resources to correct hazards that contributed to falling in the home environment.

   3. Reinforce the need to use prescribed eyeglasses to prevent further injury from falls.

   4. Provide information about medications, side effects, and interactions.

8. Which of these health promotion screenings should be completed annually for the older adult patient who is over age 65?

   1. Chest x-ray.

   2. Pneumococcal vaccination.

   3. Colonoscopy.

   4. Stool guaiac test.

9. While teaching a class to a group of senior citizens, which would be most important for the family nurse practitioner to consider during the presentation?

   1. Provide increased overhead lighting to enhance visualization.

   2. Provide handouts on blue paper with black print.

   3. Review a video narrated by a woman.

   4. Recognize that past life experiences are beneficial in learning new information.

10. **QSEN** What is the most common occupationally related health problem?

    1. Repetitive motion injury.

    2. Hearing loss.

    3. Lung disease.

    4. Cancer.

11. Which of the following best describes the benefit of sports screening physicals?

    1. Screening for undiagnosed cardiomyopathy.

    2. Assessment of drug and alcohol use.

    3. Estimation of aerobic capacity.

    4. Identification of risk for an adverse cardiovascular event.

12. A 48-year-old male presents to the clinic after having his cholesterol checked at a health fair. He states that his results were over 300 and that he needed to see his primary care provider for further testing. Appropriate interventions for the family nurse practitioner include:

    1. Prescribing a cholesterol-lowering agent.

    2. Ordering an electrocardiogram and an exercise stress test.

    3. Starting the patient on an exercise program.

    4. Performing a thorough history and physical and drawing a lipid profile.

13. In preparing a patient for a colorectal screening, the family nurse practitioner should instruct the patient to:

    1. Eat at least two servings of meat daily before collecting samples.

    2. Avoid antibiotics, aspirin, iron, and antiinflammatory medications.

    3. Avoid taking extra vitamin and mineral supplements before the test.

    4. Eat extra servings of high-fiber foods and water to ensure good samples.

14. Teaching testicular self-examination should be targeted to which age group?

    1. 10–14 years.

    2. 15–25 years.

    3. 30–40 years.

    4. 45–65 years.

15. According to ChooseMyPlate, what foods are included in the vegetable group? Select two responses.

    1. Chickpeas.

    2. Quinoa.

    3. Beans.

    4. Popcorn.

    5. Wild rice.

16. At what age should a routine screening mammography begin for women who have no increased risk of breast cancer?

    1. Before 30 years old.

    2. At age 35.

    3. At age 40.

    4. Before age 50.

17. Which of the following components should be included when taking a history from a patient who is new to the clinic?

    1. Past medical and surgical history, family medical and surgical histories, psychosocial history, diet and exercise habits, chemical use, sexual practices, and review of systems.

    2. Interval history, past medical history, family medical history, dietary habits, substance use, and sexual practices.

    3. Past medical and surgical histories, family medical history, psychosocial history, physical activity, tobacco and other substance use, and sexual practices.

    4. The history listed on the form provided to patients for completion before the physical examination is sufficient, and no interview needs to be done.

18. A 50-year-old female presents to the clinic for a first-visit checkup. She states she is in good health and takes no medications. She was adopted and does not know her family history. She is 62 inches tall and weighs 175 lb. She is a secretary and admits to a sedentary lifestyle. She does not smoke and drinks 4–5 alcoholic beverages per week. Which of the following interventions would be most appropriate for the family nurse practitioner to recommend in this patient's plan of care?

    1. Recommend that she start an exercise program that includes jogging and weight training.

    2. Prescribe vitamin supplements to incorporate into her diet while she eliminates alcoholic beverages.

    3. Discuss possible job changes that that will increase her daily amount of exercise.

    4. Suggest that she keep a daily record of her food intake and bring it to her next visit.

19. Which group is at greatest risk for alterations in immune functions related to nutritional status?

    1. Young adults.

    2. Adults.

    3. Premature infants.

    4. Older adults.

20. The most common cause of infant deaths worldwide is:

    1. Pneumonia.

    2. Malnutrition.

    3. Acquired immunodeficiency syndrome (AIDS).

    4. Beta-streptococcal infections.

21. The family nurse practitioner is discussing making lifestyle changes that will decrease the older adult's risks for cardiovascular disease. Which of the following is most important to include in this discussion?

    1. Decrease smoking, increase vitamin supplements, and increase protein intake.

    2. Control hypertension, stop smoking, maintain normal weight, and exercise regularly.

    3. Maintain normal levels of serum blood sugar and decrease cholesterol intake.

    4. Have a yearly physical examination, increase fiber in the diet, and exercise regularly.

22. The family nurse practitioner is discussing anticipatory guidance with the parents of a 26-week-gestation premature infant who is now 2 months old and being discharged from the neonatal intensive care unit (NICU). Which of the following would be most important to include in the discussion?

    1. Fluoride supplement due to lack of breast-feeding.

    2. Lights to be on 24 hours a day.

    3. Decreased handling and stimulation.

    4. Bright colors and continuous music for stimulation.

23. Which of the following is an example of a community health promotion activity?

    1. High school–based family planning clinic.

    2. Work-site urgent care clinic.

    3. Asthma follow-up clinic in an elementary school.

    4. Employer-sponsored multiphasic health screening.

24. Which of the following is most important for the family nurse practitioner to do each time a child comes in for a health maintenance clinic visit?

    1. Order routine laboratory tests.

    2. Perform vision and auditory screening.

    3. Plot height and weight on charts.

    4. Review immunization record.

25. Which of the following guidelines should the family nurse practitioner follow when developing educational materials? Select two guidelines.

    1. Present the most important material first using all capital letters for emphasis.

    2. Provide the information in English along with three other languages.

    3. Keep sentences short and to the point using graphic images for clarification.

    4. Keep a readability level no higher than an eighth grade level.

    5. Use only brightly colored paper and a bold typeface to enhance learning.

26. In explaining the purpose of primary prevention programs to a group of nursing students, the family nurse practitioner states that primary prevention programs:

    1. Work to lower the incidence of birth defects.

    2. Emphasize early diagnosis and treatment of pediatric anomalies.

    3. Minimize the handicapping effect of mental retardation.

    4. Focus on the prevention of complications and rehabilitation.

27. A healthy 4-month-old infant weighing 13 lb 3 oz has started waking up at night after previously sleeping for periods of 9–11 hours. The infant takes 32 oz of formula in a 24-hour period. The family nurse practitioner recommends:

    1. Increase the formula to 38 oz in a 24-hour period.

    2. Start introducing one food item at a time, beginning with vegetables.

    3. Maintain current formula intake and introduce small amounts of rice cereal.

    4. Switch to whole milk instead of formula.

28. The family nurse practitioner understands that the infant mortality rate is:

    1. The number of infant deaths per 1000 live births.

    2. The total number of infant deaths per 1000 persons in the population.

    3. The number of infant deaths attributed to specific illnesses.

    4. The monthly infant death rate per 100 live births.

29. A father (height 74 inches; onset of puberty was at age 16) is concerned that his 15-year-old son is going to be short. On physical exam, the family nurse practitioner finds Tanner stage II, height 62 inches, and physical exam essentially normal for a well-nourished adolescent. After reviewing his growth records, which indicate a growth pattern of height at the fifth percentile, the most likely diagnosis is:

    1. Constitutional growth delay.

    2. Familial short stature.

    3. Hypopituitarism.

    4. Idiopathic gonadotropin deficiency.

30. Which of the following is most important to include in the anticipatory guidance of a family with a 9-month-old child?

    1. Keep buttons, beads, and coins out of the child's reach.

    2. Turn the handles of pots on the stove inward.

    3. Encourage self-feeding with silverware.

    4. Encourage weaning to a cup and eliminating pacifier use.

31. Anticipatory guidance for the family with a 6-year-old includes:

    1. Avoid fluoride supplements to prevent staining of teeth and dental caries.

    2. Continue to use a belt-positioning booster seat until the child has reached 4 ft 9 inches tall and is between 8 and 12 years of age.

    3. Instruct parents to use bottled drinking water when traveling to different parts of the country.

    4. Serve only three regular meals with no snacks to prevent development of poor nutrition habits.

32. In teaching a new mother about fevers, the family nurse practitioner knows that:

    1. Fevers over 104°F (40°C) can cause brain damage.

    2. Most fevers over 104°F (40°C) are usually of bacterial origin.

    3. Children under 6 months of age are especially susceptible to brain damage from a fever.

    4. Fevers may precipitate convulsions in children between 6 months and 5 years of age.

33. A new mother asks about the differences between human milk and cow's milk. The family nurse practitioner explains that:

    1. Human milk has more lipase and linoleic acid.

    2. Human milk has more calcium, phosphorus, sodium, and potassium.

    3. Cow's milk has low protein and casein content.

    4. Cow's milk has high linoleic acid and low saturated fatty acids.

34. The nurse recognizes the following as correct for the frequency and quantity of formula feedings:

    1. 1 month: 9–10 feedings/24 hr of 2–3 oz.

    2. 6 months: 8–10 feedings/24 hr of 4–5 oz.

    3. 10 months: 3–4 feedings/24 hr of 7–8 oz.

    4. 12 months: 6–8 feedings/24 hr of 8–9 oz.

35. According to the American Academy of Pediatrics (AAP), infants may be fed whole cow's milk once they reach:

    1. 6 months of age.

    2. 8 months of age.

    3. 12 months of age.

    4. 18 months of age.

36. A mother states that the iron-fortified formula her 3-month-old is on has been causing the infant constipation. The family nurse practitioner recommends:

    1. Discontinuing the iron-fortified formula.

    2. Starting the infant on rice cereal.

    3. Adding 1–2 tsp of dark corn syrup to the formula.

    4. Adding ½ teaspoon of mineral oil to daily intake.

37. Which of the following best describes lactose intolerance?

    1. Symptoms typically include intestinal dilation, bloating, increased flatulence, and pain followed eventually by diarrhea; occurs in children 4–6 years of age.

    2. An abrupt onset of nausea, vomiting, and diarrhea within 30 minutes after consuming milk products; occurs in children 12–18 months of age.

    3. Its presentation is the same as cow's milk intolerance.

    4. Its prevalence is highest among the Caucasian population.

38. A 1-year-old child who had a normal physical exam has a lead level of 15 µg/dL. Which of the following actions should the family nurse practitioner take?

    1. Repeat the test because it may be a false result.

    2. Hospitalize for immediate chelation therapy.

    3. Investigate possible sources of lead and repeat in 3–4 months.

    4. Repeat the test in 1 year.

39. The recommended time for the introduction of solid foods into an infant's diet is:

    1. Age 2 months.

    2. Age 3 months.

    3. Age 4–6 months.

    4. Age 6–8 months.

40. A 20-day-old infant is brought to the clinic by her parents. She has not been eating well and has a temperature of 100.8°F (38.2°C). Exam data reveals no focal bacterial infection; laboratory tests indicate white blood cell (WBC) count of 12,000/mm^3 with 1480 bands/mm^3; urinalysis is normal; and no diarrhea is noted. Which of the following is the most appropriate management plan for this infant?

    1. Treat at home with antipyretics and fluids.

    2. Hospitalize for a septic workup.

    3. Treat at home with antipyretics and ampicillin.

    4. Do a urine culture and have the infant return in 24 hours.

41. Which of the following is most important to remember when teaching children in grades 5 through 8 about health promotion behaviors?

    1. Girls are more extrinsically motivated than boys.

    2. Both boys and girls are highly influenced by family.

    3. Boys are more extrinsically motivated than girls.

    4. High maternal education levels affect both.

42. In the preparation of reading and education materials for patients and parents, the family nurse practitioner is aware that the reading level of most adults is at the:

    1. Twelfth-grade level.

    2. Tenth-grade level.

    3. Sixth-grade level.

    4. Fourth-grade level.

43. A child presenting with vague symptoms and a serum lead level of 28 µg/dL would be managed by:

    1. Removal of the child from the lead source.

    2. Removal of the environmental lead hazard.

    3. Chelation therapy treatment.

    4. Rescreening and referral to a physician.

44. Which of the following should be included when discussing primary injury prevention with the parents of a 2-month-old child?

    1. Set water heater thermostat at <120°F.

    2. Make sure crib rails are no more than 3¼ inches apart.

    3. Use a rear-facing car seat until the child is >40 lb.

    4. Apply sunscreen when child is outside and the temperature is 75°F.

45. A Hispanic child presents with symptoms of weakness, irritability, weight loss, constipation, and mild ataxia, and a history of elevated lead level. Which of the following homeopathic substances would the family nurse practitioner suspect had been used?

    1. White willow bark.

    2. Arnica root.

    3. Mexican yam root.

    4. Azarcon and greta.

46. Which lifestyle modifications are most effective in controlling hypertension in the older adult patient?

    1. Maintain normal weight, decrease sodium in diet, and exercise regularly.

    2. Increase dietary protein, decrease weight, and use stress-reduction techniques.

    3. Consume a high-complex carbohydrate, low-sodium diet and decrease stress.

    4. Reduce weight, increase vitamin supplements, and exercise regularly.

Immunizations

47. A child is in first grade. How many doses of inactivated poliovirus vaccine (IPV) will he have received?

    1. 2 doses.

    2. 3 doses.

    3. 4 doses.

    4. 5 doses.

48. Before giving a child the measles, mumps, rubella trivalent vaccine, it is recommended to wait how long after cancer chemotherapy has stopped?

    1. 30 days.

    2. 2 months.

    3. 3 months.

    4. 6 months.

49. The National Childhood Vaccine Injury Act requires standardized consent forms for the administration of vaccines to children. The content on the form for the medical record includes the vaccine lot number, nurse signature, injection/inoculation site, and:

    1. Signature of parent or legal guardian.

    2. Education provided.

    3. Absence of contraindications.

    4. Vaccine expiration date.

50. The mother of a 15-year-old who has not had chickenpox is concerned and wants her daughter to be vaccinated. The recommendations are:

    1. Not recommended for children over age 12.

    2. One-time dose.

    3. Two doses at least 28 days apart apart.

    4. Three doses at 2 months apart.

51. Consultation with the mother of an 18-month-old who has received no immunizations reveals that the child was exposed to measles 48 hours before the visit. At this time, the family nurse practitioner would:

    1. Discharge the patient with care instructions.

    2. Administer the live attenuated measles vaccine.

    3. Administer 0.5 mL/kg immunoglobulin G (IgG).

    4. Administer half the regular measles vaccine dose.

52. Which statement about the polyvalent pneumococcal vaccine is true?

    1. It is recommended for children older than 2 years of age with chronic diseases, including diabetes.

    2. It is recommended to prevent otitis media (OM) and other pneumococcal infections in children younger than 2 years of age.

    3. It may not be given concurrently with other vaccines.

    4. Severe systemic reactions are common after immunization.

53. The influenza vaccination is recommended annually for high-risk groups. The family nurse practitioner knows that the greatest need for this vaccination would be for:

    1. Adults with chronic disease.

    2. Residents of long-term care facilities.

    3. Dialysis patients.

    4. Health care employees.

54. The family nurse practitioner understands that the only contraindication to hepatitis B vaccination is:

    1. Pregnancy and lactation.

    2. History of poliomyelitis.

    3. Prior anaphylaxis or severe hypersensitivity.

    4. Mild viral illness.

55. Immunizations and chemoprophylaxis offered routinely to patients 65 years of age or older are:

    1. Tetanus toxoid, diphtheria toxoid, and acellular pertussis (Tdap); influenza; and pneumococcal vaccine.

    2. Tetanus toxoid and diphtheria (Td), varicella, or shingles vaccine.

    3. Td and influenza; for those with a weakened immune system, offer the shingles vaccine.

    4. Influenza and Td to those who have not had vaccine in the past 10 years.

56. The family nurse practitioner understands that the following is considered an attenuated live-virus vaccination:

    1. Rubella and measles.

    2. Mumps and hepatitis B.

    3. Poliomyelitis and hepatitis B.

    4. Rubella and rabies.

57. The family nurse practitioner understands that children who should not receive the measles vaccine are children who have severe allergic reactions to:

    1. Fungi.

    2. Pollen.

    3. Pets.

    4. Neomycin.

58. What type of immunity does a child develop after contracting chickenpox?

    1. Active natural immunity.

    2. Active artificial immunity.

    3. Passive natural immunity.

    4. Passive artificial immunity.

59. The family nurse practitioner is assessing an 8-month-old infant in an immunization clinic. By this time, the infant should have received which immunizations?

    1. All three hepatitis B injections, all RV series, 3 doses of the PCV series, and at least 2 doses of IPV.

    2. Hepatitis B first and second dose, all the DTaP, the polio series, and MMR.

    3. DTaP first and second dose, MMR first dose, all hepatitis B series.

    4. Varicella, Tdap first dose, and hepatitis B first dose.

60. Which of the following patient situations requires the use of inactivated (not live) vaccines?

    1. History of nonspecific allergies.

    2. Immunocompromised adult.

    3. Concurrent antimicrobial therapy.

    4. Mild acute illness.

61. In taking the history of a healthy 50-year-old man, the family nurse practitioner determines the patient is an avid gardener and spends much of his time enjoying outdoor activities. A health maintenance recommendation for this patient is to obtain a:

    1. Pneumococcal vaccine.

    2. Tdap/Td vaccine.

    3. Hepatitis B vaccine.

    4. Varicella vaccine.

62. The Advisory Committee on Immunization Practices (ACIP) recommends that healthy older adults receive the Tdap booster vaccination:

    1. Every 5 years.

    2. Every 10 years.

    3. At age 65.

    4. At age 50.

63. Which statement most correctly describes tetanus toxoid?

    1. Tetanus toxoid (Td) is a bacterial toxin that has been changed to a nontoxic form.

    2. DTaP and DT are safe to give to adults.

    3. The recommended dose of tetanus toxoid for adults is 1 mL IM.

    4. Tetanus toxoid provides immunity from *Corynebacterium diphtheriae.*

64. Immunizations recommended for healthy young adults include:

    1. Measles, rubella, varicella, and hepatitis B.

    2. Pneumovax, influenza, and rubella.

    3. Tetanus, influenza, varicella, Pneumovax, and hepatitis B.

    4. Influenza, hepatitis B, rubella, measles, and tetanus.

65. A 2-month-old infant received his immunizations, and 12 hours later, the mother calls and says the infant has a fever of 101°F (38°C). What is the most likely cause of the fever?

    1. Vaccination for measles, mumps, and rubella.

    2. Combination of the diphtheria and the polio vaccinations.

    3. Presence of an infection when immunizations were given.

    4. Pertussis immunization.

66. Primary prevention of Neonatal Abstinence Syndrome (NAS) includes:

    1. Prescribing a reliable form of birth control for a patient being treated for chronic pain with opioids.

    2. Universally screen pregnant women for substance abuse and make referrals to treatment when appropriate.

    3. Never prescribe opioids to a woman of child-bearing age.

    4. Obtain a patient's records from the state prescription drug monitoring program if you suspect she is getting opioids from another provider.

67. In caring for youth, the family nurse practitioner should be aware that the number one reason for school absenteeism is:

    1. Sports injuries.

    2. Influenza.

    3. Asthma.

    4. Lack of sleep.

68. The human papillomavirus (HPV) vaccine should be recommended to all of the following except:

    1. A 25-year-old man who did not finish the vaccine series as a teen.

    2. Only young men through the age of 21.

    3. Any man who has sex with men.

    4. Men with compromised immune systems (including HIV) through age 30, if they did not get the HPV vaccine when they were young.

69. When screening for intimate partner violence (IPV), it is important for the family nurse practitioner to understand that the following statement is true:

    1. Only men with psychological problems abuse women.

    2. IPV occurs in a small percentage of the population.

    3. Only people who come from abusive families end up in abusive relationships.

    4. One fourth of all women experience IPV.

70. The following person should not receive the shingles vaccine:

    1. A 62-year-old patient who previously had chickenpox.

    2. A 45-year-old patient who was exposed to chickenpox.

    3. A 60-year-old patient who had the vaccine when she was 50 years old.

    4. A person being treated with corticosteroids.

3 Health Promotion & Maintenance Answers & Rationales

1. Answer: 1

Rationale: The American Cancer Society (ACS) recommends maintenance of a desirable body weight; research has shown an association between increased mortality from various cancers and varying degrees of being overweight. Another recommendation is to eat a wide variety of foods, consistent with the ChooseMyPlate of the U.S. Department of Agriculture and U.S. Department of Health and Human Services. A variety of fruits and vegetables should be included in the daily diet (make half your plate fruits and vegetables) because research has shown an association between lower cancer rates and high fruit and vegetable consumption. High-fiber foods are also recommended; a lower risk of colon cancer is seen in those who consume a high-fiber diet. There are no recommendations to increase the amount of protein in the diet at this time. Due to the high consumption of red meat in the American diet, many people are already receiving large quantities in their current diets. The ACS recommends limiting the daily consumption of alcohol to two drinks for males, one drink for females, and no drinks for pregnant females. They also state that ideally no alcohol should be consumed; regular alcohol consumption has been shown to increase the risk of various cancers.

2. Answer: 1

Rationale: The recommendation is low-density lipoprotein (LDL) <100 mg/dL and triglyceride levels <200 mg/dL for individuals with risk factors for coronary heart disease. All other choices have inaccuracies of goals.

3. Answer: 2

Rationale: The American Diabetes Association recommends screening adults starting at least by age 45 and repeating the fasting plasma glucose (FPG) every 3 years.

4. Answer: 2

Rationale: The physical therapy program will assist the older adult woman in restoring her optimum level of functioning after a stroke. An annual influenza vaccination is a primary prevention activity nonspecific to the care of a patient with a stroke. An annual mammogram and ophthalmologic examination to evaluate for glaucoma are examples of secondary prevention activities nonspecific to the care of a patient with a stroke.

5. Answer: 3

Rationale: The patient needs an increased intake of protein and vitamin C to promote healing. Red meat, citrus fruits, and green vegetables will give the highest amounts of these elements from the selections offered.

6. Answer: 3

Rationale: Shouting increases the pitch of the voice. In presbycusis, or hearing loss in older adults, high-pitched consonant sounds are the first to be affected, and the change may occur gradually. The family nurse practitioner should face the patient when speaking. If the nurse needs to stand behind the patient, touch is used to get the patient's attention. Simple sentences should be used to facilitate understanding.

7. Answer: 4

Rationale: The information about side effects and interactions of medication will prevent complications that may result in a fall. Evaluating for assistive devices following a fall and providing resources to correct hazards in the home are appropriate for tertiary prevention. Reinforcing the need to wear prescribed eyeglasses is appropriate for secondary prevention, which is to prevent the patient from experiencing another fall.

8. Answer: 4

Rationale: The stool guaiac test will assist in identifying any problems with intestinal bleeding. Option #1 is not necessary. Option #2 is not a screening and would not be administered annually. A colonoscopy is recommended at age 50 and then every 10 years thereafter.

9. Answer: 4

Rationale: Using past life experiences applies the concept of adult educational principles. Overhead lighting may produce an increase in the glare, which can decrease visualization. There is an alteration of color perception (e.g., blue appears green-blue) as an individual ages. As individuals age, the ability to hear women's and children's voices decreases because these are generally at a higher pitch. The video would not enhance the program if the patients frequently have presbycusis as a result of the normal aging process.

10. Answer: 3

Rationale: All these disorders can be associated with workplace exposure, but currently, lung disease is still the most common occupationally related disease. Representing approximately 10% of the chronic occupational diseases, lung disease has been named as one of 10 leading work-related disease and injury categories by the National Institute for Occupational Safety and Health (NIOSH). Musculoskeletal injuries are on the rise.

11. Answer: 4

Rationale: The primary goal and benefit of a sports screening physical is to identify athletes at risk for an adverse cardiovascular event. The physical also screens for athletes at risk for orthopedic injuries secondary to previously unresolved injuries; however, this is not the primary benefit. Even with a thorough history from the screening exam, it is unlikely to completely eliminate injuries or be able to identify all underlying health problems. The other options (assessing drug and alcohol use and estimating aerobic capacity) are not the benefit of the sports screening physical.

12. Answer: 4

Rationale: The patient's history and physical will reveal the presence of any coronary heart disease (CHD) risk factors (age, family history of CHD, diabetes, current cigarette smoking, blood pressure, height/weight, cardiovascular exam). A lipid profile is also recommended to assess the level of risk and consists of total cholesterol, high-density lipoprotein (HDL), low-density liproprotein (LDL), and triglyceride levels. It would be prudent to have a precise cholesterol level done because the previous result was from a screening health fair and no written record was taken. These parameters should be assessed first before a cholesterol-lowering agent, ECG, or stress test is ordered. An exercise program is also important but should only be done after a history and physical are taken, and after lipid profile results are known. If the lipid profile or the history and physical results are abnormal, stress testing may be appropriate before undertaking a new exercise program.

13. Answer: 2

Rationale: Screening for colorectal cancer includes annual fecal occult blood screening for individuals over age 50. Avoiding medications that can cause gastrointestinal irritation and bleeding can help avoid false-positive results. Rare meat and vegetables that are high in peroxidase will cause false-positive results, whereas vitamin C can cause false-negative results.

14. Answer: 2

Rationale: The 15- to 25-year-old group is most often affected by testicular cancer.

15. Answer: 1, 3

Rationale: Beans and peas are legumes, which are included in the vegetable group and are excellent sources of plant proteins. Quinoa, popcorn, and wild rice belong to the grains group.

16. Answer: 3

Rationale: In the summer of 1997, the National Institutes of Health (NIH) and American Cancer Society changed the recommendation to begin yearly mammography screenings at age 40. This was supported by the U.S. Preventive Services Task Force (USPSTF) in implementing the 2002 recommendation on breast cancer screening.

17. Answer: 1

Rationale: All areas are important to probe in the initial interview of a new patient. The history will help determine the necessary components of the physical examination and laboratory or radiologic studies that are ordered and the counseling that is done during the appointment.

18. Answer: 4

Rationale: An account of the patient's usual intake is necessary so that problem areas can be identified. Before beginning any exercise program, a physical examination should be done to assess the patient's physical condition and to aid in the proper selection of a specific exercise plan. A dietary assessment needs to be completed before recommending vitamin and protein supplements; the patient may already be receiving adequate amounts in her diet. A more active job would be ideal; however, most people do not have options regarding their choice of job, so increasing her activity outside of work would be most appropriate.

19. Answer: 4

Rationale: The older adult is at greatest risk for altered immune function related to nutrition. The older adult often does not receive enough nutrition for a variety of reasons, including altered taste, eating alone, ability to prepare meals, and malabsorption. Adequate nutrition in the older adult has been shown to improve immune status and antibody response to influenza vaccine.

20. Answer: 2

Rationale: Malnutrition results in the deaths of more infants worldwide than any other syndrome.

21. Answer: 2

Rationale: Hypertension, smoking, and hyperlipidemia are the major risk factors in the development of cardiovascular disease. Controlling hyperglycemia, increasing high dietary fiber intake, and taking vitamin supplements assist in maintaining a healthy lifestyle but are not as important in preventing cardiovascular disease.

22. Answer: 2

Rationale: Premature infants who have spent an extended period in the neonatal intensive care unit (NICU) take 6–10 months to be deinstitutionalized to the noise and light. These must be decreased slowly over time.

23. Answer: 4

Rationale: Multiphasic health screening is a form of periodic health surveillance in which participants undergo a battery of laboratory or diagnostic tests to determine risk factors and disease detection. The other three settings described are not examples of community health promotion activities; they are secondary care settings. The locations of the two clinics are in community settings.

24. Answer: 4

Rationale: It is essential that the immunization record be reviewed. The other options are important but not essential for a health maintenance visit.

25. Answer: 3, 4

Rationale: The average adult in the United States reads at about the sixth to eighth grade level. Printed materials must be written to a level of readability so that they can be understood. Do not use all capital letters or all bolding because such words are difficult to read. In addition, it is helpful to write in the active versus the passive voice, to use one- and two-syllable words, to avoid complex grammatical structures, and to express only one idea in each sentence. Well-chosen and easily understood graphics can significantly enhance the literature, as does the selection of paper on which to print the material.

26. Answer: 1

Rationale: Primary prevention programs exist to prevent disease, malfunctioning, or maladaptation from occurring (e.g., work to lower the incidence of birth defects). Examples of these types of programs include the promotion of a healthy diet, practice of safe sex, and avoidance of alcohol and tobacco. Secondary prevention is early diagnosis and treatment (e.g., screening for tuberculosis or sickle cell disease, breast and testicular self-examination). Tertiary prevention is the prevention of complications and rehabilitation after the disease or condition has occurred (e.g., cardiac rehabilitation; complete blood count done before chemotherapy).

27. Answer: 3

Rationale: If the infant has been satisfied up to this point (by sleeping for long intervals), the infant probably needs additional calories in the form of rice cereal. Adding increased amounts of formula can lead to iron-deficiency anemia.

28. Answer: 1

Rationale: This frequently used ratio is calculated as follows:

$$\frac{\text{No. of deaths} < 1 \text{ year of age in a year}}{\text{No. of live births in the same year}} \times 1000 = \text{Infant mortality rate}$$

29. Answer: 1

Rationale: Familial short stature is not indicated in this case because the father is of normal height. Hypopituitarism would be associated with other findings (micropenis, small testes, immature facies, olfactory defects). Gonadotropin deficiency might be a possibility, but considering all findings in the situation and based on the father having a pubertal onset at age 16 and achieving an average height, the more likely diagnosis is constitutional growth delay.

30. Answer: 4

Rationale: Children should be using a cup and ideally not using a pacifier at 12 months of age. At 9 months of age, the child does not have the mobility to reach the pot handles on the stove. Self-feeding should be encouraged at this age, but silverware is not used until the second year of life. Keeping buttons, beads, and coins out of the child's reach should have been done since the child was about 4 months of age.

31. Answer: 2

Rationale: Car safety and use of a forward-facing car seat continues to be a priority for the 6-year-old. Belt-positioning booster seats are used until the child is 4 ft 9 inches tall and is between 8 and 12 years of age. Bottled drinking water is not necessary when traveling, unless it is outside of the United States. A fluoridated dentifrice should be used in a small amount (pea size), and children under age 6 should be supervised so that they do not swallow too much toothpaste, which would put them at risk for fluorosis. Three regular meals and two snacks are recommended for the busy 4-year-old. Snacks should be rich in complex carbohydrates and low in fat, such as in yogurt; children should avoid candy, chips, and soft drinks.

32. Answer: 4

Rationale: Febrile seizures are benign and do not lead to brain damage. Most febrile illnesses in children result from a virus rather than bacteria and are associated with a high fever.

33. Answer: 1

Rationale: Human milk has more lipase and linoleic acid. Cow's milk is not as good of a nutritional source as human milk because cow's milk has more mineral content (calcium, phosphorus, sodium, potassium), which causes a larger renal solute load. In addition, cow's milk is high in protein, casein, and saturated fat and is lower in carbohydrates than human milk.

34. Answer: 3

Rationale: Usual frequency and quantity of formula feedings are as follows:

0–1 month	6–8 feedings/24 hr of 2–4 oz
2 months	4–5 feedings/24 hr of 5 oz
3 months	4–5 feedings/24 hr of 5–6 oz
4 months	4–5 feedings/24 hr of 6–7 oz
7–10 months	3–4 feedings/24 hr of 8 oz
11–12 months	3 feedings/24 hr of 8 oz

35. Answer: 3

Rationale: At 1 year of age, infants may be fed whole cow's milk. The purpose for waiting is that it has been shown that cow's milk is low in iron, linoleic acid, and vitamin E as well as being high in protein, sodium, and potassium.

36. Answer: 3

Rationale: The American Academy of Pediatrics does not recommend low-iron formulas but does recommend, if stools are hard, to treat for constipation. Typical treatment includes giving 1–2 tsp of dark corn syrup, including fruit juices (prune, pineapple, apricot), nonstarchy vegetables, and water and avoiding rice cereal. Mineral oil is not recommended at this age.

37. Answer: 1

Rationale: These are characteristics of lactose intolerance. Symptoms occur from 2 hours up to 12 hours after milk or milk product ingestion. The prevalence is highest in African Americans, Native Americans, and Asians. Cow's milk intolerance occurs in infancy with symptoms of blood in the stools that is often accompanied by allergies (e.g., eczema, hives, asthma).

38. Answer: 3

Rationale: Although 15 μg/dL is an elevated lead level (normal is <10 μg/dL), chelation therapy in children with a normal exam is not usually conducted until the lead level is >25 μg/dL. It is important at this level to identify the source of the elevation and to monitor the child frequently.

39. Answer: 3

Rationale: Solid food does not need to be introduced before 4–6 months of age. The first foods introduced are cereals. New foods are introduced one at a time at weekly intervals. In this way, the infant's digestive system can adapt to the food, and any reaction can be easily detected.

40. Answer: 2

Rationale: Practice guidelines recommend that even if they meet low-risk criteria, febrile infants younger than 28 days of age should have a sepsis evaluation.

41. Answer: 1

Rationale: Girls in grades 5 through 8 are more motivated by peers and family than are boys. Boys are more intrinsically motivated, with family and peers having less influence. Peers are also more influential for girls in the high school years. High maternal education level is not an influential factor for boys.

42. Answer: 3

Rationale: The reading level of most American adults is from grade 6 to 8; therefore, the sixth grade level would be the most appropriate answer among the choices given.

43. Answer: 4

Rationale: Recommendations of the Centers for Disease Control and Prevention (CDC) for a serum lead level greater than 10 μg/dL are for rescreening and referral to a physician. Rescreening is done before the removal of the child/family from the hazard, although a thorough environmental assessment is essential at rescreening.

44. Answer: 1

Rationale: The water heater should not be set over 120°F to prevent scald burns. Crib rails should be no more than 2⅜ inches apart. The rear-facing infant seat is applicable to 20 lb of weight or 1 year of age. Sunscreen should be applied whenever there is sun exposure.

45. Answer: 4

Rationale: Azarcon and greta are traditional Hispanic remedies that contain lead, which can result in increased lead levels and eventual poisoning. The other substances will not cause the symptoms described. Arnica root is used as a topical preparation to reduce inflammation, muscle pain, and bruising. The Mexican yam root is used for menopausal symptoms and is a source of natural progesterone. White willow bark action is similar to that of aspirin and is used for the relief of pain.

46. Answer: 1

Rationale: Maintaining normal weight, decreasing sodium in the diet, and exercising regularly are three modifications that are most effective in maintaining normal blood pressure in the older adult.

Immunizations

47. Answer: 3

Rationale: It is recommended that the child receive the inactivated poliovirus vaccine (IPV) at 2 months, 4 months, the third dose between 6 and 18 months, and the fourth dose between 4 and 6 years of age.

48. Answer: 3

Rationale: The measles mumps rubella (MMR) is a live-virus vaccine. Children severely immunosuppressed because of cancer therapy should not receive live-virus vaccines for 3 months after chemotherapy has been stopped.

49. Answer: 1

Rationale: The law calls for the parental signature to be maintained in the clinical record.

50. Answer: 3

Rationale: Children over the age of 13 years who have not had chickenpox and have not been previously immunized are recommended to have two doses at least 28 days apart for effective immunity.

51. Answer: 2

Rationale: If given within 72 hours of exposure, the live attenuated measles vaccine will provide protection in most cases. The dose of immunoglobulin G (IgG) would be 0.25 mL/kg, given within 6 days of exposure.

52. Answer: 1

Rationale: Polyvalent pneumococcal vaccine is recommended for children with chronic diseases. It is not recommended for use to prevent otitis media (OM) and other pneumococcal diseases. It can be given concurrently with other vaccines, and it does not cause severe systemic reactions. It will occasionally cause mild local reactions.

53. Answer: 2

Rationale: Influenza outbreaks may affect 60% of those in long-term care, and mortality rates are high. All the other groups listed are appropriate for the influenza vaccine but are not as high a priority.

54. Answer: 3

Rationale: Prior anaphylaxis and severe hypersensitivity would be considered a contraindication; a mild viral illness would not. The patient who is pregnant or lactating may be immunized.

55. Answer: 1

Rationale: Pneumococcal and annual influenza immunizations are recommended for those who are age 65 and older. Tdap (tetanus toxoid, reduced diphtheria toxoid, and acellular pertussis) for all adults aged 65 years and older is recommended. Boostrix should be used for adults aged 65 years and older; however, the Advisory Committee on Immunization Practices (ACIP) concluded that either vaccine (Adacel or Boostrix) administered to a person 65 years or older is immunogenic and would provide protection. Shingles vaccine is contraindicated in women who are pregnant and in individuals who have a weakened immune system.

56. Answer: 1

Rationale: Attenuated live-virus vaccines are available for the following communicable diseases: measles, mumps, rubella, poliomyelitis, yellow fever, and smallpox. Rabies vaccine is a killed virus, and hepatitis B is a purified viral antigen obtained from the blood of an infected patient and then inactivated when manufactured into a vaccination.

57. Answer: 4

Rationale: Children who have a severe allergy to neomycin are at increased risk for the development of an allergic reaction to the measles vaccine.

58. Answer: 1

Rationale: A child who contracts chickenpox for the first time develops antibodies during the period of infection. These antibodies create a naturally acquired, lifelong type of active immunity. Artificially acquired active immunity occurs with immunizations. Natural passive immunity occurs with placental transfer. Artificial passively acquired immunity occurs with an injection of human or animal serum (antitoxin).

59. Answer: 1

Rationale: Hepatitis B first dose should be given at birth. By 8 months of age, all 3 doses of the hepatitis B series should have been given. Rotavirus (RV) should be given at 2, 4, and 6 months. Inactivated poliovirus (IPV) should be given at 2 and 4 months, and the 3rd dose anytime from 6 months to 18 months. Measles, mumps, and rubella (MMR) first dose is given at 12 months and again at 4–6 years of age. Tetanus toxoid, diphtheria toxoid, and acellular pertussis (Tdap) is given to children who are age 11 years and older; however, if children who are age 7 years and older are not fully immunized with the DTaP vaccine, they should receive the Tdap vaccine as 1 dose (preferably the first) in the catch-up series.

60. Answer: 2

Rationale: The live vaccine can produce serious disseminated disease in patients with immunocompromised status (e.g., leukemia, lymphoma, HIV/AIDS) and in those undergoing cancer chemotherapy. Mild acute illness, concurrent antimicrobial therapy, and a history of nonspecific allergies are not contraindications for use of a live vaccine.

61. Answer: 2

Rationale: Older adults who enjoy gardening and outdoor activities should have a Tdap/Td booster once, as recommended by the Advisory Committee on Immunization Practices (ACIP). As part of standard wound management care to prevent tetanus, a tetanus toxoid-containing vaccine might be recommended for wound management in adults aged 19 years and older if 5 years or more have elapsed since last receiving Td. If a tetanus booster is indicated, Tdap is preferred over Td for wound management in adults aged 19 years and older who have not received Tdap previously. A pneumococcal vaccine is recommended for adults aged 65 or older and for those with a chronic illness or in an immunosuppressed state. Most older adults had chickenpox as a child and do not require the vaccine.

62. Answer: 3

Rationale: On February 22, 2012, the Advisory Committee on Immunization Practices (ACIP) approved the use of Tdap (tetanus toxoid, reduced diphtheria toxoid, and acellular pertussis) for all adults aged 65 years and older. Boostrix should be used for adults aged 65 years and older; however, ACIP concluded that either vaccine (Boostrix or Adacel) administered to a person 65 years or older is immunogenic and would provide protection.

63. Answer: 1

Rationale: Tetanus toxoid is a bacterial toxin that has been changed to nontoxic form and produces persistent antitoxin antibody titers because the patient's immune system is stimulated to manufacture antitoxins (i.e., antibodies directed against the bacterial toxin). *Corynebacterium diphtheriae* is the organism that causes diphtheria, not tetanus. DTaP and DT are for use in children under age 7 years and should *not* be used in adults. DT does not contain pertussis and is given as a substitute for children who cannot tolerate the DTaP that contains pertussis. The recommended dose of tetanus toxoid alone for an adult is 0.5 mL IM. To help you remember, look closely at the letters and keep the following in mind:

- Uppercase "T" means there is about the same amount of tetanus in DTaP, Tdap, and Td. (DTaP is given to children, usually infants, under age 7.)

- Uppercase "D" and "P" means there is more diphtheria and pertussis in DTaP than in Tdap and Td; lowercase letters ("d" and "p") means there is less. (Tdap is a booster given at age 11 and throughout life, usually every 10 years, and is recommended as a booster after age 65.)

64. Answer: 4

Rationale: A percentage of young adults (5% to 20%) are susceptible to measles and/or rubella. Influenza and hepatitis B are recommended for students who have exposure to a large number of people. Tetanus is recommended every 10 years, especially in high-risk situations (young adults who participate in outdoor sports). Pneumovax is indicated in a young adult who has a chronic disease (e.g., diabetes, chronic pulmonary disease, chronic cardiovascular disease) and is also indicated for young adults who are immunocompromised.

65. Answer: 4

Rationale: The most common cause of fever at the 2-month immunization series is the pertussis. This vaccine causes reactions in about 75% of infants. The MMR vaccine is not given until 12–15 months of age.

66. Answer: 1

Rationale: Pregnancy prevention is the primary prevention for Neonatal Abstinence Syndrome (NAS). Universal screening and referrals to treatment are recommended, but they do not prevent NAS. There will be times when child-bearing-age women must be prescribed opioids. While consulting the drug monitoring program does help decrease doctor shopping, it does not prevent NAS.

67. Answer: 3

Rationale: In 2013, the Centers for Disease Control and Prevention reported that asthma was the number one reason children were absent from school.

68. Answer: 2

Rationale: All boys and girls ages 11 or 12 years should get vaccinated. Catch-up vaccines are recommended for males through age 21 and females through age 26. The vaccine is also recommended for gay and bisexual men (or for any man who has sex with a man) through age 26. It is also recommended for men and women with compromised immune systems (including people living with HIV/AIDS) through age 26, if they did not get fully vaccinated when they were younger.

69. Answer: 4

Rationale: One fourth of all women do experience intimate partner violence (IPV). IPV can occur in any family. Most abused women report that their partner was the first person to abuse them. Many batterers are successful professionals, including politicians, ministers, physicians, and lawyers.

70. Answer: 4

Rationale: A person should not receive the shingles vaccine if he is immunosuppressed or receiving medications that suppress the immune system, such as corticosteroids. Other situations when a person should not receive the immunization include if she is pregnant, has untreated tuberculosis, is allergic to gelatin or neomycin, and if he or she is receiving chemotherapy or radiation therapy. Anyone 60 years of age or older should receive the vaccine, regardless of whether he or she can recall having the vaccine or not. Exposure to chickenpox in a 45-year-old patient does not warrant vaccination at this time. Adults receiving the vaccine before the age of 60 might not be protected when their risk for shingles and its complications are greatest.

4

Cardiovascular

Physical Examination & Diagnostic Tests

1. The family nurse practitioner is performing a physical examination on a healthy adult male. On auscultation, the stethoscope would be placed in what areas to best hear the characteristic heart sounds S_1 and S_2?

   1. S_1 is best heard at the apex and S_2 at the base of the heart.

   2. Both are heard equally well at the right midclavicular line.

   3. On the left side, S_1 is at the area of the pulmonic valve and S_2 at the aortic valve.

   4. Both sounds are best heard at Erb's point.

2. On the general assessment of an adult patient, the family nurse practitioner determines the presence of the apical impulse at the PMI on the patient's chest wall. Where on the chest wall is the PMI normally found?

   1. Second intercostal space at the midclavicular line on the left side.

   2. Right lower sternal border, fifth intercostal space.

   3. Left side at the fifth intercostal space on the midclavicular line.

   4. Left fifth intercostal space, lateral to the midclavicular line.

3. The family nurse practitioner is auscultating the carotids. What is the correct procedure?

   1. Use the diaphragm of the stethoscope.

   2. Use the bell of the stethoscope.

   3. Place the stethoscope 1 inch off the area above the sternocleidomastoid muscle.

   4. Position the patient at a 30-degree angle, and press firmly using the bell of the stethoscope.

4. When inspecting the precordium, the family nurse practitioner is checking for:

   1. Scars and anatomic landmarks.

   2. Pulsations and retractions.

   3. Heaves and cardiac dullness.

   4. Pericardial friction rub and lifts.

5. While examining a patient in a left lateral position, the family nurse practitioner auscultates a third heart sound (S_3). The family nurse practitioner knows:

   1. This sound is considered normal in children and young adults.

   2. This rarely is associated with myocardial failure in the older adult.

   3. This patient should be immediately referred to a cardiologist for evaluation.

   4. This is considered a normal splitting of the S_2 during inspiration.

6. The family nurse practitioner knows that the correct ausculatory site for the aortic area is the:

   1. Midclavicular line, fifth interspace, left side.

   2. Left fourth interspace close to the sternum.

   3. Right second interspace close to the sternum.

   4. Midclavicular line, second interspace, left side.

7. The family nurse practitioner should include which statement in patient teaching when ordering a lipid profile on a patient?

   Eat a typical diet over the next week and:

   1. Eat a normal breakfast the morning of the lipid profile blood draw.

   2. Fast for 12 hours before the lipid profile is drawn.

   3. There are no restrictions on alcohol for this blood test.

   4. Take any current medications with a few sips of water before the blood test.

8. When auscultating the heart sounds of a 72-year-old patient with a history of hypertension, the family nurse practitioner notes an S_4. This finding could indicate:

   1. Normal variant in people 65 years and older.

   2. Beginning of ventricular failure.

   3. Decreased resistance to ventricular filling.

   4. Severely failing heart.

9. Which of the following is an appropriate blood pressure goal for a 65-year-old male with no comorbidities?

   1. SBP <150/DBP <90

   2. SBP <140/DBP <90

   3. SBP <140/DBP <80

   4. SBP <150/DBP <90

10. The family nurse practitioner is examining a patient with a history of rheumatic fever who is being followed for the development of carditis. During cardiac auscultation, where on the chest wall is the stethoscope placed to determine the most common murmur associated with this condition?

    1. At the left sternal border, fourth left intercostal space.

    2. Fifth intercostal space, left side, at the midclavicular line.

    3. Second or third intercostal space at the left of the sternal border.

    4. Second intercostal space on the right of the sternal border.

11. A patient presents with unusual coolness in the left hand compared with the right hand. What is the next step in the exam?

    1. Palpate the radial pulse on both hands for a full minute.

    2. Perform Allen's test on both hands.

    3. Feel the forearms with the backs of the fingers.

    4. Hold the hand in a dependent position, and then reexamine.

12. S_1 and S_2 are identified when the family nurse practitioner auscultates for cardiac sounds. The physiology responsible for the production of these heart sounds is:

    1. Closure of atrioventricular (AV) valves produces S_1; closure of semilunar valves forms S_2.

    2. Closure of the aortic valve produces S_2; opening of mitral valve produces S_1.

    3. Opening of AV valves produces S_1; closure of semilunar valves produces S_2.

    4. Opening of the tricuspid valve produces S_1; closure of the pulmonic valve forms S_2.

13. The family nurse practitioner is assessing a cardiac patient who is experiencing an atrial dysrhythmia. The pulse rate is irregular at 110 beats/min, and there is concern regarding a pulse deficit. How is a pulse deficit determined in this patient?

    1. A 12-lead electrocardiogram (ECG) is necessary to determine the presence and length of the PR intervals.

    2. The apical pulse is counted, and then the radial pulse is counted; the pulse deficit is determined by the difference in the two rates.

    3. The apical pulse is counted, and an increase or decrease is correlated with the phases of the respiratory cycle.

    4. The apical pulse and radial pulse are determined simultaneously; a pulse deficit is established if the apical rate is higher than the radial rate.

14. The family nurse practitioner notes a grade V systolic murmur while examining a patient's precordium. Which characteristics describe this type of murmur?

    1. Barely audible; faintly heard with the bell of the stethoscope.

    2. Heard only with the diaphragm of the stethoscope.

    3. Heard with the stethoscope partly off the chest.

    4. Heard without the aid of the stethoscope.

15. Normal physiologic changes in the geriatric population that affect conductivity and contractility of the myocardium include:

    1. Increased automaticity and excitability.

    2. Increased contractility and conductivity.

    3. Decreased excitability and conductivity.

    4. Decreased automaticity and contractility.

16. When assessing the temperature of an extremity as part of a patient's peripheral vascular assessment, which part of the hand is the most sensitive?

    1. Palm.

    2. Fingertips.

    3. Back of the wrist.

    4. Back of the fingers.

17. A 45-year-old male patient's lipid profile results are sent to the family nurse practitioner with levels as follows: total cholesterol = 287 mmol/L; HDL = 30 mg/dL; and LDL = 165 mg/dL. Based upon the interpretation of these findings, the family nurse practitioner should do which of the following?

    1. Initiate treatment with low-dose statins.

    2. Discuss adherence to a heart-healthy diet and regular aerobic physical activity.

    3. Assess the 10-year arteriosclerotic cardiovascular disease (ASCVD) risk.

    4. Refer to cardiologist.

18. A patient returns to the chest pain clinic 3 weeks post MI complaining of pericardial pain and elevated temperature. Physical exam reveals a pericardial friction rub. What diagnostic studies are indicated?

    1. 24-hour Holter monitoring.

    2. Echocardiogram.

    3. Complete blood count (CBC) with differential.

    4. Cardiac enzymes with myoglobin.

19. On assessment of an older adult patient, the family nurse practitioner notes bilateral pulsations and distention of the jugular veins when the patient's head is elevated 45 degrees. What further assessment needs to be done at this time?

    1. Estimate the level of venous pressure by measuring from the sternal angle to the highest level of venous pulsations.

    2. Place the patient in a supine position and determine the effect of position change on distention and pulsations of the jugular vein.

    3. Measure carotid pulses because of the increased left ventricular pressure.

    4. Have the patient hold his or her breath to facilitate evaluation for the presence of carotid bruits.

20. The family nurse practitioner is examining a woman with a known history of mitral valve disease. What type of murmur heard on auscultation supports a history of mitral stenosis?

    1. Diastolic murmur, heard loudest at the apex with the patient on her left side.

    2. Midsystolic ejection murmur heard loudest over the left lower sternal border.

    3. Holosystolic murmur, heard loudest over the apex and left axillary area.

    4. Diastolic murmur, heard loudest with patient in a sitting position, leaning forward.

21. The family nurse practitioner is doing an assessment of a patient who is 2 weeks post MI affecting the left ventricle. The family nurse practitioner would pay particular attention to what area of the physical assessment?

    1. Lower extremities and the jugular vein.

    2. Area on the chest where the post MI is heard.

    3. Presence of dyspnea and auscultation of crackles in the lungs.

    4. Level of dependent edema and fluid intake over the past 24 hours.

22. Which symptoms would indicate to the family nurse practitioner that the patient is experiencing intermittent claudication?

    1. Petechiae and itching of the lower part of the leg.

    2. Extensive discoloration and edema of the upper leg.

    3. Profuse rash and discoloration from the trunk down to the feet.

    4. Complaints of pain on walking, relieved by sitting down.

23. Stress testing, or the exercise tolerance test, is the most widely used diagnostic test in ischemic heart disease. It is most accurate, up to 98%, in what patient population?

    1. Males under age 40 with atypical angina pectoris.
    2. Asymptomatic premenopausal females without risk factors.
    3. Males over age 50 with typical angina pectoris.
    4. Males receiving digitalis with typical angina pectoris.

24. When palpating for the apical impulse of a 46-year-old female, the family nurse practitioner feels a hyperkinetic impulse. The nurse would auscultate for which additional finding?

    1. Pericardial friction rub.
    2. Pansystolic murmur.
    3. Pulsus paradoxus.
    4. Decreased intensity of heart sounds.

25. While assessing a patient with a history of recent MI, the family nurse practitioner notes pulsus alternans. The nurse would assess for other assessment changes caused by:

    1. Unstable angina.
    2. Cardiogenic shock.
    3. Recurrent MI.
    4. Left-sided heart failure.

Disorders

26. A 70-year-old woman comes to the clinic with the complaint of severe aching of her legs after standing for 10 minutes. What other assessment finding of the lower extremities would support the family nurse practitioner's tentative diagnosis of chronic venous insufficiency?

    1. Pitting edema of 3+ and cyanosis on dependency.
    2. Shiny skin and dusky red on dependency.
    3. Minimal hair and pallor on elevation.
    4. Pulses 1+ and ulceration involving the toes.

27. The diagnosis of hypertension (HTN) should be established on the basis of:

    1. At least three hypertensive readings in a week.
    2. At least five readings 1 month apart.

3. One reading of 140 mm Hg systolic and 90 mm Hg diastolic or higher.
4. One reading taken in three different positions.

28. A patient has a 2-year history of hypertensive heart disease. The family nurse practitioner expects the major pathophysiologic change to be:

    1. Right ventricular hypertrophy.
    2. Left atrial dilation.
    3. Left ventricular hypertrophy.
    4. Right atrial dilation.

29. Of the following descriptions, which data most clearly describe atrial tachycardia?

    1. Heart rate of 96 beats/min, P waves present on each QRS complex, T wave every other beat.
    2. P waves present on every other beat, heart rate of 100 beats/min, and irregular.
    3. Heart rate of 110 beats/min, P waves present before each QRS complex, and regular.
    4. P waves for every third QRS complex, adequate PR interval, heart rate of 90 beats/min.

30. What clinical manifestation of a myocardial infarction is frequently not present in the older adult cardiac patient?

    1. Prolonged severe chest pain.
    2. Diaphoresis, pallor, and syncope.
    3. Dyspnea and increasing anxiety.
    4. Gastrointestinal distress and orthopnea.

31. The family nurse practitioner is performing an assessment on a patient who is having difficulty controlling his left-sided heart failure. The family nurse practitioner understands that the primary symptoms associated with this type of heart failure are:

    1. Systemic venous congestion.
    2. Dyspnea and pulmonary congestion.
    3. Increased peripheral edema and anorexia.
    4. Atrial fibrillation with a heart rate around 110 beats/min.

32. The family nurse practitioner is concerned a patient that is post MI is developing a problem of constrictive pericarditis. What is a characteristic finding with constrictive pericarditis, and how is it evaluated?

    1. Cardiac tamponade, identified by muffled heart sounds and a paradoxical pulse.

    2. Pericardial triphasic friction rub, best heard at the apical area of the heart.

    3. Mitral valve prolapse, characterized by late systolic murmur at apex and left sternal borders.

    4. Altered waves on jugular venous pulse, as determined with a light directed tangentially to illuminate the shadows of the pulsations.

33. An older adult patient has a diagnosis of left-sided heart failure. The family nurse practitioner would identify what common condition associated with heart failure?

    1. Peripheral vascular disease.

    2. Untreated hypertension.

    3. Ventricular dysrhythmias.

    4. Chronic obstructive pulmonary disease.

34. In evaluating the effectiveness of cardiopulmonary resuscitation (CPR) on the adult patient, the family nurse practitioner would note:

    1. Dilated pupils.

    2. Palpable carotid pulse.

    3. Capillary refill.

    4. Pink and warm skin.

35. The family nurse practitioner is evaluating an ECG of a patient who presented at the clinic with complaints of weakness and fainting. The patient's ECG reveals a cardiac rate of 68 beats/min, absent P waves, regular QRS complex, and T waves present after each QRS complex. What is the best interpretation of this information?

    1. Normal ECG; need to further evaluate patient's complaints of weakness.

    2. Third-degree block with junctional rhythm; transfer patient to emergency room for cardiology consult.

    3. First-degree block; need to further evaluate patient related to cardiac medications.

    4. Administer sublingual nitroglycerin and refer patient for a cardiology consult.

36. The family nurse practitioner is conducting a follow-up examination on a patient with coronary artery disease and a history of pericarditis. What is a characteristic physical finding in pericarditis, and how is it evaluated?

    1. Paradoxical pulse, identified by evaluating the changes in the amplitude of arterial pulse pressure associated with the respiratory cycle.

    2. Pulse deficit, as determined by counting the radial pulse and apical pulse at the same time and evaluating the difference.

    3. Pericardial friction rub, best heard using the diaphragm of the stethoscope and loudest to the left of the sternum at the fourth or fifth intercostal space.

    4. An S_4 present, usually heard at the apex with the bell of the stethoscope and patient in a left lateral position.

37. The symptoms of MI usually experienced by the older adult patient include:

    1. Dyspnea and diaphoresis.

    2. Back pain and muscle cramping.

    3. Numbness and tingling of the left arm.

    4. Epigastric pain and nausea.

38. What are the cardiovascular risk factors predisposing females to cardiovascular disease?

    1. Absence of estrogen adversely affects lipoprotein metabolism.

    2. Fat deposited on the hips mobilizes, raising serum cholesterol.

    3. Coronary arteries are longer and wider in diameter.

    4. Resting ejection fraction is lower.

39. The family nurse practitioner is planning the treatment of an older adult patient newly diagnosed with hypertension. What parameters are most important in determining the appropriate pharmacologic therapy?

    1. Determine medications and dosage based on the patient's weight, age, and drug availability.

    2. Begin step method utilizing diuretics and beta-adrenergic blockers.

    3. Initiate lifestyle changes before beginning medications.

    4. Determine other medical conditions for which the patient is being treated.

40. Which statement accurately describes coronary artery disease (CAD) in geriatric patients?

    1. Cardiovascular disease is increased in the female patient receiving estrogen replacement.

    2. A major risk factor for cardiovascular disease in females and males is chronic hypertension.

    3. The majority of geriatric patients with CAD also have type 2 diabetes.

    4. Males over 60 years old continue to experience the highest level of CAD.

41. A patient with a history of COPD comes to the clinic for his annual checkup with complaints of increasing difficulty breathing. Assessment findings include S_3 gallop, early systolic ejection click, and increased P-wave amplitude in leads II, III, and aVF of the ECG. The family nurse practitioner would expect to observe which change on the chest x-ray film?

    1. Hypertrophy of the left ventricle.

    2. Hypertrophy of the right ventricle.

    3. Hypertrophy of the left atrium and ventricle.

    4. Hypertrophy of the right atrium and ventricle.

42. When cardiac output falls in heart failure, the body attempts to compensate. What electrolyte imbalances result from this response?

    1. Hypernatremia and hyperkalemia.

    2. Hyponatremia and hypokalemia.

    3. Hypophosphatemia and hypercalcemia.

    4. Hyperphosphatemia and hypocalcemia.

43. When assessing the carotid pulse of a 72-year-old patient at a community-based clinic, the family nurse practitioner notes a bounding pulse with rapid rise and sudden collapse. The family nurse practitioner would include which additional assessment to support this finding?

    1. Auscultation for a diastolic murmur.

    2. Auscultation for paradoxical pulse.

    3. BP in both arms lying, sitting, and standing.

    4. BP for an auscultatory gap.

44. The family nurse practitioner understands that the pain experienced with angina pectoris or MI is caused by irritation of the myocardial nerve fibers by the increase in:

    1. Blood glucose.

    2. Lactic acid.

    3. Serum potassium.

    4. Serum magnesium.

45. New York Heart Functional Class III for patients with cardiac disease is characterized by:

    1. Symptoms present at rest, with any activity leading to increased discomfort.

    2. Slight limitation in ordinary activity, resulting in fatigue, palpitations, dyspnea, or angina.

    3. No physical limitation in activity.

    4. Marked limitation in activity, comfortable at rest, but ordinary activity leads to symptoms.

46. During the history and physical examination of a patient with suspected early heart failure, which is the most prominent finding?

    1. Moist crackles in the lung bases bilaterally.

    2. Anorexia with weight loss of 3 lb in 1 week.

    3. Increased urine output and peripheral edema.

    4. Facial edema and distended neck veins.

47. Chest pain that is sudden and severe, described as "tearing," and accompanied by a decrease in peripheral pulses may indicate a diagnosis of:

    1. Angina.

    2. Acute MI.

    3. Aortic dissection.

    4. Pericarditis.

48. Which of the following would be appropriate dietary therapy recommendations for a patient with hyperlipidemia?

    1. Limiting intake of salt, sweets, and sugar-sweetened beverages.

    2. Increasing the average daily protein intake to 70 g/day.

    3. Decreasing total fat to <37% of the daily total calories per day.

    4. Limiting carbohydrate intake.

49. The most frequent life-threatening dysrhythmia experienced by a patient with an acute MI is:
    1. Atrial fibrillation.
    2. Ventricular tachycardia.
    3. Third-degree heart block.
    4. Ventricular fibrillation.

50. In an overweight older adult female patient with an elevated cholesterol level and abnormal lipoprotein profile, the first step in treatment includes:
    1. Prescribing a bile acid sequestrant agent.
    2. Initiation of a diet and exercise program.
    3. Estrogen replacement therapy.
    4. Referral to a cardiologist.

51. Patients with chronic atrial fibrillation are at risk for which condition?
    1. Sudden cardiac death.
    2. Stroke.
    3. Ventricular tachycardia.
    4. Acute myocardial infarction.

52. The family nurse practitioner understands that the most common symptom of heart failure in adults is:
    1. Anorexia.
    2. Dependent edema.
    3. Dyspnea.
    4. Weakness.

53. The family nurse practitioner teaches the cardiac patient to avoid foods high in saturated fats, which include:
    1. Nuts, legumes, and seeds.
    2. Fish, shellfish, and mussels.
    3. Palm oil, coconut oil, and butter.
    4. Peanut oil, soybean oil, and olive oil.

54. An older adult male patient is complaining of chest pain. A parameter to assist the family nurse practitioner to differentiate the chest pain of angina from that of a myocardial infarction is:
    1. Myocardial pain with an infarction is more severe.
    2. Anginal pain is more substernal and does not radiate to other areas.
    3. Anginal pain is frequently relieved by nitroglycerin.
    4. Pain from an infarction is always associated with other symptoms.

55. The family nurse practitioner is evaluating a patient in the office who is complaining of chest pain. The patient's BP is 86/52 mm Hg, and ECG results show some signs of ischemia. The patient is to be transferred to the emergency department. What drug might the family nurse practitioner give the patient while awaiting transfer?
    1. Furosemide (Lasix) 40 mg IV.
    2. Morphine sulfate 25 mg IV.
    3. Nitroglycerin 0.3 mg SL.
    4. Aspirin 81 mg PO.

56. Which would not be considered as contributing to the development of thrombophlebitis?
    1. Excessive use of oral anticoagulants.
    2. Blow to the leg or arm.
    3. Recent IV therapy.
    4. Secondary to pregnancy.

57. An older adult patient is being evaluated for a complaint of dizziness. What symptom/observation will make the family nurse practitioner consider that this is a life-threatening event?
    1. The dizziness occurs in certain positions.
    2. It is accompanied by tinnitus.
    3. The symptoms worsen when standing.
    4. It is preceded by rapid breathing.

58. A 28-year-old male presents to the family nurse practitioner with a history of chest pain that has been increasing over the past several days. The patient states that the pain worsens on lying down and denies any shortness of breath, cough, or radiation of the pain. The patient gives a history of a recent infection with coxsackievirus. Examination shows that the patient has a cardiac friction rub. One probable diagnosis considered by the family nurse practitioner is:
    1. Acute myocardial infarction.
    2. Pleural effusion.
    3. Pericarditis.
    4. Esophageal reflux.

59. The family nurse practitioner would most likely suspect which differential diagnosis for an older adult patient presenting with atrial fibrillation and functional decline?

    1. Hyperthyroidism.

    2. Hypothyroidism.

    3. Sick sinus syndrome.

    4. Heart failure.

60. Which assessment made by the family nurse practitioner for an older patient would be a deviation from the normal changes of aging?

    1. Decreased exercise tolerance.

    2. Grade II/VI systolic ejection murmur.

    3. Prolongation of PR intervals on ECG.

    4. Jugular venous pressure (JVP) of 4 cm H_2O.

61. Cardiac auscultation of an older patient reveals a grade II/VI murmur that is heard best at the second right intercostal space. The murmur is louder with squatting. There is a small carotid pulse with a delayed upstroke. The patient's history is benign, and his activity tolerance is within normal limits for his age. The family nurse practitioner would interpret this murmur to be indicative of:

    1. Aortic regurgitation.

    2. Aortic stenosis.

    3. Mitral valve prolapse.

    4. Mitral regurgitation.

62. What is the most frequently diagnosed valvular heart problem in older adult patients?

    1. Aortic stenosis.

    2. Mitral stenosis.

    3. Mitral regurgitation.

    4. Aortic regurgitation.

63. A middle-aged man with no known risk factors for coronary artery disease presents with a total cholesterol level of 255 mg/dL. The family nurse practitioner would:

    1. Start him on an HMG CoA reductase inhibitor.

    2. Reevaluate the total cholesterol in 8 weeks.

    3. Repeat the total cholesterol and obtain HDL and calculated LDL levels.

    4. Do nothing because this patient demonstrates no coronary risk factors other than male gender.

Pharmacology

64. A 75-year-old patient presents to the office complaining of "not feeling well." He has a history of chronic lung disease and heart failure. His vital signs are pulse 78 beats/min and irregular, respirations 26 breaths/min, and BP of 158/100 mm Hg. An ECG indicates sinus rhythm and confirms the rate. The PR interval is 0.28 second, P waves are present, and each is followed by a QRS complex. There are frequent premature atrial beats. The patient is taking digitalis, potassium, theophylline, hydrochlorothiazide, and a calcium channel blocker. What is the next best action to take?

    1. Obtain serum theophylline, digitalis, and potassium levels.

    2. Increase dosage of calcium blocker and diuretic.

    3. Order pulmonary function studies.

    4. Refer the patient to a cardiologist.

65. A 49-year-old female was started on a thiazide diuretic for hypertension 1 month ago. She arrives in the clinic complaining of muscle cramps and dizziness. Physical exam findings are BP 132/88 mm Hg (previous 186/112 mm Hg); pulse 112 beats/min; respirations 24 breaths/min; tenting positive; skin turgor decreased; neck veins flat; sodium 114 mEq/L; chloride 92 mEq/L; potassium 3.0 mEq/L; and blood glucose 201 mg/dL. Initial treatment for this patient should include fluid replacement:

    1. Orally with free water and a potassium supplement.

    2. Intravenously with normal saline and regular insulin subcutaneously.

    3. Intravenously with 1000 mL of normal saline with 40 mEq KCl at 50 mL/hr.

    4. Intravenously with 1000 mL of lactated Ringer's solution at 250 mL/hr.

66. A patient is recovering from an acute episode of thrombophlebitis and is being treated with warfarin (Coumadin) 5 mg PO daily. In reviewing medication information, the family nurse practitioner would include what information in her teaching?

    1. Do not take a multivitamin supplement.

    2. Limit dairy products.

    3. Aerobic exercises are the most effective.

    4. Maintain a daily record of intake and output.

67. The family nurse practitioner is evaluating a patient who is "not feeling good." He has a history of coronary artery disease (CAD) and heart failure. Vital signs are pulse 72 beats/min; respirations 20 breaths/min; BP 130/88 mm Hg; and temperature normal. The patient has no complaints of chest pain or difficulty breathing. The patient had some nausea but no vomiting over the past 2 days. Lower extremities are negative for edema. The patient states he has been able to take his medications. His current medications are digoxin (Lanoxin) 0.25 bid, hydrochlorothiazide (HydroDiuril) 100 mg bid, potassium (Micro-K) 10 mEq daily, and nitroglycerin transdermal patches. What is the priority of care for this patient?

    1. STAT electrocardiogram (ECG) and white blood cell count (WBC).

    2. Arterial blood gases and oxygen at 4 L/min.

    3. Serum digoxin and potassium levels.

    4. Serial cardiac enzymes now and q6h ×2.

68. The family nurse practitioner has prescribed losartan (Cozaar) 50 mg PO qd. This medication promotes vasodilation by:

    1. Blocking the action of angiotensin II.

    2. Promoting release of aldosterone.

    3. Promoting synthesis of prostaglandin.

    4. Inhibiting calcium influx into smooth muscle cells.

69. A patient with a history of hypertension is started on spironolactone (Aldactone) 50 mg PO qd. The family nurse practitioner instructs the patient to call the clinic if which symptoms are experienced?

    1. Increased irritability, abdominal cramping, and lower extremity weakness.

    2. Decreased reflex response, nausea, and vomiting.

    3. Muscle twitching, numbness, tingling, burning sensations of the limbs, and diarrhea.

    4. Weight gain, excessive thirst, and fever.

70. A patient with a history of unstable angina is seen in the cardiac clinic for a checkup. The assessment reveals increased weight of 10 lb, distended jugular neck veins, and an S_3. What changes in the pharmacologic treatment should be initiated?

    1. Discontinue beta-blockers and calcium channel blockers.

    2. Initiate thrombolytic therapy.

    3. Discontinue nitrate and aspirin therapy.

    4. Initiate diuretic and vasoconstrictor therapy.

71. A patient arrives at the emergency room of a small rural hospital complaining that he "feels like my heart is racing." He is connected to a cardiac monitor, which reveals supraventricular tachycardia at a rate of 184 beats/min, QRS complex of <0.10 second, and BP 112/62 mm Hg. Which treatment modality is indicated?

    1. Synchronized cardioversion with 50 joules.

    2. Defibrillation with 100 joules.

    3. Adenosine 6 mg IV push.

    4. Lidocaine 1 mg/kg IV push.

72. An 80-year-old patient with a history of glaucoma develops unstable angina. He is started on diltiazem (Cardizem) 30 mg PO qid and aspirin 325 mg PO qd in addition to timolol ophthalmic solution (Timoptic) 1 gtt right eye bid. This patient would have an increased risk for:

    1. Bleeding episodes.

    2. Fainting episodes and falls.

    3. Rebound supraventricular tachycardia.

    4. Blurred vision.

73. A patient with a serum cholesterol level of 256 mg/dL, HDL of 38 mg/dL, and LDL of 172 mg/dL is instructed on dietary modifications and niacin (nicotinic acid) 1 gm PO tid. Specific instructions include:

    1. Limiting daily fluid intake.

    2. Taking measures to minimize orthostatic hypotension.

    3. Administering the drug an hour after eating.

    4. Avoid exposure to direct sunlight.

74. When monitoring for the therapeutic effects of verapamil (Calan SR), the family nurse practitioner would assess for:

    1. Increase in heart rate.

    2. Decrease in systemic vascular resistance.

    3. Increase in blood pressure.

    4. Decrease in ventricular premature beats.

75. A 45-year-old African American male patient with essential hypertension is treated by the family nurse practitioner with sodium restriction and hydrochlorothiazide (Diuril) 25 mg PO daily. After 3 months of therapy, the patient's blood pressure is measured at 160/110 mm Hg. At this point, the family nurse practitioner would:

    1. Begin enalapril (Vasotec) 5 mg qd.

    2. Begin with 50 mg of metoprolol (Toprol XL) qd.

    3. Add 5 mg of amlodipine (Norvasc) daily.

    4. Discontinue Diuril and change to captopril (Capoten) 50 mg tid.

76. When prescribing antihypertensive drug therapy for older adult patients, the family nurse practitioner recognizes that which class of antihypertensive agents should be avoided in the older adult?

    1. Calcium channel blockers.

    2. Diuretics.

    3. Beta-blockers.

    4. ACE inhibitors.

77. Medications used in managing ischemic heart disease include:

    1. Beta-blockers, sedatives, and aspirin.

    2. Nitrates, beta-blockers, calcium channel blockers, and aspirin.

    3. Vasoconstrictors, aspirin, and anxiolytics.

    4. Nitrates, ACE inhibitors, aspirin, and lipid-lowering drugs.

78. The family nurse practitioner initiates antihypertensive therapy for a middle-aged nonsmoking male. One week later, the patient returns for a follow-up visit and complains of a recurrent dry cough since initiating the medications. This is most likely a side effect of:

    1. Beta-blocker.

    2. Thiazide diuretic.

    3. ACE inhibitor.

    4. Calcium channel blocker.

79. The role of digoxin in the management of heart failure (HF) is indicated with:

    1. Atrial fibrillation.

    2. Mitral stenosis.

    3. Normal ejection fraction.

    4. Pericarditis.

80. The family nurse practitioner should monitor the older adult patient for which of the most common adverse reactions of digoxin?

    1. Blurred vision.

    2. Confusion.

    3. Diarrhea.

    4. Eating disorder.

81. The family nurse practitioner has been successfully treating an older patient's hypertension with diet, exercise, and hydrochlorothiazide (HydroDiuril) 25 mg PO qd for 5 months. During today's clinic visit, the patient's BP was 154/90 mm Hg and temperature was 99.9°F (37.7°C). The physical exam revealed clear breath sounds, S_1 and S_2 with no murmurs, gallops, or rubs, and no JVD. The patient denied syncope, headaches, or visual changes; there was a tender and edematous right ankle. Which laboratory values would be most appropriate for evaluation?

    1. Blood urea nitrogen and sodium.

    2. Serum cholesterol and serum calcium.

    3. Serum potassium and blood count.

    4. Serum uric acid and complete blood count.

82. An older adult white male with a long history of COPD has recently developed hypertension. Which class of antihypertensive agents should the family nurse practitioner avoid for this patient?

    1. ACE inhibitors.

    2. Beta-blockers.

    3. Calcium channel blockers.

    4. Diuretics.

83. Which class of pharmacologic agents would the family nurse practitioner select for an older adult patient who has hypertension and is newly diagnosed with heart failure (HF)?

    1. ACE inhibitors.

    2. Beta-blockers.

    3. Calcium channel blockers.

    4. Diuretics.

84. A male patient who is mildly hypertensive presents with red, painful swelling of the great toe. In addition to treating the gout, the family nurse practitioner also knows to:

    1. Order laboratory studies for diabetes.

    2. Explore for possible alcohol abuse.

    3. Advise him to lose weight.

    4. Change his thiazide antihypertensive medication.

85. An older adult male was diagnosed 3 months ago with systolic hypertension and presents for follow-up care. He is on a no-added-salt diet and has lost 8 lb in 3 months. Weekly BP checks at a senior center average in the 180s/70s. The health history includes benign prostatic hyperplasia, diet-controlled type 2 diabetes, and CAD with an MI 8 years ago. His chief complaint includes periodic angina, occasional heartburn, slowed urine stream with some dribbling, and decreasing energy level. The BP today is 188/78 mm Hg. Current medications are cimetidine (Tagamet) 200 mg prn, aspirin 325 mg qd, nitroglycerin, and Maalox prn. The patient is married and sexually active. Which medication would the family nurse practitioner initiate after a complete physical, including an ECG, and all indicated blood work?

    1. ACE inhibitor.

    2. Diuretic.

    3. α_1-Adrenergic blocker.

    4. β-Adrenergic blocker.

86. An older adult patient has been on procainamide (Pronestyl) for 4 years to control his cardiac dysrhythmias. The family nurse practitioner would evaluate for what side effect in the chronic use of this medication?

    1. Elevated liver function tests.

    2. Appearance of antinuclear antibodies.

    3. Shortened AV interval.

    4. Tachycardia.

87. Secondary prophylaxis for acute rheumatic fever (ARF) in a 25-year-old schoolteacher includes:

    1. Penicillin V 125–250 mg PO bid indefinitely.

    2. Erythromycin 800 mg PO bid.

    3. One-time dose of 2.0 million units of benzathine penicillin G, combined with penicillin G procaine (Bicillin C-R) IM.

    4. No medication prophylaxis is needed after patient reaches the early 20s.

88. A patient has been prescribed lisinopril (Prinivil) 5 mg PO qd for hypertension. He has developed an intractable cough that is unrelated to heart failure. Which of the following medications can be substituted for this medication?

    1. Calcium channel blocker.

    2. Digoxin.

    3. ACE inhibitor.

    4. Angiotensin II receptor blocker (ARB).

89. A 60-year-old male with a history of unstable angina comes to the clinic complaining of increased pain that is not relieved by his nitroglycerin. During the assessment, the family nurse practitioner notes elevation of the ST segment on the ECG. Oxygen therapy is administered and an IV line inserted. What other therapy should be initiated while arranging transfer to an acute care facility?

    1. Lidocaine drip at 2 mg/min.

    2. Metoprolol (Toprol) 100 mg PO.

    3. Morphine 2 mg IV push.

    4. Aspirin 162 mg PO.

90. A 54-year-old patient with type 2 diabetes has been diagnosed with hypertension. Which antihypertensive drug is the recommended choice to treat hypertension in patients with diabetes?

    1. Beta-blocker.

    2. Diuretic.

    3. Calcium channel blocker.

    4. ACE inhibitor.

91. A 68-year-old with a history of MI who has experienced atrial fibrillation for 2 years comes to the clinic with a complaint of "increasing difficulty breathing and occasionally awakening at night with a feeling of smothering." Which pharmacologic therapy would be appropriate?

    1. Digitalis and ACE inhibitor.

    2. Loop diuretic and beta-blocker.

    3. Thiazide diuretic and calcium channel blocker.

    4. α_1-adrenergic blocker and nitrate.

92. A patient with coronary artery disease has a cholesterol count of 278 mg/dL and a triglyceride level of 300 mg/dL. The family nurse practitioner initiates therapy with lovastatin (Mevacor) 20 mg daily. The patient is instructed to take the lovastatin daily:

    1. In the morning with breakfast.
    2. 30 minutes before eating breakfast.
    3. In the evening.
    4. Around noon.

93. A toddler has ingested some of his grandfather's pills. The toddler is vomiting, feels weak, and has a first-degree atrioventricular (AV) block pattern on the ECG. The grandfather brings in four medication bottles. Which medication did the toddler most likely ingest?

    1. Amitriptyline (Elavil).
    2. Digoxin (Lanoxin).
    3. Furosemide (Lasix).
    4. Aspirin.

94. A 70-year-old white female is a resident of a long-term care facility where the family nurse practitioner makes rounds on a weekly basis. The nurse is reviewing recent laboratory results and notices the following: serum potassium of 5.9 mEq/L; serum sodium of 144 mEq/L; serum of chloride 111 mEq/L; BUN of 28 mg/dL; and creatinine of 1.8 mg/dL. Her current medications include furosemide (Lasix) 20 mg PO qd, potassium chloride (K-Dur) 16 mEq PO qd, captopril (Capoten) 25 mg PO qd, and citalopram (Celexa) 10 mg PO qd. There have been no changes in her medications. What is the likely cause of the elevated serum potassium?

    1. Furosemide.
    2. Potassium chloride.
    3. Captopril.
    4. Citalopram.

4 Cardiovascular Answers & Rationales

Physical Examination & Diagnostic Tests

1. Answer: 1

Rationale: S_1 is heard loudest at the apex (characteristic "lub"), S_2 at the base (characteristic "dub"). Each sound should be carefully assessed as to the intensity of the sound in each area. The S_2 second heart sound has two components: A_2 is produced by aortic valve closure, and P_2 is produced by pulmonic valve closure.

2. Answer: 3

Rationale: The point of maximal impulse (PMI) represents the thrust and contraction of the left ventricle (LV). The LV lies behind the right ventricle (RV) and extends to the left, forming the left border of the heart.

3. Answer: 2

Rationale: The correct procedure is to listen for carotid bruits with the bell of the stethoscope, which brings out low-frequency sounds and filters out high-frequency sound. The bell should be placed very lightly on the neck with just enough pressure to seal the edge.

4. Answer: 2

Rationale: The purpose of inspection and palpation of the precordium is to determine the presence and extent of normal and abnormal pulsations. A slight retraction of the chest wall just medial to the midclavicular line in the fifth interspace is a normal finding, whereas marked or active retraction of the rib is abnormal and may indicate pericardial disease. Pericardial friction rubs are heard by auscultation.

5. Answer: 1

Rationale: The splitting during inspiration refers to S_1 and S_2. The S_3 is normal in children, young adults, and pregnant women. In the older adult with heart disease, this often signifies myocardial failure.

6. Answer: 3

Rationale: The right side of the chest close to the sternal border at the second intercostal space is the correct area to auscultate the aortic valve. The mitral valve is auscultated at the fifth left intercostal space at the midclavicular line. The tricuspid value is auscultated at the fourth left intercostal space at the sternal border. The pulmonic valve is auscultated at the second left intercostal space at the sternal border.

7. Answer: 2

Rationale: A 12-hour fast is recommended because of the influence of intake on cholesterol levels, which may increase. A normal diet for the 7 days before drawing the lipid profile is recommended, so that an accurate picture of the patient's normal life is obtained. Alcohol should not be consumed for 48 hours before the test because it may increase cholesterol, HDL, LDL, and triglyceride levels. If possible, all medication should be withheld until the blood test is drawn, especially corticosteroids, diuretics, beta-blockers, oral contraceptives, and estrogens.

8. Answer: 1

Rationale: An S_4 is a normal variant in people 65 years and older and may result from increased resistance to ventricular filling during atrial contraction.

9. Answer: 1

Rationale: Based on the Joint National Committee 8 report (JNC8) hypertension treatment guidelines, an appropriate blood pressure goal for a patient greater than or equal to age 60 is SBP <150/DBP <90. Patients of all ages with diabetes or chronic kidney disease (CKD) should have blood pressure goals set at SBP <140/DBP <90.

10. Answer: 2

Rationale: The fifth intercostal space at the midclavicular line on the left side is the best place to auscultate the closure sounds of the mitral valve. Auscultating at the left sternal border, fourth left intercostal space describes the area of the tricuspid valve. Auscultating at the second or third intercostal space at the left of the sternal border describes the pulmonic valve area. The aortic valve area is auscultated at the second intercostal space on the right of the sternal border.

11. Answer: 3

Rationale: It is important to determine whether the coolness extends proximally from the hand, so feeling the forearms with the backs of the fingers is appropriate. Next, it would be important to palpate the radial pulses.

12. Answer: 1

Rationale: Closure of the AV valves, which allows the filling of both ventricles simultaneously, produces the first heart sound (S_1); closure of the aortic and pulmonic valves produces the second heart sound (S_2).

13. Answer: 4

Rationale: The apical and radial pulses must be evaluated simultaneously to determine whether all the apical beats are being reflected in the radial pulse. If there is an apical rate of 100 and a radial rate of 94, the patient is said to have a pulse deficit of 6. This is usually done with two people counting simultaneously over the same period.

14. Answer: 3

Rationale: A grade V heart murmur is very loud and can be heard with the stethoscope partly off the chest wall with a thrill that is easily palpable. A grade VI murmur is the loudest, is audible with the stethoscope removed from contact with the chest wall, and is accompanied by a thrill that is palpable and visible. A grade I murmur is barely audible or very faintly heard with the bell of the stethoscope.

15. Answer: 4

Rationale: The normal aging process impairs automaticity, conductivity, and contractility. Ischemic changes and degeneration decrease sinus node automaticity and conduction velocity, resulting in bradycardic rhythms or atrial fibrillation. The poor myocardial contractility, usually related to hypertension or valvular disease, causes decreased ventricular emptying and increased filling pressures. These changes predispose the older adult patient to heart failure.

16. Answer: 4

Rationale: The most sensitive area on the examiner's hand is the back of the fingers.

17. Answer: 3

Rationale: The Adult Treatment Panel (ATP IV) cholesterol guidelines no longer recommend treatment adjusted to a specific target lipid value. The patient's 10-year arteriosclerotic cardiovascular disease (ASCVD) risk should be calculated and determination should be made if the patient falls into a pharmacologic treatment benefit group. A heart-healthy diet, lifestyle modifications, and regular aerobic physical activity should always be included in the treatment regimen. Referral to a cardiologist is not appropriate at this time.

18. Answer: 3

Rationale: Dressler's syndrome (post-MI syndrome) may develop 1 to 4 weeks post MI and is characterized by pericarditis with effusion and fever. Dressler's syndrome is caused by antigen-antibody reactions. Laboratory findings include elevated white blood count and erythrocyte sedimentation rate. Treatment includes NSAIDs and colchicine.

19. Answer: 1

Rationale: Jugular vein distention (JVD) is common in older adult patients. If JVD is present when the patient's head is elevated 45 degrees, further examination is necessary regarding the venous pressure, which reflects pressure in the right-side heart chambers. The supine position will increase venous pressure and does not provide valid information in this situation. Auscultation for carotid bruits is an important part of assessment but is not significant in evaluating JVD.

20. Answer: 1

Rationale: Mitral valve stenosis is a diastolic murmur of low intensity heard at the apex of the heart. Midsystolic ejection murmur heard loudest over the left lower sternal border describes characteristics of a murmur with aortic stenosis. A holosystolic murmur is characteristic of mitral regurgitation, which allows for backflow of blood from ventricles into the atrium. A diastolic murmur, heard loudest with patient in a sitting position, leaning forward best describes aortic regurgitation.

21. Answer: 3

Rationale: The patient had a left ventricular MI. One of the most common complications is left-sided failure, resulting in heart failure. This would manifest first as pulmonary congestion (crackles in lungs) and difficulty breathing.

22. Answer: 4

Rationale: Classically, intermittent claudication is described as pain in the lower extremity on activity that is relieved by stopping the activity. During exercise, there is an increased demand for blood supply to the extremity that cannot be met. Subsequently, there is a build-up of lactic acid and other metabolites in the muscle, which causes the tightening or cramping discomfort in the calf muscles.

23. Answer: 3

Rationale: A positive result on stress testing indicates the likelihood of coronary artery disease (CAD) with 98% accuracy in males over age 50. Results are progressively lower in asymptomatic persons, with false-positive results increased in asymptomatic men under age 40, premenopausal women without risk factors, and patients taking digitalis.

24. Answer: 2

Rationale: A hyperkinetic impulse (increased amplitude) is caused by pressure overload of the left ventricle. Causes include hyperthyroidism, severe anemia, or mitral regurgitation. A pansystolic murmur is a classic finding of mitral regurgitation.

25. Answer: 4

Rationale: Pulsus alternans (weak pulse alternating with strong pulse) is caused by left ventricular failure (strong and weak venticular contractions) and is usually accompanied by an S_3 heart sound and is seen in patients with left-sided heart failure. It may be present in severe acute aortic insufficiency (AI), but it is unusual in patients with chronic AI.

Disorders

26. Answer: 1

Rationale: This assessment reflects changes caused by chronic venous insufficiency, which includes edema, varicose veins, chronic skin changes, dependent cyanosis, and skin ulceration. The other assessment findings reflect chronic arterial insufficiency.

27. Answer: 1

Rationale: A diagnosis of hypertension (HTN) from a single measurement of blood pressure (BP) elevation should not be done. A minimum of three readings with an average systolic BP of 140 mm Hg and diastolic of 90 mm Hg establishes the diagnosis. An average of two or more readings taken at each of two or more visits should follow an initial screening. The patient should be seated with the arm at heart level. No caffeine or nicotine ingestion should be allowed for 30 minutes before the reading. The room should be quiet at least 5 minutes, and an appropriate cuff should be used. Another high reading should be confirmed within 2 months.

28. Answer: 3

Rationale: In the early stages of hypertensive heart disease, when there is an increased peripheral resistance to blood flow, the most significant change occurring in the heart is left ventricular hypertrophy. This is associated with an increase in the size of the myocardial cells without a corresponding increase in cell number (hyperplasia). Over time, all other options listed occur in the heart.

29. Answer: 3

Rationale: Sinus or atrial tachycardia is characterized by a heart rate of 100 beats/min or higher, P waves present for each QRS complex, PR interval below 0.20, T wave after each QRS complex, and regular rhythm.

30. Answer: 1

Rationale: The classic chest pain associated with an MI may not be present in the older adult patient because of altered pain perception and diminished pain sensation.

31. Answer: 2

Rationale: Respiratory symptoms are predominant in patients with left-sided heart failure. Venous congestion and peripheral edema are associated with right-sided heart failure.

32. Answer: 1

Rationale: Cardiac tamponade occurs as a complication of pericarditis. An excessive accumulation of fluids between the pericardium and myocardium interferes with effective cardiac contraction and produces a paradoxical pulse. The triphasic friction rub is common to pericarditis but is not indicative of a complication of constrictive pericarditis. Jugular venous pressure is used to determine levels of venous distention.

33. Answer: 2

Rationale: Untreated hypertension causes significant increased work of the left ventricle, eventually causing left-sided heart failure.

34. Answer: 2

Rationale: Palpable carotid pulse with each compression is the best sign of effective cardiopulmonary resuscitation (CPR). The other answers are appropriate but not the best indicators of effective resuscitation efforts.

35. Answer: 2

Rationale: This is a description of complete heart block with hemodynamic consequences. The patient should be seen immediately by a cardiologist for possible pacemaker insertion. First-degree block has characteristic P waves and a long PR interval.

36. Answer: 3

Rationale: A triphasic friction rub or pericardial rub occurs in the majority of patients with pericarditis. Paradoxical pulse may occur if constrictive pericarditis and cardiac tamponade are present. Pulse deficits and presence of S_4 are not characteristic of problems with pericarditis.

37. Answer: 1

Rationale: Older adults experience atypical symptoms of MI, including dyspnea, diaphoresis, vomiting, syncope, confusion, and weakness.

38. Answer: 1

Rationale: Cardiovascular risk factors predisposing women to cardiovascular disease include smaller body size, declining estrogen level, heart and thoracic cavity smaller and lighter, coronary arteries smaller in diameter, shorter PR interval, and a higher resting ejection fraction. Increased body fat percentage and fat distributed in the abdomen may be mobilized more easily in response to stress. This may raise serum cholesterol and blood glucose levels.

39. Answer: 4

Rationale: The family nurse practitioner must consider the geriatric patient's other medical problems and treatment before prescribing medications for hypertension. Frequently, geriatric patients cannot take beta-blockers because of chronic pulmonary conditions; the patient may already be taking diuretics for problems of fluid retention. Step therapy is appropriate if there is no other significant medical history. Lifestyle changes should be initiated and medications adjusted as changes are made.

40. Answer: 2

Rationale: Hypertension is considered a major factor in the development of coronary artery disease (CAD) in the geriatric patient. Female patients have an increased incidence of CAD after menopause; estrogen replacement appears to have cardioprotective effects on the heart, thus decreasing the incidence of CAD. Although diabetic patients have an increased incidence of CAD, most CAD patients are not diabetic.

41. Answer: 4

Rationale: Cor pulmonale is characterized by hypertrophy of the right ventricle secondary to pulmonary hypertension (resistance). The increased P-wave amplitude (P pulmonale) occurs as the right atrium enlarges.

42. Answer: 2

Rationale: The compensatory mechanism (activation of the renin-angiotensin-aldosterone system) causes excess secretion of aldosterone that predisposes to potassium excretion. Total body sodium content will be above normal, but the excessive secretion of antidiuretic hormone causes greater retention of water, diluting the serum level.

43. Answer: 1

Rationale: Water-hammer pulse (bounding pulse with a rapid rise and sudden collapse) results from an increase in pulse pressure and may be caused by increased stroke volume, decreased peripheral vascular resistance, or both. Because the family nurse practitioner suspects either aortic regurgitation or patent ductus arteriosus (primarily in children), auscultation for a diastolic murmur is indicated.

44. Answer: 2

Rationale: Occlusion of the coronary arteries deprives the myocardial cells of glucose needed for aerobic metabolism. Anaerobic metabolism occurs, which causes the accumulation of lactic acid. Lactic acid irritates the myocardial nerve fibers, sending pain messages to the cardiac nerves and upper thoracic posterior roots located in the left shoulder and arm.

45. Answer: 4

Rationale: Marked limitation in activity, comfortable at rest, but ordinary activity leads to symptoms is noted as Functional Class III. Symptoms present at rest, with any activity leading to increased discomfort characterizes Functional Class IV. Slight limitation in ordinary activity, resulting in fatigue, palpitations, dyspnea, or angina is Functional Class II. Functional Class I is characterized by no physical limitation in activity.

46. Answer: 1

Rationale: The moist crackles (rales) heard in the bases of the lung are the most prominent physical examination findings of early heart failure. They are caused from transudation of fluid into the alveoli and into the airways. Later findings include distended neck veins, peripheral edema, hepatomegaly, and ascites (rather than weight loss).

47. Answer: 3

Rationale: Aortic dissection almost invariably begins with a sudden onset of severe chest pain that is tearing or ripping in quality and is accompanied by absent or decreased peripheral pulses and neurologic deficits. The pain of angina and acute MI is usually described as "pressure." Pericarditis produces pain that is more gradual in onset.

48. Answer: 1

Rationale: The Adult Treatment Panel (ATP IV), the American College of Cardiology, and American Heart Association (ACC/AHA) cholesterol guidelines recommend lifestyle modifications for hyperlipidemia patients, including increasing vegetables, fruits, and whole grains and limiting sodium, sweets and sugar-sweetened drinks, red meats, and saturated fats. The amount of fat in the average diet should be between 20% and 35% of the total calories. Daily protein intake should be between 10% and 35%. Carbohydrate intake should be monitored in the maintenance of a healthy weight.

49. Answer: 4

Rationale: Although the other dysrhythmias may occur after MI, the most life-threatening is ventricular fibrillation. The vast majority of deaths due to ventricular fibrillation occurs within the first 24 hours, and more than half of these occur in the first hour. The majority of out-of-hospital deaths from MI is caused by ventricular fibrillation.

50. Answer: 2

Rationale: Diet and exercise are the mainstays of any treatment program and would be used initially in all cases. A bile acid sequestrant agent or estrogen replacement therapy may eventually be necessary if no improvement is seen with diet and exercise therapy. Referral to a cardiologist is not necessary, unless the patient develops symptoms or shows resistance to treatment.

51. Answer: 2

Rationale: A stroke is often the outcome of chronic atrial fibrillation because of the blood pooling in the quivering atria. As a result, a blood clot can be formed in this pooling blood, which then travels to the brain and causes an ischemic stroke. For this reason, warfarin (Coumadin) should be maintained at an international normalized ratio (INR) of 2 to 3.

52. Answer: 3

Rationale: Dyspnea is the most common symptom of heart failure (HF). Initially, it is present only with moderate exertion, but as severity of HF increases, dyspnea may occur on mild exertion or at rest. Fatigue is another common complaint. Right-sided heart failure is associated with weakness, anorexia, nausea, and dependent edema. Chronic left ventricular failure usually leads to right ventricular failure.

53. Answer: 3

Rationale: Palm and coconut oils, along with butter, are very high in saturated fats and should be avoided. The other selections are moderately high in fat content but are mainly unsaturated fats.

54. Answer: 3

Rationale: Anginal pain is difficult to differentiate from the pain of an infarction. One of the most characteristic symptoms of anginal pain is relief with the administration of sublingual nitroglycerin.

55. Answer: 4

Rationale: Aspirin helps prevent the formation of platelet-aggregating substances and may help the occlusion of narrowed coronary arteries. Although furosemide and morphine have a role in treating acute MI, aspirin can be readily given in the typical primary care office. Nitroglycerin should not be given because the patient's systolic blood pressure is less than 90 mm Hg.

56. Answer: 1

Rationale: Superficial inflammation of a vein may be caused by trauma (e.g., blow to the arm or leg) or recent IV therapy with irritating fluids or may occur secondary to pregnancy, especially during the postpartum period, because of the increase in clotting factors (thromboplastin). Excessive use of oral anticoagulants can lead to bleeding but not to thrombophlebitis. Deep vein thrombosis (DVT) associated with thrombophlebitis results from prolonged bed rest, major surgical procedures, injury to the blood vessel wall, and hypercoagulable states, such as use of oral contraceptives, especially in women who smoke or have cancer, and polycythemia vera.

57. Answer: 3

Rationale: Dizziness that improves when lying down and worsens when standing is symptomatic of cardiac involvement and may indicate serious cardiac dysrhythmias. If it occurs in certain positions, the dizziness suggests benign positional vertigo, which is common in older adults. Dizziness accompanied by tinnitus is common in acute labyrinthitis and, if preceded by rapid breathing, may be caused by hyperventilation.

58. Answer: 3

Rationale: The stated history of a recent coxsackievirus infection, pain that worsens when supine, and a friction rub is classic for viral pericarditis. The patient's age makes an acute MI unlikely, and the pain is not typical for pleural effusion or esophageal reflux.

59. Answer: 1

Rationale: Signs and symptoms of hyperthyroidism in the older adult include progressive functional decline, atrial fibrillation, MI, tachycardia, weakness, fatigue, weight loss, anorexia, diarrhea, nervousness, tremor, pruritus, memory loss, and heat intolerance. Symptoms of hypothyroidism include arthralgia; weakness; decreased mental function; depression; constipation; weight loss; dry, coarse skin with yellowish cast; dry sparse hair; and masklike puffy face with periorbital edema. Bradycardia would be assessed with both sick sinus syndrome and heart failure. Sick sinus syndrome is often associated with the "bradycardia-tachycardia" syndrome.

60. Answer: 4

Rationale: A jugular venous pressure of 4 cm H_2O is a sign of heart failure. Decreased exercise tolerance is a normal sign of aging. A grade II/VI systolic ejection murmur is a result of sclerosing of the aorta, which occurs with aging. Prolongation of PR intervals on an ECG is expected with the aging process.

61. Answer: 2

Rationale: This assessment is consistent with aortic stenosis. Aortic regurgitation is a diastolic murmur secondary to rheumatic heart disease, for which no history is given. Mitral valve disease is one of the most common valvular disorders. A small percentage of patients who have a mitral valve prolapse do experience autonomic dysfunction and complain of palpitations, atypical chest pain, orthostatic dizziness, near-syncope, cold extremities, throbbing headaches, and neurasthenia and manifest tachydysrhythmias. Patients who have mitral regurgitation may remain asymptomatic for many years because the left ventricle dilates and adjusts well to the increase in volume load. Onset of dyspnea and fatigue may not occur for decades.

62. Answer: 1

Rationale: Aortic stenosis is the most frequently diagnosed valvular heart problem and is caused by calcification. The symptoms include syncope, angina, and dyspnea on exertion.

63. Answer: 3

Rationale: The family nurse practitioner needs to repeat the cholesterol and obtain HDL and LDL values before initiating any treatment. The HDL and LDL will help stratify risks and aid in the determination of recommended management.

Pharmacology

64. Answer: 1

Rationale: This patient is presenting with symptoms of digitalis toxicity—first-degree block and increasing cardiac irritability. If the potassium level is low, it may be precipitating the toxicity. Also, it is important to determine that serum theophylline levels remain within the therapeutic range. No evidence indicates that the pulmonary disease is progressing. The blood pressure may be adequately controlled for this patient; further information should be obtained before adjusting the medications. Based on the information presented, referral to a cardiologist is not appropriate at this time.

65. Answer: 3

Rationale: Thiazide diuretics inhibit sodium reabsorption, promoting the excretion of sodium, chloride, and water. As the extracellular fluid volume decreases, plasma renin activity and aldosterone levels increase, resulting in potassium loss. Treatment is to restore the volume with normal saline and correct the potassium depletion. If the sodium is increased too rapidly, irreversible neurologic damage can occur.

66. Answer: 1

Rationale: Vitamin K is an antidote for warfarin. Increased intake of green leafy vegetables could cause an increase in vitamin

K levels and decrease the effectiveness of the medication. Also, multivitamin supplements may contain additional vitamin K.

67. Answer: 3

Rationale: The patient presents with the classic profile of digitalis toxicity, which is frequently related to hypokalemia, especially since the potassium replacement is rather low for an adult and there is a history of poor eating and nausea. The actions listed in the other options may be taken, but it is important to determine the presence of hypokalemia and digitalis toxicity so that these may be addressed immediately.

68. Answer: 1

Rationale: Angiotensin II receptor blockers (ARBs), such as losartan (Cozaar), block access of angiotensin II to its receptors in blood vessels, the adrenals, and all other tissues. By blocking the action of angiotensin II, losartan relaxes muscle cells and dilates blood vessels (arterioles and veins), thereby reducing blood pressure. By blocking angiotensin II receptors in the adrenals, ARBs decrease release of aldosterone, which increases renal excretion of sodium and water. Sodium and water excretion is further increased through dilation of renal blood vessels.

69. Answer: 3

Rationale: Aldactone is a potassium-sparing diuretic. Patients should be instructed on the early signs of hyperkalemia, which include muscle twitching, numbness, tingling, and burning sensations of the limbs, diarrhea, palpitations, and skipped heartbeats. Hypokalemia symptoms are characterized by irritability, confusion followed by lethargy, abdominal cramping, distention, constipation, and lower extremity weakness.

70. Answer: 1

Rationale: Beta-blockers are myocardial depressants that suppress heart rate and contraction (negative inotropic). Calcium channel blockers decrease atrioventricular conduction, which suppresses heart rate. Both drugs are contraindicated with the onset of left ventricular dysfunction. The increase in jugular vein distention (JVD) and a 10-lb gain are associated with right-sided heart failure. The presence, of an S_3 indicates left venticular dysfunction, especially when associated with signs and symptoms of right-sided heart failure.

71. Answer: 3

Rationale: The American Heart Association's Advanced Cardiac Life Support (ACLS) guidelines recommend adenosine as the drug of choice for emergency treatment of supraventricular tachycardia when a patient is hemodynamically stable.

72. Answer: 2

Rationale: The combination of calcium channel blockers and β-adrenergic blocking agents, systemic or ophthalmic, may result in bradycardia and/or hypotension.

73. Answer: 2

Rationale: Niacin can cause vasodilation, leading to orthostatic hypotension. Antihyperlipidemic drugs may cause constipation. Antihyperlipidemic effectiveness is enhanced when taken before or with meals.

74. Answer: 2

Rationale: Calcium channel blockers (a) depress the rate of discharge from the sinoatrial node and conduction velocity through the atrioventricular node, causing a decrease in heart rate; (b) relax the coronary and systemic arteries, producing vasodilation (decrease in afterload and blood pressure); and (c) decrease myocardial contractility (negative inotropic effect).

75. Answer: 3

Rationale: According to the Joint National Committee 8 report (JNC 8), African American males without diabetes or chronic kidney disease (CKD) should be prescribed calcium channel blockers alone or in combination with a thiazide-type diuretic in the treatment of hypertension. Enalapril and captopril are angiotensin-converting enzyme (ACE) inhibitors, which are not appropriate for this patient. Metoprolol is a beta blocker and not recommened in the JNC 8 guidelines for the treatment of hypertension.

76. Answer: 3

Rationale: Beta-blockers are not appropriate in normal doses for older adults because of decreased beta-receptor sensitivity in these patients. Larger doses also result in depression, impotence, fatigue, and declining mental function. Older adult patients are especially likely to experience heart failure and peripheral vascular insufficiency from beta-adrenergic blocker toxicity. Blood pressure should be lowered cautiously using smaller doses of calcium channel blockers, ACE inhibitors, or diuretics in older adult patients.

77. Answer: 2

Rationale: Nitrates are venous and arterial dilators that decrease myocardial oxygen demand. Beta-blockers have an antianginal effect and reduce myocardial oxygen demand. Calcium channel blockers relieve myocardial ischemia by reducing myocardial oxygen demand and dilate coronary arteries. Aspirin is effective for secondary prevention of MI. Unless contraindicated, small doses of aspirin (162 to 325 mg daily) should be prescribed for patients with angina. Patients remaining symptomatic when treated with nitrates, beta-blockers, or calcium channel blockers should be treated with a beta-blocker plus another agent. Appropriate combinations are a nitrate or beta-blocker plus a calcium channel blocker other than verapamil. Combination therapy does not include sedatives, vasoconstrictors, ACE inhibitors, or lipid-lowering drugs.

78. Answer: 3

Rationale: Adverse side effects of angiotensin-converting enzyme (ACE) inhibitors include cough (1%–30%), headache, and dizziness. Adverse effects of calcium channel blockers include peripheral edema, dizziness, headache, nausea, and tachycardia. Adverse effects of thiazide diuretics include nausea, vomiting, diarrhea, dizziness, and headache. Side effects of beta-blockers include fatigue, impotence, depression, and shortness of breath.

79. Answer: 1

Rationale: Digoxin, once a first-line drug for all patients with heart failure (HF), is now used in patients with atrial fibrillation, other tachycardias, and left ventricular dysfunction. By controlling the ventricular rate in the patient with atrial fibrillation or tachycardias, cardiac output increases. In cases of diastolic dysfunction with a sinus rhythm, digitalis is of no benefit. Digoxin is of relatively little value in most forms of cardiomyopathy, myocarditis, mitral stenosis, and chronic constrictive pericarditis.

80. Answer: 2

Rationale: Noncardiac adverse reactions include a change in the mental status. Although visual disturbances, diarrhea, anorexia, nausea, or vomiting are also adverse reactions, they are not the most common in older adult patients.

81. Answer: 4

Rationale: The assessments indicate gout. A side effect of hydrochlorothiazide is hyperuricemia. Blood for a complete blood count (CBC) should be drawn before therapy. The other options are not addressing the assessment of a tender and edematous right ankle. The cardiac assessments were benign. No evidence indicates a concern for hypo/hypernatremia or hypo/hyperkalemia.

82. Answer: 2

Rationale: Beta-blockers increase peripheral vascular resistance, a phenomenon that already occurs with normal aging, so these drugs can precipitate or worsen symptoms of asthma, COPD, peripheral vascular disease, sexual dysfunction, or heart failure. The other classes have no effect or decrease the effect on peripheral resistance.

83. Answer: 1

Rationale: Angiotensin-converting enzyme (ACE) inhibitors have been shown to prolong life in patients with heart failure (HF) by improving overall cardiac function. Beta blockers and calcium channel blockers should be contraindicated in HF. Although diuretics may be correct, it is not a priority over an ACE inhibitor.

84. Answer: 4

Rationale: The most likely precipitating cause of this patient's gout is the thiazide diuretic used to control his hypertension because it blocks the excretion of uric acid leading to hyperuricemia. Although gout may be more common in obese, alcoholic, and diabetic patients, these conditions are not indicated here.

85. Answer: 1

Rationale: The ACE inhibitor will preserve renal function and have less impact on sexual functioning. The family nurse practitioner must monitor potassium and carefully follow renal status for change. The ACE inhibitor has fewer negative side effects or interactions with this patient's other medical conditions.

86. Answer: 2

Rationale: Of the patients receiving long-term procainamide therapy, 80% develop antinuclear antibodies, and 23% of these develop a lupus-like syndrome.

87. Answer: 1

Rationale: Secondary prophylaxis/prevention or preventing the recurrent attacks of acute rheumatic fever (ARF) is controversial. Some authorities identify (a) reaching the early 20s and (b) 5 years since the last ARF attack as the criteria to stop the use of prophylactic penicillin, unless the patient is at increased risk of exposure to streptococcal infections, as are schoolteachers or health professionals. Other authorities recommend lifelong prophylactic drug therapy. Although erythromycin is an alternative medication for penicillin-sensitive individuals, the dose of erythromycin is for a patient having a dental or surgical procedure. The secondary prophylactic dose for erythromycin is 250 mg PO bid.

88. Answer: 4

Rationale: An annoying, untoward effect of angiotensin-converting enzyme (ACE) inhibitors is an intractable cough. Lisinopril is an ACE inhibitor. Angiotensin receptor blockers (ARB) can be substituted as long as the cough is not related to heart failure. Antidysrhythmic agents, calcium channel blockers, and nonsteroidal antiinflammatory drugs (NSAIDs) should be avoided.

89. Answer: 4

Rationale: The American Heart Association recommends that aspirin be administered ASAP, whenever a patient is suspected of having a myocardial infarction (MI). The decreased platelet aggregation effect of aspirin helps limit the size of the myocardial damage.

90. Answer: 4

Rationale: Angiotensin-converting enzyme (ACE) inhibitors enhance renal function in patients with diabetes and slow progression of kidney injury.

91. Answer: 1

Rationale: The patient with atrial fibrillation is exhibiting symptoms of left ventricular (LV) failure. Treatment recommendations include enhancing contractility with a positive inotropic agent (digitalis), and ACE inhibitors have been shown to slow LV dilation.

92. Answer: 3

Rationale: Because most cholesterol is synthesized between midnight and 3 AM, HMG CoA reductase inhibitors (lovastatin) are best taken in the evening.

93. Answer: 2

Rationale: Nausea, vomiting, and anorexia are common side effects of many medications. The first-degree atrioventricular (AV) block confirms the ingestion of digoxin in this situation. Tricyclic antidepressant toxicity is characterized by agitation and anticholingeric symptoms; furosemide toxicity by hypokalemia, weakness, and cardiac dysrhythmias; and aspirin toxicity by tinnitus, confusion, gastrointestinal symptoms, and rapid, deep respirations.

94. Answer: 2

Rationale: The likely cause of the elevated serum potassium is the potassium chloride. The family nurse practitioner should hold the potassium chloride (K-Dur) and order daily serum potassium monitoring until levels return to normal. The patient is taking furosemide, which is a potassium-wasting diuretic, and the amount of potassium given to compensate for the anticipated losses apparently was too much. This often occurs as a result of the changes of aging. Once serum potassium returns to normal, the level is monitored again at 1 week. With the low dose of furosemide and with captopril (an ACE inhibitor that may retain potassium), the patient may not need potassium chloride restarted.

Respiratory

5

Physical Examination & Diagnostic Tests

1. The family nurse practitioner knows that normal breath sounds that have a low pitch and soft intensity and that are heard best on inspiration over the posterior lung fields are called:

   1. Bronchial.

   2. Vesicular.

   3. Bronchovesicular.

   4. Rhonchi.

2. When auscultating for vocal resonance in a patient with possible consolidation of lung tissue, the family nurse practitioner tells the patient to say "ninety-nine" and the voice remains loud and distinct over the area of suspected consolidation. This is called:

   1. Tactile fremitus.

   2. Bronchophony.

   3. Whispered pectoriloquy.

   4. Egophony.

3. The family nurse practitioner understands that in percussion of the lungs, hyperresonance is:

   1. A normal finding in the adult patient.

   2. Common when the lungs are hyperinflated, like with chronic emphysema.

   3. Characterized by soft intensity, high pitch, short duration, and extremely dull quality.

   4. Characterized by loud intensity, high pitch, medium duration, and dull quality.

4. What is the correct procedure when percussing the anterior and posterior chest?

   1. Percuss the entire right side of the anterior chest and move to the left side.

   2. Begin at the upper left side of the posterior chest, and compare to the respective anterior side, moving from front to back.

   3. Percuss systematically and symmetrically the intercostal spaces of the anterior chest, moving from the left to the right side, and then percuss the posterior chest.

   4. Percuss the posterior chest, and then measure for diaphragmatic excursion on the anterior chest.

5. The family nurse practitioner understands that pleural friction rubs are:

   1. Auscultated in the lower anterolateral chest.

   2. Heard best at the end of expiration.

   3. Characterized by a continuous, low-pitched, snoring sound that is heard early in inspiration.

   4. Noted when the patient says "e-e-e" and the examiner hears through the stethoscope "a-a-a."

6. Normal physiologic changes in the respiratory system of the geriatric patient include:

   1. Increased residual volume.

   2. Increased ciliary action, resulting in a more forceful and recurrent cough.

   3. Increase in number of smaller alveoli with decreased residual capacity.

   4. Decrease in AP diameter of the rib cage with decreased lung expansion.

7. When assessing for tactile fremitus, the family nurse practitioner knows that increased fremitus:

    1. Occurs when there is an obstruction in the transmission of vibrations.

    2. Occurs with consolidation or compression of lung tissue.

    3. Is the symmetric transmission of vibration through the chest wall.

    4. Is found in emphysema.

8. On assessment of the patient's respiratory status, crepitation is felt over the third rib at the midaxillary line on the left side. What is the interpretation of this finding?

    1. There is consolidation of fluid in the left lower lobe of the lung.

    2. Severe inflammation is present on the visceral pleural surfaces of the left lung.

    3. An increase in pressure has occurred in the pleural cavity of the right lung.

    4. Air is present in the subcutaneous tissue.

9. An important anatomic landmark on the anterior thoracic wall is the angle of Louis. Where on the thorax is this landmark present?

    1. The midnipple line on either side of the manubrium.

    2. At the manubriosternal junction.

    3. Midline at the base of the suprasternal notch.

    4. Just below the clavicle but above the manubrium.

10. During the assessment of an older adult patient's respiratory status, the family nurse practitioner determines the presence of increased tactile fremitus posteriorly at the second intercostal space. The best interpretation of this finding is:

    1. Increased air trapping in the alveoli on the affected side.

    2. Presence of fluid or solid mass within the lungs.

    3. Increased pressure in the bronchial tree.

    4. Presence of hyperactive airway disease.

11. When the lateral diameter of the chest is the same size as the AP diameter, the family nurse practitioner correctly identifies this finding as a:

    1. Biot's deviated chest.

    2. Pigeon chest.

    3. Funnel chest.

    4. Barrel chest.

12. **QSEN** The family nurse practitioner is planning a community screening program for lung cancer in older adult patients. The current evidence-based practice suggests that:

    1. Bronchoscopy with biopsy for cytology should be done every 2–3 years for smokers.

    2. Low-dose computed tomography should be used in high-risk individuals.

    3. Routine screening for lung cancer does not decrease mortality in high-risk populations.

    4. Chest x-ray with comparison of previous x-ray is a sensitive test for lung cancer.

13. An adult male patient comes to the clinic with the chief complaint of "coughing up blood" and night sweats. He has no history of respiratory or cardiac problems. His vital signs are pulse of 96 beats/min, respirations of 28 breaths/min, BP of 140/92 mm Hg, and a temperature of 99°F (37.2°C) orally. The initial diagnostic evaluation of this patient includes:

    1. Electrocardiogram, pulmonary function studies, and sputum cytology.

    2. Complete blood count, chest x-ray, and sputum smear for acid-fast bacillus.

    3. ABG studies, complete blood count, and chest x-ray.

    4. Direct bronchoscopy with biopsy and complement fixation antibody titer.

14. An adult male patient comes into the clinic complaining of increased fatigue and irritability. He has gained approximately 20 pounds over the past year. Although he sleeps through the night, his spouse says he seems somewhat restless. Based on these symptoms, what else should be determined?

    1. Presence of ongoing daytime sleepiness.

    2. History of depression.

    3. Fluctuations in blood pressure.

    4. Recent changes in medications.

15. When assessing the pulmonary function studies of a patient, which assessment finding is seen in chronic airflow limitation, such as in emphysema?

    1. Decreased forced vital capacity (FVC) and decreased forced expiratory volume in 1 second (FEV_1).

    2. Decreased functional residual capacity (FRC) and residual volume (RV).

    3. Decreased RV and increased total lung capacity (TLC).

    4. Increased FEV_1 and TLC.

16. When interpreting PPD skin tests in patients at a long-term care facility, the family nurse practitioner identifies positive results in individuals with:

    1. Redness or erythema at the site.

    2. Induration reaction ≥5 mm.

    3. Induration reaction ≥10 mm.

    4. Induration reaction up to 15 mm.

17. The family nurse practitioner is auscultating a patient's chest and asks the patient to say "ninety-nine." With the stethoscope, a clear transmission of the words is heard indicating increased lung density. This describes which voice sound?

    1. Egophony.

    2. Whispered pectoriloquy.

    3. Rhonchal fremitus.

    4. Bronchophony.

Disorders

18. A patient has received a blunt trauma injury to the chest. Which assessment finding would be most indicative of further respiratory complications?

    1. Complaints of increased pain over the affected area.

    2. Oximetry readings consistently about 90%.

    3. Decreased breath sounds on the affected side.

    4. Fever of 102°F (38.9°C) and increased sputum production.

19. The family nurse practitioner understands that the following characteristic is more likely to occur when the adult patient has pneumonia (due to *Streptococcus pneumoniae*) rather than bronchitis:

    1. Purulent sputum production.

    2. Nonproductive cough.

    3. Dyspnea.

    4. Wheezing.

20. **QSEN** A young adult is recovering from tuberculosis. What information should be included in a teaching plan for home care?

    1. It is critical for the young adult to take medications at the prescribed time; do not skip doses or allow the supply to run out.

    2. Respiratory isolation procedures need to be carried out at home; the young adult should avoid contact with immediate family members.

    3. It will be necessary for the young adult to return to the clinic every week to have his or her sputum checked for viable bacteria.

    4. The young adult may experience a rash along with nausea and vomiting from the medications; if this occurs, he or she should decrease the dosage.

21. What would be a priority intervention for a patient experiencing respiratory arrest?

    1. Starting chest compressions at 15 compressions and two breaths.

    2. Opening the airway with a head tilt and chin lift.

    3. Giving oxygen using a rebreathing mask at 10 L/min.

    4. Pinching the nose and giving two breaths.

22. A patient comes to the family practice clinic complaining of difficulty breathing. What is most important to establish initially in this patient?

    1. Type of activity that produces the dyspnea.

    2. Presence of consolidation on chest x-ray.

    3. ABGs with respect to oxygen pressures.

    4. Presence of bilateral breath sounds over the lower lobes.

23. A patient is severely dyspneic, and the history strongly suggests the possibility of a foreign body in the bronchi. What observation would contribute to the documentation of this problem?

    1. Unilateral retraction of the right chest wall.

    2. Presence of crepitation on the anterior chest wall.

    3. Retraction of the lower chest wall with decreased breath sounds.

    4. A friction rub heard over the area of the bronchi.

24. The family nurse practitioner is assessing a patient who is complaining of shortness of breath and chest discomfort. His respirations are shallow at 26 breaths/min. When evaluating the diaphragmatic excursion, it is determined that the diaphragm on the right is slightly higher than on the left side. The best interpretation of these findings is:

    1. This is normal because the liver is located on the right side.

    2. There may be atelectasis in the right lower lobe.

    3. Consolidation is present in the right lower lobe.

    4. This indicates the presence of severe chronic obstructive lung disease.

25. A 22-year-old male comes to the office complaining of chest pain and shortness of breath. He states the problems started suddenly after running sprints in basketball practice. He states he has no past history of pulmonary problems. He is about 72 inches tall and 145 lb, with pulse rate of 118 beats/min, respiratory rate of 30 breaths/min, decreased breath sounds, and hyperresonance over the left lung. Based on these findings, what is the best diagnosis for the patient?

    1. Spontaneous pneumothorax.

    2. Exercise-induced asthma.

    3. Pulmonary edema.

    4. Acute bronchiectasis.

26. A young woman presents at the clinic with complaints of tingling in her face and hands, sudden shortness of breath, and vague chest discomfort. She appears very anxious and denies any history of respiratory problems. On examination, her hands are cool to the touch; her vital signs are respirations of 34 breaths/min, pulse regular at 100 beats/min, BP 110/76 mm Hg, and normal temperature. Respiratory examination reveals bilateral breath sounds with tachypnea, no adventitious sounds, and normal percussion and visual examination of the chest. What is the best immediate treatment?

    1. Relaxation techniques and encouraging controlled diaphragmatic breathing.

    2. Two puffs of short-acting bronchodilator (albuterol) with metered-dose inhaler (MDI).

    3. Oxygen at 4 L and ABGs after 30 minutes.

    4. Rebreathing into paper bag to increase $PaCO_2$ levels.

27. A patient with newly diagnosed COPD is being discharged from the hospital. The family nurse practitioner is discussing home care with the patient. What information is important for the family nurse practitioner to include in the home care teaching?

    1. Use the bronchodilator before exercising.

    2. Maintain bed rest for the first few days at home.

    3. Decrease the amount of fluid intake to prevent fluid overload.

    4. Use the inhaled corticosteroid inhaler only when significantly short of breath.

28. Age-associated changes that increase the risk for pneumonia in the older adult patient include an increase in:

    1. Compliance of the chest wall.

    2. Diameter of the trachea and bronchi.

    3. Lung parenchyma.

    4. Cough forcefulness.

29. An adult patient arrives at the clinic complaining of difficulty breathing, a cough, and chest pain. History indicates that she was discharged from the hospital 2 days ago after a cesarean section and has a 15-pack per year smoking history. What would be an appropriate action?

    1. Obtain a sputum specimen for culture and sensitivity.

    2. Order a chest x-ray, pulmonary CT scan, and angiogram.

    3. Take a pulse oximetry and obtain vital signs.

    4. Immediately transfer to the emergency department.

30. The family nurse practitioner is aware that the flu or influenza:

    1. Can be caused by receiving a live attenuated influenza vaccine when one's resistance is low.

    2. Is characterized by a slow, insidious onset of chills, fever, and muscle aches.

    3. In older adults may persist for days and increase the prevalence of bacterial pneumonia.

    4. Is primarily contagious in the early autumn and spring, with children at greatest risk.

31. An adult patient with a history of asthma calls to tell the family nurse practitioner that she is "blowing 55%" on the peak flowmeter. What advice would the family nurse practitioner give this patient?

    1. Call an ambulance immediately.

    2. Use a bronchodilator now and come in for evaluation in the office today.

    3. Use an inhaled corticosteroid inhaler now and every 4 hours as needed.

    4. Refer to a pulmonary physician.

32. An older adult patient is evaluated by the family nurse practitioner for a complaint of cough, fever, pleuritic chest pain, and sputum production. In gathering a history on this patient, it is important to know if the patient has:

    1. Received the pneumococcal vaccine.

    2. Traveled out of the country.

3. Pets in the household.

4. Recently changed or started new medications.

33. An older adult patient presents with signs and symptoms that make the family nurse practitioner suspect the diagnosis of community-acquired pneumonia (CAP). Which assessment would the family nurse practitioner most likely evaluate specific to an older adult patient during the examination?

   1. Chest pain with inspiration.

   2. Confusion/disorientation with or without a low-grade fever.

   3. Productive cough.

   4. Fever with leukocytosis.

34. In developing a plan for an older patient with typical pneumonia, the family nurse practitioner understands that 60%–65% of community-acquired pneumonia is caused by which organism?

   1. *Haemophilus influenzae.*

   2. *Klebsiella pneumoniae.*

   3. *Mycobacterium tuberculosis.*

   4. *Streptococcus pneumoniae.*

35. **QSEN** What would be most appropriate to include in the health promotion plan for an older adult patient who is at risk for developing pneumonia?

   1. Administer the pneumococcal vaccination annually.

   2. Administer the pneumococcal vaccination and yearly influenza immunization.

   3. Sputum culture annually along with a chest x-ray.

   4. PPD skin test every 3–5 years.

36. The family nurse practitioner evaluates an older adult patient with a current history of alcoholism. The patient presents with an elevated temperature, congested cough with rusty sputum, and occasional chills. The suspected diagnosis is bacterial pneumonia. The Gram-stained sputum smear would most likely reveal which organism?

   1. *Haemophilus influenzae.*

   2. *Klebsiella pneumoniae.*

   3. *Staphylococcus aureus.*

   4. *Pseudomonas aeruginosa.*

37. An older adult patient residing in a nursing home has recently been exposed to tuberculosis (TB). During the contact investigation, the family nurse practitioner interprets the initial PPD skin test to be negative. Which plan would be most appropriate at this time?

   1. Evaluate the patient in another year.

   2. Repeat PPD test in 8 to 10 weeks.

   3. Ignore results and immediately begin ethambutol.

   4. Evaluate the patient in 6 months because the patient is asymptomatic at this time.

38. The family nurse practitioner knows that Horner's syndrome, a condition that can cause unilateral pupillary constriction and anhidrosis, is often associated with:

   1. Chronic bronchitis.

   2. Pulmonary tuberculosis.

   3. Pulmonary sulcus (Pancoast) tumor.

   4. Pulmonary embolism.

39. An adult patient who smokes presents with complaints of orthopnea. The family nurse practitioner notes on examination dilated blood vessels on the chest and mild edema of the head and supraclavicular area. The family nurse practitioner recognizes this condition as:

   1. Thyroid abnormality.

   2. Chronic bronchitis with mild heart failure.

   3. Asthma with fluid retention.

   4. Superior vena cava syndrome.

40. An older adult patient presents with postural hypotension, and laboratory studies reveal hyponatremia. The patient is currently not taking any medications that may cause this. Which condition is likely the cause of these findings?

   1. Diabetic ketoacidosis.

   2. Severe trauma.

   3. Bronchogenic carcinoma.

   4. Bronchitis.

41. The family nurse practitioner knows the following about asthma in older adult patients:

   1. Subcutaneous epinephrine is standard therapy.

   2. It is usually of the allergic type.

   3. It can be confused with ischemic heart disease.

   4. Clinical presentation is usually dyspnea, costal retraction, and fever.

42. Clinical signs and symptoms of late-phase antigen exposure in asthma include:

    1. Bronchoconstriction refractory to bronchodilator therapy.

    2. Sneezing, watery eyes, and cough.

    3. Wheezing and increased sputum production.

    4. Bronchodilation secondary to the release of histamine.

43. The family nurse practitioner is assessing a patient for asthma. What is a common clinical manifestation of asthma?

    1. Pruritus.

    2. Diffuse crackles.

    3. Nocturnal exacerbation.

    4. Chronic hypoxemia.

44. During a routine follow-up visit for a patient with asthma, the patient states that she has been doing fine except that, when she goes out for dinner, she has increased bronchospasm and wheezing. Which of the following would be an appropriate response by the family nurse practitioner?

    1. "Have you been taking your medication?"

    2. "Do you usually have wine with dinner?"

    3. "I recommend you do not go out for dinner."

    4. "Does going out to dinner make you feel stressed?"

45. The family nurse practitioner is evaluating an adult with symptoms characteristic of obstructive sleep apnea. An overnight polysomnogram (PSG) is ordered. What is the characteristic result of this study that would confirm sleep apnea?

    1. Loud snoring all night long.

    2. Oxygen desaturation and 10-second periods of apnea.

    3. Frequent periods of brief arousal during sleep.

    4. Periods of 5-second apnea with brief arousal.

46. The family nurse practitioner is screening older adult patients for problems related to obstructive sleep apnea (OSA). What risk factors are typically associated with this condition?

    1. Usage of sleep aids.

    2. Weight loss.

    3. Frequent night-time sleep disturbance.

    4. Daytime hyperactivity.

47. A patient comes to the clinic complaining of difficulty breathing, lethargy, and coughing up blood in his sputum. He has no history of chronic illness or major health problems. The family nurse practitioner orders diagnostic tests to determine the problem. What diagnostic test results would require immediate treatment of this patient?

    1. Positive sputum smear for acid-fast bacillus.

    2. Sputum culture positive for *Pneumocystis carinii*.

    3. Presence of hemolysis on complement fixation test.

    4. Oxygen saturation 94%, leukocyte count >5000 WBC/mm^3.

48. When determining the classification of asthma control in an adult patient, who has symptoms less than 2 days per week, no interference with normal activity, reports nighttime awakening 1 time or less per month and using a short-acting β_2 agonist 1 time per week, the family nurse practitioner would classify the patient as:

    1. Well controlled.

    2. Not well controlled.

    3. Very poorly controlled.

    4. Out of control.

49. When examining the chest x-ray of patient with an initial tuberculosis infection, you would expect to see changes in what part of the lung?

    1. Trachea.

    2. Upper lobes.

    3. Bronchi.

    4. Lower lobes.

50. An adult, who has an FEV$_1$ greater than 80%, has been experiencing nighttime awakenings (4–5x/month) and using a short-acting β_2 agonist 3–4 times per week, and reports minimal limitation to normal activity would be classified as:

    1. Intermittent

    2. Mild persistent.

    3. Moderate persistent.

    4. Severe persistent.

Pharmacology

51. **OSEN** The family nurse practitioner is following up on a patient who is experiencing acute asthma problems. Albuterol (Proventil) by metered-dose inhaler (MDI) has been ordered as treatment. Which patient response would indicate to the family nurse practitioner that the patient understands how to take the medication?

    1. "I will take 1 puff of the medication and then wait a minute before taking the second puff."
    2. "I will take 2 puffs of the medication every 4 hours, even if I am not short of breath."
    3. "It is important for me to take this medication on a regular cycle to prevent future attacks."
    4. "I will take 2 puffs, one right after the other, whenever I begin to get short of breath."

52. A patient who was recently diagnosed with tuberculosis calls the clinic because her urine is reddish orange. She is taking isoniazid (INH), rifampin (Rifadin), and pyrazinamide (PZA). What would be an appropriate response for the family nurse practitioner to make?

    1. "This is a urinary tract infection symptom; drink plenty of fluids."
    2. "This is a normal response to the rifampin."
    3. "This often is an indication of liver toxicity. Stop the medications."
    4. "This is indicative of bleeding. You must see a physician immediately."

53. A patient with a history of bronchial asthma is seen in the clinic for increased episodes of difficulty breathing. He has been taking theophylline 100 mg PO tid. He is 40 years old and obese with an 18-pack-year history of cigarette smoking and excessive intake of coffee daily. He eats a low-carbohydrate, high-protein diet. Which identified factors decrease the therapeutic effects of the theophylline?

    1. Age and gender.
    2. Coffee intake and weight.
    3. Age and weight.
    4. Smoking history and diet.

54. **OSEN** An adult male comes to the clinic with complaints that he is experiencing increased difficulty breathing over the past few days. He has a history of asthma and coronary artery disease. He was recently diagnosed with hypertension. Examination reveals no jugular vein distention and no productive cough. Breath sounds are present, but expiratory wheezes are noted bilaterally, and he denies any chest pain. His vital signs are pulse of 72 beats/min, respirations of 34 breaths/min, and BP of 170/100 mm Hg. His current medications are albuterol (Proventil) inhaler 2 puffs every 4 hours prn for wheezing, nitroglycerin transdermal patch, and propranolol (Inderal) 60 mg PO bid. What is the best treatment for this patient?

    1. Discontinue propranolol and begin verapamil (Calan) 80 mg PO tid qd.
    2. Begin theophylline (Theo-24; methylxanthine) 200 mg q12h PO.
    3. Discontinue propranolol (Inderal) and begin atenolol (Tenormin) 50 mg PO qd.
    4. Start beclomethasone (Beclovent) inhaler 2 puffs 3 to 4 times daily.

55. The recommended range for maintaining serum theophylline levels is:

    1. 0.05 to 2 µg/mL.
    2. 10 to 20 µg/mL.
    3. 20 to 25 µg/mL.
    4. 30 to 40 µg/mL.

56. An immunocompromised patient in a long-term care facility whose roommate has been diagnosed with active tuberculosis should be started on latent tuberculosis infection (LTBI) treatment:

    1. As soon as possible and initiated at the time of the tuberculosis skin testing.
    2. In 72 hours after PPD skin test results are obtained.
    3. Only if PPD skin test results are positive.
    4. In 3 months if the repeated skin test is positive.

57. In adults with asthma, the most common reason outpatient treatment fails, resulting in hospitalization, is:

    1. Exposure to allergens.
    2. Increased use of steroids.
    3. Improper inhaler technique.
    4. Use of cromolyn inhalers.

58. Which can elevate theophylline levels?

    1. Concomitant treatment with cimetidine (Tagamet).
    2. Intravenous ampicillin.
    3. Heavy smoking.
    4. History of seizure disorder.

59. A patient with a long history of COPD has noticed an increase in dyspnea and a change in sputum over the past few days, with increased amounts of thick, yellow-green mucus and congestion. What would be the appropriate therapy?

    1. Loratadine (Claritin) 10 mg PO daily.

    2. Augmentin 500 mg/125 mg PO three times daily for 10 days.

    3. Acetaminophen with codeine 300 mg/30 mg PO every 6 hours as needed.

    4. Beclomethasone (Qvar) 40 mcg MDI 2 puffs every 4 hours as needed.

60. Which medication is most effective in promoting a decrease in airway inflammation as well as providing long-term medication coverage in a patient with asthma?

    1. Montelukast (Singulair).

    2. Beclomethasone (Vanceril; Beclovent).

    3. Albuterol (Proventil; Ventolin).

    4. Salmeterol (Serevent).

61. The family nurse practitioner is planning regular daily controller treatment for a patient with asthma. Which is the preferred medication for the asthmatic patient who is not currently experiencing an exacerbation?

    1. Antibiotic.

    2. Inhaled corticosteroid.

    3. β_2-agonist.

    4. Leukotriene receptor antagonist.

62. **QSEN** Patients with asthma need to be instructed to:

    1. Begin inhaled corticosteroids as soon as symptoms appear.

    2. Take 1 to 2 puffs of β_2-agonist as needed using MDI.

    3. Use inhaled corticosteroids when they experience bronchospasm.

    4. Start an antibiotic regimen when they experience bronchospasm.

63. An adult female patient presents in the clinic with a dry, hacking, nonproductive cough that is interfering with her sleep. The family nurse practitioner would encourage the patient to purchase an over-the-counter preparation that contains:

    1. Pseudoephedrine.

    2. Diphenhydramine.

    3. Guaifenesin.

    4. Dextromethorphan.

64. An adult patient with chronic asthma is seen in the clinic complaining of vomiting and stomach cramps. He is confused and unsure what medications he is currently taking. His vital signs are BP of 158/92 mm Hg, pulse of 152 beats/min and irregular, and respirations of 28 breaths/min and shallow. What STAT diagnostic study should be obtained?

    1. Serum electrolytes.

    2. Digoxin level.

    3. Theophylline level.

    4. Arterial blood gases.

65. An adult patient is seen in the clinic complaining of increased difficulty breathing and an intermittent productive cough that worsens in the evening. The history reveals that the patient has a 20-pack-year history of smoking. Breath sounds are clear to auscultation, there is no evidence of fever, and chest radiography is within normal limits. The family nurse practitioner instructs the patient concerning the importance of smoking cessation and fluid therapy and prescribes:

    1. Erythromycin 500 mg PO qid × 14 days.

    2. Albuterol 2 mg PO tid.

    3. Mucomyst 10 mL 10% solution nebulized q4h prn.

    4. Tetracycline 100 mg PO q12h × 14 days.

66. When initiating preventive care to decrease the incidence of pneumonia in patients in an extended-care facility, the family nurse practitioner would identify patients receiving immunosuppressive therapy, repeated antibiotic use, sedation, and:

    1. β_1-Adrenergic blockers.

    2. Calcium channel blockers.

    3. Diuretics.

    4. Histamine (H_2) antagonists.

67. An older adult patient presents with new complaints of dyspnea, cough, fatigue, and dependent edema that has been worsening over the past few days. In planning treatment, the family nurse practitioner considers:

    1. Streptokinase therapy.

    2. Referral for hospitalization for evaluation of heart function.

3. Prescription for furosemide (Lasix) 40 mg PO qd.

4. Addition of a calcium channel blocker to the patient's medications.

68. **QSEN** A patient with a history of Parkinson's disease has an initial positive tuberculosis (TB) skin test, and INH is ordered for treatment of latent tuberculosis infection. Before beginning INH, it is important for the family nurse practitioner to determine:

1. If the patient's Parkinson's condition is being treated with levodopa (Larodopa).

2. How long the patient has been diagnosed with Parkinson's disease.

3. How much respiratory compromise the patient is currently experiencing.

4. The adequacy of urine output and renal function.

69. An adult white male with a history of COPD presents to the clinic with increased dyspnea, temperature of 102°F (39°C), pulse of 104 mm Hg, respirations of 44 breaths/min, and O_2 saturation of 84%. Physical examination reveals diffuse rales and rhonchi bilaterally. Medications include atenolol (Tenormin) 25 mg PO qd, prednisone (Deltasone) 10 mg PO qd, ipratropium bromide (Atrovent) 1 to 2 puffs 18 μg qid prn, and fluticasone and salmeterol (Advair HFA) 2 puffs 100/50 bid. The family nurse practitioner's preliminary diagnosis is pneumonia, pending chest x-ray results. Which medication puts this patient at risk to become immunocompromised?

1. Atenolol.

2. Prednisone.

3. Ipratropium.

4. Fluticasone and salmeterol.

70. The pharmacologic treatment shown to be superior in multiple studies for the treatment of COPD by reducing exacerbation, lowering cost, and improving lung function and quality of life is:

1. Albuterol (Proventil) metered-dose inhaler.

2. Theophylline (Theo-24).

3. Ipratropium bromide (Atrovent) metered-dose inhaler.

4. Ipratropium bromide and albuterol (Proventil) combined.

71. An adult female comes to the clinic with complaints of cough, clear rhinorrhea, and a low-grade fever for 2 days. The family nurse practitioner diagnoses acute bronchi-

tis. The family nurse practitioner knows that with acute bronchitis:

1. The patient will likely need antibiotics.

2. A cough can last for 10 to 20 days.

3. Routine sputum cultures are helpful because of nasopharyngeal colonization.

4. Only 5% to 10% of acute bronchitis cases have a viral etiology.

72. The family nurse practitioner has diagnosed an adult patient with community-acquired pneumonia (CAP). In this healthy patient with no comorbidities and no previous antibiotic use within the past 3 months, the family nurse practitioner should prescribe:

1. Doxycycline 100 mg PO twice daily for 10 days.

2. Amoxicillin (Amoxil) 500 mg PO three times daily for 10 days.

3. Azithromycin (Zithromax) 500 mg PO once and then 250 mg daily for 4 days.

4. Ciprofloxacin (Cipro) 500 mg PO daily for 7 days.

73. An adult male comes into the family practice office with a complaint of a chronic cough. The cough has persisted for 6 weeks and continues following resolution of his upper respiratory infection. The family nurse practitioner understands that:

1. This cough is chronic and is likely caused by cigarette use or exposure to second-hand smoke.

2. This is a subacute cough and is likely post-infectious.

3. The cough has lasted longer than 3 weeks, which means it is not related to past infection.

4. The patient should be worked up for gastroesophageal reflux (GERD).

74. An adult male is started on ciprofloxacin (Cipro) 500 mg PO twice daily for possible exposure to anthrax. Five days later, upon return to the clinic, he notes increased pain in his posterior ankle. Understanding the potential complications with fluoroquinolone therapy, the family nurse practitioner understands:

1. The posterior ankle pain is an unrelated condition.

2. This is a known side effect and the ciprofloxacin (Cipro) should be continued as prescribed.

3. This is a known adverse reaction and the ciprofloxacin (Cipro) should be discontinued.

4. Ciprofloxacin (Cipro) should not be used empirically to treat anthrax exposure.

75. An adult teacher comes to the office with a loud cough starting 2 days ago. She says that several children in her fourth grade class have been out sick because of whooping cough. There is a high probability of exposure to *Bordetella pertussis*. The family nurse practitioner elects the best treatment option to be:

    1. Watchful, waiting to see if the cough clears up in the next few days.

    2. Doxycycline 100 mg PO twice daily for 7 days.

    3. Azithromycin (Zithromax) 500 mg PO once, and then 250 mg PO daily for 4 days.

    4. Oseltamivir (Tamiflu) 75 mg PO twice daily for 5 days.

76. According to the Global Initiative for Chronic Obstructive Lung Disease (GOLD), a clinical diagnosis of COPD is likely when a patient presents with (select 3 responses that apply):

    1. Smoking history.

    2. Chronic cough.

    3. Family history of COPD.

    4. FEV_1/FVC of 0.8.

    5. History of alcohol and drug abuse.

77. The family nurse practitioner sees an adult female with a history of asthma during a first-time office visit. She had been using albuterol (Proventil) metered-dose inhaler (MDI) one inhalation twice monthly over the past several years. More recently, she has been using her MDI inhaler 5 to 7 times per week. Based on the Global Initiative for Asthma (GINA) guidelines, the family nurse practitioner diagnoses mild persistent asthma and starts her on "Step 2" therapy, which includes:

    1. Fluticasone and salmeterol (Advair) 250 mg/50 mg one inhalation twice daily.

    2. Fluticasone (Flovent) 44 mcg, two inhalation daily.

    3. Fluticasone and salmeterol (Advair) 100 mg/50 mg, one inhalation twice daily.

    4. Salmeterol (Serevent) 42 mcg one inhalation twice daily.

78. An adult female comes in for a follow-up for COPD. She notes an increased frequency of morning headaches and daytime somnolence. A complete blood count notes that her hematocrit is 52%. The family nurse practitioner understands that a common, but not always recognized, complication of COPD this patient could have is:

    1. Acute respiratory failure.

    2. Cor pulmonale.

    3. Depression.

    4. Nocturnal oxygen desaturation.

79. An adult patient in the family nurse practitioner's office has been diagnosed with community-acquired pneumonia (CAP). According to the Infectious Diseases Society of America and American Thoracic Society (IDSA/ATS) joint guidelines for CAP, criteria indicating the probable need for immediate admission to an inpatient facility includes (select three that apply):

    1. White blood cell count of 2500 cells/mm^3.

    2. Temperature of 98.2°F (36.8°C).

    3. Respiratory rate of 30 breaths/min.

    4. Platelet count of 165,000 cells/mm^3.

    5. BUN of 32 mg/dL.

80. Which three statements relate to pregnancy considerations with asthma?

    1. Pregnant patients with poorly controlled asthma have low birth-weight infants, increased prematurity, and perinatal mortality.

    2. Albuterol is the preferred short-acting β_2 agonist (SABA) for pregnant patients.

    3. The ICS budesonide is the preferred ICS due to its excellent safety profile.

    4. All ICS should be avoided as they can cause fetal defects.

    5. Long-acting β_2 agonists (LABA) should be used only as monotherapy in pregnancy.

    6. Montelukast and zafirlukast are Category X and should be used in pregnancy.

81. The family nurse practitioner is teaching a patient about the role of medications in the treatment of asthma. Which statement by the patient would require further teaching?

    1. "My albuterol is my quick-relief medication."

    2. "The salmeterol that I take provides me with long-term control."

    3. "I do not need to use a spacer with my MDI."

    4. "I need to use my peak flow meter to self-monitor how I am doing."

5 Respiratory Answers and Rationales

Physical Examination & Diagnostic Tests

1. Answer: 2

Rationale: Vesicular breath sounds are heard over peripheral lung fields where air is flowing through the smaller bronchioles. The inspiratory phase of these low-pitched soft sounds is heard better and is about 2.5 times longer than the expiratory phase. Bronchial breath sounds, normally heard over the trachea and larynx, are high-pitched loud sounds with a shortened inspiratory and lengthened expiratory phase. Bronchovesicular breath sounds that are heard mainly where fewer alveoli are located, which is over the second interspace anteriorly and between the scapulae posteriorly, have an moderate pitch and intensity with equal duration of expiratory and inspiratory sounds. Rhonchi are abnormal breath sounds that are low pitched with a snoring quality.

2. Answer: 2

Rationale: Tactile fremitus is a palpable vibration of the thoracic wall that is produced when the patient speaks. Bronchophony is abnormal, lung sounds are normally soft, muffled, and indistinct. Bronchophony occurs when you ask the patient to say "ninety-nine," during auscultation, you hear a clear distinct sound of "ninety-nine," if there is lung consolidation. Whispered pectoriloquy is exaggerated bronchophony and is heard through a stethoscope when the patient whispers a series of words (e.g., "one-two-three"). In egophony, the spoken voice has a nasal or bleating quality (sounds like a goat) when heard through a stethoscope, and the spoken "e-e-e" sounds like "a-a-a."

3. Answer: 2

Rationale: Hyperresonance is an abnormal percussion tone in adults suggesting an obstructive condition or disease with hyperinflation, like emphysema. It is characterized by very loud intensity, very low pitch, long duration, and a booming quality.

4. Answer: 3

Rationale: Both the anterior and posterior chest should be percussed systematically and symmetrically, moving from left to right. Care is needed to ensure percussion is done in the intercostal spaces. Diaphragmatic excursion is usually only measured on the posterior chest.

5. Answer: 1

Rationale: Pleural friction rubs are loud, dry, creaking or grating sounds produced by the rubbing together of inflamed and roughened pleural surfaces. Rubs are heard best during the latter part of inspiration and the beginning of expiration and in the lower anterolateral chest where the lung expands the most. A continuous, low-pitched, snoring sound that is heard early in inspiration is characteristic of sonorous rhonchi. Egophony is noted when the patient says "e-e-e" and the examiner hears through the stethoscope "a-a-a."

6. Answer: 1

Rationale: With aging, the number of alveoli decreases. The alveoli become rigid and lose their recoil and elasticity, which affects the patient's ability to exhale effectively. This increases a patient's residual volume (the amount of air left in the chest after expiration). Residual volume increases, whereas basilar inflation and ability to expel foreign matter decrease. The anteroposterior (AP) diameter of the chest increases, as seen in patients with kyphosis.

7. Answer: 2

Rationale: Consolidation or compression of lung tissue will cause an increase in fremitus, which is noted with lobar pneumonia. Decreased fremitus occurs with obstruction of vibration, like in emphysema, pneumothorax, or obstructed bronchus. Symmetric transmission of vibration is a normal finding.

8. Answer: 4

Rationale: Crepitation or crepitus (also called subcutaneous emphysema) usually results from air bubbles under the skin caused by a leakage of air into the subcutaneous tissue. Infection by a gas-producing organism is a less common cause. Crepitation always requires attention. Severe inflammation of the pleural surface would not have a palpable abnormality. Fluid consolidation would cause an increased asymmetric fremitus on palpation.

9. Answer: 2

Rationale: This landmark can be used to determine the position of the second rib and intercostal space and corresponding spaces below that level. The angle of Louis is a visible and palpable angle of the sternum at the point where the second rib attaches to the sternum.

10. Answer: 2

Rationale: Fluid or a solid mass transmits more vibrations, so tactile fremitus may be increased at that location on the exterior chest wall. Increased air trapping decreases or masks fremitus. A reactive airway results in wheezing because of an edematous airway.

11. Answer: 4

Rationale: The adult chest is somewhat asymmetric and the AP diameter is often half the transverse diameter. Pigeon chest (pectus carinatum) is a forward protrusion of the sternum with the ribs sloping back. Funnel chest (pectus excavatum) is a depression of the sternum. Barrel chest occurs when the AP diameter equals the transverse diameter.

12. Answer: 2

Rationale: The U.S. Preventive Services Task Force (USP-STF) recommends an annual screening for lung cancer with a low-dose computed tomography (LDCT) in adults aged 55 to 80 years who have a smoking history of 30 packs per year and currently smoke or have quit within the past 15 years. Current evidence-based research does support routine screening for lung cancer in high-risk populations. There is insufficient evidence that lung cancer screening by x-ray or sputum cytology reduces mortality. Bronchoscopy with biopsy is a diagnostic test, not a screening test.

13. Answer: 2

Rationale: The patient should be initially evaluated for tuberculosis, which includes a chest x-ray, sputum smear for acid-fast bacillus, and a CBC. Pulmonary function studies, arterial blood gas (ABG) studies, and bronchoscopy are not indicated initially. Complement fixation studies are done to diagnose atypical pneumonia.

14. Answer: 1

Rationale: A male patient with recent weight gain and restless sleep is at risk for having obstructive sleep apnea (OSA). Ongoing daytime sleepiness is the hallmark sign of OSA. Fluctuations in blood pressure, including hypertension, can be seen in OSA but would not cause the fatigue and nighttime restlessness. Recent changes in medication should be evaluated but are unlikely to cause all his symptoms.

15. Answer: 1

Rationale: Hyperinflation due to air trapping causes an increase in functional residual capacity (FRC), residual volume (RV), and total lung capacity (TLC), which may be twice normal. A corresponding decrease in forced vital capacity (FVC) and forced expiratory volume in 1 second (FEV1) occurs. This causes a flattening of the diaphragm, decreased inspiratory efficiency, and increased work of breathing.

16. Answer: 3

Rationale: Positive interpretation of purified protein derivative (PPD) skin test results are as follows, based on the 2012 criteria from the Centers for Disease Control and Prevention:

INDURATION	POSITIVE PPD SKIN TEST RESULT
≥5 mm	Individuals with human immunodeficiency virus (HIV) infection
	Individuals in recent close contact with persons who have active tuberculosis (TB)
	Individuals with chest x-ray indicating healed TB
≥10 mm	Medically underserved individuals
	Intravenous drug users
	Residents in long-term care facilities and health care workers
≥15 mm	All individuals

17. Answer: 4

Rationale: When you ask the patient to repeat "ninety-nine" while you listen with the stethoscope over the chest wall, bronchophony is the voice sound being tested. With normal voice transmission the sound is soft, muffled, and indistinct; however, the sound can be heard through the stethoscope but cannot be distinguished as to what is exactly being said. When there is increased lung density due to pathology, then the words are heard clearly and bronchophony is present. When testing for egophony, ask the patient to say a long set of "e-e-e" sounds, and normally the sounds are clearly heard through the stethoscope; however, with consolidation or compression the "e-e-e" sounds change to a bleating long "a-a-a" sound, which is similar to how a goat sounds. When checking for whispered pectoriloquy, ask the patient to whisper "1-2-3" as you auscultate. The normal response is faint and muffled; however, with minimal consolidation, the whispered voice is heard clearly. Rhonchal fremitus is vibration felt when inhaled air passes through thick secretions in the larger bronchi.

Disorders

18. Answer: 3

Rationale: The most common respiratory complication after a traumatic injury to the chest is pneumothorax caused from a fractured rib. Oximetry readings at 90% and increased pain are expected at this point and may not be indicative of a problem. Although fever and increased sputum are problems, they are not associated with early manifestations of blunt trauma chest injury.

19. Answer: 1

Rationale: Community-acquired pneumonia (CAP) due to *Streptococcus pneumoniae* often presents abruptly with high fever, shaking chills (rigor), cough productive of purulent sputum, and pleuritic chest pain. In acute bronchitis, cough is the primary symptom and initially is dry and nonproductive. Fever, dyspnea, wheezing, and possible mucoid sputum production are also characteristic of acute bronchitis.

20. Answer: 1

Rationale: On discharge, a patient must understand the importance of taking medications as prescribed. Missed doses increase mutation of the tubercule bacillus and decrease the medication's effectiveness. Respiratory isolation at home is not necessary, and if the patient experiences problems of rash, nausea, and vomiting, he or she should contact the health care provider. A patient should never change a medication dosage without first consulting with a health care provider. Weekly sputum checks are not necessary.

21. Answer: 2

Rationale: According to the American Heart Association, the protocol for cardiopulmonary resuscitation (CPR; rescue breathing) due to respiratory arrest would be to open the airway by tilting the head and lifting the chin.

22. Answer: 1

Rationale: It is most important to obtain information about the dyspnea. Is it present during rest or does it occur with activity? What level of activity precipitates dyspnea? This information is necessary to determine the severity of the patient's complaint. A chest x-ray gives only limited information and may be normal in conditions like asthma. An ABG result is abnormal when the symptoms are severe. Presence of bilateral breath sounds over the lower lobes is a normal finding.

23. Answer: 1

Rationale: The most common area for a foreign body obstruction is the right bronchus, which produces a unilateral retraction of the right chest wall and diminished breath sounds to that area. Retraction of the lower chest occurs with lower respiratory problems, such as asthma. A pleural friction rub is heard when there is inflammation between the viscera and parietal pleura. Crepitation is present when air is leaking into the subcutaneous tissue.

24. Answer: 1

Rationale: This is a normal finding because of the bulk of the liver. Atelectasis and consolidation present with normal diaphragmatic movement but with dullness to percussion over the affected area. Severe obstructive lung disease results in hyperinflation and limited diaphragmatic excursion but is bilateral.

25. Answer: 1

Rationale: Spontaneous pneumothorax occurs in healthy, thin young adults, especially after strenuous exercise; predominant symptoms include sudden pain, dyspnea, and asymmetric chest expansion. The clinical hallmark of asthma is wheezing; with pulmonary edema, there are frequently coughing, frothy sputum, and crackles heard on auscultation. Bronchiectasis is most often chronic and is characterized by moist crackles and wheezing on auscultation; cough is usually present.

26. Answer: 1

Rationale: The situation described is hyperventilation syndrome (HVS); treatment should be concentrated on patient education through reassurance and suggested breathing and relaxation techniques. Albuterol, oxygen, and arterial blood gases (ABGs) are not appropriate initial treatments. Breathing into a paper bag is not recommended because significant hypoxemia and death have occurred in the past from this treatment.

27. Answer: 1

Rationale: To prevent dyspnea on activity, the bronchodilator should be used before walking or increased physical activity. The patient should not stay in bed and should be encouraged to increase activity gradually. Fluid intake of 2–3 L/day should be encouraged, unless there are cardiac problems. A corticosteroid inhaler should be used at regular intervals as ordered and is not meant for rescue during periods of acute dyspnea.

28. Answer: 2

Rationale: Age-associated physiologic changes include:
    Decreased compliance of the chest wall, making deep inspiration difficult.
    Increased trachea and bronchi diameters that increase dead space and result in a decreased volume of air reaching the alveoli. An increase in a small airway closure results in decreased vital capacity and increased residual volume.
    Less elastic lung parenchyma, which decreases function of the alveoli.
    Shallow breathing and less forceful coughs because respiratory muscles weaken.

29. Answer: 4

Rationale: The patient is at risk for a pulmonary embolism as a result of hypercoagulation related to giving birth, smoking, and vascular injury (recent surgery). Immediate testing and treatment are critical to survival of someone with a pulmonary embolism, so he or she should be referred or transferred to the emergency department. Assessment reveals common symptoms of a pulmonary embolism: dyspnea, cough, and pleuritic pain. Diagnostic tests include D-dimer test, chest x-ray, ventilation/perfusion (V/Q) scan, CT scan, and/or pulmonary angiogram, which would be ordered at the emergency department.

30. Answer: 3

Rationale: The flu, or influenza, is a highly contagious respiratory infection that occurs epidemically during the winter months and may increase the prevalence of bacterial pneumonia. It is characterized by a sudden onset of chills, elevated temperature (101°–104°F [38.3-40°C]), headache, fatigue, muscle pain, dry cough, laryngitis, rhinorrhea, and red eyes occurring 24 to 48 hours after exposure directly through respiratory droplets from an infected person or indirectly by drinking from a contaminated glass. Flu vaccines do not cause the flu; they are made with a live attenuated (nasal vaccine) or killed virus (injection).

31. Answer: 2

Rationale: This patient is considered to be in the "yellow" zone of personal best peak flow but is close to the "red" zone (50% or less of personal best). The patient should use her bronchodilator immediately and if not improved may need emergency intervention by the family nurse practitioner. Inhaled corticosteroids are used for maintenance therapy and are a poor choice when someone needs immediate relief of symptoms. A referral to a pulmonologist may be necessary at some point, but not immediately.

32. Answer: 1

Rationale: The pneumococcal vaccine is recommended for older adult patients because their immune system is less efficient. The symptoms of fever, chest pain, and sputum production suggest pneumonia.

33. Answer: 2

Rationale: Confusion/disorientation with or without a low-grade temperature may be the first sign that the older adult patient has severe community-acquired pneumonia (CAP) or sepsis. The patient may not have a fever or leukocytosis. Leukopenia may be caused by severe CAP and require hospitalization. The patient may not experience any discomfort or a cough.

34. Answer: 4

Rationale: *Streptococcus pneumoniae* is the most common cause of community-acquired and nursing home-acquired bacterial pneumonia. *Haemophilus influenzae* is common in older adult patients with underlying chronic diseases (e.g., COPD; diabetes). *Klebsiella pneumoniae* and other gram-negative bacteria are pathogens in patients with alcoholism, immunocompromised hosts, and hospitalized patients. *Mycobacterium tuberculosis* is an infrequent cause of pneumonia.

35. Answer: 2

Rationale: The pneumococcal vaccination given as directed and yearly influenza immunization will decrease complications and hospitalizations for the older adult patient. The pneumococcal vaccination is not administered annually. There is no evidence to support the use of an annual sputum culture or chest x-ray for pneumonia prevention. The purified protein derivative (PPD) skin test should be done annually for high-risk patients and only detects exposure to tuberculosis.

36. Answer: 2

Rationale: *Klebsiella pneumoniae* is an important pathogen in patients with alcoholism. *Staphylococcus aureus* generally affects older adult patients recovering from influenza and is also common in hospitalized, diabetic patients and in IV drug users. *Pseudomonas aeruginosa* is most likely found in someone with structural lung disease (e.g., bronchiectasis).

37. Answer: 2

Rationale: If a person is infected, a delayed-type reaction may occur 2 to 8 weeks after infection. In a contact exposure, if the initial purified protein derivative (PPD) skin test is negative, a repeat PPD test 8 to 10 weeks later is recommended in all patients. A patient should not be treated empirically for tuberculosis (TB) exposure. Six months is too long to wait for someone who could have active TB. A yearly evaluation should be reserved for those who work or live in high-risk environments but have not been exposed.

38. Answer: 3

Rationale: Horner's syndrome, which is a paralysis of the cervical sympathetic nerves that result in ptosis, loss of sweating, pupillary, and sometimes anophthalmos, is often associated with malignant tumors in the upper lung, leading to nerve compression—for example, pulmonary sulcus (Pancoast) tumor or superior sulcus tumor.

39. Answer: 4

Rationale: Over 70% of the cases of superior vena cava syndrome (SVCS) occur as a complication of lung malignancy involving the mediastinum. This is considered an oncologic emergency and requires immediate referral. Although chronic bronchitis or heart failure may cause orthopnea, upper extremity edema is usually not present. A thyroid abnormality usually results in unilateral or bilateral thyroid enlargement in the neck. Asthma does not cause fluid retention.

40. Answer: 3

Rationale: Hyponatremia results from an overproduction of antidiuretic hormone and can be caused by ectopic production from a bronchogenic tumor. Ketoacidosis and trauma result in fluid loss, causing hypernatremia. Bronchitis does not usually cause sodium abnormalities.

41. Answer: 3

Rationale: In older individuals, asthma can be confused with ischemic heart disease or left ventricular failure. Asthma symptoms can be discounted as old age or a lack of fitness. It is rarely allergic, and costal retraction and fever are not usually seen. Subcutaneous epinephrine is not standard treatment for asthma at any age but may be indicated in emergency situations.

42. Answer: 1

Rationale: Late-phase asthma occurs at 8–12 hours after the initial or acute bronchoconstrictive phase. The inflammatory response is the result of mast cell degranulation and the release of inflammatory mediators, including histamines and leukotrienes. The mediators act on the lung by causing bronchoconstriction, vascular permeability, and vasodilation. In late-phase asthma, bronchoconstriction is refractory to most bronchodilator therapy.

43. Answer: 3

Rationale: Nocturnal exacerbation of asthma is a clinical sign. It is linked to variations in circulating cortisol, epinephrine, inflammatory mediators, and vagal tone. Chronic hypoxemia and diffuse crackles are seen in the patient with chronic bronchitis. Pruritus is often seen in contact allergic reactions.

44. Answer: 2

Rationale: Asking the patient about the consumption of wine with dinner is the most appropriate response. Many wines, especially white wines, contain sulfites, which can trigger a mild allergic response.

45. Answer: 2

Rationale: Desaturation and 10-second periods of apnea are diagnostic of sleep apnea. Loud snoring at night, frequent arousals during the night, and sleeping during the day are characteristic of the problem but are not diagnostic.

46. Answer: 1

Rationale: Frequent substance use, including alcohol, benzodiazepines, sleep aids, opiates, and muscle relaxants, can exacerbate obstructive sleep apnea. Obesity, weight gain, nasal allergies, and polyps are common factors associated with this condition. Most patients with sleep apnea will not report nighttime sleep disturbances even though a spouse may witness nighttime restlessness. Snoring, daytime sleepiness, and fatigue are frequently reported symptoms. Men are more likely than premenopausal women to have obstructive sleep apnea.

47. Answer: 1

Rationale: The positive sputum for acid-fast bacillus is indicative of active tuberculosis. *Pneumocystis carinii* is a common organism in healthy respiratory tracts; it becomes a problem if the patient is immunocompromised. Hemolysis on a complement fixation test is a negative finding. When oxygen saturation is low and white blood cell (WBC) count is within normal range, treatment is not as important as it is with tuberculosis.

48. Answer: 1

Rationale: The level of control is based on the most severe impairment or risk category. This patient is well controlled. The components of well-controlled asthma are exacerbations less than 1 per year and symptoms ≤2 days/week, nighttime awakening ≤2x/month, no interference with normal activity, using a short-acting β_2-agonist ≤2 days/week.

49. Answer: 4

Rationale: The initial tuberculosis infection is seen more often in the lower lobes of the lung. The local lymph nodes are infected and enlarged. An asymptomatic period usually follows the primary infection and can last for years or decades before clinical symptoms develop. When there a reactivation of the disease in a previously infected person, this scenario is more likely to occur in situations when defenses are lowered, such as with older adults and people with HIV disease. The upper lobes are the most common site of reactivation.

50. Answer: 2

Rationale: The criteria for mild persistent asthma is symptoms >2 days/week but not daily, nighttime awakenings 3–4×/month, short-acting β-agonist use >2 days/week but not daily, minor limitations in normal activity, and FEV1 (predicted) >80% and FEV1/FVC >80%.

Pharmacology

51. Answer: 1

Rationale: A 1-minute lapse between the two puffs is necessary for the medication to be most effective. The first puff opens the upper airways, allowing more effective penetration of the lower tract with the second puff. Albuterol (Proventil) should not be used as maintenance therapy. Only inhaled corticosteroids should be taken on a regular schedule.

52. Answer: 2

Rationale: The patient would not stop taking the medications because this is a common side effect of rifampin. Also, soft contact lenses may become discolored.

53. Answer: 4

Rationale: Because tobacco increases the metabolism of theophylline, a higher dose is required in smokers than in nonsmokers. A high-protein, low-carbohydrate diet increases the metabolism of theophylline and decreases serum concentrations. Coffee (and other xanthine-containing beverages) may increase the central nervous system effects of xanthine derivatives.

54. Answer: 1

Rationale: Beta-blockers (propranolol, atenolol) are known to exacerbate chronic respiratory problems, especially reactive airway disease. Another antihypertensive, such as a calcium channel blocker (verapamil), should be considered. The patient's pulse is 74 beats/min and blood pressure remains elevated, which indicates the beta-blocker is probably not effective in decreasing blood pressure in this patient. Theophylline derivatives are not indicated unless other medications are not effective. Although beclomethasone may be appropriate to start, discontinuing the beta-blocker, which is likely exacerbating the problem, is the better choice.

55. Answer: 2

Rationale: Therapeutic plasma levels range from 10 to 20 μg/mL. Drug levels of ≥20 μg/mL are associated with toxicity.

56. Answer: 1

Rationale: Latent tuberculosis infection (LTBI) treatment is initiated at the time of the tuberculosis skin testing (TST). TST testing should be repeated in 3 months if initial test results are negative. If the second TST is negative, LTBI treatment can be discontinued.

57. Answer: 3

Rationale: One of the most common causes of outpatient treatment failure is improper inhaler technique. Exposure to allergens may trigger an asthma attack, but proper use of inhalers will control the attacks in many cases. Use of both steroids and cromolyn inhalers has decreased the severity of asthma attacks.

58. Answer: 1

Rationale: Theophylline is used in the treatment of chronic lung disease and can accumulate in toxic levels. Cimetidine decreases the hepatic clearance of theophylline. Nicotine and some antiseizure drugs may actually increase clearance, and ampicillin does not change the clearance.

59. Answer: 2

Rationale: In someone with COPD, antibiotic therapy is indicated when there is a change in color, consistency, or amount of sputum and increased symptoms of COPD exacerbation. Antitussives are not recommended in stable COPD. Inhaled corticosteroids should be taken on a schedule and not ordered as needed.

60. Answer: 2

Rationale: Beclomethasone is a long-acting corticosteroid that stabilizes mast cells and greatly reduces mast-cell degranulation when exposed to allergens. Albuterol is a short-acting bronchodilator used as a rescue medication. Salmeterol is a long-acting bronchodilator most useful in controlling nocturnal asthma symptoms. Montelukast, a leukotriene receptor antagonist, inhibits bronchoconstriction and is used as an adjunct to bronchodilators and corticosteroids.

61. Answer: 2

Rationale: Preferred, regular daily controller treatment (long-term treatment) of the patient with asthma includes inhaled corticosteroids for their anti-inflammatory effects. Antibiotics are indicated if there is a concurrent infection, such as acute bronchitis. β2-agonists are used for their bronchodilator effects and rapid onset of action when a patient may need "rescue" or acute treatment of symptoms with quick-relief medications. A leukotriene receptor antagonist is another option but is not preferred to inhaled corticosteroids for regular daily treatment.

62. Answer: 2

Rationale: Patients with asthma should be instructed to keep their inhaled β_2-agonists with them at all times in case of bronchospasm and use them as necessary (prn). The β_2-agonists are effective in reversing bronchospasm. Inhaled corticosteroids are long acting and will not give immediate relief, so the patient should be instructed to use them as prescribed. Antibiotics are not indicated for acute bronchospasm.

63. Answer: 4

Rationale: Dextromethorphan is specific for the control of coughing. Guaifenesin is an expectorant, pseudoephedrine a decongestant, and diphenhydramine an antihistamine.

64. Answer: 3

Rationale: The drug therapy regimen for chronic asthma may include theophylline. Symptoms of toxicity include anorexia, nausea, vomiting, confusion, restlessness, tachycardia, dysrhythmias, and seizures.

65. Answer: 2

Rationale: The hallmark clinical presentation of acute bronchitis is a productive cough. The family nurse practitioner should rule out pneumonia, which was done with this patient as noted by the normal chest x-ray and breath sounds. Bronchodilators (albuterol) have been found to eliminate the cough of acute bronchitis. Antibiotic therapy (erythromycin and tetracycline) is not recommended. Research has demonstrated that antibiotic-susceptible organisms rarely cause acute bronchitis.

66. Answer: 4

Rationale: Histamine H_2 antagonists neutralize the normal gastric acid barrier, allowing for an increased colonization of gram-negative bacilli and *Staphylococcus aureus*.

67. Answer: 2

Rationale: Worsening dyspnea and fatigue with increasing cough may indicate early pulmonary edema. Patients with pulmonary edema require hospitalization with oxygen therapy, IV furosemide (Lasix), and morphine. Patients suspected of having new-onset pulmonary edema **should not** be treated as outpatients. Calcium channel blockers are of little benefit in heart failure. Streptokinase is for the acute treatment of a myocardial infarction (MI). There is no indication that this patient is experiencing an acute MI.

68. Answer: 1

Rationale: INH requires concurrent administration of vitamin B6 to prevent problems of optic neuritis. Vitamin B6

will decrease the effectiveness of levodopa. If the patient is to receive INH, his anti-Parkinson medication needs to be re-evaluated.

69. Answer: 2

Rationale: Prednisone is a corticosteroid that suppresses immune response and puts the patient in an immunocompromised state, increasing susceptibility to infections. Patients on prednisone therapy should be educated about the risk for developing infections and the need to seek medical attention if they suspect illness. Atenolol is a beta-blocker used as an antihypertensive. Ipratropium is a bronchodilator used as a rescue inhaler. Fluticasone propionate and salmeterol is a combination of inhaled corticosteroid and a long-acting β-agonist. Although inhaled corticosteroids can suppress immune response, absorption is considerably less than oral prednisone.

70. Answer: 4

Rationale: Multiple studies show that the combination of anticholinergic and β-agonist, particularly ipratropium bromide and albuterol, reduce exacerbation, lower cost, and improve lung function and quality of life.

71. Answer: 2

Rationale: Most cases of acute bronchitis are of viral etiology and do not require antibiotic therapy. Approximately 5% to 10% of acute bronchitis is bacterial. A cough can last for 10 to 20 days, but routine sputum cultures are not helpful.

72. Answer: 3

Rationale: In the absence of drug-resistant *Streptococcus pneumoniae* (DRSP) or other comorbidities, azithromycin (Zithromax) is the best choice with Level I evidence. Doxycycline is a weak recommendation (Level III), according to the Infectious Diseases Society of America (IDSA) guidelines. If a beta-lactam like amoxicillin is used, a macrolide should also be prescribed for better coverage. A respiratory fluoroquinolone is recommended in instances of comorbid conditions or the presence of additional risk factors for DRSP, and ciprofloxacin (Cipro) is not a respiratory fluoroquinolone. Moxifloxacin, levofloxacin, gemifloxacin are respiratory fluoroquinolones.

73. Answer: 2

Rationale: The patient most likely has a subacute, post-infectious cough, which can last up to 8 weeks. After 8 weeks, it would more likely be a chronic cough related to environmental factors like smoking, asthma exacerbation, or gastroesophageal reflux.

74. Answer: 3

Rationale: Posterior ankle pain is suggestive of Achilles tendonitis. Tendon ruptures are a known adverse reaction to fluoroquinolone therapy, and there have been a significant number of cases in the United States. If tendon inflammation or pain occurs, the fluoroquinolone should be discontinued immediately. Ciprofloxacin (Cipro) is recommended for empiric treatment of anthrax exposure.

75. Answer: 3

Rationale: In patients with high probability of exposure to *Bordetella pertussis,* first-line therapy with a macrolide antibiotic will improve symptoms if started within 5 to 7 days of symptom onset. Doxycycline is not a first-line choice for *Bordetella pertussis.* Waiting delays the possibility of limiting the spread and treatment of *Bordetella pertussis.* Oseltamivir (Tamiflu) is an antiviral and will not be effective against *Bordetella pertussis.*

76. Answer: 1, 2, 3

Rationale: The presence of risk factors that include tobacco use, chronic cough, and family history all suggest chronic obstructive pulmonary disease (COPD). A post-bronchodilator fixed ratio FEV1/FVC of >0.70 is NOT diagnostic; however, a post-bronchodilator fixed ratio FEV1/FVC of <0.70 is diagnostic.

77. Answer: 2

According to the Global Initiative for Asthma (GINA) guidelines, "Step 2" therapy should start with a low-dose inhaled corticosteroid (ICS). Flovent is an ICS and would be the most appropriate therapy to start, based on GINA guidelines. Fluticasone and salmeterol (Advair) is a combination product. ICS and a long-acting β_2-agonist (LABA) should not be used for initial therapy. Salmeterol (Serevent) is an LABA and should not be used initially.

78. Answer: 4

Rationale: Although acute respiratory failure, cor pulmonale, and depression are common complications of (COPD), they are less likely to cause the patient's current symptoms. Elevated hematocrit, morning headaches, and daytime somnolence are all potential signs of decreased oxygen saturation at night and would be an indication for home overnight oxygen monitoring or sleep disorder specialist referral.

79. Answer: 1, 3, 5

Rationale: Criteria for severe community-acquired pneumonia (CAP) includes white blood cell count less than 4000 cells/mm^3, temperature less than 36°C, respiratory rate greater than or equal to 30 breaths/min, arterial oxygen pressure/fraction of inspired oxygen (PaO$_2$/FiO$_2$) ratio less than 250, platelet count less than 100,000 cells/mm^3, and uremia (blood, urea, and nitrogen) greater than 20 mg/dL.

80. Answer: 1, 2, 3

Rationale: Pregnant women with poorly controlled asthma have low birth-weight infants, increased risk of prematurity, and perinatal mortality. Albuterol is the preferred SABA, and budesonide is the preferred ICS due to excellent safety profile. SABA is the most effective rescue therapy for acute asthma symptoms. ICSs are the preferred long-term control therapy for patients of all ages. Other ICS agents are labeled in pregnancy as Category C, but no data indicate that they are unsafe in pregnancy. Montelukast and zafirlukast are Category B and have not been studied extensively in pregnancy. Long-acting β_2-agonists (LABA), such as salmeterol or formoterol, should not be used as monotherapy, as doing so leads to an increased risk of severe outcomes, including death.

81. Answer: 3

Rationale: It is important to emphasize how to take medications correctly. The MDI usually has 3 parts: mouthpiece, cap that goes over the mouthpiece, and a canister of medicine. A spacer device will help to avoid getting less medication in the mouth. The spacer connects to the mouthpiece. The inhaled medicine goes into the spacer tube first. The patient takes two deep breaths to get the medicine into the lungs; waiting a full minute between the two breaths. Using a spacer wastes a lot less medicine than spraying the medicine into the mouth. MDI technique is important, as well as understanding the use of the devices, such as the prescribed valved holding chamber (VHC), spacer, and nebulizer.

Immune & Allergy

Physical Examination & Diagnostic Tests

1. When taking the history of a patient with known atopic disorder, what is the most important information to determine?

   1. Specific reaction.

   2. Drug allergies.

   3. Food allergies.

   4. Environmental exposure.

2. Which test is used to determine the concentration of gamma globulins that contain the majority of the immunoglobulins?

   1. Immunofixation electrophoresis.

   2. Complement fixation.

   3. Protein electrophoresis.

   4. Antinuclear antibody (ANA).

3. Which diagnostic studies are typically abnormal when ruling in systemic lupus erythematosus (SLE) as a differential diagnosis?

   1. CBC, SMA-12, and ESR.

   2. Chest radiograph and coagulation profile.

   3. ANA, ESR, and C-reactive protein.

   4. CBC, urinalysis, and chest radiograph.

4. Which tests are appropriate for the family nurse practitioner to order in an initial workup for asymptomatic patients at risk for HIV infection?

   1. CD4 count and HIV enzyme-linked immunosorbent assay (ELISA).

   2. Serology for cytomegalovirus, herpes simplex, and Epstein-Barr virus.

   3. HIV ELISA followed by a Western blot.

   4. Hepatitis C screen and Western blot.

5. The family nurse practitioner would identify which laboratory findings as most significant in a patient with joint pain, "butterfly rash," photosensitivity, weight loss, and fever? Select two laboratory findings.

   1. Presence of antinuclear antibodies (ANAs).

   2. Positive serum complement level.

   3. Decreased red blood cells (RBCs).

   4. Thrombocytopenia.

   5. Glycosuria.

   6. Negative LE cell preparation.

6. When assessing a patient for angioedema, the family nurse practitioner would examine the:

   1. Neck and ears.

   2. Lower extremities.

   3. Torso.

   4. Eyes and mouth.

7. How soon after exposure should patients who believe they have been exposed to HIV have an HIV antibody test?

   1. The next day and 2 months later.

   2. 6 months after exposure and again at 12 months.

   3. 6 to 12 weeks after exposure and again at 6 months.

   4. 4 weeks and 12 weeks.

8. Which two tests are the most reliable for the presence of specific immunoglobulin E (IgE) antibody?

    1. Skin testing.

    2. Radioallergosorbent testing (RAST).

    3. Nasal smear for eosinophils.

    4. Complete blood count.

    5. Serum ImmunoCAP testing.

9. To diagnose allergic rhinitis from vasomotor rhinitis in the primary care office setting, the family nurse practitioner would consider performing:

    1. Nasal smear for eosinophils.

    2. Total serum IgE.

    3. Skin prick testing.

    4. Serum radioallergosorbent test (RAST).

Disorders

10. A young adult presents to the clinic with a 10-day history of fever, myalgia, sore throat, and measles-like rash. The patient is not taking any medications. Which of the following viral syndromes is characterized by a measles-like rash?

    1. Influenza.

    2. Varicella.

    3. HIV.

    4. Mononucleosis.

11. A young woman presents to the urgent care center reporting that a male "date" vaginally raped her last night. She is treated today for *Chlamydia* infection, gonorrhea, and syphilis and is started on a 1-month course of medications to prevent HIV. She wants to know why she needs the HIV therapy since no one she knows has "AIDS." What is the basis for the family nurse practitioner's counseling?

    1. The patient should assume that the man was not HIV positive.

    2. She probably does not need the therapy, but it is a good idea to take the medications.

3. More than 30% of HIV-infected individuals are unaware that they are infected.

4. HIV is not easily transmitted.

12. A patient tells the family nurse practitioner that her husband's sister has HIV but now she is "cured." She takes medications, and "her doctor cannot find the virus in her blood." Which response would be appropriate?

    1. "Oh, I'm so sorry, but she must be mistaken; AIDS is not curable."

    2. "That is wonderful news, but are you sure?"

    3. "You must be very happy; I didn't know that was possible."

    4. "I've heard that the new medications are very good at lowering the virus counts."

13. **QSEN** A co-worker has just stuck herself with a needle while performing a phlebotomy. She asks the family nurse practitioner for help and requests that the nurse manager is not informed about the incident. What should be the family nurse practitioner's initial response?

    1. Send the co-worker to the nurse manager.

    2. Sit with her and calm her down.

    3. Put on gloves, run water, and make her "bleed" the site under running water for several minutes.

    4. Put on gloves and pour povidone-iodine (Betadine) on the area.

14. An adult patient presents to the clinic with fatigue, sore throat, and myalgia. On examination, the family nurse practitioner finds axillary lymphadenopathy and a slightly enlarged spleen. Based on the history, the nurse adds acute HIV infection to the differential diagnosis. Which STAT laboratory result increases concern about HIV infection?

    1. Hypochromic, normocytic anemia (HC/NC).

    2. Leukopenia and thrombocytopenia.

    3. Elevated lymphocyte count.

    4. Elevated neutrophil count.

15. A woman comes to the clinic for the first time in the seventh month of her pregnancy. She knows that she has HIV disease but has not been receiving care. Physical examination includes Doppler ultrasound of the fetal heart, prenatal panel, and urine specimen. The family nurse practitioner discusses the patient's urgent need for obstetric and prenatal care, and the patient refuses, saying that it is too late and that she "knows" her baby is infected. The family nurse practitioner's response is based on the following information:

    1. All infants contract HIV from their mother, unless the mother takes medications.

    2. It is not too late to begin antiviral medications to decrease the risk to the baby.

    3. The mother's viral load is probably high, and the baby may already be HIV positive.

    4. HIV is nearly always fatal to infants who contract it.

16. A new mother tells the clinic nurse that her infant was born HIV positive. She asks the family nurse practitioner how long her baby has to live. Which of the following should be the basis of the family nurse practitioner's response?

    1. The antibodies present in the infant's blood may reflect the antibodies received from the mother at birth.

    2. If antibodies are present at birth, the infant has AIDS in an active form.

    3. Because the infant is HIV positive, the child will develop full-blown AIDS within 3 years.

    4. The antibodies detected at birth indicate presence of the HIV; the test does not indicate when the child will develop AIDS.

17. **QSEN** Patient education regarding common antigens of anaphylaxis includes:

    1. Wheat.

    2. Egg albumin.

    3. Dust mites.

    4. Animal dandruff.

18. The family nurse practitioner understands that an HIV infection results in a reduction of:

    1. Helper T cells.

    2. Suppressor T cells.

    3. Killer T cells.

    4. Suppressor B cells.

19. Which assessment findings are typically associated with a diagnosis of systemic lupus erythematosus (SLE)?

    1. Excitability, diarrhea, and vomiting.

    2. High fever, measles-like rash on limbs, and weight loss.

    3. Joint pain, malar rash, and photosensitivity.

    4. Weight loss, diarrhea, and generalized abdominal pain.

20. After a repeat HIV antibody test, a patient continues to test positive but is asymptomatic. Which of the following is important for the family nurse practitioner to understand regarding the transmission of the virus by this patient?

    1. The patient is infectious when symptoms are active.

    2. The patient may remain infectious for life.

    3. The dormant virus is not infectious while the patient is asymptomatic and the T-cell count is high.

    4. Laboratory tests should be done every 4 to 6 weeks to identify the infectious periods of the disease process.

21. **QSEN** A young woman has just received news of a positive HIV test. She does not want her sexual partner to be informed. What is the family nurse practitioner's most appropriate response?

    1. Respect for her decision because she is the patient.

    2. Informing her now that the nurse has a legal responsibility to inform her partner.

    3. Counseling her about the nurse's ethical responsibility to inform all sexual partners.

    4. Documenting her decision in the record for future reference.

22. The family nurse practitioner has been assigned a new patient. The problem list indicates this patient has CREST syndrome. The family nurse practitioner will be following this patient for what condition?

    1. Scleroderma.

    2. Dental caries.

    3. Systemic lupus erythematosus.

    4. Rheumatoid arthritis.

23. A patient presenting with complaints of fatigue, malaise, arthralgias, oral ulcers, malar rash, and positive ANA test would most likely be diagnosed as having:

    1. Chronic fatigue syndrome.

    2. Fibromyalgia.

    3. Scleroderma.

    4. Systemic lupus erythematosus (SLE).

24. What are the most common clinical manifestations of Sjögren's syndrome?

    1. Corneal dryness and lack of saliva.

    2. Increased urination and hunger.

    3. Abdominal discomfort and thickening of the epidermis.

    4. Joint destruction and alopecia.

25. An older adult female patient presents to the family nurse practitioner with low-grade temperature and a unilateral throbbing headache. She also reports scalp sensitivity and some visual disturbances. Laboratory results show a greatly elevated ESR and anemia. She has been relatively healthy except for a recent history of polymyalgia rheumatica (PMR). Which of the following conditions should be diagnosed based on this clinical presentation?

    1. Bacterial meningitis.

    2. Primary angle closure glaucoma (PACG).

    3. Temporal (giant cell) arteritis.

    4. Subdural hematoma.

26. A middle-aged female patient presents with weight loss, heartburn, dysphagia, dry cough, pain, stiffness of the fingers and knees, and Raynaud's phenomenon. The family nurse practitioner recognizes these as the symptoms of:

    1. Rheumatoid arthritis.

    2. Systemic lupus erythematosus (SLE).

    3. Barrett's esophagus.

    4. Scleroderma.

27. The erythematous confluent macular eruption of the face known as the "butterfly rash" is characteristic of:

    1. Allergic drug eruption.

    2. Systemic lupus erythematosus (SLE).

    3. Rosacea.

    4. Seborrheic dermatitis.

28. The family nurse practitioner is discussing general health care with a female patient who has systemic lupus erythematosus (SLE) and is in remission. What are important points to include in the teaching?

    1. Daily weight checks to assess for fluid retention.

    2. Decrease physical and psychological stress.

    3. Avoid isometric exercise.

    4. Maintain diet low in fat and high in carbohydrates.

29. A 50-year-old male patient presents with complaints of frequent sinus infections, decrease in ability to hear, and arthralgias. Laboratory findings are mild normochromic/normocytic anemia, elevated ESR, mild hypergammaglobulinemia (elevated IgA), proteinuria, and hematuria with granular or cellular casts. Physical findings include mild conjunctivitis, vasculitic dermatitis, chronic cough, chest pain, dyspnea, paranasal sinus pain, occasional epistaxis, and imbalance of intake and output. What would be a tentative diagnosis?

    1. Connective tissue disease.

    2. Wegener's granulomatosis.

    3. Pulmonary neoplasm.

    4. Infectious granulomatous disease.

30. A patient presents with sneezing, watery eyes, postnasal drip, and sore throat. What diagnosis do these symptoms most likely suggest?

    1. Acute sinusitis.

    2. Allergic rhinitis.

    3. Vasomotor rhinitis.

    4. Influenza.

31. A 70-year-old woman presents with complaints of morning headache, malaise, and anorexia. What condition would the family nurse practitioner suspect?

    1. Pneumonia.

    2. Temporal arteritis.

    3. Anemia of chronic disease.

    4. Acute sinusitis.

32. When teaching a patient about risk factors and prevention of transmission of HIV, which statement is most appropriate?

    1. HIV can be transmitted by casual kissing.

    2. Unprotected oral sex with an infected partner may result in transmission.

    3. Sharing an office with an HIV-positive person increases the risk of HIV exposure.

    4. Using the same bathroom as an infected family member puts one at risk of HIV exposure.

33. Signs and symptoms that alert the family nurse practitioner to identify a patient who is at an increased risk for HIV infection include:

    1. Frequent emergency department visits for urinary tract infections (UTIs).

    2. Malaise and fatigue.

    3. Frequent sexually transmitted infections (STIs).

    4. Swollen glands and diarrhea.

34. What is an appropriate classification for HIV?

    1. Cytomegalovirus.

    2. Herpetic virus.

    3. Papillomavirus.

    4. Retrovirus.

35. What are the most frequently occurring symptoms of systemic lupus erythematosus (SLE)?

    1. Splenomegaly and Raynaud's syndrome.

    2. Pulmonary effusions and hepatomegaly.

    3. Butterfly rash on face and lymphadenopathy.

    4. Fever, arthritis, arthralgia, and weight loss.

36. A systemic IgE-mediated antigen-antibody response resulting in a life-threatening massive release of mediators is:

    1. Recurrent urticaria.

    2. Allergic rhinitis.

    3. Anaphylaxis.

    4. Contact dermatitis.

37. The release of histamine results in:

    1. Bronchospasm, vasodilation, and vascular permeability.

    2. Bronchodilation, vasodilation, and vascular permeability.

    3. Smooth muscle contraction, decreased vascular permeability, and vasoconstriction.

    4. Pain, increased vascular permeability, and bronchodilation.

38. After a bone marrow transplant (BMT), the family nurse practitioner can expect the peak onset of an acute graft-versus-host disease (GVHD) to occur between:

    1. 10 and 15 days post transplant.

    2. 30 and 50 days post transplant.

    3. 1 and 5 days post transplant.

    4. 90 and 100 days post transplant.

39. A patient has a history of recent bone marrow transplant (BMT). The family nurse practitioner identifies signs and symptoms of graft-versus-host disease (GVHD) to include:

    1. Fever, headache, and mental status changes.

    2. Chills, fever, and urticaria over flank area.

    3. Increased serum bilirubin, maculopapular rash, and abdominal cramping.

    4. Decreased red blood cells (RBCs), hematocrit, hemoglobin, and petechiae.

40. The pathogenesis of systemic lupus erythematosus (SLE) is characterized by autoantibody development. This results in:

    1. Increased T suppressor cell.

    2. B cell decrease.

    3. Polyclonal hypogammaglobulinemia.

    4. Decreased T suppressor cells and inhibited cell activity.

41. What blood cell is responsible for the activation of the immune response?

    1. Band neutrophil.

    2. T4 lymphocyte.

    3. Segmented neutrophil.

    4. B lymphocytes.

42. A 22-year-old male presents with breathlessness, weight loss, nonproductive cough, temperature of 100.4°F (38°C), pulse of 124 beats/min, respirations of 36 breaths/min, BP of 120/78 mm Hg, and a history of positive HIV serum test. Based on this information, which is the most accurate diagnosis?

    1. *Klebsiella pneumoniae* infection.

    2. *Mycoplasma pneumoniae* infection.

    3. *Pneumocystis carinii* pneumonia.

    4. Community-acquired pneumonia.

43. A nurse at the clinic experiences a needlestick from a patient with known hepatitis C. What immunoglobulin (Ig) should be administered to provide passive immunity?

    1. IgE.

    2. IgA.

    3. IgG.

    4. IgC.

44. Which sign/symptom is indicative of a type I hypersensitivity reaction?

    1. Contact dermatitis.

    2. Immediate wheal-and-flare reaction.

    3. Hematuria.

    4. High fever.

45. Which patients are at risk for developing HIV/AIDS?

    1. Immunocompromised patients.

    2. Sexually active teenagers.

    3. Middle-aged adults.

    4. Marijuana users.

46. What are the cardiovascular effects of anaphylaxis?

    1. ST-segment and T-wave changes.

    2. Hypertension.

    3. Prolonged PR intervals with elevated QT segment.

    4. Elevated serum cardiac enzymes.

47. When assessing a patient for systemic lupus erythematosus (SLE), what ophthalmologic findings would the family nurse practitioner determine to be consistent with this condition?

    1. Retinal hemorrhages.

    2. Conjunctivitis.

    3. Cotton-wool spots.

    4. Arteriovenous (AV) nicking.

48. What information does the family nurse practitioner include in the education for the patient with allergic rhinitis?

    1. Monitor air quality and the allergy index.

    2. Use a surgical-type mask when going outdoors.

    3. Remain inside during allergy season.

    4. Avoid working in the garden or yard.

49. **QSEN** A nurse from the operating room (OR) comes into the clinic with complaints of shortness of breath, itching, reddened hands, and wheezing. He says that he does not seem to have the symptoms when he is not working. Based on the history and symptoms, the family nurse practitioner would evaluate for:

    1. Indoor toxic mold exposure.

    2. Bronchitis.

    3. Latex allergy.

    4. Contact dermatitis.

50. Which statement is true regarding latex allergy?

    1. It usually only produces symptoms of contact dermatitis and allergic rhinorrhea.

    2. It is a progressive disorder that worsens with continued exposure.

    3. It affects less than 5% of the health care population.

    4. It is an autoimmune response.

Pharmacology

51. An adult patient comes to the urgent care clinic with nausea, vomiting, and acute abdominal pain. His history is significant for HIV disease, and for the past month he has been taking didanosine (Videx) 400 mg qd, Kaletra (400 mg LPV/100 mg RTV) 2 tablets bid, and lamivudine (Epivir) 150 mg bid. After the examination, the family nurse practitioner determines that didanosine can cause pancreatitis and lactic acidosis. What laboratory tests would be ordered?

    1. CBC, CD4 count, viral load, and electrolytes.

    2. CBC with differential, lipase, lactic acid, electrolytes, BUN, creatinine, and liver function tests (LFTs).

    3. Amylase, lipase, and lactic acid.

    4. Lipase, amylase, and liver function tests (LFTs).

52. Which drugs have been associated with a lupus-like syndrome?

    1. Sulfonamides (Septra DS) and penicillin (Pen-Vee K, Penicillin G).

    2. Progestin/estrogen oral contraceptives.

    3. Nonsteroidal anti-inflammatory drugs (NSAIDs; Motrin).

    4. Procainamide (Pronestyl) and hydralazine (Apresoline).

53. A patient is diagnosed with temporal (giant cell) arteritis. What is the medication of choice?

    1. Prednisone (Deltasone).

    2. Ibuprofen (Motrin).

    3. Indomethacin (Indocin).

    4. Azathioprine (Imuran).

54. What medications are used for malaria prophylaxis? Select 4 medications.

    1. Ampicillin (Omnipen).

    2. Doxycycline (Vibramycin).

    3. Ceftriaxone (Rocephin).

    4. Chloroquine phosphate (Aralen).

    5. Mefloquine (Lariam).

    6. Primaquine.

55. Which medications are used in the treatment of allergic rhinitis?

    1. Antihistamines, corticosteroids, and environmental control.

    2. Antihistamines, analgesics, and allergen control.

    3. Anticholinergics, antibiotics, and oral prednisone.

    4. Nasal saline rinses, corticosteroids, and antibiotics.

56. Development of an adverse drug reaction depends on which factors?

    1. Patient age, prior drug reactions, genetic factors, and degree of exposure.

    2. Patient gender, oral route of administration, and history of atrophic disease.

    3. Patient age, gender, and genetic factors.

    4. Genetic factors, prior drug reactions, and patient gender.

57. A medication frequently used for the prophylaxis as well as initial treatment of *Pneumocystis carinii* pneumonia (PCP) is:

    1. Fluconazole (Diflucan).

    2. Amphotericin B (Fungizone).

    3. Trimethoprim-sulfamethoxazole (TMP-SMX; Septra).

    4. Acyclovir (Zovirax).

58. When instructing patients with allergic rhinitis about the use of nasal decongestants, it is important for them to understand:

    1. The condition is self-limiting and will resolve in a matter of weeks whether or not the patient is reexposed to the allergen.

    2. A nasal decongestant used continuously for greater than 3 days can result in a worsening of the symptoms.

    3. It is not necessary to avoid exposure to the allergen once therapy has been initiated.

    4. Allergic rhinitis is only seen in the spring and fall; the condition requires treatment during these seasons only.

59. What is the major advantage of using second-generation antihistamines, such as cetirizine (Zyrtec) and loratadine (Claritin)?

    1. Decreased cost.

    2. Increased anticholinergic activity.

    3. Delayed absorption.

    4. Do not cross the blood-brain barrier.

60. What is the desired action of sympathomimetics (adrenergics) when used in the treatment of allergic rhinitis?

    1. Promote vasoconstriction in nasal mucosa.

    2. Block mast cell degranulation.

    3. Decrease the effect of histamines.

    4. Increase mast cell degranulation.

61. In the older adult patient, histamine H1 blockers may cause which side effects?

    1. Ataxia.

    2. Nausea.

    3. Bradycardia.

    4. Gastrointestinal upset.

62. What information is important for the family nurse practitioner to include when teaching a patient about the use of antihistamines?

    1. Use of topical antihistamines is safe and has relatively few side effects.

    2. Do not use over-the-counter (OTC) medications without consulting the health care provider.

    3. Constipation and urinary retention are expected side effects and do not need to be reported.

    4. Once antihistamine therapy has been taken for 3 days, avoidance of allergens is not necessary.

63. A primary advantage of using loratadine (Claritin) in treating a patient with seasonal allergies is that it:

    1. Is prudent to take only as needed.

    2. May be prescribed for once-a-day (daily) dosing.

    3. Costs considerably less than other medications.

    4. Effectively decreases nasal secretions.

64. What medications are drugs of choice for the secondary treatment of patients with an anaphylactic reaction?

    1. Antibiotics and anticholinergics.

    2. NSAIDs and decongestants.

    3. Decongestants and expectorants.

    4. Antihistamines and corticosteroids.

65. Patients newly presenting with signs and symptoms of systemic lupus erythematosus (SLE) should have their medication profile reviewed to determine whether they are taking any medication that may have caused a drug-induced lupus. Which drug should the family nurse practitioner most suspect?

    1. Digoxin (Lanoxin).

    2. Procainamide (Pronestyl).

    3. Trimethoprim-sulfamethoxazole (TMP-SMX).

    4. Cimetidine (Tagamet).

66. An adult patient presents at the clinic, and his family states he has a history of anaphylactic reactions. What signs and symptoms indicate to the family nurse practitioner that the patient is experiencing another reaction?

    1. Cough, wheezing, and urticaria.

    2. Severe malaise, pallor, stridor, and dyspnea.

    3. Anxiety, nasal congestion, and tachycardia.

    4. Rhinorrhea, nausea, and gastrointestinal pain.

6 Immune & Allergy Answers and Rationales

Physical Examination & Diagnostic Tests

1. Answer: 1

Rationale: The reaction to each allergen is most important to know. Often patients state they have an "allergy" to a particular food or medication, such as nausea, stomach pain, or diarrhea, which they regard as an allergy. The signs and symptoms of the reaction, speed of onset, duration, and successful treatments used in the past are also important information. Medication side effects must be distinguished from true allergic reactions to drugs, so patient statements of drug or food allergies should be thoroughly explored.

2. Answer: 3

Rationale: In protein electrophoresis, proteins are electrically separated on a strip. It is a screening test to measure various proteins in body fluids, usually serum or urine. It assists in screening for diseases characterized by an increase or decrease in immunoglobulins. Serum protein electrophoresis is also used to identify occult malignancy in a patient with failing health when no cause can be found. Complement fixation and antinuclear antibody (ANA) are diagnostic studies for rheumatoid problems.

3. Answer: 3

Rationale: Although all tests listed may be included in a complete physical examination, laboratory tests specific to the diagnosis of systemic lupus erythematosus (SLE) include antinuclear antibody (ANA), erythrocyte sedimentation rate (ESR), and C-reactive protein. During flares, ESR and C-reactive protein are elevated. The ANA titer in a patient with SLE is positive at a 1:80 ratio.

4. Answer: 3

Rationale: The initial screening test for HIV is enzyme-linked immunosorbent assay (ELISA). If the test is positive, antibodies are confirmed with Western blot. Although serology and hepatitis screening with complete blood count (CBC) and tuberculosis skin test are routinely performed, the initial workup starts with an ELISA test. The CD4 count is performed during the active disease process.

5. Answer: 1, 4

Rationale: The majority of patients with systemic lupus erythematosus (SLE) have antinuclear antibodies (ANAs) present in their blood with leukopenia, thrombocytopenia, lymphopenia, anemia, positive LE cell preparation, elevated

sedimentation rate (ESR), and positive C-reactive protein. Proteinuria with cellular casts is often noted.

6. Answer: 4

Rationale: Angioedema is edema of the mucous membrane tissue and is most easily seen in the eyes and mouth. It also affects the tongue, feet, hands, and genitalia. Diffuse erythema may be seen in the upper body parts. Gastrointestinal symptoms (e.g., vomiting, cramping, diarrhea) may occur. African-American patients are more likely to experience angioedema when given ACE inhibitors (e.g., lisinopril, captopril, etc.).

7. Answer: 3

Rationale: The HIV antibody develops between 6 and 12 weeks after exposure. Because of the variability of antibody development, it is recommended that the test be repeated in 6 months to confirm the findings.

8. Answer: 1, 5

Rationale: The most reliable tests for the presence of the specific immunoglobulin E (IgE) antibody is the skin test and the serum ImmunoCAP test that can provide quantitative measurement of IgE and accurately determine whether patients have allergies and determine what they are allergic to. Radioallergosorbent testing (RAST) is an earlier and less sensitive blood allergy test than skin testing and is difficult to standardize and reproduce results. The smear for eosinophils and complete blood count (CBC) are not specific for IgE antibody.

9. Answer: 1

Rationale: A nasal smear for eosinophils is a simple office procedure. Many patients who have uncomplicated allergic rhinitis have a normal serum immunoglobulin E (IgE). Skin-prick testing should be performed by allergy-trained providers only. Radioallergosorbent testing (RAST) testing is higher in cost and lower in sensitivity.

Disorders

10. Answer: 3

Rationale: Acute HIV infection is characterized by a history of prolonged fever and a red, raised, discrete skin eruption described as morbilliform ("measles-like"). Neither influenza nor mononucleosis typically presents with a rash. Varicella (chickenpox) presents with a vesicular skin eruption.

11. Answer: 3

Rationale: Treating a woman who has been raped requires time for patient education. The patient should not assume that the man was HIV negative. Evidence based on postexposure prophylaxis (PEP) in health care workers and infants supports its effectiveness. Traumatic sex increases the risk of sexually transmitted disease (STD), including HIV.

12. Answer: 4

Rationale: Repeating what the patient has said along with more information about how HIV medications can lower viral counts is appropriate. The other responses do not address the patient's comments.

13. Answer: 3

Rationale: Bleeding the site under running water is more effective than using topical antiseptics (Betadine). Sending the co-worker to the nurse manager does not address the medical need of washing the needlestick site. Talking with the co-worker and providing support is necessary, but not until the family nurse practitioner addresses the need to wash the site immediately.

14. Answer: 2

Rationale: Acute, primary HIV infection depletes the CD4 cells, which produces leukopenia and depletes platelets. A hypochromic, normocytic (HC/NC) anemia is present more often in advanced HIV. Elevated lymphocyte counts are more likely in other viral illnesses, and elevated neutrophil counts are seen in bacterial infections.

15. Answer: 2

Rationale: Not all infants contract HIV from their mothers during pregnancy. It is recommended that the woman be placed on antivirals for the pregnancy. Also, HIV may not be fatal in children with access to effective antiretroviral therapy. The immune system of some individuals with HIV keeps the viral load under control for many years.

16. Answer: 4

Rationale: It is important to give the mother as much hope as possible but still be realistic about the infant's condition. There is no way to tell when or if the infant will convert to active AIDS. Many infants seroconvert to HIV-negative status.

17. Answer: 2

Rationale: Egg albumin is one of many identified common antigens that may result in an anaphylactic reaction. Others include vaccines, allergen extracts, sulfonamides, penicillins, hormones, legumes (especially peanuts), berries, nuts, seafood, and venom bites (bee, wasp, yellow jacket). Wheat ingestion and dust mite exposure rarely result in anaphylaxis.

18. Answer: 1

Rationale: There is a severe, life-threatening reduction of helper T cells, along with an increase in suppressor T cells. The helper T cells help amplify or increase the production of antibody-forming cells from B lymphocytes after an encounter with an antigen. Killer T cells are produced after mature helper T cells interact with an antigen. Suppressor T cells suppress the formation of antibody-forming cells from B lymphocytes, which, when their numbers are increased, have a detrimental effect on the immunity and ability of the HIV patient to make antibody-forming cells.

19. Answer: 3

Rationale: The symptoms most often experienced are joint pain, fatigue, Raynaud's phenomenon, chronic low-grade or recurrent fever, sun sensitivity, hair loss, weakness, butterfly (malar) facial rash, and weight loss. Typically, the pulmonary, cardiac, renal, and central nervous systems are involved, which may cause multisystem failure and contribute to mortality in patients with systemic lupus erythematosus (SLE).

20. Answer: 2

Rationale: HIV infection creates a chronic infectious state in the body that is transmitted through blood or body fluids and transplacentally throughout the patient's life.

21. Answer: 3

Rationale: Ethical response includes notification of all persons at risk so that early intervention and treatment can be initiated.

22. Answer: 1

Rationale: CREST (**C**alcinosis, **R**aynaud's phenomenon, **E**sophageal dysfunction, **S**clerodactyly, **T**elangiectasia) is associated with a slow, progressive form of scleroderma.

23. Answer: 4

Rationale: The patient is presenting with 4 of the 11 criteria necessary for diagnosing systemic lupus erythematosus (SLE). No single test exists for SLE, but these characteristics plus laboratory results (antinuclear antibody (ANA), erythrocyte sedimentation rate (ESR), C-reactive protein) can differentiate the diagnosis.

24. Answer: 1

Rationale: Corneal dryness and lack of saliva are the most common clinical manifestations of Sjögren's syndrome. Patients may also have joint inflammation, but this rarely leads to joint destruction.

25. Answer: 3

Rationale: About 40% of patients with temporal (giant cell) arteritis have a history of polymyalgia rheumatica (PMR). The other diagnoses may have some of these symptoms, but only arteritis has all symptoms listed in the situation. It is especially crucial to note visual disturbances because these patients can develop sudden blindness. Definitive diagnosis is confirmed by biopsy. Treatment typically consists of increasing the patient's prednisone to 60 mg daily in divided doses for 4 weeks, and then gradually decreasing ESR monitoring.

26. Answer: 4

Rationale: The symptom of Raynaud's phenomenon differentiates this as scleroderma. The esophageal dysfunction is often an initial complaint in scleroderma, which affects women four times more often than men. Barrett's esophagus is diagnosed in patients with long-term gastroesophageal reflux disease (GERD) and is associated with an increased risk of developing esophageal cancer.

27. Answer: 2

Rationale: The butterfly (malar) rash is one of the characteristic symptoms of systemic lupus erythematosus (SLE). Allergic drug eruptions are characterized by an erythematous rash or hives. Rosacea is characterized by redness and small, red, pus-filled bumps. Seborrheic dermatitis is characterized by scaly patches and red skin, mainly on the scalp.

28. Answer: 2

Rationale: Because systemic lupus erythematosus (SLE) is considered an autoimmune disorder, psychological and physical stress can exacerbate the condition. A balanced diet helps limit the side effects of some medications, and regular exercise helps reduce arthralgia and myalgia associated with SLE. It is not necessary to check daily weights.

29. Answer: 2

Rationale: Wegener's granulomatosis is a multisystem disorder that occurs equally in both genders. Peak occurrence is between 40 and 60 years of age. The disease usually targets the upper respiratory tract and the kidneys. Connective tissue disease, pulmonary neoplasm, and infectious granulomatous disease would be considered in the differential diagnosis.

30. Answer: 2

Rationale: The signs and symptoms presented are classic for allergic rhinitis. Acute sinusitis would present with sinus pressure and pain, perhaps tooth pain and fever. Vasomotor rhinitis typically does not present with ocular symptoms and occurs in response to environmental triggers, such as cold air, strong smells, irritants, changes in weather, some medications (ACE inhibitors, beta blockers), stress, exercise, and certain foods. Influenza presents with acute onset, fever, chills, and general malaise.

31. Answer: 2

Rationale: The family nurse practitioner should suspect temporal arteritis, an inflammatory disorder of unknown etiology that affects large and medium-sized arteries. It occurs two times more frequently in women than in men and most frequently in older adults, but rarely in the African-American population. The clinical findings would reveal temporal tenderness and temporal bruits. About 40% of the patients who have been diagnosed with polymyalgia rheumatica (PMR) also have temporal arteritis, and the older adult patient may be relating some of her arthralgia and myalgias to normal changes of aging versus PMR. The family nurse practitioner should also check an ESR and consider referring the patient to a rheumatologist.

32. Answer: 2

Rationale: Unprotected oral sex with an HIV-positive person puts one at risk for exposure to the virus. Human contact, such as casual kissing or sharing an office or bathroom, does not transmit the virus. The virus is transmitted in body fluids and secretions.

33. Answer: 3

Rationale: Frequent sexually transmitted infections (STIs) would alert the family nurse practitioner to the patient's lack of protected sex and the possibility of multiple partners. Night sweats, malaise, fatigue, swollen glands, and diarrhea may be associated with many other illnesses. Urinary tract infections (UTIs) are not always diagnostic of frequent sexual activity.

34. Answer: 4

Rationale: HIV is a retrovirus. It contains an enzyme, reverse transcriptase, that copies ribonucleic acid (RNA) into deoxyribonucleic acid (DNA). When it binds to a CD4 receptor, the virus inserts its RNA and enzymes into the cell, where a copy of its RNA is made and enters the cell nucleus. As the infected host cell reproduces, HIV DNA is duplicated and passed on in the infectious cycle.

35. Answer: 4

Rationale: Although any of the clinical symptoms listed may be present in patients with systemic lupus erythematosus (SLE), fever, weight loss, arthritis, and arthralgias occur most often. Butterfly rash of the face and lymphadenopathy occur in less than half the cases. Pulmonary effusion, hepatomegaly, splenomegaly, and Raynaud's syndrome occur in less than a third of SLE patients.

36. Answer: 3

Rationale: The massive release of mediators triggers a series of events in target organs. Prior sensitization to the antigen must have occurred to trigger an anaphylactic reaction. Anaphylaxis may result from injection of an antigen, ingested food or drugs, or inhaled antigens.

37. Answer: 1

Rationale: The release of histamine results in bronchospasm, vasodilation, and vascular permeability, leading to wheezing, increased mucus production in the lung, and edema of the airway.

38. Answer: 2

Rationale: The onset of acute graft-versus-host disease (GVHD) occurs between 30 and 50 days after bone marrow transplant (BMT). It results from immunocompetent donor T lymphocytes attacking the host tissues.

39. Answer: 3

Rationale: The signs and symptoms of graft-versus-host disease (GVHD) include maculopapular rash, generalized erythroderma with desquamation, increased bilirubin, increased AST and SGOT, and/or increased alkaline phosphatase, abdominal cramping, and diarrhea. Infection is characterized by fever, mental status changes, and headaches. Decreased RBCs, hematocrit, hemoglobin, and petechiae are signs of anemia. Fever, chills, and urticaria are indications of a reaction to white blood cells (WBCs) in the bone marrow.

40. Answer: 4

Rationale: T lymphocytes are the white blood cells (WBCs) responsible for control of the immune response. In systemic lupus erythematosus (SLE), T suppressor cells are decreased and cell activity is inhibited, leading to hypergammaglobulinemia and B cell proliferation.

41. Answer: 2

Rationale: The T4 lymphocyte is known as the T helper cell. These cells are responsible for the proliferation of lymphocytes and macrophages, causing activation of the cells in response to an antigen. The B lymphocytes are effector cells that mediate humoral responses by production of antibodies. The band neutrophil and segmented neutrophil are slightly mature and fully mature neutrophils, respectively. Neutrophils are the most abundant cells in the bone marrow and blood.

42. Answer: 3

Rationale: Based on the history of an HIV-positive test and the symptoms presented, the patient is at risk for *P. carinii* pneumonia. Further examination would include a chest radiograph

and pulse oximetry (for oxygen saturation). The lack of purplish lesions is considered in ruling out Kaposi's sarcoma. *Klebsiella pneumoniae* is a nosocomial infection, not community acquired. *Mycoplasma pneumoniae* infection is typically seen in teenagers and older adult patients with an insidious onset of symptoms.

43. Answer: 3

Rationale: The nurse should be given IgG because it is the major antibody against viruses and bacteria. IgG is the principal mediator of the secondary immune response, which requires repeated response to the same antigen to increase the immune response. There is no IgC antibody. IgA is the secretory immunoglobulin found in tears, saliva, and mucous secretions of the lung and gastrointestinal tract. IgE mediates allergic reactions.

44. Answer: 2

Rationale: Type I hypersensitivity reaction causes an immediate wheal-and-flare reaction. Contact dermatitis is seen in type IV (delayed) reaction. Hematuria is seen in type II reaction that is caused by preformed circulating cytotoxic antibodies, as in a blood transfusion reaction or autoimmune hemolytic anemia. High fever may be seen in type III hypersensitivity reaction when large quantities of antigen-antibody complexes are released in the body.

45. Answer: 2

Rationale: Sexually active teenagers are the fastest growing group of HIV-positive patients because of unprotected sexual activity. Immunocompromised patients and elderly adults are at no greater risk for developing HIV than any other group. However, an increasing number of middle-aged males are becoming HIV positive from their association with prostitutes after the loss of their partners. Risk factors for HIV include unprotected sexual contact with persons of unknown HIV status, multiple sexual partners, intravenous drug use, hemophilia, and blood transfusions received before 1985.

46. Answer: 1

Rationale: Changes in the electrocardiogram (ECG) are associated with coronary and myocardial ischemia. Although ECG changes suggest myocardial injury, there is no change in the serum enzymes. Other signs and symptoms include hypotension and tachycardia.

47. Answer: 3

Rationale: Cotton-wool spots are the most common ophthalmologic problem associated with systemic lupus erythematosus (SLE). Retinal hemorrhages and AV nicking may be seen in patients with hypertension. Conjunctivitis is an infection of the conjunctiva.

48. Answer: 1

Rationale: Patients with allergic rhinitis should monitor the air quality and allergy index in their area and understand their allergy triggers. A surgical-type mask will not filter out small allergens. Remaining inside during allergy season is an unrealistic expectation and can lead to decreased socialization and increased depression for the patient. Patients can enjoy a summer garden if they are careful about the choice of plants and flowers. For example, the patient with an allergy to ragweed should avoid daisies, dahlias, and chrysanthemums.

49. Answer: 3

Rationale: The operating room (OR) nurse likely has a latex allergy. The incidence of latex allergies has increased dramatically since the onset of standard precautions and increased use of latex gloves. In an effort to meet the increased demand for gloves, changes in the manufacturing process have resulted in a higher protein count in the gloves. The increased exposure to the protein has led to a proliferation of health care workers being diagnosed with a latex allergy.

50. Answer: 2

Rationale: Latex allergy is a progressive disorder that worsens with continual exposure. The symptoms range from contact dermatitis to anaphylaxis. Currently, latex allergy affects 17% of health care workers and 39% of dental professionals. Latex allergy is an acquired immune response to the latex protein allergen. No vaccine is available; the only defense is to avoid contact with latex.

Pharmacology

51. Answer: 2

Rationale: The laboratory tests ordered would be complete blood count (CBC) with differential, lipase, lactic acid, electrolytes, BUN, creatinine, and liver function tests (LFTs). Assessment of immune function (CD4 count, viral load) is unnecessary at this point and would not change the management of the acute illness. Having the amylase, lipase, lactic acid, and LFTs would assist in the diagnosis of pancreatitis, but would not provide information on the patient's hydration status, the status of the biliary system, or presence of acute infection.

52. Answer: 4

Rationale: Procainamide, hydralazine, and isoniazid have been shown to induce a lupus-like syndrome. Discontinuation of the medication results in the disappearance of the clinical signs and symptoms. Antibiotics (e.g., sulfonamides, penicillin) have been associated with anaphylactic reactions in some patients. Oral contraceptives may increase blood pressure and the risk for thromboemboli. NSAIDs (e.g., ibuprofen) have been associated with gastrointestinal upset and gastric pain, especially when taken on an empty stomach, and are contraindicated in patients with renal disease.

53. Answer: 1

Rationale: Temporal arthritis, seen primarily in elderly patients, can lead to blindness if not treated immediately with corticosteroids. The usual daily dose of prednisone is 60 mg in divided doses initially, and then a single morning dose (every-other-day steroids are not used). A slow taper is initiated after 4 weeks if the patient is asymptomatic and the ESR is decreased. Tapering of the dose is individualized, and the patient may be on drug therapy for several months to years. Average time for disease remission is 3–4 years (range 1–10 years).

54. Answer: 2, 4, 5, 6

Rationale: Chloroquine phosphate, doxycycline, mefloquine, and primaquine are medications used for malaria prophylaxis. Ceftriaxone is used for bacterial septicemia and respiratory and urinary tract infections caused by gram-negative bacilli. Ampicillin is used to treat infections from a variety of organisms and as prophylaxis for bacterial endocarditis.

55. Answer: 1

Rationale: Unless there is a secondary bacterial infection, antibiotics are contraindicated. Antihistamines and reduction of exposure to the allergen will help reduce the symptoms. For continued control and stabilization of the mast cell, corticosteroids are indicated.

56. Answer: 1

Rationale: Adults are at greater risk for the development of adverse drug reactions, probably because of the increased number of medications used and the amount of exposure and effects of aging on the immune system. Patients with prior drug reactions are more likely to develop reactions to new drugs. The risk of an adverse drug reaction occurs in the first 2 to 3 weeks of therapy. Prolonged course of therapy, high dosage, and intermittent therapy increase the risk of an adverse reaction. Genetic factors may increase mediator and metabolic pathway activity. Gender has no effect except with muscle relaxants and chymopapain, when women are at greater risk of an adverse drug reaction. Route of drug administration contributes to the risk, with IV, IM, SC, PO, and topical, ranked in the order of greatest to least risk.

57. Answer: 3

Rationale: Trimethoprim-sulfamethoxazole (TMP-SMX) is used to treat as well as prevent *P. carinii* pneumonia, usually with a 21-day course, with up to 7 to 10 days for a clinical response. Fluconazole and amphotericin B are antifungal drugs. Acyclovir is an antiviral used primarily to treat the herpes simplex virus, types 1 and 2, and herpes zoster (shingles).

58. Answer: 2

Rationale: The chronic use of nasal decongestants for more than 3 days can result in a rebound effect when discontinued, leading to increased nasal congestion from reflex vasodilation. The condition may take as long as 2 to 3 weeks to resolve. Allergic rhinitis is not a self-limiting illness associated only with spring and fall. Even though therapy is initiated, the patient should be instructed to avoid exposure to the allergen as much as possible.

59. Answer: 4

Rationale: The major advantage of the second-generation antihistamines is that they do not cross the blood-brain barrier and therefore do not cause sedation and psychomotor dysfunction. There is little anticholinergic activity and less dry mouth and constipation. The cost of these antihistamines is 15–30 times greater than for the first-generation antihistamines. The medications are rapidly absorbed in 1–2 hours of PO administration on an empty stomach.

60. Answer: 1

Rationale: Sympathomimetics (adrenergics) cause vasoconstriction, thereby reducing edema and secretions. Inhaled corticosteroids stabilize mast cells and block degranulation.

61. Answer: 1

Rationale: The use of H1 blockers can cause paradoxical central nervous system (CNS) stimulation, resulting in ataxia in older adult patients. Antihistamines can cause many simultaneous side effects in older adults, such as impaired vision and gait, which can lead to falls, and impaired thinking, which can interfere with functional skills (cognition) and could necessitate unnecessary hospitalization or nursing home stay. Antihistamines also may interact with the older adult patient's numerous medications and exacerbate the side effects (e.g., dry mouth, constipation).

62. Answer: 2

Rationale: The patient should be instructed not to use over-the-counter (OTC) medications without consulting the family nurse practitioner or pharmacist. The nurse should explain that OTC drugs and herbal supplements are considered medications and that they may interact with prescribed medications. To avoid possible interactions, the patient should inform the family nurse practitioner of all the OTC drugs and herbals the patient is taking. The patient should be cautioned on the extended use of topical antihistamines. Antihistamines do not affect circulating histamine, so the patient must avoid exposure to a known allergen. Constipation and urinary retention are adverse effects that should be reported to the family nurse practitioner.

63. Answer: 2

Rationale: An advantage of using loratadine is that once-a-day dosing helps with patient compliance. The cost is greater than for some first-generation antihistamines. Loratadine with pseudoephedrine (Claritin D) is an antihistamine/decongestant with bid or extended-release (daily) dosing.

64. Answer: 4

Rationale: Medications, such as antihistamines and corticosteroids, are used to counter mediator release and block release of additional mediators. NSAIDs, antibiotics, and decongestants are contraindicated in the treatment of anaphylactic reaction.

65. Answer: 2

Rationale: Of patients receiving procainamide, 20% develop clinical drug-induced systemic lupus erythematosus (SLE). The other drugs listed have not been associated with SLE.

66. Answer: 2

Rationale: Severe malaise, pallor, stridor, and dyspnea are signs and symptoms associated with a severe anaphylactic reaction. Symptoms may occur immediately or up to 2 hours after exposure to the allergen. Severe reactions require immediate intervention.

7

Head, Eyes, Ears, Nose, & Throat (HEENT)

Physical Examination & Diagnostic Tests

Head

1. The family nurse practitioner is examining lymph nodes in the neck. Which nodes are palpated in the anterior triangle of the neck?

   1. Posterior cervical chain.

   2. Anterior superficial chain.

   3. Periauricular lymph nodes.

   4. Supraclavicular lymph nodes.

Eyes

2. When using an ophthalmoscope, the family nurse practitioner:

   1. Holds the ophthalmoscope in the right hand (uses right eye) while examining the patient's left eye.

   2. Starts the examination with the ophthalmic lens set at zero.

   3. Begins in a position 1 inch from the eye to check the red light reflex.

   4. Examines the anterior chamber in a well-lighted room and asks the patient to focus on an object.

3. The family nurse practitioner checking for strabismus would use which test?

   1. Cover-uncover test.

   2. Vertical prism test.

   3. Ishihara's test.

   4. Snellen's test.

4. The family nurse practitioner observes lid lag in a patient with:

   1. Myasthenia gravis.

   2. Hyperthyroidism.

   3. Hordeolum.

   4. Chalazion.

5. The family nurse practitioner is examining an older adult patient. There is a glossy white circle around the pupils of the eyes, yellowing of the sclera, and the pupils have a decreased reaction to the direct light reflex. The patient has a history of presbyopia. What is the correct interpretation of these findings?

   1. Beginning development of cataracts with a significant decrease in visual acuity.

   2. Expected changes in the eyes as a result of the aging process.

   3. Decrease in depth perception and early eye changes associated with glaucoma.

   4. Visual changes secondary to long-term treatment with digitoxin and corticosteroids.

6. The family nurse practitioner is preparing to examine the eyes of an adult patient. To examine the retinal vessels and assess for hemorrhages, the family nurse practitioner uses which aperture on the ophthalmoscope?

   1. Small aperture.

   2. Red-free filter.

   3. Slit.

   4. Grid.

7. When testing the eyes for the presence of a normal consensual response, the family nurse practitioner:

   1. Shines the light into the patient's pupil and observes the rate of pupillary constriction.

   2. Directs the light into one pupil and observes for the constriction or response of the other pupil.

   3. Holds a card in front of one eye and has the patient focus on a fixed object, removes the card, and observes movement of the newly uncovered eye.

   4. Asks the patient to focus on an object and then directs a light source to the bridge of the nose while observing for symmetric reflection in both eyes.

8. On ophthalmic examination, there appears to be a narrowing or blocking of the vein at the point where an arteriole crosses over it. The significance of this finding is:

   1. The need to evaluate the patient for chronic hypertension.

   2. The possibility of increased ocular pressure associated with glaucoma.

   3. Its association with papilledema, causing decreased venous drainage.

   4. It may represent a small embolus in the retinal vessels.

9. When examining the eyes, the family nurse practitioner determines that the pupils constrict when a patient shifts her gaze from a far object to a near one. This is interpreted as:

   1. Accommodation.

   2. Intact extraocular motor nerves.

   3. Appropriate consensual response.

   4. Visual acuity within normal limits.

10. During a physical exam, the family nurse practitioner notes xanthelasma. What laboratory test will the nurse order?

    1. ESR.

    2. CBC.

    3. Thyroid profile.

    4. Lipid profile.

Ears

11. When examining the ears of an adult patient, the family nurse practitioner determines that the tympanic membrane (TM) is pearl gray, shiny, and translucent. This is interpreted as:

    1. Scarring from previous infections.

    2. Decreased circulation to the membrane.

    3. Presence of serous fluid behind the membrane.

    4. Normal characteristics of the adult ear.

12. The Rinne test compares bone conduction (when the tuning fork is placed on the mastoid bone) with air conduction (when the tuning fork is held near the ear). A normal Rinne test is described as:

    1. Equal conduction through mastoid bone and ear canal.

    2. Air conduction is greater than bone conduction.

    3. Bone conduction is twice as long as air conduction.

    4. Sound is clearer with bone conduction than air conduction.

13. When assessing the tympanic membrane (TM), specific landmarks are determined and described according to the face of a clock. Where are the normal landmarks for the right TM located?

    1. Direct light reflex located at 5- to 6-o'clock position and malleus at 1 to 2 o'clock, with the umbo in the center.

    2. Manubrium slanted to the left, with malleus at 10-o'clock position.

    3. Direct light reflex in center of membrane, with malleus at 9-o'clock position.

    4. Umbo is to the left of the center, with anterior malleolar folds at the 10-o'clock position.

Nose

14. The family nurse practitioner understands that the nasal mucosa:

    1. Is dark pink, smooth, and moist.

    2. Is pale and translucent in appearance.

    3. Is pale and boggy.

    4. Is red and swollen.

Throat

15. A throat culture is indicated for the following suspected cause of pharyngitis:

    1. Rhinovirus and coronavirus infection.

    2. Group A β-hemolytic streptococci (GABHS).

    3. Mononucleosis.

    4. *Candida albicans.*

Disorders

Head

16. An adult patient presents to the office with a white plaque near the base of the tongue. The family nurse practitioner notes that the plaque does not wipe off and assesses it as:

    1. Hemangioma.

    2. Leukoplakia.

    3. Papilloma.

    4. Erythroplasia.

17. Which of the following are predominant risk factors for oral carcinoma?

    1. History of dental infections and age <40.

    2. Tobacco use and alcohol use.

    3. Infection with human papillomavirus and tobacco use.

    4. Alcohol use and history of dental abscess.

18. The hallmark of early oral cancer is:

    1. Tissue retraction.

    2. Thickening oral tissues.

    3. Persistent red and/or white patch and nonhealing ulcer.

    4. Halitosis and cough.

19. An adult male patient is being evaluated for a complaint of a sore throat. He states that he has difficulty swallowing and has mild oral pain. On examination, the family nurse practitioner finds that the patient's mouth, tongue, and pharynx are coated with white curdlike plaques that are difficult to remove and leave a red surface when scraped with a tongue blade. What would be the best next action for the family nurse practitioner to take at this time?

    1. Refer the patient to an ear, nose, and throat specialist for evaluation.

    2. Prescribe amoxicillin 500 mg PO tid × 10 days.

    3. Encourage the patient to have HIV screening.

    4. Recommend only clear liquids for the next few days.

20. The family nurse practitioner knows that the most common site for head and neck cancer is the:

    1. Sinuses.

    2. Oral cavity.

    3. Larynx.

    4. Nasal cavity.

Eyes

21. A patient is being prepared for cataract surgery. What information is important for the family nurse practitioner to explain to the patient?

    1. The procedure is short, and the patient usually goes home the morning after the surgery.

    2. Both eyes will be patched for the first 24 hours, and it is important for the patient to stay in bed.

    3. The patient may have problems with headache and eye pain for the first 24 hours and should take the pain medication provided.

    4. Patients usually go home 2–3 hours after the surgery; the patient will have increased tearing, but it should not be painful.

22. A patient, who is a sheet metal worker, reports a foreign body sensation in his right eye that began shortly after working this morning. Initial assessment would most likely be to:

    1. Instill topical anesthetic.

    2. Assess the visual acuity.

    3. Examine the eye using a penlight.

    4. Examine the eye using fluorescein.

23. A patient works as a welder. He finished work about 8 hours ago and discovered the protective glass on his welding hood was cracked. He is complaining of severe left eye pain and photophobia. The most likely diagnosis and next best action are:

    1. Chemical keratitis; dilate with atropine twice daily.

    2. Viral conjunctivitis; supportive treatment with artificial tears.

    3. Corneal abrasion; oral analgesics and an ophthalmic antibiotic ointment.

    4. Ultraviolet keratitis; ophthalmic antibiotic, and oral analgesics.

24. An older adult patient presents at the clinic with complaints of bilateral blurred vision that has increasingly worsened over the past 2 years. The patient also has a problem with night driving but denies eye pain. The family nurse practitioner would first evaluate for the presence of:

    1. Glaucoma.

    2. Retinal detachment.

    3. Degeneration of the macula.

    4. Cataracts.

25. An adult patient presents to the family nurse practitioner for evaluation of a "red," right eye for 24 hours. The patient states that when he awoke, the eye was matted shut. The patient denies trauma to the eye, eye pain, and any changes in vision. During the exam, it is noted that the pupils are equal and reactive, there is mild conjunctival hyperemia bilaterally, and a significant amount of yellowish discharge. The family nurse practitioner treats this patient for:

    1. Allergic conjunctivitis.

    2. Corneal abrasion.

    3. Viral conjunctivitis.

    4. Bacterial conjunctivitis.

26. Which assessment of the eye is a deviation from common age-related physiologic changes?

    1. Arcus senilis.

    2. Presbyopia.

    3. Sensitivity to glare.

    4. Sustained nystagmus.

27. During a routine physical examination of a 30-year-old patient, the family nurse practitioner identifies arcus senilis. What is the significance of this disorder?

    1. High potential for future blindness.

    2. None, because this is a normal variant of the aging process.

    3. Abnormal lipid metabolism requiring further evaluation.

    4. Hereditary variant of no consequence.

28. A 70-year-old patient comes to the clinic complaining of an increased sensitivity to glare, difficulty adapting to darkness, and altered depth perception. The family nurse practitioner should suspect:

    1. Cataract.

    2. Macular degeneration.

    3. Glaucoma.

    4. Normal age-related physiologic changes.

Ears

29. In teaching patients how to avoid acoustic trauma because of noise in the very loud range, the family nurse practitioner knows that noise is loudest from a:

    1. Vacuum cleaner.

    2. Power lawn mower.

    3. Clothes washer.

    4. Food blender.

30. A geriatric patient is complaining of difficulty hearing in both ears and states that the problem seems to have steadily worsened over the past few years. What finding would support a diagnosis of presbycusis?

    1. Complaint that he can hear voices but that everyone mumbles.

    2. Rinne test indicating air conduction greater than bone conduction.

    3. History of long-term tetracycline therapy for chronic infections.

    4. Long-term family history of chronic hearing loss.

31. Which of the following organisms is **least likely** to cause otitis media?

    1. *Moraxella catarrhalis.*

    2. *Streptococcus pneumoniae.*

    3. *Staphylococcus aureus.*

    4. *Haemophilus influenzae.*

32. Which assessment finding of the ear would indicate a deviation from the normal aging process?

    1. A dull, retracted, and white tympanic membrane.

    2. An elongated lobule.

    3. A sensorineural hearing loss.

    4. A bulging tympanic membrane with a distorted cone of light.

33. Which statement by the family nurse practitioner indicates an understanding of conductive hearing loss in the older patient?

    1. "This has occurred because of damage of the eighth cranial nerve from gentamicin."

    2. "This is a result of an inner ear infection."

    3. "This is a normal part of aging and is referred to as presbycusis."

    4. "This may be reversible after the cerumen is removed from the ear canal."

34. Sensorineural hearing loss is common in industrial settings and preventable with the use of adequate hearing protection. This type of hearing loss is usually first noted with changes at what level?

    1. 500 Hz.

    2. 200 Hz.

    3. 1000 to 2000 Hz.

    4. 3000 to 6000 Hz.

Nose

35. An adult patient presents to the family nurse practitioner's office with the following complaints for the past 10 days: fever and complaints of right facial pain, copious yellow nasal discharge, and acute pain and headache primarily when bending over. The physical exam is significant for right maxillary sinus tenderness upon palpation. The most likely diagnosis is:

    1. Chronic sinusitis.

    2. Acute sinusitis.

    3. Dental abscess.

    4. Temporal arteritis.

36. The family nurse practitioner notes a nasal septal perforation on a young adult. What does the family nurse practitioner suspect as the cause?

    1. Deviated nasal septum.

    2. Chronic epistaxis.

    3. Nose picking.

    4. Cocaine use.

Throat

37. A 20-year-old patient presents to the family nurse practitioner's office with a chief complaint of "severe sore throat" for 3 days. The patient states he also "ran a fever,

but does not know how high it got," and has been very fatigued. Physical examination reveals enlarged tonsils with large patchy exudate, erythematous pharynx, and nontender posterior cervical lymphadenopathy. The remainder of the exam was unremarkable. The family nurse practitioner would most likely make the diagnosis of:

    1. Infectious mononucleosis.

    2. Leukemia.

    3. Scarlet fever.

    4. Oral candidiasis.

38. Which of the following clinical findings are most likely associated with bacterial streptococcal pharyngitis?

    1. Rhinorrhea.

    2. Cough.

    3. Enlarged erythematous tonsils with exudate.

    4. Small oral vesicles.

Pharmacology

39. When the nurse practitioner decides to prescribe an antibiotic for the treatment of acute sinusitis, which antibiotic is recommended as first-line empiric therapy for nonpenicillin allergic adults?

    1. Azithromycin (Zithromax).

    2. Doxycycline (Vibramycin).

    3. Trimethoprim-sulfamethoxazole (TMP/SMX).

    4. Amoxicillin-clavulanate (Augmentin).

40. A geriatric patient is diagnosed with chronic open-angle glaucoma. She has a past history of bradycardia and first-degree atrioventricular block. In consideration of her treatment, what medication is to be avoided?

    1. Pilocarpine (Isopto Carpine).

    2. Timolol (Timoptic).

    3. Hydrochlorothiazide (HydroDIURIL).

    4. Acetazolamide (Diamox).

41. The treatment plan for a patient diagnosed with infectious mononucleosis includes which of the following?

    1. Resting during acute phase.

    2, Avoiding exercise during acute phase.

    3, Corticosteroids during acute phase.

    4. Ampicillin orally for 10 days.

Physical Examination & Diagnostic Tests

Head

1. Answer: 2

Rationale: The conceptualization of triangles is useful in determining the location of palpable lymph nodes in the neck. The sternocleidomastoid muscle is the division between the anterior (containing the anterior superficial cervical chain) and the posterior (containing the posterior cervical chain) triangles. The trapezius muscle marks the posterior border of the posterior triangle. The supraclavicular nodes are palpated in the angle formed by the clavicle and the sternocleidomastoid muscle.

Eyes

2. Answer: 2

Rationale: The correct use of the ophthalmoscope involves using the right hand and right eye to examine the patient's right eye. The room should be semidarkened for best visualization. The examiner initially inspects the lens and vitreous body from a distance of about 12 inches (at zero setting) and moves closer to the eye, usually rotating the lenses to the positive numbers (+15 to +20), which assists in focusing on near objects.

3. Answer: 1

Rationale: The cover/uncover test is used to detect latent strabismus. The vertical prism test assesses for amblyopia. The Ishihara's test examines color perception. The Snellen's test assesses for far vision.

4. Answer: 2

Rationale: Lid lag occurs in patients with hyperthyroidism and is evaluated by having the patient follow the examiner's finger as it is moved up and down. The patient has lid lag if sclera can be seen above the iris as the patient looks downward. Ptosis is a drooping lid margin that falls at the pupil or below and may indicate an oculomotor lesion or myasthenia gravis. A chalazion is a chronic, sterile lipogranulomatous inflammatory lesion of the meibomian gland. A hordeolum is an acute inflammation of one of the glands in the eyelid.

5. Answer: 2

Rationale: Yellowing of the sclera and arcus senilis (also known as corneal arcus) is a benign whitish ring around the limbus and is seen in the older adult due to age-related physi-

ologic changes. Cataracts occur as a result of an opacity of the lens of the eye that causes partial or total blindness. The visual acuity and depth perception of the patient cannot be determined from the information provided.

6. Answer: 2

Rationale: The red-free filter is used to visualize the vessels and hemorrhages in better detail by improving contrast. This setting will make the retina look black and white. The small aperture is used when the pupil is very constricted; the slit is to examine contour abnormalities of the cornea, lens, and retina; and the grid is for estimating the size of lesions found in the fundal area.

7. Answer: 2

Rationale: A light beam shining onto one retina causes pupillary constriction in both that eye, termed the *direct reaction* to light, and in the opposite eye, the *consensual reaction*.

8. Answer: 1

Rationale: Chronic hypertension stiffens and thickens arteries, resulting in arteriovenous nicking. Intraocular pressure cannot be determined from an ophthalmic examination. Papilledema is associated with swelling around the optic disc with blurred margins. Small emboli are represented by an abrupt impediment or severe narrowing of an arteriole not associated with where the retinal veins and arteries cross.

9. Answer: 1

Rationale: Accommodation is the ability of the lens to change shape. Changes in pupil size when focusing from near to distant objects (and vice versa) tests for accommodation. Extraocular movements refer to the ability to move the eye in six cardinal directions. Consensual response is constriction of the eye in response to light being shined in the opposite eye. The Snellen eye chart is used to determine visual acuity.

10. Answer: 4

Rationale: Xanthelasma are soft or hard yellow plaques on the inside corners of the eyelids (near the inner canthus), which are made up of cholesterol and are found more often on the upper lid than the lower lid. Xanthelasma is a type of xanthoma and is associated with hyperlipidemias, so a lipid profile would be an appropriate test to order.

Ears

11. Answer: 4

Rationale: The normal tympanic membrane (TM) is thin, translucent, shiny, and slightly concave with a pearl gray or pale pink appearance. This describes the normal characteristics of the TM. There is no evidence indicating scarring, fluid, or decreased circulation to the membrane.

12. Answer: 2

Rationale: The Rinne test is positive (or normal) when air conduction is greater than bone conduction (AC>BC). If the patient hears the tuning fork better by bone conduction, the Rinne test is negative, which suggests a conductive hearing loss.

13. Answer: 1

Rationale: Direct light reflex located at 5- to 6-o'clock position and malleus at 1 to 2 o'clock, with the umbo in the center describes the correct position for the landmarks on the right ear. The manubrium slants to the right with the malleus at the 1- to 2-o'clock position for the right ear. The direct light reflex in the center of the membrane with the malleus at the 9-o'clock position describes the correct position for the left ear. The umbo is in the center with the anterior folds at the 1- to 2-o'clock position for the right ear.

Nose

14. Answer: 1

Rationale: The nasal mucosa is normally dark pink, smooth, and moist. A pale, boggy mucosa suggests chronic allergy. A red and swollen mucosa suggests acute allergic rhinitis. The normal secretion is mucoid. Purulent, crusty, or bloody secretions are abnormal.

Throat

15. Answer: 2

Rationale: Diagnostic studies used to detect group A β-hemolytic streptococci (GABHS) infection include a throat culture and a rapid antigen detention test (RADT). Throat culture has been considered the gold standard method to establish the microbial cause of acute pharyngitis. RADT is often used because it is rapid and convenient; however, RADT is less sensitive (true positive) than a throat culture. A positive Monospot test result reveals heterophil antibodies. The Monospot test is highly specific and sensitive. *Candida albicans* and rhinovirus are not diagnosed by bacterial cultures. Rhinovirus is one of the most common viral causes of pharyngitis. Oral candidiasis, a fungal infection, can be diagnosed with a potassium hydroxide smear.

Disorders

Head

16. Answer: 2

Rationale: Oral leukoplakia is a precancerous lesion that presents as white patches or plaques of the oral mucosa that cannot be rubbed off. Hemangiomas are usually a benign tumor made up of blood vessels that typically appear as a purplish or reddish, slightly elevated area of skin that can include the lips, tongue, and buccal mucosa. Erythroplasia is an asymptomatic, red, velvety lesion on the oral or genital mucosa that is considered a precancerous lesion. Papillomas are benign verrucous lesions that are manifestations of human papillomavirus (HPV) infection.

17. Answer: 2

Rationale: Tobacco use and alcohol use are among the greatest risk factors for oral cavity and oropharyngeal cancers. Smokers are many times more likely than nonsmokers to develop these cancers. Tobacco smoke from cigarettes, cigars, or pipes can cause cancers anywhere in the mouth or throat. Drinking alcohol increases the risk of developing oral cavity and oropharyngeal cancers, as about 7 out of 10 patients with oral cancer are heavy drinkers. The disease is age related, occurring in those over 40 years of age and increasing with age. Infection with cancer-causing types of human papillomaviruses (HPV), especially HPV-16, is a risk factor for some types of head and neck cancers, particularly oropharyngeal cancers that involve the tonsils or the base of the tongue.

18. Answer: 3

Rationale: Erythroplasia is accompanied by an inflammatory reaction in a patient with suspected oral cancer. Lesions persisting over 14 days strongly suggest early oral cancer. Tissue retraction and thickening of the oral tissues are later signs of oral cancer. Halitosis (odor) may be associated with dysfunction within the oral cavity (dental caries), nasal cavity, sinuses, or esophageal disorders. Cough is the primary symptom of respiratory disorders such as acute bronchitis or pneumonia.

19. Answer: 3

Rationale: Adults who present with thrush (oral candidiasis) may be immunologically impaired. It is important to make the diagnosis of HIV early to start treatment modalities. Treatment with amoxicillin is not the appropriate action since the presenting disorder describes a fungal infection.

20. Answer: 2

Rationale: The family nurse practitioner knows that the risk factors for head and neck cancer include tobacco and alcohol use, poor oral hygiene, and occupational exposure to asbestos, coke, nickel, wood, or leather. The most common site is in the oral cavity, accounting for 48% of head and neck cancer diagnoses.

Eyes

21. Answer: 4

Rationale: Patients go home almost immediately after the procedure. The eye may be patched, depending whether anesthesia was local or topical. There is some discomfort, but pain should not be a problem. The patient can be mobile and active as tolerated.

22. Answer: 2

Rationale: Initial assessment of visual acuity would provide the basis for comparison in the event of complications. Visual acuity should be measured before the instillation of a topical anesthetic or fluorescein. Following acuity, an examination of the eye using a penlight is performed to assess for a penetrating foreign body.

23. Answer: 4

Rationale: Photokeratitis, also known as ultraviolet keratitis or UV keratitis, is an acute syndrome that occurs after ultraviolet irradiation of the eyes and can be intensely painful. Although the exposure may not be initially apparent to the patient, there is a latent period of approximately 6 to 12 hours between exposure and onset of symptoms. Photokeratitis is generally a self-limited condition with complete resolution. Initial treatment consists of oral analgesics and lubricant antibiotic ointments. An eye injury from a welder's arc is commonly known as flash burn, welder's flash, or arc eye.

24. Answer: 4

Rationale: A cataract is an opacity of the lens of the eye that causes partial or total blindness. Cataracts are characterized by painless loss of visual acuity over time. Retinal detachment most often occurs suddenly, with partial loss of the field of vision. Glaucoma results in the loss of peripheral vision, and macular degeneration primarily involves the central vision field.

25. Answer: 4

Rationale: Bacterial conjunctivitis presents with injection of the conjunctiva, no pain, and a history of purulent discharge. The chief complaint of a corneal abrasion is pain. Unlike conjunctivitis with infectious causes, allergic conjunctivitis typically presents simultaneously in both eyes with the predominant feature of itching. Viral conjunctivitis will usually present with acute onset of a red eye with itching, photophobia, and excessive watery discharge.

26. Answer: 4

Rationale: Sustained nystagmus is indicative of a neurologic complication. The other options include normal age-related changes.

27. Answer: 3

Rationale: Arcus senilis is the deposit of lipids at the junction of the cornea and sclera that is present in many people over age 50. When identified in younger individuals, it may be related to a disorder of lipid metabolism. High cholesterol is more likely associated with a similar gray or white arc visible around the entire cornea (circumferential arcus) in younger adults.

28. Answer: 4

Rationale: These findings are normal age-related physiologic changes. Signs and symptoms of cataracts include reduced visual acuity, painless progressive loss of vision, and sensitivity to light, especially at night (night driving). Reduced color discrimination and presbyopia may also develop. Macular degeneration presents with a loss of the central vision. Primary open-angle glaucoma presents with occasional headaches and halos around lights but may be asymptomatic in its early stages. Primary angle-closure glaucoma can present with decreased vision, halos around lights at night, and conjunctival redness.

Ears

29. Answer: 2

Rationale: Although all identified household appliances are noisy, the patient should wear a protective ear device when using a power lawn mower regularly for long periods.

30. Answer: 1

Rationale: In presbycusis the ability to hear high-frequency sounds is diminished. These patients have difficulty distinguishing consonant sounds, so words such as "shoe" and "true" are heard as "oo." The Rinne test helps distinguish whether a patient hears better by air or bone conduction. Air-conducted sound should be heard twice as long as bone-conducted sound. Tetracyclines are not ototoxic, and the family history may or may not contribute to the problem.

31. Answer: 3

Rationale: The key factor that contributes to acute otitis media (AOM) is a dysfunctional eustachian tube. The actual cause is unknown, but it may be sequelae of upper respiratory tract infections or allergies that result in edema of the eustachian tube or it may also result from reflux of nasopharynx bacteria into the eustachian tube. The most frequent bacterial organisms that infect the middle ear, especially in children, are similar to those of the nasopharynx: *S. pneumoniae, H. influenzae,* and *M. catarrhalis. Staphylococcus aureus* is one of the most common causative organisms in otitis externa.

32. Answer: 4

Rationale: A bulging tympanic membrane with a distorted cone of light would be indicative of an acute inflammation of the middle ear (AOM). The other options indicate age-related physiologic changes.

33. Answer: 4

Rationale: Conductive hearing loss may result from acute otitis media (AOM), perforation of the eardrum, and obstruction of the ear canal, as by cerumen. The other options result in sensorineural hearing loss.

34. Answer: 4

Rationale: Noise-induced hearing loss is a sensorineural hearing deficit that begins at the higher frequencies (3000–6000 Hz) and develops gradually as a result of chronic exposure to excessive sound levels.

Nose

35. Answer: 2

Rationale: The patient is experiencing the classic characteristics of acute sinusitis. Chronic sinusitis continues 12 weeks or longer. Dental abscess can have pain that radiates to the sinuses but more often causes constant, severe, tooth-associated pain and jaw tenderness. Temporal arteritis causes pain in the jaw, tongue, and face but no nasal discharge.

36. Answer: 4

Rationale: Nasal snorting of cocaine results in nasal congestion and discharge. Because cocaine is a potent sympathomimetic, the nasal passages appear similar to what is found on physical exam of patients who abuse nasal decongestants (e.g., Afrin). Chronic use of cocaine causes the nasal septal mucosa to become ischemic, which leads to tissue atrophy and eventual septal perforation, which is noted on physical exam and should be followed up with questions about snorting cocaine.

Throat

37. Answer: 1

Rationale: Mononucleosis is often seen in adolescents and young adults. It often presents with fever, exudate on the tonsils, generalized lymphadenopathy, malaise, posterior cervical adenopathy, and palatine petechiae. Leukemia presents with anorexia, irritability, lethargy, and bone pain, with peak incidence in 3- to 5-year-olds. Scarlet fever presents in children 2 to 10 years old with fever, abdominal pain, headache, sore throat, rash, and strawberry tongue. Oral candidiasis presents with white curdlike plaques on erythematous mucosa. The tongue is red with a white coat.

38. Answer: 3

Rationale: The clinical presentation of pharyngitis varies and depends on the causative agent. Characteristics of bacterial pharyngitis include headache, mild to severe erythema of tonsils with white or yellow exudate, dysphagia, tender anterior cervical nodes, sore throat with dysphagia, fever higher than 101°F (38°C), and nausea. Viral organisms that cause herpangina present with small oral vesicles. Cough is typically the primary symptom of acute bronchitis. Rhinorrhea is associated with allergic rhinitis.

Pharmacology

39. Answer: 4

Rationale: Amoxicillin has been recommended as a first-line agent in the past because of its narrow spectrum and relative low cost. However, there is increasing emergence of antimicrobial resistance among respiratory pathogens, including pneumococci and *H. influenzae.* Amoxicillin-clavulanate rather than amoxicillin is recommended as empiric therapy for nonpenicillin-allergic adults. Doxycycline is a reasonable alternative for first-line therapy and can be used in patients with a penicillin allergy. Azithromycin is not recommended for empiric therapy because of its high rates of resistance of *S. pneumoniae.* Trimethoprim-sulfamethoxazole (TMP/SMX) is not recommended due to high rate of resistance.

40. Answer: 2

Rationale: Topical beta blockers, such as timolol, lower intraocular pressure but can be absorbed systemically. The major side effects are similar to those associated with systemic beta-blocker therapy, which can include a worsening of heart failure, bradycardia, and heart block. Topical beta blockers are contraindicated in some patients with cardiac or pulmonary disease.

41. Answer: 1

Rationale: Treatment of mononucleosis includes bed rest while the patient has fever and myalgia (10–14 days), supportive acetaminophen or ibuprofen, warm saline gargles, and throat lozenges or spray. The patient must avoid strenuous exercise and contact sports for 2 months because of the risk of splenic rupture. Splenomegaly is seen in 50% to 60% of all patients with infectious mononucleosis. Corticosteroids are recommended only in patients with impending airway obstruction, and an immediate referral to an otolaryngologist is warranted. Ampicillin is not recommended because of the viral etiology of this disease. Additionally, rashes are common in patients with infectious mononucleosis and are treated with amoxicillin or ampicillin. About 95% of patients with mononucleosis recover uneventfully with supportive treatment.

Integumentary

8

Physical Exam & Diagnostic Tests

1. The family nurse practitioner describes an annular skin lesion as usually arranged in:

    1. Groups of vesicles erupting unilaterally.
    2. A line.
    3. A pattern of merging together, not discrete.
    4. A circle or ring shaped.

2. A patient has pitting of the nails. The family nurse practitioner understands this is associated with:

    1. Psoriasis.
    2. Iron-deficiency anemia.
    3. Malnutrition.
    4. Hyperthyroidism.

3. The family nurse practitioner is inspecting a dark-skinned individual for signs of jaundice. The best place to observe skin color in dark-skinned individuals is:

    1. Sclera of the opened eye.
    2. Palms and soles of the hands and feet.
    3. Oral mucosa.
    4. Nail beds.

4. When assessing an adult's hydration status, the best place to evaluate skin turgor on an adult is:

    1. Just below the clavicle.
    2. Below the scapula on the back.
    3. On the inside of the forearm.
    4. On the back of the hand.

5. The Wood's lamp may be used to evaluate skin lesions. When the light is shone on the patient's skin, a green-yellow fluorescence indicates:

    1. Presence of fungi.
    2. Lichenification.
    3. Keratinized cells.
    4. Bacterial colonies.

6. On exam of a patient's skin, the family nurse practitioner finds a lesion that is about 0.75 cm in diameter, brown, circumscribed, flat, and nonpalpable. What is the correct term for this lesion?

    1. Macule.
    2. Papule.
    3. Nodule.
    4. Wheal.

7. The history and physical of a patient indicate past occurrences of lichenification. The family nurse practitioner identifies the characteristics of this lesion as:

    1. Dried, crusty exudate, slightly elevated.
    2. Rough, thickened epidermis, accentuated skin markings.
    3. Keratinized cells shaped in an irregular pattern with exfoliation.
    4. Loss of epidermis with hollowed-out area and dermis exposed.

8. Clubbing of the nails commonly occurs in patients with chronic respiratory conditions. The family nurse practitioner assesses for this condition by:

   1. Evaluating the nail for transverse depressions and ridges.

   2. Placing the patient's hands together with palms inward and index fingers aligned.

   3. Placing nail beds of each index finger together to determine angle of nail plate.

   4. Determining if there is diffuse discoloration of the nail bed from decreased oxygenation.

9. A circumscribed, elevated lesion >1 cm in diameter and containing clear serous fluid is best described as a:

   1. Papule.

   2. Vesicle.

   3. Bulla.

   4. Pustule.

10. In performing a skin assessment, the family nurse practitioner understands that the following characteristic of a mole would necessitate immediate intervention:

    1. A 5-mm, symmetric, uniformly brown mole on the thigh that has not changed in appearance for more than 5 years.

    2. Multiple small (1–3 mm) flat moles across the upper back that are dark brown in color, round, and have smooth edges.

    3. A 3-cm, waxy papule with a "stuck-on" appearance, noted on the face.

    4. A new, 2-mm brown mole with an irregular red border that is occasionally pruritic.

11. Dermatophyte skin infections can be diagnosed from skin scrapings and prepared with which solution for microscopic exam?

    1. Hydrochloric acid.

    2. 10% or 20% potassium hydroxide (KOH) solution.

    3. Gram's stain.

    4. Distilled water.

12. When administering skin tests to an immunocompromised patient, the family nurse practitioner must consider:

    1. The importance of not applying more than one skin test at a time.

    2. That the skin test may react more aggressively than expected.

    3. Identifying a known allergen for the patient and using it as a control.

    4. That an immunocompromised patient should not have skin testing.

13. The nurse is examining a 6-week-old infant of Latin American descent. There are irregular areas of deep-blue pigmentation across the infant's buttocks. The nurse would identify this as characteristic of:

    1. Child abuse.

    2. Telangiectatic nevi.

    3. Cutis marmorata.

    4. Mongolian spots.

Skin Disorders

14. A patient complains of intolerable itching in the pubic hair. On exam, the family nurse practitioner notes erythematous papules and tiny white specks in the pubic hair. The differential diagnosis includes all except:

    1. Pediculosis pubis.

    2. Scabies.

    3. Impetigo.

    4. Atopic dermatitis.

15. An older adult woman has an area of vesicles in clusters with an erythematous base that extend from her spine, around and under her arm and breast, to the sternum on her left side. She states that the area was very tender last week and that the vesicles started erupting yesterday. She is complaining of severe pain in the area. What is the probable diagnosis for this condition?

    1. Psoriasis.

    2. Herpes zoster.

    3. Contact dermatitis.

    4. Cellulitis.

16. What is a chronic skin condition that is sometimes associated with arthritis?

    1. Eczema.

    2. Psoriasis.

    3. Neurodermatitis.

    4. Pityriasis rosea.

17. Which is a true statement about psoriasis?

    1. It is usually worse in the summer.

    2. It is highly contagious.

    3. It can be aggravated by stress.

    4. All patients have accompanying pruritus.

18. What information should be provided to a patient with actinic keratosis?

    1. The affected areas are a normal part of aging and are benign.

    2. These lesions can develop into squamous cell carcinomas.

    3. This is part of an allergic reaction, and the offending allergen needs to be identified.

    4. This skin condition responds well to sunlight, which will help alleviate the symptoms.

19. The following are all true statements regarding urticaria except:

    1. Most cases of acute urticaria involve IgE-mediated mast cell degranulation.

    2. Chronic urticaria may be related to occult infections.

    3. Urticaria is characterized by red, itchy wheals a few millimeters to a few centimeters in size.

    4. Laboratory studies are necessary to identify the causative agent.

20. A patient known to be positive for HIV presents with several painless, persistent, raised purple lesions on the face. What is the most likely diagnosis of the lesions?

    1. Seborrheic dermatitis.

    2. Molluscum contagiosum.

    3. Kaposi's sarcoma.

    4. Fungal infection.

21. In making a differential diagnosis between nummular eczema (dermatitis) and dyshidrotic eczematous dermatitis, the family nurse practitioner knows:

    1. Nummular eczema is characterized by flushing and clusters of papulopustules on the cheek and forehead.

    2. Dyshidrotic eczematous dermatitis is a chronic vesicular type of hand-and-foot eczema characterized by vesicles (tapioca-like), scaling, lichenification, and pruritus.

    3. Nummular eczema is a hereditary disorder characterized by chronic, usually bilateral scaly plaques on exposed areas (knees, elbows).

    4. Dyshidrotic eczematous dermatitis affects primarily young adults, is contagious, and is characterized by firm papules with a cleft surface and multiple conical vegetations.

22. A middle-aged male patient presents to the clinic with a complaint of being bitten last night by another individual during a fight. He has a bite mark on his forearm, and the skin has been broken. He reports he has had a tetanus shot about 8 years ago. Recommended treatment by the family nurse practitioner should include all the following **except**:

    1. Administer Tdap (Adacel).

    2. Instruct patient to watch for signs of infection.

    3. Initiate treatment with a β-lactam penicillin.

    4. Close the wound with sutures or Steri-Strips.

23. Nail involvement secondary to primary foot-and-hand tinea, characterized by accumulation of subungual keratin that produces thickened, distorted, crumbling nails, is termed:

    1. Hippocratic nails.

    2. Onychomycosis.

    3. Koilonychia.

    4. Anonychia.

24. A middle-aged patient presents for an office visit with a complaint of a measles-like rash on his trunk and spreading to his extremities. He was seen several days ago for bronchitis and started on trimethoprim-sulfamethoxazole (TMP-SMX; Septra) DS 1 tab PO bid. What is the recommended action for the family nurse practitioner?

    1. Instruct patient to continue medication and see if any change occurs in the rash.

    2. Discontinue TMP-SMX.

    3. Take the patient off medication for 3 days, and then restart the drug.

    4. Decrease TMP-SMX to half-dose.

25. A patient complaining of hyperhidrosis should be counseled that:

    1. This is a normal occurrence.

    2. There are no therapies for this complaint.

    3. Bathing in 20% alcohol solution of aluminum chloride hexahydrate (Drysol) may be beneficial.

    4. A history and physical need to be completed to rule out any medical etiologies.

26. During the physical exam, the family nurse practitioner assesses a maculopapular skin lesion on a patient's back that is warty, scaly, greasy in appearance, and light tan in color. What would be the probable diagnosis?

    1. Actinic keratosis.

    2. Basal cell carcinoma.

    3. Seborrheic keratosis.

    4. Senile lentigines.

27. The family nurse practitioner is assessing an older patient diagnosed with herpes zoster (shingles) in the prodromal stage. What would the practitioner expect to find on the assessment of this patient?

    1. Erythematous lesions present over four different parts of the body.

    2. Red, pinpoint, painless rash.

    3. Burning pain in a line on only half the patient's chest that does not cross the midline.

    4. Painless purulent lesions for 2 days followed by complaints of itching, burning, and nausea.

28. What would be the appropriate management for a patient with herpes zoster (shingles)?

    1. Acyclovir (Zovirax).

    2. Miconazole (Monistat-Derm).

    3. Clotrimazole (Lotrimin).

    4. Corticosteroid (prednisone).

29. A retired farmer presents with a dome-shaped, pearly, firm nodule with telangiectasia on his nose. In making a diagnosis, the family nurse practitioner recognizes this to be:

    1. Compound nevus.

    2. Melanoma.

    3. Bullous pemphigoid.

    4. Basal cell carcinoma.

30. An adult female presents with an irregular, variegated nevus on her lower left back that has doubled in size in the past 3 months. What would be an appropriate action for the family nurse practitioner?

    1. Do a punch biopsy to confirm the diagnosis.

    2. Take a photograph of the lesion and recheck it in 1 month.

    3. Refer immediately to a dermatologist.

    4. Reassure the patient that these are normal changes related to hormone variations.

31. An older adult patient presents with pain in the right chest wall for the past 48 hours. On exam, the family nurse practitioner notices a vesicular eruption along the dermatome and identifies this as herpes zoster. The family nurse practitioner informs the patient that:

    1. All symptoms will disappear in 3 days.

    2. Oral medication can dramatically reduce the duration and intensity of symptoms.

    3. The patient has chickenpox and may be contagious to grandchildren until the lesions are completely gone.

    4. The eruptions will recur at regular intervals.

32. A young adult female presents to the family nurse practitioner's office stating that she has a red rash over her trunk for 2 weeks that does not itch. She has tried over-the-counter lotions and creams, but the rash is still there. The rash started as a small, round red patch on her chest and has since spread across her chest, back, arms, and legs. Physical exam reveals a generalized distribution of erythematous and scaly macular lesions that run parallel to each other, creating a "Christmas tree" pattern. The family nurse practitioner should:

    1. Do a thorough medication history, investigate any potential allergens, and send the patient to an allergy specialist.

    2. Prescribe triamcinolone 0.025% cream (Aristocort A) bid for 2 weeks.

    3. Teach the patient this viral disease is self-limiting, lasting 6-8 weeks, and to avoid prolonged or excessive exposure to sunlight.

    4. Refer the patient to a dermatologist for a biopsy.

33. An adult male patient presents to the family nurse practitioner's office complaining of flulike symptoms, a large red spot in the right groin, headaches, and generalized muscle pain. These symptoms have persisted for about 4–5 weeks. In taking the history, it would be most important to determine whether the patient:

    1. Was using new skin care products.

    2. Was taking any new medications, such as vitamins, herbal therapies.

    3. Has had a recent insect bite or was potentially exposed to insects such as ticks.

    4. Has been exposed to a person with tuberculosis.

34. When do bites from insects, spiders, snakes, and bees most often occur?

    1. High humidity months.

    2. Spring to early fall.

    3. Winter.

    4. Any time of the year.

35. Medical management for a brown recluse spider bite includes:

    1. Warm moist soaks to the affected area.

    2. Ice pack and elevation and immobilization of the area.

    3. Active and passive range of motion (ROM) to area.

    4. Avoidance of antihistamines.

36. A scout leader is explaining about snakes and snake bites and says to his group about the coral snake, "Red on yellow, kill a fellow; red on black, venom lack." Later, one of the boys is bitten by a snake described as having broad rings of red and black, separated by narrow rings of yellow. The family nurse practitioner understands that this patient will probably experience all the following except:

    1. Numbness and change in sensation.

    2. Local swelling at the fang mark site.

    3. Dizziness and diplopia.

    4. No symptoms, as the snake was not venomous.

37. The family nurse practitioner is examining a patient with a diagnosis of pityriasis rosea. Which three statements are correct about the condition?

    1. Pruritus is not present.

2. Vesicles progressing to pustules occur within 2–3 days of eruption.

3. Salmon-colored patch with fine scales is commonly noted on face, hands, and feet.

4. Typical Christmas tree pattern of lesion distribution is observed.

5. Presence of a herald patch before onset of generalized rash.

38. What diagnostic test would be appropriate to order for a patient who has acanthosis nigricans?

    1. Skin biopsy.

    2. Liver function tests (LFT).

    3. Fasting blood glucose (FBS).

    4. IgE electrophoresis.

Pharmacology

39. An obese woman presents to the clinic with complaints of tenderness and irritation under both of her breasts. The exam reveals a very irritated, moist, inflamed area with macules and papules present. What is the best treatment for the woman?

    1. Nystatin cream bid/tid × 10 days, with thorough drying of area and exposure to light and air.

    2. Systemic antistaphylococcal antibiotics (dicloxacillin) and soaking with moist pads of normal saline three times daily.

    3. Gentle washing of the area and removal of crusts, then application of antibiotic ointment.

    4. Antiviral treatment (acyclovir) and topical ointment to prevent secondary infection.

40. Which classification of drugs has the potential to aggravate psoriasis?

    1. Beta blockers.

    2. Thiazide diuretics.

    3. Vasodilators.

    4. Tricyclic antidepressants.

41. All the following are true of postherpetic neuralgia except:

    1. Capsaicin cream (Zostrix) may alleviate some of the discomfort.

    2. In most patients the postherpetic pain gradually subsides over several weeks.

    3. Acyclovir (Zovirax) 200 mg 5 caps qd PO in divided doses is an effective therapy.

    4. It is more common in patients over age 60.

42. When treating genital warts with topical podophyllin, it is important for the family nurse practitioner to:

    1. Apply preparation directly to the wart and approximately 5 mm around the base.

    2. Cover with a dressing so that solution remains moist, and caution patient not to remove for 24 hours.

    3. Instruct patient to wash off medication in 4–6 hours.

    4. Treat with liquid nitrogen before applying podophyllin.

43. What is the recommended treatment of rosacea?

    1. Oral hydrocortisone.

    2. Oral ketoconazole.

    3. Low-dose tetracycline.

    4. Topical 5-fluorouracil.

44. When using lidocaine with epinephrine 1%–2% as a local anesthetic in the repair of an injury, it is essential to remember that the maximum allowable dose is:

    1. 7 mg/kg.

    2. 2 mg/kg.

    3. 10 mg/kg.

    4. 5 mg/kg.

45. An older adult patient presents to the family nurse practitioner complaining of a painful, tingling rash across the right side of the abdomen. Exam reveals vesicles with erythematous bases; some of the vesicles are draining cloudy fluid, whereas others are crusted. The family nurse practitioner makes the diagnosis of herpes zoster infection, and the patient is prescribed antiviral therapy. The patient states that the painful rash has caused difficulty sleeping for the past 4 nights. What would be appropriate therapy for this patient's pain?

    1. Amitriptyline (Elavil) 10 mg PO hs and nonsteroidal anti-inflammatory drugs (NSAIDs) prn as directed.

    2. High-dose corticosteroid therapy.

    3. Application of heat directly to the area involved.

    4. No appropriate therapy is currently available to treat neuropathic pain.

46. On a return visit to the clinic, a patient receiving sulfonamide therapy exhibits generalized rash, mucous membrane lesions, skin sloughing on the palms and feet, high fever, and generalized malaise. These findings would alert the family nurse practitioner to consider:

    1. Hepatitis B.

    2. Stevens-Johnson syndrome.

    3. HIV infection/AIDS.

    4. *Pneumocystis carinii* pneumonia.

Physical Exam & Diagnostic Tests

1. Answer: 4

Rationale: The term *annular* stems from the Latin word *annulus*, meaning ringed. Lesions are circular or ovoid patches with a red periphery and central clearing (e.g., tinea corporis). Multiple groups of vesicles erupting unilaterally following the course of cutaneous nerves are described as herpetiform or zosteriform (herpes zoster). Linear lesions are arranged in a line (allergic contact dermatitis to poison ivy). Confluent lesions merge and are not discrete (scarlet fever rash).

2. Answer: 1

Rationale: Psoriasis, peripheral vascular disease, diabetes, tuberculosis, and other infectious diseases, such as syphilis, are associated with pitting deformities of the nail that may vary from pinpoint to pinhead size and may be linear or irregular in distribution. Iron-deficiency anemia, eczema, malnutrition, and pellagra are associated with koilonychia (spoon nails). Hyperthyroidism and hypothyroidism are associated with onycholysis, which is a separation of the nail from the nail bed starting at the free edge and progressing proximally.

3. Answer: 1

Rationale: The place to inspect is in that portion of the sclera that is observed when the eye is open. If jaundice is suspected, the posterior portion of the hard palate should be examined for a yellowish cast. Pallor and cyanosis can be noted in the nail beds, palms, and soles. Oral mucosa may be affected by surface stains.

4. Answer: 1

Rationale: On an adult, the best place is just below the clavicle or on the abdomen. The best place to evaluate skin turgor for hydration status in children is the fleshy part of arms or legs because a child with a distended abdomen may have a tight abdomen, which appears to have adequate turgor, even though the child may actually be dehydrated.

5. Answer: 1

Rationale: Fungal lesions will be visualized as a green-yellow fluorescence when viewed with the Wood's lamp in a dimly lit room.

6. Answer: 1

Rationale: A macule is less than 1 cm in diameter, nonpalpable, flat, and brown, red, purple, or tan (freckles, flat moles, rubella). A papule is elevated and palpable (warts, pigmented nevi). A nodule is 1–2 cm in diameter, solid, elevated, and deeper (lipoma). A wheal is elevated and irregular and has a variable diameter (insect bites, urticaria).

7. Answer: 2

Rationale: Lichenification occurs with chronic irritation, often of an exposed extremity (chronic dermatitis). Crusts are dried exudate; scales are heaps of keratinized cells from exfoliation (psoriasis); and loss of epidermis is excoriation, as seen in an abrasion.

8. Answer: 3

Rationale: The angle between the nail plate and the proximal nail fold when viewed from the side is >180° and should form a diamond in clubbed nails. Normal nails form a 160° angle and should form a diamond shape between them when the nail beds of the index fingers are placed together. Transverse ridges and grooves may occur from trauma. Placing the palms together provides no assessment data. Diffuse discoloration may be from a fungal infection or an injury.

9. Answer: 3

Rationale: Bulla is the correct term. A papule is solid. A vesicle is less than 1 cm in diameter, and a pustule contains a purulent exudate.

10. Answer: 4

Rationale: The appearance of a new mole with high-risk features, including irregular border, color changes, and changes in sensation (e.g., pruritus), would necessitate immediate biopsy and/or referral to a dermatologist. Uniform moles, those that are symmetric and have smooth borders, and those not showing signs of change can be followed with annual skin assessments. Seborrheic keratosis is a benign skin growth, usually on sun-exposed areas, and appearing as waxy or "stuck-on" that requires no treatment.

11. Answer: 2

Rationale: Under microscopic exam, fungal scrapings in potassium hydroxide (KOH) solution will appear as threadlike hyphae crossing cell walls. The other solutions are not indicated to identify dermatophytes.

12. Answer: 3

Rationale: It is important to remember to apply controls when skin testing the immunocompromised patient. A positive control test is used to determine whether the patient reacts to histamine. If there is not an immediate reaction to histamine, the results of allergy skin tests can be difficult to interpret. A negative control test contains a solution that does not contain allergens. If a reaction occurs, the skin is too sensitive to allow for correct interpretation of allergy skin tests.

13. Answer: 4

Rationale: This best describes mongolian spots that are characteristic in newborns of African, Asian, or Latin descent. When closely evaluated, these spots do not resemble the ecchymoses that occur with trauma. Telangiectatic nevi are commonly known as "stork bites" and are deep-pink lesions that are most often found on the back of the neck. Cutis marmorata is the transient mottling that occurs when an infant is cold.

Skin Disorders

14. Answer: 3

Rationale: Intense itching is characteristic of pediculosis pubis, scabies, and atopic dermatitis. Impetigo starts out as a tender erythematous papule and progresses through a vesicular to a honey-crusted stage with no itching.

15. Answer: 2

Rationale: Herpes zoster typically presents with a history of tenderness followed by eruptions and vesicles that follow a dermatome on one side of the body. The condition is very painful. Other symptoms may include fever, headaches, and malaise. Psoriasis is characterized by thick, white, silvery, or red patches of skin. Contact dermatitis is a rash caused by touching something. Cellulitis is a skin infection characterized as red, hot, swollen, and tender skin.

16. Answer: 2

Rationale: Approximately 10%–30% of people with psoriasis develop an accompanying form of arthritis called psoriatic arthritis. The other options are dermatologic conditions that are not directly associated with arthritis.

17. Answer: 3

Rationale: Stress can aggravate psoriasis. Sunlight helps psoriasis, so it is usually better in the summer. It is not contagious, and only about 30% of patients with psoriasis itch.

18. Answer: 2

Rationale: Actinic keratoses are potentially precancerous lesions that are found in areas of skin exposed to sunlight.

19. Answer: 4

Rationale: Laboratory studies are not likely to be helpful in evaluation of urticaria. Identification of causes is usually based on history and physical findings. The other statements are true of urticaria.

20. Answer: 3

Rationale: Although any of these conditions can affect the skin, particularly of a patient who is HIV-positive, the description relates most closely to Kaposi's sarcoma and warrants a biopsy.

21. Answer: 2

Rationale: Despite the name "dyshidrotic" eczematous dermatitis (bullous form called pompholyx), there is no evidence of sweating. Most patients have an atopic history, and emotional stress is often a precipitating factor in the appearance of the vesicles. Nummular (discoid) eczema is a chronic, pruritic, inflammatory dermatitis that occurs as coin-shaped plaques composed of papules and vesicles on an erythematous base. Rosacea is characterized by flushing and clusters of papulopustules on the cheek and forehead. Psoriasis is a hereditary disorder characterized by chronic, usually bilateral scaly plaques on exposed areas (knees, elbows). A verruca or common wart affects primarily young adults, is contagious, and is characterized by firm papules with a cleft surface and multiple conical vegetations.

22. Answer: 4

Rationale: Delay wound closure until determination of no infection in approximately 24 to 48 hours. Mouth flora of humans is abundant, and a bite carries the risk of heavy bacterial inoculum and severe infection. A Td booster should be given every 10 years. Tdap may be given as one of these boosters if the patient has never received Tdap before. Typically, one dose of Tdap is routinely given at age 11 or 12. People who did not get Tdap at that age should get it as soon as possible. Tdap may also be given after a severe cut or burn to prevent tetanus infection.

23. Answer: 2

Rationale: Onychomycosis is the correct term. Hippocratic nails are clubbed nails and fingers associated with chronic heart and lung disorders. Koilonychia is a concavity of the nail plate often associated with iron-deficiency anemia. Anonychia is a total congenital absence of the nail.

24. Answer: 2

Rationale: In case of suspected drug reactions, it is recommended that the drug be eliminated and documented in the patient's record so it is not reintroduced.

25. Answer: 4

Rationale: Excessive sweating may be normal, but history and physical are needed to rule out underlying causes. Therapies can be offered. Drysol is for use only on the feet and axilla.

26. Answer: 3

Rationale: The assessment describes a seborrheic keratosis. The actinic keratosis is an irregular, rough, scaly, white-to-erythematous macular lesion found most often on sun-exposed areas, such as on the dorsal surface of the hands, arms, neck, and face. It has malignant potential. The basal cell carcinoma is a smooth, round nodule with a pearly gray border and central induration. Senile lentigines are gray-brown, irregular, macular lesions on sun-exposed areas of the face, arms, and hands.

27. Answer: 3

Rationale: Herpes zoster (shingles) is a vesicular dermatomal eruption related to a reactivation of latent varicella virus. It increases with advanced age and is characterized by burning pain and paresthesia along one or two dermatomes, not crossing the midline, and may be accompanied by fever, malaise, or headache. The vesicular stage lasts 2–3 weeks. The vesicles are initially clear or blood filled and become purulent. The area along the dermatome is erythematous, and the vesicles crust and then scab, which may leave hypopigmented scars. The other options discuss painless lesions and are not specific to this prodromal stage.

28. Answer: 1

Rationale: Antiviral therapy with acyclovir 800 mg 5 times daily for 7 days may expedite healing if started within 2–3 days of onset, especially in immunocompromised individuals. Miconazole and clotrimazole are antifungal creams. Prednisone would only be used to decrease the incidence of postherpetic neuralgia and may increase the incidence of disseminated infection, so it is not recommended during the acute phase.

29. Answer: 4

Rationale: These are classic signs of a basal cell carcinoma, also supported by the patient's employment history. Melanoma would be pigmented; compound nevus would not be firm or have telangiectasia; and bullous pemphigoid results in bullous lesions.

30. Answer: 3

Rationale: Refer immediately to a dermatologist because the findings are highly suspicious for a melanoma. A biopsy should never be done on a melanoma, and any delay could be detrimental to the outcome.

31. Answer: 2

Rationale: Oral acyclovir is very effective in reducing the intensity and duration of the symptoms if started early in the course of the disease. Herpes zoster does not usually recur at regular intervals but frequently lasts for several weeks. Once the rash has developed crusts, the person is no longer contagious. Shingles is less contagious than chickenpox, and the risk of a person with shingles spreading the virus is low if the rash is covered.

32. Answer: 3

Rationale: The patient presents with a classic case of pityriasis rosea, a benign, self-limiting skin eruption of unknown etiology. Although a medication/allergen history would be warranted, referral to an allergy specialist or dermatologist would not be necessary. Triamcinolone would not be indicated because the treatment is mainly symptomatic. Sunlight in moderate amounts has been shown to hasten healing in some patients.

33. Answer: 3

Rationale: The signs and symptoms presented are classic for Lyme disease, which is transmitted by ticks. Therefore, it would be important to inquire about potential exposure to ticks before the signs and symptoms developed. Exposure to new skin care products would be important if the practitioner suspected an allergic reaction, which is not consistent with the signs and symptoms. Although always important, a thorough medication history probably will not reveal the cause of the signs and symptoms in this case. Tuberculosis does not present in this manner.

34. Answer: 2

Rationale: Insects reproduce, are more active, and are present in greater numbers in the warm months of spring to early fall.

35. Answer: 2

Rationale: Heat application is contraindicated; ice packs are preferred, as is elevation, to decrease the edema. The area should be immobilized. Tdap or Td may be given along with antihistamines to reduce swelling and relieve itching.

36. Answer: 4

Rationale: This was a venomous coral snake bite. The typical symptoms are those listed, as well as nausea, vomiting, and muscle fasciculations.

37. Answer: 3, 4, 5

Rationale: A "herald patch" usually appears on the skin first. This is usually an oval- or round-shaped patch that can vary from 2–5 cm in diameter and is salmon-colored with fine scales. It is followed within days by a regional outbreak of numerous smaller erythematous patches, thus providing a key diagnostic clue with smaller lesions oriented along skin cleavage areas (Langer's lines) in a "Christmas tree" pattern. It most commonly appears on the chest or upper back, although it can sometimes appear on the abdomen, neck, back, thigh or upper arms. Mild pruritus occurs, which typically causes the patient to seek medical assistance.

38. Answer: 3

Rationale: Acanthosis nigricans (AN) typically occurs in patients who are obese or have diabetes and is a benign dermatosis characterized by velvety, hyperpigmented, hyperkeratotic plaques in body folds and creases (armpits, groin, and neck), which is associated with hyperinsulinemia and insulin resistance. A fasting blood glucose would be an appropriate diagnostic test to order.

Pharmacology

39. Answer: 1

Rationale: The description is consistent with intertriginous candidiasis, which is treated with an antifungal ointment or oral medication. It is not a staphylococcal infection; the area needs to be kept dry, not moist. An antibiotic ointment will not relieve the problem. Herpes zoster is treated with antiviral medications; this case is not described as particularly painful, and it is bilateral.

40. Answer: 1

Rationale: Beta blockers can exacerbate psoriasis. They are believed to decrease cAMP-dependent protein kinase, an inhibitor of cell proliferation. Drugs in the other classifications have no known effect on psoriasis.

41. Answer: 3

Rationale: Acyclovir treats the acute phase during initial eruption of vesicular lesions and offers no benefit for postherpetic pain.

42. Answer: 3

Rationale: Patients need to be instructed to wash off podophyllin. It should be applied sparingly, only to the wart and avoiding normal skin, and allowed to dry thoroughly before the patient dresses. No rationale exists to treat with both liquid nitrogen and podophyllin.

43. Answer: 3

Rationale: Systemic treatment with low-dose tetracycline is very effective for rosacea; topical treatment with metronidazole or low-dose hydrocortisone may also be useful. Oral cortisone and antifungal agents are not known to be effective. Topical 5-fluorouracil is used in the treatment of actinic keratosis, a precancerous skin condition.

44. Answer: 1

Rationale: The maximum allowable dose for adults is 7 mg/kg of lidocaine with epinephrine and 5 mg/kg of lidocaine without epinephrine. Although local anesthetics are often used, the maximum allowable doses are rarely emphasized, and overdose can result in anaphylactic shock.

45. Answer: 1

Rationale: Amitriptyline in low doses is effective in treating neuropathic pain. Nonsteroidal antiinflammatory drugs (NSAIDs) may also be effective in treating the inflammatory component of herpes zoster pain. The most effective nonpharmacologic method of treating pain from shingles is the application of cool compresses. Heat may exacerbate neuropathic pain in some patients. Antidepressants and anticonvulsants are effective adjuvant therapies in the treatment of neuropathic pain.

46. Answer: 2

Rationale: Stevens-Johnson syndrome is a severe form of erythema multiforme that can be fatal. The clinical picture is mucous membrane lesions, conjunctival and corneal lesions, fever, malaise, arthralgia, and sloughing of the skin of the hands and feet. Distinguishing characteristics of the syndrome are eruption of vesicles, mucosal ulcerations, and sloughing skin.

Endocrine

9

Physical Exam & Diagnostic Tests

1. What is the correct procedure for palpation of a patient's thyroid gland?

   1. Stand behind the patient, hyperextend the head, and palpate both sides simultaneously.

   2. Have the patient lower the chin and tilt head slightly toward the side being evaluated.

   3. Hyperextend the head and have the patient lean away from the side being evaluated.

   4. Have the patient lean away from the side being examined and take a swallow of water.

2. When a patient sips water and swallows, the thyroid gland:

   1. Moves downward and slightly posterior and feels smooth on palpation.

   2. Elongates and enlarges during the swallow and immediately returns to a resting position.

   3. Moves slightly out during the sipping and backward during the swallowing.

   4. Moves upward during the swallow and feels symmetric and smooth to palpation.

3. Which four questions are part of the five-question Carville Diabetic Foot Screen? Select 4 responses.

   1. Has there been a change in the foot since the last evaluation?

   2. Does the foot hurt when walking?

   3. Does the foot have an abnormal shape?

   4. Are the nails thick, too long, or overgrown?

   5. Have you purchased new shoes in the past 6 months?

   6. Do you have a foot ulcer now or a history of a foot ulcer?

4. While conducting the interview for a physical exam, the family nurse practitioner identifies which finding in the patient's history as being commonly associated with thyroid carcinoma?

   1. Family history of thyroid cancer.

   2. History of hyperthyroidism.

   3. Irradiation of the neck.

   4. Smoking for 15 years.

5. When doing a physical exam on a patient with hyperthyroidism, a common neurologic finding is:

   1. Memory, attention, and problem-solving deficits.

   2. Diminished deep tendon reflexes.

   3. Severe cognitive impairment.

   4. Delusions and psychosis.

6. The treatment goal for glycemic control in a person with type 2 diabetes is to achieve and maintain hemoglobin A1C level (HgbA1C) of:

   1. <10%.

   2. 6%–9%.

   3. <7%.

   4. >8%.

7. Which finding would alert the family nurse practitioner that a patient might be experiencing a problem with the endocrine system?

   1. Coagulation abnormalities and fatigue.

   2. Growth abnormalities and glucose intolerance.

   3. Hypoxia and jaundice.

   4. Steatorrhea and abdominal distention.

8. The family nurse practitioner notes a solitary thyroid nodule on a patient during a routine physical exam. The next step for diagnostic testing is:

   1. Thyroid scan and antibody level.

   2. TSH level and ultrasound.

   3. X-ray film of the thyroid.

   4. Fine-needle aspiration (FNA) biopsy.

9. An adult female patient presents to the family nurse practitioner's office complaining of fatigue, weakness, and weight gain over the past 4 months. Physical exam reveals elevated blood pressure (BP), facial and supraclavicular fullness, hirsutism noted on the face, proximal muscle weakness, and facial and truncal distribution of acne. Appropriate laboratory tests the family nurse practitioner should order include:

   1. Antinuclear antibody (ANA) and rheumatoid factor (RF).

   2. Three-hour glucose tolerance test and lipid profile.

   3. RBC count and a calcium level.

   4. Dexamethasone suppression test, urinary-free cortisol level, and TSH and T_4.

10. The family nurse practitioner would anticipate which laboratory values in the patient with Graves' disease?

    1. TSH levels to be increased.

    2. TSH levels to be decreased.

    3. TSH levels to be within normal limits (WNL).

    4. T_4 levels to be decreased.

11. Which information is correct regarding foot screening using a nylon filament (5.07 Semmes-Weinstein)?

    1. Use a 25-g filament and apply along perimeter of any scar or ulcer tissue.

    2. Apply the filament at a 45-degree angle to the skin surface.

    3. Apply sufficient force for approximately 1.5 seconds to cause the filament to bend.

    4. Slide the filament across the skin and make repetitive contact to each of the 10 sites.

12. To make the diagnosis of diabetes, the patient must have two fasting plasma glucose levels documented on two occasions greater than or equal to ($\geq$):

    1. 200 mg/dL

    2. 140 mg/dL

    3. 126 mg/dL

    4. 110 mg/dL

Disorders

13. The etiology of type 1 diabetes can be best described as:

    1. An autosomal dominant genetic disorder.

    2. Autoimmune destruction of the beta cells.

    3. Overnutrition and resulting obesity as the major risk factor.

    4. Prevented by exercise, which increases the concentration of insulin receptors.

14. A patient has been diagnosed with diabetes for more than 5 years. To whom should the family nurse practitioner maintain an annual referral for this patient?

    1. Cardiologist.

    2. Dietitian.

    3. Vascular surgeon.

    4. Ophthalmologist.

15. Hirsutism presenting in a female with normal menstruation and normal plasma androgens is most likely:

    1. An ovarian tumor.

    2. Cushing's syndrome.

    3. Idiopathic.

    4. Polycystic ovary disease.

16. Pathophysiologic causes of decreased testosterone levels develop in the:

    1. Hypothalamus.

    2. Anterior pituitary.

    3. Testes.

    4. All the above.

17. **QSEN** When counseling a diabetic patient on foot care, it is important to emphasize:

    1. Daily foot soaks in warm, soapy water.

    2. Careful daily foot inspections.

    3. Trimming corns and calluses regularly.

    4. Trimming toenails close to the nail bed.

18. An adult patient presents to the family nurse practitioner for evaluation of polyuria, polydipsia, and weight loss. Which laboratory result would require immediate intervention by the family nurse practitioner?

    1. A1C of 14%.

    2. Serum glucose of 150 mg/dL.

    3. A1C of 6.0%.

    4. Serum glucose of 65 mg/dL.

19. An adult patient is being evaluated for hypoglycemia because of a blood sugar of 58 mg/dL. The family nurse practitioner would begin the differential diagnosis by:

    1. Deciding if the hypoglycemia is fasting or postprandial.

    2. Ascertaining if it is related to alcohol use.

    3. Deciding if the patient has other medical problems.

    4. Reassuring the patient that it is a benign problem.

20. An older adult male patient complains of lethargy, cold intolerance, weight gain, and yellowing of the palms. The most important laboratory study ordered by the family nurse practitioner in diagnosing this condition is:

    1. Complete blood count.

    2. Liver enzymes.

    3. Thyroid panel.

    4. Cardiac enzymes.

21. A middle-aged, normally healthy female presents for evaluation of intermittent palpitations. She also reports mood variability, tremulousness, difficulty falling asleep, and a 10-lb weight loss despite a normal appetite. She feels warm most of the time and wonders if she is perimenopausal. She has no history of heart disease. The objective data that would yield the most useful information would be:

    1. Electrocardiogram (ECG).

    2. TSH, free T_4.

    3. Electrolytes.

    4. Holter monitor.

22. An adult woman presents to the clinic complaining of fatigue, weakness, weight gain despite lack of appetite, and feelings of depression. Physical exam reveals an obese, alert patient with thinning hair, bilateral chest puffiness, increased facial hair, supraclavicular fat pad, thin arms and legs, purple striae on the abdomen, and multiple ecchymotic areas on extremities. Her vital signs are BP of 158/96 mm Hg, pulse of 88 beats/min, and respirations of

22 breaths/min. Laboratory results show FBS of 200 mg/dL, electrolyte panel within normal limits (WNL), except for potassium of 3.0 mEq/L, hemoglobin of 11.8 g, and hematocrit of 34%. This assessment information would support the family nurse practitioner's diagnosis of:

    1. Addison's disease.

    2. Pheochromocytoma.

    3. Cushing's syndrome.

    4. Hypoaldosteronism.

23. Which of the following is the best alternative for treating hyperthyroidism diagnosed during the first trimester of pregnancy?

    1. Radioactive iodine in smaller than usual dose during first trimester.

    2. Propylthiouracil (PTU) during first trimester, subtotal thyroidectomy during second trimester, no thyroid replacement.

    3. PTU during first trimester, subtotal thyroidectomy during second trimester, thyroid replacement.

    4. No treatment until after delivery.

24. Clinical findings in a patient with hypothyroidism include:

    1. Hyperactive bowel sounds.

    2. Oily skin and acne.

    3. Postural tremors of the hands.

    4. Edema of the face and eyelids.

25. A young adult male reports anxiety, tremulousness, headaches, palpitations, and sweating 2–4 hours after eating. Physical exam is normal. No lab results are currently available. No medical conditions are noted in the history. What is the most likely diagnosis?

    1. Dumping syndrome.

    2. Hypoglycemia.

    3. Alcohol abuse.

    4. Hyperthyroidism.

26. Which of the following is the most likely etiology for hypercalcemia in the medically well asymptomatic adult?

    1. Hyperthyroidism.

    2. Hyperparathyroidism.

    3. Hyperpituitarism.

    4. Hypothyroidism.

27. A middle-aged male with no previous medical history presents with a 30-lb weight gain in 2.5 months. He denies any medication use or allergies. He was recently laid off of a very active job and has been sedentary. Physical exam reveals BP of 172/111 mm Hg, central obesity, FBS of 200 mg/dL. What is the most likely cause of the patient's weight gain?

   1. Cushing's disease.

   2. Hypothyroidism.

   3. Depression.

   4. Diabetes.

28. A middle-aged woman presents with agitation, confusion, fever, tachycardia, and diaphoresis. Her daughter states that nausea, vomiting, and abdominal pain preceded these symptoms. The patient has no history of cardiac disease, diabetes, or substance abuse. She was started on some "anti- drug" 2 weeks ago and is scheduled for some form of throat surgery next week (per daughter). Based on this history, the family nurse practitioner immediately orders:

   1. TSH, T_4.

   2. Urinalysis.

   3. Spinal tap.

   4. Computed tomography of head.

29. A 45-year-old female patient presents to the office complaining of a 6-month history of fatigue, 15-lb weight gain, lethargy, an inability to tolerate cold temperatures, forgetfulness, hair loss, and constipation. Physical findings include dry, coarse skin, periorbital edema and puffy facies, bradycardia, hyporeflexia and muscle weakness, and a smooth, goitrous thyroid. The family nurse practitioner would make the diagnosis of:

   1. Heart failure.

   2. Diabetes mellitus.

   3. Hypothyroidism.

   4. Thyroid cancer.

30. A diabetic patient has been taking 6 U of regular insulin and 12 U of NPH insulin in the morning. In the evening, she has been taking 3 U of regular insulin and 8 U of NPH insulin. The patient has been monitoring her blood glucose levels (mg/dL) and shows the family nurse practitioner the following chart:

	7 am	Noon	5 pm	Bedtime
Monday	100	76	98	109
Tuesday	119	75	88	110
Wednesday	119	66	86	100
Thursday	123	70	111	122
Friday	128	60	99	110

The family nurse practitioner adjusts the patient's insulin by:

   1. Increasing the regular insulin.

   2. Decreasing the regular insulin.

   3. Decreasing the NPH insulin.

   4. Increasing both insulins.

31. The role of the family nurse practitioner in the initial management of a patient with a thyroid nodule involves:

   1. Referring the patient to an endocrinologist for further evaluation.

   2. Obtaining fine-needle aspiration (FNA) biopsy of the nodule and sending it to cytology.

   3. Ordering an ultrasound and a thyroid scan.

   4. Ordering levothyroxine (Synthroid) to reduce the size of the nodule.

32. When teaching a patient with diabetes about "sick day" guidelines, the family nurse practitioner explains that the patient should:

   1. Stop measuring blood glucose and only check urine for ketones.

   2. Not take the usual dose of insulin at the usual time.

   3. Be sure to take metformin (Glucophage) and acarbose (Precose), even if nausea and vomiting are present.

   4. Administer extra doses of regular insulin according to instructions for blood glucose levels above 240 mg/dL.

33. A young adult female patient presents to the clinic with complaints of nervousness, tremulousness, palpitations, heat intolerance, fatigue, weight loss, and polyphagia. After a complete history and physical, along with thyroid function tests, the family nurse practitioner makes the diagnosis of hyperthyroidism, recognizing that the most common cause of this condition is:

   1. Thyroid cancer.

   2. Graves' disease.

   3. Pituitary adenoma.

   4. Postpartum thyroiditis.

34. A young adult male patient presents to office stating that he found a lump in his neck while shaving. Physical exam reveals a firm, 2-cm nodule that is fixed, nontender, and located on the right lobe of the thyroid gland. Right posterior cervical lymphadenopathy is also noted. The family nurse practitioner should:

    1. Order a TSH level to determine thyroid function, and refer to a surgeon for a fine-needle aspiration (FNA) biopsy of the nodule.

    2. No intervention is necessary at this time; schedule a follow-up visit in 6 months.

    3. Prescribe levothyroxine (Synthroid) 0.1 mg PO daily, and schedule a 6-week follow-up visit.

    4. Immediately ablate the patient's thyroid with radioactive iodine, and refer to an endocrinologist.

35. A patient with Graves' disease is to have radioactive iodine (^{131}I) therapy. Which information is important for the family nurse practitioner to include when teaching about this treatment?

    1. Patients are highly radioactive for approximately 7 days after treatment and need to be isolated.

    2. Patients should not become pregnant during or after receiving this therapy because of the teratogenic effects to the fetus that occur due to chromosomal abnormalities.

    3. Patients may become hypothyroid after this treatment and, therefore, need to have regular TSH and T_4 levels drawn, with the potential for thyroid hormone replacement therapy.

    4. This therapy is contraindicated in patients with cardiac disease.

36. During an evaluation of a patient with prediabetes (glucose intolerance), the family nurse practitioner identifies what finding in the patient's objective data as being associated with the increasing insulin resistance?

    1. Triglycerides >150 mg/dL.

    2. High-density lipoprotein >40 mg/dL in men and >50 mg/dL in women.

    3. Blood pressure <130/85 mm Hg.

    4. Fasting blood sugar <110 mg/dL.

37. While taking a history on a patient, the family nurse practitioner identifies what finding that may be associated with osteopenia/osteoporosis?

    1. High calcium intake.

    2. Minimal alcohol intake.

    3. Smoking 1 pack/day for 20 years.

    4. Walking 30 minutes 4 days a week.

38. Of the following risk factors for osteoporosis, which would the family nurse practitioner see primarily with men?

    1. Smoking 2 packs of cigarettes a day.

    2. Excessive use of alcohol.

    3. Low testosterone level.

    4. Minimal exercise.

39. When prescribing a meal plan for a patient with type 2 diabetes, the family nurse practitioner tells the patient that the macronutrient with the most influence on postprandial glucose levels is:

    1. Fiber.

    2. Fat.

    3. Protein.

    4. Carbohydrate.

Pharmacology

40. When prescribing oral medications for an overweight patient with type 2 diabetes who also has a voracious appetite, the family nurse practitioner is likely to prescribe which medication to encourage weight loss and reduce appetite?

    1. Exenatide (Byetta).

    2. Pioglitazone (Actos).

    3. Metformin (Glucophage).

    4. Glyburide (Micronase).

41. Glargine (Lantus) is an insulin analog that essentially has no peak and is usually administered:

    1. Before meals.

    2. With lispro insulin (Humalog) in one injection.

    3. Before breakfast and dinner.

    4. Once a day.

42. An adult male patient with type 2 diabetes has a creatinine level of 1.8 mg/dL. Which of the following drugs is contraindicated?

    1. Pioglitazone (Actos).

    2. Metformin (Glucophage).

    3. Rapaglinide (Prandin).

    4. Acarbose (Precose).

43. Patients started on metformin (Glucophage) need to be monitored closely for what potential side effect?

    1. Significant increase in weight.

    2. Elevation of LDL level.

    3. Lactic acidosis.

    4. Increase in insulin requirements.

44. A patient with type 2 diabetes is taking glipizide (Glucotrol) 10 mg PO bid. In evaluating the medication's effectiveness, the family nurse practitioner knows that glipizide reduces blood glucose by:

    1. Delaying the cellular uptake of potassium and insulin.

    2. Stimulating insulin release from the pancreas.

    3. Decreasing the body's need for and utilization of insulin at the cellular level.

    4. Interfering with the absorption and metabolism of fats and carbohydrates.

45. The family nurse practitioner would expect which symptom to be a side effect of metformin (Glucophage)?

    1. Gastrointestinal (GI) upset.

    2. Photophobia.

    3. Hypoglycemia.

    4. Skin eruptions.

46. A patient is receiving antithyroid medication. The family nurse practitioner understands that:

    1. Lifelong daily treatment is necessary to keep TSH levels within the normal range.

    2. Antithyroid medications do not cross the placenta.

    3. The drugs are somewhat expensive and have serious cardiac and hematologic side effects.

    4. Patients remain on drug therapy for 1–2 years, and then the medication is gradually withdrawn.

47. When prescribing an antihypertensive medication for a type 2 diabetic patient, the drug classifications that would tend to reduce insulin sensitivity are:

    1. Diuretics and calcium channel blockers.

    2. Diuretics and beta blockers.

    3. Calcium channel blockers and ACE inhibitors.

    4. Alpha blockers and ACE inhibitors.

48. A 35-year-old female sees the family nurse practitioner with a complaint of cold intolerance, fatigue, dry skin, weight gain, and heavy menstrual periods. Physical exam shows a pulse of 58 beats/min, a "waxy" sallow complexion, and a firm goiter. Her TSH level is 36 mU/L. What is the best treatment choice for this patient?

    1. Begin levothyroxine (Synthroid) at 0.025 mg PO qd and repeat TSH in 2 weeks.

    2. Administer loading dose of PO levothyroxine and start full replacement dose.

    3. Administer loading dose of IV levothyroxine and start on half replacement dose.

    4. Begin levothyroxine at 0.1 mg PO qd and recheck TSH in 6 weeks.

49. The family nurse practitioner is performing the preoperative evaluation of a man scheduled to undergo coronary artery bypass grafting. Physical exam shows mild facial puffiness, hoarse voice, and dry skin. Thyroid function results show that the patient has a TSH level of 34 mU/L. What is the recommended treatment for the patient?

    1. Give loading IV bolus of levothyroxine (Synthroid) 0.5 mg and proceed with surgery.

    2. Cancel surgery and send him home to begin levothyroxine PO 0.1 mg. Reschedule surgery.

    3. Begin PO levothyroxine and monitor in the hospital until he is euthyroid.

    4. Proceed with surgery and treat hypothyroidism postoperatively.

50. The family nurse practitioner is seeing an obese, middle-aged female patient for a follow-up visit. She was diagnosed with type 2 diabetes 3 months ago and started on a regimen of diet and exercise. Today, her fasting plasma glucose is 200 mg/dL and A1C is 10%. She has lost 2 lb. She reports her home glucose monitoring has ranged from 180–300 mg/dL. The rest of her chemistry profile is within normal limits (WNL). What is the best treatment choice for the patient?

    1. Review her diet and exercise plan, increase exercise regimen, and reduce caloric intake. Schedule her for another follow-up in 3 months.

    2. Start her on sliding-scale insulin and instruct her on recording glucose and insulin requirements. Schedule her to return in 1 week for reevaluation regarding long-acting insulin.

    3. Initiate treatment with metformin (Glucophage).

    4. Initiate treatment with an oral sulfonylurea agent (e.g., glyburide).

51. What is associated with chronic overtreatment with levothyroxine (Synthroid)?

    1. Tachycardia.

    2. Osteoporosis.

    3. Insomnia.

    4. Sweating.

52. A middle-aged male presents for a diabetes follow-up exam. He has been in good health without identified complications of diabetes. His FBS is 100 mg/dL, and his personal records indicate that he is taking insulin in the prescribed amounts and times. Vital signs are BP 142/98 mm Hg, pulse 80 beats/min, and respirations 20 breaths/min. Today's plan would include:

    1. Begin diuretics and a beta blocker.

    2. Begin ACE inhibitor and consider a diuretic.

    3. Obtain ECG and chest x-ray.

    4. Return for BP check in 5–7 days.

53. An adult male has recently been started on insulin. His regimen is two daily injections with two thirds of the total daily insulin in the morning and one third in the evening. He is using the 70/30 mixture of intermediate- and short-acting insulin in both injections. He presents for a follow-up visit with his FBS log. The family nurse practitioner notes that his recorded glucose levels before the evening meal have been 60–70 mg/dL. Other checks during the day are 100–120 mg/dL. What adjustment needs to be made?

    1. Intermediate insulin: change 70/30 combination to self-mix and reduce AM dose.

    2. Regular insulin: reduce AM dose of 70/30.

    3. Intermediate insulin: reduce AM dose of 70/30.

    4. Regular insulin: change 70/30 combination to self-mix and reduce AM regular dose.

54. A patient on antithyroid drug therapy for hyperthyroidism presents with complaints of palpitations and dry mouth for the past 2 days. He has had a cough and cold symptoms for the past 3 days, which he has been treating with over-the-counter medications. Which medication would the family nurse practitioner encourage the patient to avoid?

    1. Benzocaine (Chloraseptic) lozenges.

    2. Guaifenesin (Robitussin).

    3. Ibuprofen (Advil).

    4. Pseudoephedrine (Sudafed).

55. What is the most frequent complaint of patients who use insulin pumps?

    1. Problems with elevated glucose after changing the catheter-type (nonneedle) infusion set.

    2. Skin and site problems with dressing adhesive not sticking; redness and pain at infusion site.

    3. Mechanical problems with the pump's digital readout.

    4. Understanding "sick day" management modifications.

56. The family nurse practitioner understands that pioglitazone (Actos) or rosiglitazone (Avandia) is indicated for:

    1. Prenatal patients with gestational diabetes.

    2. "Brittle" type 1 diabetic patients.

    3. Type 2 diabetic patients requiring insulin who have poor glycemic control and insulin resistance.

    4. Type 2 diabetic patients, to prevent the rapid postprandial blood glucose surges by delaying carbohydrate absorption.

57. An older patient with a history of hypertension and coronary bypass surgery has been diagnosed with hypothyroidism. Appropriate medication management is:

    1. Levothyroxine (Synthroid) 0.1 mg qd and return in 6 weeks for follow-up.

    2. Desiccated thyroid extract 2 grains qd and return in 6 weeks for follow-up.

    3. Levothyroxine (Synthroid) 0.025 mg qd for 6 weeks with gradual increase in dosage every 4–6 weeks until therapeutic level is obtained.

    4. Methimazole (Tapazole) 15 mg daily in three divided doses, gradually increasing dose every 4 weeks until therapeutic level is obtained.

58. A patient is newly diagnosed as being hypothyroid and is placed on levothyroxine (Synthroid) 0.1 mg PO qd. What should be the family nurse practitioner's approach to follow-up?

    1. No follow-up visits are necessary.

    2. The patient should return to the clinic in 4–6 weeks for TSH measurement and determination of any symptomatic improvement.

    3. The patient should have weekly levothyroxine levels drawn.

    4. The patient should have monthly CBCs while on levothyroxine (Synthroid) because the medication has been found to be myelosuppressive.

59. Classes of medications typically used to treat hyperthyroid conditions include:

    1. Antibiotics and corticosteroids.

    2. ACE inhibitors, anxiolytics, and antithyroid medications.

    3. Beta blockers, NSAIDs, and antithyroid medications.

    4. Calcium channel blockers and corticosteroids.

60. A patient with hypothyroidism receiving daily levothyroxine (Synthroid) for 3 weeks presents to the clinic with complaints of intermittent chest pain. What is the appropriate therapeutic response?

    1. Discontinue levothyroxine because chest pain is a contraindication to its continuance.

    2. Schedule the patient for a stress test.

    3. Decrease dose of levothyroxine, order an electrocardiogram (ECG), and consult immediately with endocrine and/or cardiology health team members.

    4. Prescribe an anxiolytic agent for the patient.

61. The family nurse practitioner understands that lispro insulin (Humalog):

    1. Can be injected just before eating.

    2. Is less costly than regular insulin.

    3. Increases the likelihood of late postprandial hypoglycemia due to its length of action.

    4. Causes teratogenic effects.

62. When prescribing sulfonylureas, the family nurse practitioner educates the patient that the most common side effect of therapy is:

    1. Upset stomach.

    2. Diarrhea.

    3. Angina.

    4. Hypoglycemia.

63. The primary action of pioglitazone (Actos) and rosiglitazone (Avandia) is to:

    1. Decrease hepatic glucose output.

    2. Increase secretion of insulin from the pancreas.

    3. Increase glucose uptake into the muscle and fat.

    4. Increase postprandial uptake of glucose into the intestine.

64. A patient has been discharged home on DDAVP (desmopressin acetate) for diabetes insipidus after removal of a pituitary tumor. On exam, the family nurse practitioner notes that the patient is lethargic, but has 4+ deep tendon reflexes. The family nurse practitioner suspects:

    1. Noncompliance with therapy.

    2. Water intoxication.

    3. Increased vasopressor effect.

    4. Interaction with over-the-counter (OTC) cough medicine products.

65. During a retrospective review of an established patient, the family nurse practitioner notes that the photographs of the person show more than just typical aging. They include increased spacing of teeth without loss of dentition, a deep furrowing of the brow, and a widening of the nose. These acromegaly signs are:

    1. Treated without intervention until they become of symptomatic concern.

    2. Investigated with an oral glucose tolerance test (OGTT).

    3. Initially reviewed with an MRI test.

    4. Tested first to rule out a thyroid disorder.

66. Primary Cushing's disease is linked to suppression of pituitary control over steroid homeostasis. Secondary Cushing's disorder must be considered in which of the following patient groups?

    1. Type 1 diabetics.

    2. Chronic hypertensive patients who respond to medications.

    3. Patients with cancers, especially of small cell variety.

    4. Any patient who is obese.

67. Some diabetic medication groups are being associated with a link to cancer. Which of the following drugs and link to possible cancer type is correct? Select two responses that identify the pairs of drugs and link to possible cancer.

    1. The thiazolidinediones (TZD group) and bladder cancer.

    2. The biguanides and pancreatic cancer.

    3. The glucagon-like peptide agonists (GLP-1) and thyroid cancer.

    4. The sulfonylureas and prostate cancer.

    5. The incretin mimetics and stomach cancer.

68. Which of the following osteoporosis medications does not carry the critical warning that the patient must take the medication with a full glass of water and remain upright 30–60 minutes after dosing?

    1. Alendronate (Fosamax).

    2. Ibandronate (Boniva).

    3. Risedronate (Actonel).

    4. Zoledronic acid (Zometa).

69. A young adult is taking DDAVP (desmopressin) nasally. The patient also has allergies to the local plants, which creates a good amount of nasal congestion. What medication education is important to emphasize?

    1. If the patient is taking an antihistamine, the patient cannot take the DDAVP.

    2. If the patient's nasal passages are full of mucus, the patient should blow the nose to clear prior to taking the DDAVP.

    3. The congestion makes the use of inhaled DDAVP ineffective, so the dose will have to be taken orally until the allergies diminish.

    4. The patient needs to take the DDAVP at least 1 hour apart from any oral antihistamine.

70. Education concerning home blood sugar testing with a personal glucometer includes the following key point:

    1. Use the matching test strips designed for the particular glucometer, as different brands are not interchangeable.

    2. When opening a new canister of test strips, recalibration or setting control codes is no longer needed.

    3. The values obtained from self-monitoring glucometers matches serum blood values.

    4. Remember to cleanse the fingertip or alternative testing site with alcohol prior to using the lancing-type device.

71. What blood test can be drawn to help identify whether the patient is a type I or type 2 diabetic?

    1. Hemoglobin A1C.

    2. Glycosylated fructose.

    3. C-peptide level.

    4. Apo A vs Apo B.

72. Which group of hypertensive agents have some positive impact on the development of diabetic nephropathy?

    1. Alpha blockers.

    2. Beta blockers.

    3. Calcium channel blockers.

    4. ACE inhibitors.

73. Which of the following diabetic medication groups is linked with higher risks for hypoglycemia when given as a solo medication? Select two diabetic medication groups.

    1. Biguanides.

    2. Insulins.

    3. Sulfonylureas.

    4. Incretin mimetics.

    5. DDP-4 inhibitors (Gliptins).

9 Endocrine Answers and Rationales

Physical Exam & Diagnostic Tests

1. Answer: 2

Rationale: When examining the thyroid, it is important that the patient relax the sternocleidomastoid muscles, which is done by having the patient tilt toward the side being evaluated.

2. Answer: 4

Rationale: The thyroid gland is fixed to the trachea and thus ascends during swallowing. This assists the family nurse practitioner to distinguish thyroid structures from other neck masses. The gland's size, degree of enlargement, consistency, surface characteristics, and the presence of nodules or bruits are noted during the exam.

3. Answer: 1, 3, 4, 5

Rationale: The five questions in the Carville Diabetic Foot Screen are as follows:

- Has there been a change in the foot since the last evaluation?
- Is there a foot ulcer now or a history of foot ulcer?
- Does the foot have an abnormal shape?
- Is there weakness in the ankle or foot?
- Are the nails thick, too long, or overgrown?

There is no reference to pain on this screening or whether new shoes have been purchased.

4. Answer: 3

Rationale: Papillary carcinoma, the most common form of thyroid cancer, is associated with a history of exposure to radiation. Family history, history of hyperthyroidism, and smoking are not considered significant risk factors for this malignancy.

5. Answer: 1

Rationale: Memory, attention, and problem-solving deficits are often noted symptoms with hyperthyroidism. The high level of thyroid hormone affects the nervous system, causing sympathomimetic symptoms such as brisk deep tendon reflexes, fine rapid tremor of the hands, restlessness, irritability, insomnia, dreams, nightmares, and rarely severe cognitive impairment and psychosis.

6. Answer: 3

Rationale: The American Diabetes Association recommends an A1C of <7% as an important treatment goal to decrease risk of long-term complications. A lab result of >8% A1C is an indication that action needs to be taken, either by a change in medication or a reinforcement of education.

7. Answer: 2

Rationale: Growth abnormalities are associated with anterior pituitary dysfunction and glucose intolerance with diabetes related to pancreatic dysfunction. Coagulation abnormalities and fatigue would be associated with hematologic dysfunction. Hypoxia would be associated with oxygenation problems and jaundice with liver or biliary problems. Steatorrhea is associated with malabsorption syndrome, cystic fibrosis, and other issues of the exocrine pancreas.

8. Answer: 2

Rationale: The primary care provider may obtain TSH, T_3, T_4, and T_7 levels and an ultrasound. Ordering antibody levels, thyroid scans, or fine-needle aspiration (FNA) biopsy should be done after coordination with the endocrine team. FNA aspirate is sent for cytology and interpretation.

9. Answer: 4

Rationale: The dexamethasone suppression test is the best screening test, and the 24-hour urine test for free cortisol is the best confirmatory test to use for Cushing's disease. Thyroid-stimulating hormone (TSH) and thyroxine (T_4) may also be appropriate to rule out a thyroid condition because some of the patient's signs and symptoms are consistent with thyroid dysfunction. Antinuclear antibody (ANA) and rheumatoid factor (RF) are ordered when rheumatoid arthritis or systemic lupus erythematosus (SLE) is suspected; however, the patient's clinical picture is not consistent with these conditions. The red blood cell (RBC) count would be done to rule out anemia, a potential problem for this patient based on the history of fatigue, but the rest of the clinical picture indicates more than anemia. No clinical findings support a calcium level being drawn.

10. Answer: 2

Rationale: Thyroid-stimulating hormone (TSH) levels should be decreased in a patient with Graves' disease because thyroid-stimulating immunoglobulins bind to TSH receptors, which increase thyroxine (T_4) synthesis and release, subsequently suppressing TSH levels.

11. Answer: 3

Rationale: The correct procedure is to use a 10-g (5.07 Semmes-Weinstein) filament and apply it to 10 sites on the foot (one on the top of the foot, nine on the heel, sole, and toes). The filament is applied perpendicular (90-degree angle) to the skin surface with sufficient force for 1.5 seconds to cause the filament to bend. The filament should not be allowed to slide across the skin or make repetitive contact with each test site. Randomizing the selection of test sites (start with great toe→heel→instep area→5th metatarsal) and the time between successive tests to reduce patient guessing and having the patient close the eyes is also helpful.

12. Answer: 3

Rationale: The American Diabetes Association has defined the diagnostic criteria for diabetes to include any one of the three following methods, which must be confirmed on a subsequent day:

- Random plasma glucose ≥200 mg/dL and acute symptoms (polyuria, polydipsia, polyphagia)

- Fasting plasma glucose ≥126 mg/dL

- Two-hour plasma glucose ≥200 mg/dL

- Hemoglobin A1C >6.5%

Disorders

13. Answer: 2

Rationale: Type 1 diabetes is caused by destruction of the beta cells mediated through the immune system. The other three choices refer to type 2 diabetes.

14. Answer: 4

Rationale: An annual eye exam with the pupils dilated should be done by a specialist who can recognize subtle abnormalities. Diabetic retinopathy is the most common eye disease for people with diabetes. Although the other referrals can offer important contributions to diabetic care, these would be done on an as-needed basis rather than annually.

15. Answer: 3

Rationale: Because of the normal menstrual periods and androgen plasma level, the hirsutism would be considered idiopathic. Diseases related to the ovaries would cause changes in the menstrual cycle and, with Cushing's syndrome, would be associated with adrenal androgen overproduction.

16. Answer: 4

Rationale: Testosterone production is regulated by the hypothalamic-pituitary-testicular (HPT) axis, so abnormalities in any of these areas can affect the production of testosterone.

17. Answer: 2

Rationale: It is important for patients with diabetes to have their feet inspected daily either by self-exam or by a family member. Feet should be washed daily but never soaked. Corns and calluses should receive a professional's care. Nails should be trimmed straight across to avoid injury to the nail beds.

18. Answer: 1

Rationale: An A1C of >8.0% indicates poor glucose control over the past few months. According to American Diabetic Association (ADA), an A1C of > 8.0% is equal to an average daily blood glucose of 355 mg/dL. The normal serum glucose for adults ranges from 70–120 mg/dL. Diabetic acidosis is not of concern until the glucose is >300 mg/dL.

19. Answer: 1

Rationale: True hypoglycemia can be organized around whether it is fasting or postprandial. Postprandial hypoglycemia may be caused by early adult-onset diabetes or postgastrectomy syndrome. Fasting hypoglycemia is most often caused by excessive doses of insulin, sulfonylureas alone, or with biguanides and thiazolidinediones.

20. Answer: 3

Rationale: The symptoms of lethargy, cold intolerance, weight gain, and yellowing of the palms suggest hypothyroidism, and thyroid studies (TSH) would be most useful.

21. Answer: 2

Rationale: This middle-aged female patient presents with many of the classic symptoms of early hyperthyroidism, e.g., tremulousness, racing pulse, difficulty falling asleep, weight loss despite a normal appetite, and feeling warm. A suppressed thyroid-stimulating hormone (TSH) with an elevated free T_4 establishes the diagnosis of hyperthyroidism.

22. Answer: 3

Rationale: The patient's physical findings and habitus, along with hypertension and hypokalemia, are associated with Cushing's syndrome, which is a state of excessive cortisol production due to a pituitary tumor. A Cushing's-like syndrome is often associated with prolonged glucocorticoid administration. Obesity is the primary finding in Cushing's syndrome, along with the "moon face," lipoma growths on the upper back, truncal obesity, hirsutism in women, and impotence and loss of body hair in men. Addison's disease is characterized by hyperkalemia, hyponatremia, hypoglycemia, anemia, and hypercalcemia. Patients with hypoaldosteronism (impaired renin secretion) have hyperkalemia. Pheochromocytoma would be in the differential diagnosis of this patient because of the hypertension; the other findings are not consistent with this diagnosis.

23. Answer: 3

Rationale: Low-dose antithyroid drugs are considered a good alternative to prevent the effects of hyperthyroidism on the mother and developing fetus until surgery can be performed. Another option is using an antithyroid drug until after delivery and then having surgery. Removal of the thyroid during the second trimester can be performed safely and is the usual recommendation. Replacement is essential after removal of the gland.

24. Answer: 4

Rationale: Accumulation of hyaluronic acid in interstitial tissues increases capillary permeability to albumin and causes the interstitial edema of the face and eyelids in patients with hypothyroidism.

25. Answer: 2

Rationale: Although alcohol abuse may be a cause of hypoglycemia, the patient is presenting with classic symptoms of postprandial hypoglycemia. Assessment for alcohol abuse as the etiology of the hypoglycemia would be advisable.

26. Answer: 2

Rationale: Hyperparathyroidism accounts for more than 60% of patients with hypercalcemia and is likely to be the explanation for elevated serum calcium levels.

27. Answer: 1

Rationale: Although depression may explain the weight gain, Cushing's disease is correct for the constellation of symptoms of rapid weight gain, hypertension, and elevated blood sugar. These symptoms suggest adrenal dysfunction. Serum cortisol and adrenocorticotropic hormone (ACTH) levels should be checked.

28. Answer: 1

Rationale: The woman is likely experiencing the life-threatening syndrome that can occur in decompensated hyperthyroidism. The clues are her symptom presentation and progression, the new "antidrug," and upcoming throat surgery. Although other possible causes of delirium are eventually considered, the family nurse practitioner needs to go with the probabilities of occurrence within the given context.

29. Answer: 3

Rationale: The symptoms (weight gain, lethargy, inability to tolerate cold temperatures, forgetfulness, hair loss, and constipation) describe the classic presentation of a patient with hypothyroidism. A patient with heart failure would have jugular venous distention, rales, and peripheral edema. The criteria for diagnosing diabetes mellitus are polydipsia, polyphagia, polyuria, and weight loss. Thyroid cancer typically presents without physical symptoms, and often the only physical finding is a hard, fixed nodule on the thyroid gland.

30. Answer: 2

Rationale: The patient's blood sugar levels are low around lunchtime, which is when the regular insulin is peaking (3–4 hours), so a reduction in the regular insulin would address this problem.

31. Answer: 1

Rationale: The family nurse practitioner's role in primary care for a patient with a thyroid nodule involves initially the early identification of the thyroid nodule on physical exam, referring the patient to an endocrinologist for further evaluation, and possibly obtaining some preliminary thyroid-stimulating hormone (TSH) and antibody testing. The endocrinologist performs the fine-needle aspiration (FNA). Levothyroxine may or may not be used to diminish the size of the nodule based on the findings from the FNA and the endocrinologist's chosen treatment plan.

32. Answer: 4

Rationale: Patients with diabetes must understand that when they are sick, blood glucose levels will probably increase, even when they are not eating. They need to monitor blood glucose levels every 2–4 hours. The medications metformin and acarbose should not be given until the patient's nausea and vomiting have subsided and the patient has resumed a normal diet (blood glucose monitoring is important during this time). Dehydration will increase the risk of metabolic acidosis for patients on metformin.

33. Answer: 2

Rationale: Graves' disease, an autoimmune condition also known as diffuse toxic goiter, is the most common cause of hyperthyroidism in this age group. Much less common causes include cancer of the thyroid, adenoma of the pituitary gland, and postpartum (or silent) thyroiditis.

34. Answer: 1

Rationale: The thyroid-stimulating hormone (TSH) level should be ordered to determine whether the patient is euthyroid, hypothyroid, or hyperthyroid. The patient should also be sent to an endocrinologist or surgeon because all nodules of the thyroid should be biopsied to rule out malignancy. "Watching and waiting" is inappropriate without having a biopsy performed. Thyroid hormone replacement therapy would be indicated only in patients found to be hypothyroid and in whom thyroid cancer has been ruled out. Thyroid ablation may be indicated in patients whose fine-needle aspiration (FNA) biopsy results are positive for thyroid cancer, but this cannot be determined without a surgeon's intervention.

35. Answer: 3

Rationale: Hypothyroidism often follows this treatment, with 50% of patients requiring replacement therapy in the first year and almost 100% requiring therapy in 10 years. For this reason, regular monitoring of thyroid-stimulating hormone (TSH) and T_4 levels should be performed. Patients emit a small amount of radioactivity after receiving the dose used to treat this condition and do not require isolation for 7 days. Radioactive iodine is very safe, without an increased risk of chromosomal abnormalities; therefore, no contraindication exists to becoming pregnant after therapy, although patients are counseled to avoid pregnancy during treatment and to avoid children and pregnant women after receiving the oral ablation dose. This therapy is recommended for patients who have cardiac disease associated with their thyroid condition.

36. Answer: 1

Rationale: Improper use of glucose increases the release of free fatty acids, which elevates triglycerides. The other values are still within normal limits.

37. Answer: 3

Rationale: Smoking causes thinning of the bones and can lead to osteopenia/osteoporosis. A diet high in calcium with minimal alcohol intake and walking are all self-care practices that may prevent or delay the onset of osteopenia/osteoporosis.

38. Answer: 3

Rationale: Low testosterone levels may result from prostate cancer treatment and longstanding liver disease. Smoking, excessive use of alcohol, and minimal exercise are risk factors of osteoporosis that can occur in both men and women.

39. Answer: 4

Rationale: Carbohydrate is the macronutrient with the greatest impact on the postprandial glucose levels. Ingested protein has minimal effect on the blood glucose levels. A diet high in fat may be associated with cardiovascular disease. Fiber has little effect on the plasma glucose response, but may result in decreased low-density lipoprotein (LDL) cholesterol.

Pharmacology

40. Answer: 1

Rationale: Incretin mimetic medications, such as exenatide, are associated with weight loss. Metformin is associated with weight neutrality and appetite suppression, although some patients may possibly lose weight. Glyburide is considered a second-generation sulfonylurea, which tends to stimulate insulin secretion from the pancreas, thus causing a weight gain.

Pioglitazone is an insulin sensitizer and increases glucose uptake in the muscle and fat. Common side effects include fluid retention and an increase in central adiposity.

41. Answer: 4

Rationale: Glargine is a long-acting basal insulin usually given once daily and lasts almost 24 hours without a peak. This clear insulin must be given alone and not mixed with other insulins in the same syringe. Lispro insulin is a rapid-acting insulin usually given 3 times daily with meals. A basal insulin can be used at the same time with a different injection. In rare cases, basal insulins are given more than once a day, but this is not usual practice.

42. Answer: 2

Rationale: Metformin should not be given to men with a serum creatinine level of ≥1.5 mg/dL and women with a serum creatinine level of ≥1.4 mg/dL, because it can predispose the patient to lactic acidosis. Pioglitazone and rapaglinide are metabolized primarily in the liver and require monitoring of liver function tests. Acarbose is metabolized mainly in the gastrointestinal tract.

43. Answer: 3

Rationale: Lactic acidosis is a potentially severe and fatal reaction to metformin. Metformin does not contribute to weight gain; it often helps with weight loss due to appetite suppression and decreases low-density lipoprotein (LDL), triglyceride levels, and insulin requirements.

44. Answer: 2

Rationale: Sulfonylureas reduce blood glucose by stimulating insulin release from the pancreas. Over time, these drugs also may actually increase insulin effects at the cellular level and decrease glucose production by the liver, which is why sulfonylureas are used in patients with type 2 diabetes who still have a functioning pancreas.

45. Answer: 1

Rationale: Anorexia, nausea, and a metallic taste in the mouth are common side effects. Over time, gastrointestinal (GI) symptoms subside and can be relieved by taking the medication with food or by starting at a lower dose. Metformin has a safety profile that does not include hypoglycemia unless mixed with other agents that trigger it.

46. Answer: 4

Rationale: Antithyroid medications (propylthiouracil; methimazole) are relatively inexpensive and do cross the placenta. The patient remains on the medications for 1–2 years with the hope of a permanent remission of symptoms when they are withdrawn.

47. Answer: 2

Rationale: Both of these drug classifications (diuretics and beta blockers) tend to reduce insulin sensitivity and can cause hyperglycemia. Angiotensin-converting enzyme (ACE) inhibitors, calcium channel blockers, and selective alpha blockers are metabolically neutral; some may actually have a beneficial effect.

48. Answer: 4

Rationale: The patient's symptoms indicate hypothyroidism, as does the elevated thyroid-stimulating hormone (TSH) level (normal levels are 0.5–4.7 mU/L). A full replacement dose of levothyroxine should be started based on the patient's age, and TSH level should be checked in 6 weeks, the time it may take for a given dose to become effective. Loading doses should never be given except for coma, which is treated by IV medication in the hospital.

49. Answer: 4

Rationale: Coronary disease patients found to be mildly to moderately hypothyroid can safely undergo urgent surgery (including bypass procedures) without prior replacement. The rate of complications is no greater than for nonhypothyroid patients, and the cardiac risks are less compared with initiating replacement therapy preoperatively.

50. Answer: 3

Rationale: Metformin is a better option in an obese patient because it is frequently associated with weight neutrality or even some weight loss, whereas sulfonylureas may actually cause weight gain. Insulin is now considered an option, but the use of a sliding scale is no longer current practice. Diet and exercise were unsuccessful, and the longer her blood sugar remains elevated, the greater the risk for end-organ damage. An A1C levels in this range (10%) requires aggressive treatment to decrease vascular complications.

51. Answer: 2

Rationale: Chronic overtreatment is associated with osteoporosis; the other options are related to acute overdose of levothyroxine and can be relieved by omitting the dose for 3 days and then starting on a lower dose.

52. Answer: 4

Rationale: To initiate treatment for elevated blood pressure (BP), it is recommended that three elevated readings be recorded on three separate occasions. No evidence suggests that this patient had increased BP on prior visits.

53. Answer: 1

Rationale: This is the best answer because the AM intermediate dose will affect the glucose level before dinner. Altering the regular insulin will affect levels before lunch and before bedtime; however, these levels are acceptable. To reduce the intermediate dose while maintaining the level of regular insulin, the patient will need to self-mix the intermediate and regular insulin, using less of the intermediate. A more modern approach is to use basal insulin plus mealtime rapid-acting insulins.

54. Answer: 4

Rationale: Pseudoephedrine and other decongestant medications that contain sympathomimetics lead to adverse reactions of central nervous system (CNS) overstimulation, palpitations, headache, hypertension, and nervousness. Guaifenesin in combination with dextromethorphan and phenylpropanolamine (Robitussin-CF) or pseudoephedrine (Robitussin-PE) can also cause palpitations and CNS overstimulation. Guaifenesin with dextromethorphan (Robitussin-DM) may cause gastrointestinal (GI) upset, drowsiness, headache, and rash. Many over-the-counter (OTC) medications also have an iodine component that may alter thyroid levels.

55. Answer: 2

Rationale: Infusion site problems and skin irritation are by far the most frequent complaints of patients who use an insulin pump and often why the pump is discontinued. Patients also find it is more time consuming and costly. However, the Diabetes Control and Complications Trial (DCCT, 1993) reported a reduced risk of microvascular complications when insulin pumps and multiple daily injections were used.

56. Answer: 3

Rationale: Pioglitazone and rosiglitazone act by decreasing peripheral insulin resistance in skeletal muscle and adipose tissue without enhancing insulin secretion and improving glucose tolerance in patients with type 2 diabetes. Prenatal patients are managed with insulin or metformin, not an insulin sensitizer. The action of α-glucosidase inhibitors, such as acarbose (Precose) and miglitol (Glyset), prevents the rapid postprandial blood glucose surges by delaying carbohydrate absorption (known as "starch blockers").

57. Answer: 3

Rationale: Older patients, especially with heart disease, need to be started on the smallest amount of thyroid medication replacement (0.025 mg, not 0.1 mg) and gradually increased until a therapeutic level is achieved. If thyroid replacement occurs too quickly, the heart may decompensate; 2 grains of thyroid extract is too much. Methimazole is an antithyroid medication used to treat hyperthyroidism.

58. Answer: 2

Rationale: The response to therapy is based on a clinical symptomatology and a thyroid-stimulating hormone (TSH) assay, approximately 4–6 weeks after the initiation of therapy. This is continued until a stable dose is obtained. TSH and a free T_4 level are the two standard tests that can be used to monitor the status of the thyroid; a levothyroxine level cannot be drawn. Levothyroxine is not a myelosuppressive.

59. Answer: 3

Rationale: Beta blockers are initially prescribed to reduce the signs and symptoms of the condition and to reduce the peripheral conversion of T_4 to triiodothyronine (T_3); nonsteroidal antiinflammatory drugs (NSAIDs) are indicated for reducing inflammation associated with thyroiditis; and antithyroid medications (propylthiouracil (PTU), methimazole) are used to treat severe hyperthyroidism. Corticosteroids are sometimes used in the treatment of thyroiditis, but the remaining classes (antibiotics, angiotensin-converting enzyme (ACE) inhibitors, calcium channel blockers, and anxiolytics) are not routinely used in the management of hyperthyroidism.

60. Answer: 3

Rationale: Decreasing the dose of levothyroxine and evaluating the patient's cardiac status are the appropriate interventions in this situation, in addition to quickly involving the other health care team members. Discontinuing the thyroid replacement would be inappropriate because the patient remains hypothyroid and requires therapy for life. An anxiolytic may be a helpful adjunct but is not appropriate as the sole intervention because it ignores the cardiac symptoms.

61. Answer: 1

Rationale: Lispro (Humalog) was the first analog of human insulin and has several advantages over regular insulin, including more rapid onset and shorter duration of action. It reaches peak activity in 1–2 hours and has a 4-hour duration, versus 6–8 hours for regular insulin. It is convenient because it can be injected immediately before eating (10–15 minutes). It is also more expensive than insulin, and some third-party payers may not reimburse patients.

62. Answer: 4

Rationale: Hypoglycemia and weight gain are the most common side effects of sulfonylurea therapy.

63. Answer: 3

Rationale: Pioglitazone and rosiglitazone are insulin sensitizers, which increase the glucose uptake in the muscle and fat. Metformin decreases hepatic glucose output. Oral sulfonylureas increase insulin secretion in the pancreas. The α-glucosidase inhibitors increase postprandial glucose uptake in the intestine.

64. Answer: 2

Rationale: DDAVP (desmopressin acetate) promotes reabsorption of water in the renal tubules, which can lead to water intoxication. The signs of water intoxication are lethargy, behavioral changes, disorientation, and neuromuscular excitability.

65. Answer: 2

Rationale: The earlier the intervention, the better the outcome for the patient with acromegaly. Although not a pancreatic-centered disorder, the oral glucose tolerance test (OGTT) is considered the best first-line diagnostic evaluation, except in patients with known diabetes who are uncontrolled. In normal patients, the values fall into normal ranges; in patients with acromegaly, growth hormone (GH) is suppressed by the blood sugar load. The GH level is drawn at the same time. Although thyroid enlargement can be part of a general organomegaly presentation, it is not the typical cause of this clinical presentation.

66. Answer: 3

Rationale: Although abnormal glucose control is a hallmark of Cushing's disease, it is typically in diabetic patients with a metabolic syndrome presentation, not in the type 1 group. Hypertension under good control is not linked to a steroid overproduction; it is the patient who does not respond to medication who is evaluated for adrenal issues. Bronchogenic and other small cell types of cancers have been known to produce "ectopic" steroids. The "moon face" of Cushing's is not the same as someone who is simply overweight.

67. Answer: 1, 3

Rationale: Bladder cancer, although rare, is linked with the selective sodium glucose cotransporters (SGLT-2) and the thiazolidinediones (TZD). Medullary cancer risk has prompted a black box for the glucagon-like peptide agonist (GLP-1) medications. The biguanides, incretin mimetics, and sulfonylureas do not have these black box warnings.

68. Answer 4

Rationale: Zoledronic acid (Zometa) is administered as an intravenous (IV) infusion. The others are all oral medications that carry the need to remain sitting upright to decrease the risk for esophageal irritation. The IV medication does require good hydration to decrease renal risks.

69. Answer: 2

Rationale: Nasally inhaled DDAVP (desmopressin) must have direct contact with the nasal mucosa for absorption. Secretions, especially those that are thicker, prevent this, so clearing the nasal passages with an effective nasal clearing blow will provide some additional time for "topical" absorption. There are no major problems with concurrent antihistamine use that would decrease the amount of secretions. The DDAVP is not taken orally, so the precaution about separation by 1 hour is not needed.

70. Answer: 1

Rationale: Test strips are proprietary to the specific monitor. Test strips are frequently not interchangeable, even in monitors from the same manufacturer. Similarly, lancets are specific to the device used to provide a skin puncture. Some newer monitors do not require frequent calibrations or a code number. Alcohol is not used to cleanse the digits, unless medically indicated. Serum, capillary, and deeper puncture glucose values do vary, especially over time.

71. Answer: 3

Rationale: Naturally occurring insulin has a C-peptide bond, which is removed during the processing of exogenous insulin as a drug. Classically, a type 1 patient has no C-peptide bonds because all circulating insulin is from exogenous sources. In comparison, a type 2 patient is expected to have some innate insulin production so C-peptides should be present. The hemoglobin A1C or glycosylated fructose can be used for either patient group. The Apo A and B levels deal with lipid values, not sugars. It should be noted that newer research states that some type 1 patients actually produce a bit of natural insulin, especially after the initial period, so the C-peptide laboratory is not the absolute determinant of disease status.

72. Answer: 4

Rationale: Although the reduction of hypertension is important to renal health, the angiotensin-converting enzyme (ACE) inhibitors and some selected angiotensin II receptor blocker (ARBs) agents have a "renal protective" effect apart from the vascular tension issue. This does not extend to their direct renin inhibitor "cousins." There may be some positive impact from the sodium glucose co-transporter (SGLT-2) group, but more research is needed.

73. Answer: 2, 3

The risk of low blood sugar is greatest with the oldest of the diabetic remedies. This is especially true when insulins are mixed with sulfonylureas. The relative lack of hypoglycemic episodes with the other drug groups makes them a safer alternative.

Musculoskeletal

10

Physical Exam & Diagnostic Tests

1. A goniometer is a measurement device used in the musculoskeletal exam of a patient. The family nurse practitioner uses this tool to determine:

   1. Strength of the muscles in the extremities.

   2. Degree of joint flexion and extension.

   3. Range of motion of the extremities.

   4. Point of joint flexion that is painful.

2. The family nurse practitioner places a patient in the prone position with the knee flexed 90 degrees. The tibia is firmly opposed to the femur by exerting downward pressure on the foot. The leg is rotated externally and internally. If locking of the knee occurs, this is accurately called a positive:

   1. Drawer sign.

   2. McMurray's test.

   3. Apley's sign.

   4. Bulge sign.

3. A patient has numbness and tingling in the thumb and first two fingers when pressing the backs of the hands together (flexes wrists at 90 degrees) for 60 seconds. This is a positive:

   1. Tinel's sign.

   2. Drawer sign.

   3. McMurray's test.

   4. Phalen's maneuver.

4. What is the sign that occurs when compressing the suprapatellar pouch back against the femur and feeling for fluid entering the spaces?

   1. Drawer sign.

   2. Kernig's sign.

   3. Balloon sign.

   4. Bulge sign.

5. De Quervain's tenosynovitis can be diagnosed in part by a positive:

   1. Finkelstein's sign.

   2. Tinel's sign.

   3. Phalen's maneuver.

   4. Lachman's sign.

6. The primary exam techniques used for assessing the musculoskeletal system are:

   1. Inspection and percussion.

   2. Auscultation and palpation.

   3. Inspection and palpation.

   4. Palpation and percussion.

7. What criteria can the family nurse practitioner use to confirm a diagnosis of polymyalgia rheumatica (PMR)?

   1. Chest radiograph showing pulmonary hyperinflation, asymmetric joint pain, and an elevated serum C-reactive protein (CRP).

   2. Serum protein electrophoresis, clonal bone marrow plasma cells ≥10% or biopsy-proven bony or soft tissue plasmacytoma, and presence of related organ or tissue impairment.

   3. Corticosteroid challenge, ESR >40 mm/hr, proximally and bilaterally distributed aching, morning stiffness (lasting at least 30 minutes or more) persisting for at least 2 weeks, and age 50 years or older.

   4. ESR <40 mm/hr, emitting seronegative symmetric synovitis with pitting edema and tremor with rigidity

8. When performing an assessment, the family nurse practitioner understands that the metacarpophalangeal (MCP) joints are frequently involved with:

    1. Gout.

    2. Rheumatic fever.

    3. Rheumatoid arthritis (RA).

    4. Osteoarthritis (OA).

9. In the evaluation of polyneuropathy, which study would **not** be recommended?

    1. ESR.

    2. CBC.

    3. HgbA1C.

    4. EMG.

10. In accurately assessing a patient who reports a back injury, it is critical to question:

    1. Family history of back problems.

    2. Previous injury.

    3. Personal history of chronic illness.

    4. Mechanism of injury.

11. Tinel's sign and Phalen's maneuver are used in identifying a common workplace condition that the family nurse practitioner recognizes as:

    1. Lateral epicondylitis.

    2. Carpal tunnel syndrome.

    3. Dupuytren's disease.

    4. Thoracic outlet syndrome.

12. An older adult patient complains of fatigue, weakness, lightheadedness, and anorexia. He also complains of hot, swollen proximal interphalangeal (PIP) and metacarpophalangeal (MCP) joints. These symptoms occurred 5 months ago and recurred a few days ago. Which laboratory findings would be most conclusive of these assessments?

    1. High mean corpuscular volume (MCV), low serum ferritin.

    2. Normal mean corpuscular volume (MCV), high serum ferritin.

    3. Elevation in uric acid level.

    4. Elevation in white blood cell (WBC) count.

13. How is the talar tilt test conducted?

    1. The tibia is grasped with one hand, and backward pressure is applied to the heel.

    2. The ankle is gently inverted, and laxity of the ligament is graded.

    3. The examiner passively inverts, everts, dorsiflexes, and plantar-flexes the ankle.

    4. The patient actively inverts, everts, dorsiflexes, and plantar-flexes the ankle.

14. Varus pressure on a knee that is slightly flexed (30 degrees) tests:

    1. Medial collateral ligament stability.

    2. Lateral collateral ligament stability.

    3. Medial cruciate ligament stability.

    4. Lateral meniscus tear.

Disorders

15. The family nurse practitioner realizes that the most common cause of shoulder pain is:

    1. Frozen shoulder.

    2. Thoracic outlet syndrome.

    3. Impingement syndrome.

    4. Osteoarthritis.

16. A 45-year-old female complains of knee pain when kneeling and a "clicking" noise when walking up steps. The family nurse practitioner notes slight knee effusion and tenderness when palpating the patella against the condyles. The diagnosis for this patient is:

    1. Anterior cruciate tear.

    2. Dislocated patella.

    3. Chondromalacia patella.

    4. Patellar tendonitis.

17. A patient has been diagnosed with a complete rotator cuff tear of the left shoulder. The nurse would expect the patient to have difficulty in:

    1. Abducting the left arm.

    2. Supinating the left forearm.

    3. Shrugging the shoulders.

    4. Touching the left hand to the right shoulder.

18. A patient has been diagnosed with polymyalgia rheumatica (PMR). The family nurse practitioner understands that this disorder is:

    1. An autoimmune, multisystem problem in which the body makes antibodies to its own proteins.

    2. A degenerative disorder with no inflammatory changes in which joint cartilage wears away with age and eventually causes bone spurs.

    3. An inflammatory disorder involving the axial skeleton and large peripheral joints.

    4. An inflammatory connective tissue disorder that primarily affects older women and is associated with giant cell (temporal) arteritis.

19. In teaching a patient about fibromyalgia, the family nurse practitioner includes what information?

    1. Diagnostic studies such as ESR and CBC are important tools to confirm disease progression.

    2. Avoid stretching exercises and daily low-impact aerobics.

    3. Take ibuprofen (Motrin) 200 mg q4–6h prn for pain and amitriptyline (Elavil) 10 mg 1–2 hours before bedtime.

    4. Apply heat or massage "trigger points" to reduce pain.

20. The family nurse practitioner understands that chronic synovitis with pannus formation is the basic pathophysiologic finding in patients with:

    1. Systemic lupus erythematosus (SLE).

    2. Ankylosing spondylitis (AS).

    3. Rheumatoid arthritis (RA).

    4. Osteoarthritis (OA).

21. The family nurse practitioner is examining a patient who is complaining of pain in her hips and knees. She has a history of osteoarthritis. On exam, the joints are painful to movement and are warm to touch. The best immediate therapy for this patient is:

    1. Physical therapy for range of motion of affected areas.

    2. Decreased physical activity and immobilizing splints for affected joints.

    3. Moist heat and/or cold therapy on painful joints.

    4. ESR to determine level of activity.

22. The history of a patient who may have contracted Lyme disease may include what characteristic?

    1. Erythematous rash on bridge of nose and cheeks with discoid patches on the trunk.

    2. Immediate development of arthritis symptoms, especially in the knees.

    3. Expanding rash with central clearing within a month of being bitten.

    4. Early symptoms of meningitis and myocarditis.

23. The family nurse practitioner understands that finding Heberden's nodes on physical exam of a patient is a cardinal sign of:

    1. Septic arthritis.

    2. Rheumatoid arthritis (RA).

    3. Gouty arthritis.

    4. Osteoarthritis.

24. Competing diagnoses for an adult male patient who presents with acute onset of unilateral inflammation, pain, and erythema of the first metatarsophalangeal (MTP) joint could be:

    1. Gout, cellulitis, and osteoporosis.

    2. Cellulitis, rheumatoid arthritis, and gout.

    3. Osteoporosis, fibromyalgia, and cellulitis.

    4. Septic arthritis, rheumatoid arthritis, and osteoarthritis.

25. Diseases that often present as polyarthritic disorders include:

    1. Lyme arthritis, rheumatic heart disease, ankylosing spondylitis, and psoriatic arthritis.

    2. Rheumatoid arthritis (RA), gout, Reiter's syndrome, and osteoarthritis.

    3. Gonococcal arthritis, systemic lupus erythematosus (SLE), and septic arthritis.

    4. Polymyalgia rheumatica (PMR), Lyme arthritis, pseudogout, and psoriatic arthritis.

26. A common injury can most often cause a meniscus tear under which circumstances?

    1. The knee is almost completely extended, and the tibia is externally rotated.

    2. An applied external force is sufficiently strong to cause external rotation or hyperextension of the knee.

    3. Valgus or varus pressure on the knee occurs at full extension and at 30 degrees of flexion.

    4. The knee is simultaneously twisted and flexed during an injury.

27. Pain in a lumbosacral strain typically begins:

    1. Immediately with the injury.

    2. 1–2 hours after injury.

    3. 6–8 hours after injury.

    4. 12–36 hours after injury.

28. An acute onset of pain that descends down to the lower leg and foot of a 25-year-old obese adult is likely to be a symptom of:

    1. Lumbosacral strain.

    2. Herniated intervertebral disc injury.

    3. Osteomyelitis.

    4. Osteoporosis.

29. The family nurse practitioner sees a patient with trauma to the knee that caused it to "give out," followed by severe pain and effusion. Later, he had "locking" of the knee with pivoting or turning. This patient has probably suffered:

    1. Patellofemoral stress syndrome.

    2. Growing pains.

    3. Shin splints.

    4. Patellar subluxation.

30. A patient with patellofemoral syndrome has quadriceps setting as a recommended exercise. The family nurse practitioner would teach the patient to:

    1. Lie supine on the floor with legs extended, dorsiflex the foot, and push the thigh into the floor.

    2. Sit on the floor leaning back on the elbows, flex one knee to 90 degrees, and extend the other completely and hold for 5 seconds.

    3. Lie on the floor and flex both knees to about 20 degrees with a rolled towel underneath them, and extend one leg and hold for 5 seconds.

    4. Use resistive exercises with an elastic band.

31. Which risk factor is associated with gout?

    1. Female gender.

    2. Age 20 years.

    3. Ingestion of salicylate medications.

    4. Overuse of extremity.

32. A third-degree ankle sprain is associated with:

    1. Minimal ecchymosis, moderate edema, and a stable joint.

    2. Moderate ecchymosis, moderate edema, and an unstable joint.

    3. Marked ecchymosis, marked edema, and a stable joint.

    4. Marked ecchymosis, marked edema, and an unstable joint.

33. A patient with rheumatoid arthritis presents for follow-up. What is the best evaluative question the family nurse practitioner can ask that will help determine the severity of the disease?

    1. "Were you able to drive the car to your appointment today?"

    2. "Were you able to fix your dinner last night?"

    3. "How long does it take for your joints to loosen up after you get up in the morning?"

    4. "How many pounds can you carry?"

34. A 35-year-old woman is seen with a complaint of diffuse musculoskeletal pain, stiffness, and fatigue for the past 3 months. The pain is worse in the morning and also with changes in weather. She states she wakes up in the morning feeling tired. Physical exam is normal except for pain on digital palpation in 12 tender points. Laboratory results are unremarkable. The most likely diagnosis is:

    1. Fibromyalgia.

    2. Myofascial syndrome.

    3. Rheumatoid arthritis (RA).

    4. Depression.

35. When counseling a postmenopausal female patient on prevention of osteoporosis, all of the following are therapeutic recommendations except:

    1. Cessation of smoking.

    2. Daily intake of 200 mg of calcium and 40 IU of vitamin D.

    3. Continue hormone therapy.

    4. Monitor bone loss by dual-energy x-ray absorptiometry (DEXA) every 1–2 years.

36. A patient tells the family nurse practitioner that she has a "whiplash." The family nurse practitioner understands that this is:

    1. Cervical facet joint dysfunction.

    2. Cervical disc injury.

    3. Zygapophyseal joint injury.

    4. Cervical strain.

37. A patient presents with a complaint of sudden pain and swelling in the knee unrelated to an injury. He also has chills and fever. On exam, the knee is warm, tender, and swollen with evidence of effusion. What action would the family nurse practitioner take?

    1. Splint the affected joint.

    2. Obtain aspiration of synovial fluid from the affected joint.

    3. Initiate treatment with nonsteroidal anti-inflammatory drugs (NSAIDs).

    4. Recommend rest, ice, compression, and elevation of affected joint.

38. When determining the specific etiology of polyarticular complaints, which clinical clues are most helpful for diagnosis?

    1. Laboratory identification of antinuclear antibodies (ANA) and ESR.

    2. Radiograph of affected joints.

    3. Affected joint pattern and presence or lack of inflammation.

    4. Sexual history of patient.

39. A patient with ankylosing spondylitis (AS) is receiving education on managing her disease. The family nurse practitioner would teach the patient all of the following except:

    1. Regular exercise program.

    2. Maintenance systemic corticosteroid therapy.

    3. Use of indomethacin (Indocin) for discomfort.

    4. Observation for signs and symptoms of iritis.

40. An adult patient comes to the office complaining of foot pain. He can recall no specific injury but gives a history of being an occasional runner who drinks 6 to 10 beers on weekends. What physical findings would the family nurse practitioner expect to find?

    1. Redness, swelling, and warmth of first metatarsophalangeal joint.

    2. Swelling, ecchymosis, and decreased range of motion of ankle.

    3. Swelling of foot and decreased circulation.

    4. Decreased range of motion of ankle and obvious bone deformity.

41. Which of the diet selections indicate that the older patient understands the health education regarding the prevention of osteoporosis?

    1. Chicken and baked potato.

    2. Glass of skim milk and toasted cheese sandwich.

    3. Hamburger and salad.

    4. Fruit with whipped cream.

42. During the history, which of the following questions would best assist the family nurse practitioner in diagnosing osteoarthritis (OA) versus rheumatoid arthritis (RA)?

    1. "Is your joint pain symmetric and localized?"

    2. "Does your morning stiffness usually last several hours?"

    3. "Have you experienced fatigue, weakness, and weight loss?"

    4. "Is your joint pain asymmetric and worse with movement and relieved by rest?"

43. The number-one cause of disability in adults under age 45 is:

    1. Cancer.

    2. Fracture.

    3. Low back pain.

    4. Migraines.

44. Primary treatment of joint injury involves:

    1. Rest, ice, compression, and elevation.

    2. Narcotic pain control and radiograph.

    3. Specialist referral and magnetic resonance imaging.

    4. Nonsteroidal anti-inflammatory drugs (NSAIDs) and exercise.

45. The most common complaint in a patient with back injury who had cauda equina syndrome, a surgical emergency, is:

    1. Urinary retention.

    2. Numbness below the level of injury.

    3. Weakness in the lower extremities.

    4. Leg pain.

46. Recognition of annular tears is important in the diagnosis of back pain because:

    1. They require immediate surgery.

    2. They are often misdiagnosed as strain or sprain, leading to herniation.

    3. They result in rapid paralysis.

    4. Radiograph would reveal them, but x-rays are usually not ordered initially.

47. What chronic musculoskeletal problem may occur after an injury, is characterized by a 3-month history of pain on both sides of body (above and below waist), and tenderness in at least 11 of 18 specified points?

    1. Chronic osteoarthritis.

    2. Reflex sympathetic dystrophy.

    3. Tendinitis.

    4. Fibromyalgia.

48. Which patient is at highest risk for osteoporosis?

    1. A 55-year-old male smoker and retired athlete.

    2. A 60-year-old, 105-lb, postmenopausal white female switchboard operator.

    3. A 42-year-old black female intensive care nurse who is lactose intolerant.

    4. A 50-year-old obese white woman with three children living on a farm.

49. A 38-year-old secretary complains of pain in her hands at night. On exam, the family nurse practitioner notes wasting of the thenar eminence of both hands and dry skin on the thumb, index, and middle fingers. The family nurse practitioner suspects:

    1. Carpal tunnel syndrome.

    2. Transient ischemic attack.

    3. Osteoarthritis.

    4. Raynaud's phenomenon.

50. A 53-year-old woman presents with complaints of morning stiffness in the neck and back. She has pelvic and shoulder pain and fatigue. Her laboratory studies reveal elevated ESR, normal rheumatoid factor, normal creatine phosphokinase, and normochromic normocytic anemia. Physical exam reveals an elevated temperature, bilateral pain, and stiffness of the pectoral and pelvic muscles. Based on this information, the most appropriate diagnosis is:

    1. Polyarteritis nodosa.

    2. Wegener's granulomatosis.

    3. Polymyalgia rheumatica (PMR).

    4. Rheumatoid arthritis.

51. A 55-year-old woman with a prior diagnosis of polymyalgia rheumatica (PMR) presents with headache, low-grade fever, aching, stiffness, fatigue, malaise, and anorexia. Based on the information, the family nurse practitioner would make a preliminary diagnosis of:

    1. Influenza.

    2. Pneumonia.

    3. Temporal arteritis.

    4. Rheumatoid arthritis.

52. A man comes into the clinic complaining of low back pain that radiates down the lateral thigh. The pain began suddenly on the job after lifting a heavy object. The family nurse practitioner would further evaluate the patient for which three conditions:

    1. Compression fracture of lower lumbar vertebrae.

    2. Piriformis syndrome.

    3. Spinal cord injury.

    4. Compression of a lumbar disc.

    5. History of spinal cord injury.

53. An 80-year-old resident of a long-term care facility with a history of multiinfarct dementia (MID) is alert but disoriented to person, place, and situation. His only health problems are MID and osteoarthritis. Over the past 2 weeks he has become agitated and exit seeking and is constantly rubbing his knees. The family nurse practitioner suspects that the patient is experiencing:

    1. Worsening dementia.

    2. Pain.

    3. Urinary tract infection (UTI).

    4. Acute cerebral infarct.

Pharmacology

54. The family nurse practitioner is seeing a middle-aged, severely arthritic woman receiving maintenance therapy of prednisone 10 mg/day for the past 6 weeks. She now presents as acutely ill with signs and symptoms of acute pneumonia. She is fatigued and weak with loss of appetite, and blood pressure (BP) is lower than on previous visits. Which action should be taken in regard to prednisone?

    1. Immediately discontinue the medication.

    2. Increase dosage to 60 mg/day, then taper back to 10 mg/day.

    3. Gradually taper from 10 to 1 mg/day.

    4. Maintain dose at 10 mg/day.

55. What is the initial drug of choice for a patient with rheumatoid arthritis (RA)?

    1. NSAIDs.

    2. Aspirin.

    3. Methotrexate.

    4. Hydrocortisone.

56. A patient with rheumatoid arthritis (RA) is placed on prednisone 5 mg PO qd. In teaching the patient about her medication, it would be important for the family nurse practitioner to include what information?

    1. When the symptoms of arthritis subside, she will be able to quit taking her medication.

    2. It is important to take the medication as prescribed, even after the redness and swelling decrease.

    3. Increased fluid intake is important to prevent renal damage by the steroids.

    4. The medication should be taken about 30 minutes before eating.

57. What is the correct drug therapy for an adult with an acute episode of gout?

    1. Indomethacin (Indocin) 25 mg PO prn.

    2. Naproxen (Naprosyn) 100 mg PO bid.

    3. Colchicine 0.6 mg 2 tablets PO × 1, then repeat in 1 hour × 1.

    4. Indomethacin (Indocin) 50 mg q8h × 6–8 doses, then 25 mg q8h until resolution.

58. If a 24-hour urine test indicates that a patient is secreting too much uric acid (>900 mg/day), the family nurse practitioner would prescribe:

    1. Aspirin 325 mg PO qd.

    2. Tylenol 325 mg PO q4–6h prn.

    3. Indomethacin (Indocin) 25 mg PO q8h, then increase at weekly intervals by 25 mg daily.

    4. Allopurinol (Zyloprim) 100 mg PO qd × 1 week, then increase daily dose by 100 mg to a maximum of 300 mg/day.

59. Disease-modifying drugs for rheumatoid arthritis in adults include:

    1. Ibuprofen (Motrin, Advil), sulindac (Clinoril), and salicylates (aspirin, Disalcid).

    2. Corticosteroids (prednisone, methylprednisolone).

    3. Misoprostol (Cytotec).

    4. Hydroxychloroquine (Plaquenil), sulfasalazine (Azulfidine), methotrexate, and gold sodium thiomalate (Myochrysine).

60. Gold compounds are contraindicated in patients with all of the following conditions except:

    1. Renal disease.

    2. Hepatic disease.

    3. Rheumatoid arthritis.

    4. Blood dyscrasia.

61. The most appropriate medication used to control pain for a patient with osteoarthritis would be:

    1. Acetaminophen.

    2. Systemic corticosteroids.

    3. Gold salts.

    4. Misoprostol.

62. What is a serious side effect of ibuprofen in the older adult patient?

    1. Rebound headaches.

    2. Impairment of renal function.

    3. Neuropathy.

    4. Pancreatic failure.

63. A patient has been on methotrexate (Rheumatrex) for 6 weeks. This was the medication of choice for her severe refractory rheumatoid arthritis (RA). What parameters should the family nurse practitioner monitor?

    1. Monthly platelet count, CBC with differential.

    2. Urinalysis, blood sugar, and ECG every 2 weeks.

    3. Monthly CBC, urinalysis, and electrolytes.

    4. Coagulation studies, electrolytes, and CBC every week.

64. A middle-aged male patient presents with a complaint of waking up yesterday morning with a swollen and painful big toe. The patient reports he has "never had anything like this before" and has not had previous health problems. On exam, the big toe is red, hot, and tender in the joint with inflammation extending into the surrounding tissue. His temperature is 99.8°F (37.7°C) and WBC count is mildly elevated. Needle aspiration of joint fluid reveals urate crystals. What is the best treatment choice that the family nurse practitioner could recommend for the patient?

    1. Bed rest, very-low-calorie diet, and increased fluid intake.

    2. Allopurinol (Zyloprim) 200 mg PO qd, continuing dose for maintenance therapy once symptoms resolve.

    3. Naproxen (Naprosyn) 500 mg PO tid, continuing full-dose until symptoms resolve, then tapering and discontinuing over 72 hours.

    4. Injection of intra-articular corticosteroid to the affected joint.

65. An older adult woman comes into the clinic complaining of "sores" in her mouth. The family nurse practitioner observes several inflamed ulcers on her gums and lips. Which medication would the nurse identify as most likely to cause this problem?

    1. Propranolol (Inderal).

    2. Spironolactone (Aldactone).

    3. Fexofenadine (Allegra).

    4. Alendronate (Fosamax).

Physical Exam & Diagnostic Tests

1. Answer: 2

Rationale: The goniometer is used to determine the degree of joint flexion and extension or joint range of motion.

2. Answer: 3

Rationale: Apley's sign, locking of the knee, or the sound of clicks and pain may indicate a torn meniscus. The drawer sign tests the cruciate ligaments with the patient in a sitting and lying, not prone, position. McMurray's test assesses for medial meniscus injury when the knee is fully flexed and the tibia is externally rotated, with varus pressure applied to the knee while extended. For medial meniscus tear, the test is performed while applying valgus pressure to the knee.

3. Answer: 4

Rationale: Phalen's maneuver, when present, suggests carpal tunnel syndrome. Tinel's sign also tests for carpal tunnel syndrome but is performed by lightly percussing over the median nerve on the volar (palmar) side of the wrist, with characteristic tingling or shocklike sensations across the palm, thumb, and first two fingers. Drawer sign and McMurray's test are used to assess the knee.

4. Answer: 3

Rationale: The balloon sign occurs when considerable fluid is in the suprapatellar pouch, with possible ballottement of the patella. The bulge sign is for testing fluid in the knee joint and is elicited with the knee extended by applying pressure to the medial aspect and watching for a bulge or fluid wave. A patellar tap suggests fluid in the knee as the patella clicks against the femur. The drawer sign tests the cruciate ligaments with the patient in a sitting and lying position. Kernig's sign for meningeal irritation is the inability to extend the lower leg when that leg is flexed at the hip, or there may be resistance or pain during elicitation of the sign.

5. Answer: 1

Rationale: Pain with gentle deviation of a fist (thumb tucked under other four fingers) to the ulnar side is a positive Finkelstein's sign and an indication of De Quervain's disease, which is swelling and tenderness over the volar portion of the "snuffbox" resulting from chronic tenosynovitis. A positive Tinel's sign (tapping gently over carpal tunnel causing tingling in thumb, index finger, and middle and radial half of ring finger) and positive Phalen's maneuver (holding dorsum of hands

flexed 90 degrees back to back with the same distribution of tingling) are indicative of carpal tunnel syndrome. Lachman's sign indicates stability of the cruciate ligament of the knee.

6. Answer: 3

Rationale: The musculoskeletal system is examined by a visual inspection and palpation of the bones, joints, and surrounding musculoskeletal soft tissue. Percussion is generally not done, and auscultation is not appropriate to the system being examined.

7. Answer: 3

Rationale: Patients with polymyalgia rheumatica (PMR) have a rapid, dramatic clinical response to corticosteroid therapy. The serum protein electrophoresis is used to rule out myeloma. The erythrocyte sedimentation rate (ESR) is elevated in a number of diseases and is not specific to PMR. The chest radiograph is used to diagnose diseases affecting the lungs and thorax. The serum C-reactive protein (CRP) would be elevated in PMR.

8. Answer: 3

Rationale: The wrist, metacarpophalangeal (MCP), proximal interphalangeal (PIP) joints, and other small joint of the hands and feet are involved with rheumatoid arthritis (RA). The great toe is most often involved with gout. The large joints of the hip, knee, and shoulder along with the distal interphalangeal (DIP) joint and base of the thumb are involved with degenerative joint disease (osteoarthritis).

9. Answer: 2

Rationale: It would not be necessary to obtain a complete blood count (CBC). The hemoglobin A (HgbA1C) would be ordered to evaluate the relative control of diabetes. The electromyography (EMG) is most often performed to evaluate both nerve conduction and needle electrode exam. Many toxins and inflammatory processes are involved with polyneuropathy, so erythrocyte sedimentation rate (ESR) would be a helpful diagnostic tool for identifying the inflammatory process, even though it is a nonspecific test for the condition.

10. Answer: 4

Rationale: A thorough history is very important in assessing any patient with an injury, but with a back injury, the mechanism will provide the best indication as to the extent of the injury and the proper diagnostic and treatment approach. Determining loss of bowel or bladder control could indicate an emergent condition, cauda equina syndrome.

11. Answer: 2

Rationale: Carpal tunnel syndrome, a compression neuropathy of the median nerve at the wrist, is commonly caused by repetitive finger and wrist motion and results in positive Tinel's sign and Phalen's maneuver. Tinel's sign is considered positive when tapping over the nerve with a reflex hammer causes tingling in the distribution of the nerve. Phalen's maneuver is performed by fully flexing the wrist passively and noting tingling in the thumb or fingers.

12. Answer: 2

Rationale: The clinical assessments point to a chronic inflammatory process, such as rheumatoid arthritis (RA). The dizziness, fatigue, lightheadedness, and weakness may be a problem with anemia. The anemia of chronic disease is either a microcytic or normocytic anemia. The value that differentiates the anemia of chronic disease from other anemias is the serum ferritin (iron stores). The value will be either normal or high. The mean corpuscular volume (MCV) of 104 indicates a macrocytic anemia, which would not include the anemia of chronic disease. The low serum ferritin would not be considered a possibility with this disorder. The uric acid level would be elevated in gout. The white blood cell (WBC) count does not address the signs of anemia.

13. Answer: 2

Rationale: The talar tilt test detects excessive ankle inversion. Anterior ankle stability is tested in the anterior drawer test, in which the tibia is grasped by the examiner's one hand while the heel is firmly grasped, and backward pressure is applied to the tibia with the examiner's other hand. In passive range of motion, the examiner inverts, everts, dorsiflexes, and plantarflexes the foot and ankle. The patient puts the foot and ankle through the complete range in active range of motion.

14. Answer: 2

Rationale: Varus pressure on a slightly flexed knee tests for lateral collateral ligament stability. Valgus pressure tests for medial collateral ligament stability. Cruciate ligaments are tested with the anterior drawer test. McMurray's test assesses for medial meniscus injury when the knee is fully flexed and the tibia is externally rotated, with varus pressure applied to the knee while extended.

Disorders

15. Answer: 3

Rationale: Impingement syndrome is usually caused by rotator cuff tendinitis, which occurs when internal/external rotation is impaired. Frozen shoulder can occur after a rotator cuff injury, especially if a sling is used for a prolonged period. With Adson's or Wright's maneuver, thoracic outlet syndrome would indicate a decrease or loss of the radial pulse when the patient abducts the arm and holds a deep breath while simultaneously hyperextending the neck and turning the chin toward the raised arm.

16. Answer: 3

Rationale: These are common symptoms of chondromalacia patella. With anterior cruciate tears, the patient generally cannot bear weight on the extremity without its buckling or giving way. With a dislocated patella, the patient would have severe pain associated with considerable effusion (loss of normal knee hollow on sides of patella) and possible patellofemoral compartment. Patellar tendonitis, or jumper's knee, causes pain, weakness, and swelling of the knee joint, but no "clicking" noises.

17. Answer: 1

Rationale: With a complete rotator cuff tear (rupture of supraspinatus tendon), the patient would have difficulty abducting the arm and impaired internal/external rotation. Touching the hand to the opposite shoulder is adduction.

18. Answer: 4

Rationale: Polymyalgia rheumatica (PMR) is an inflammatory connective tissue disorder that primarily affects older women and is associated with giant cell (temporal) arteritis. Anemia is common in PMR, along with an elevated erythrocyte sedimentation rate (ESR). There is a common complaint of morning stiffness; rheumatoid factor is negative. An autoimmune, multisystem disorder is characteristic of systemic lupus erythematosus (SLE). A degenerative joint disorder is characteristic of osteoarthritis. An inflammatory disorder involving the axial skeleton and large peripheral joints is characteristic of ankylosing spondylitis.

19. Answer: 3

Rationale: Diagnostic studies are of little value and benefit, except to rule out other causes, such as polymyalgia rheumatica (PMR) or hypothyroidism. Treatment is symptomatic; the usual drugs are amitriptyline (Elavil), nonsteroidal antiinflammatory drugs (NSAIDs), tramadol (Ultram), cyclobenzaprine (Flexeril), temazepam (Restoril), zolpidem (Ambien), pregabalin (Lyrica), duloxetine (Cymbalta), and triazolam (Halcion). Daily, slow, low-impact aerobics, preferably in the late afternoon or early evening, is encouraged. Heat and massage are helpful but not on the "trigger points."

20. Answer: 3

Rationale: The chronic inflammatory disorder of rheumatoid arthritis (RA) has synovial hypertrophy from chronic synovitis and pannus formation that results in progressive destruction of the cartilage, ligament, tendons, and bone. Ankylosing spondylitis (AS) usually involves the large peripheral joints (e.g., sacroiliac) and is characterized by extreme kyphosis. There is no inflammation with osteoarthritis (OA). Systemic lupus erythematosus (SLE) has a distribution of symptoms similar to that of RA but no pannus formation.

21. Answer: 3

Rationale: Moist heat or cold, whichever relieves the pain more effectively, is appropriate to use on acutely affected joints. Physical therapy is recommended after the acute involvement of the joint; care must be taken to decrease repetitive movements. Immobilization is avoided because it tends to increase the stiffness of the joint. The erythrocyte sedimentation rate (ESR) is not an appropriate indicator to determine the level of activity in patients with osteoarthritis.

22. Answer: 3

Rationale: Expanding rash with central clearing may also be described as the "bull's-eye rash," which is associated with Lyme disease. An erythematous rash on the bridge of the nose and checks describes the malar or "butterfly" rash of systemic lupus erythematosus (SLE). The arthritis symptoms and other complications (meningitis and myocarditis) occur later in the disease process, especially if the patient is not treated with antibiotics, usually tetracycline, doxycycline, or amoxicillin.

23. Answer: 4

Rationale: Deformities (bony protuberances) of the distal interphalangeal joints (DIP) are called Heberden's nodes and are cardinal signs of osteoarthritis. The DIP joints are seldom involved with rheumatoid arthritis (RA). Gouty arthritis most often affects the great toe. Joints are warm, red, tender, and swollen with septic arthritis.

24. Answer: 2

Rationale: Cellulitis usually presents with warm, erythematous, painful areas of the skin. Symptoms of erythema, edema, and pain of the first metatarsophalangeal (MTP) joint are a common presentation for gout. Symptoms present in rheumatoid arthritis (RA) are similar: red, swollen, and painful joint(s). The inflammation of RA is usually symmetric but can present as erythematous, swollen joints. Systemic symptoms may also be present. Osteoporosis most often occurs in postmenopausal women because of bone loss that occurs with the decline of the estrogen in the blood. Bone thinning leads to fractures, not inflammation of joints or skin. Osteoarthritis presents as pain and stiffness with decreased range of motion, stiffness in the morning for a few minutes that relieves with movement, and occasionally joint effusions. Point tenderness in 11 of 18 sites with digital palpation is present in fibromyalgia. Joint swelling and erythema are not present. In septic arthritis, joint pain, inflammation, and erythema would be accompanied by systemic symptoms of fever and chills. It would be considered in the differential for this patient.

25. Answer: 1

Rationale: Lyme arthritis, rheumatic heart disease, ankylosing spondylitis, psoriatic arthritis, rheumatoid arthritis (RA), Reiter's syndrome, osteoarthritis, gonococcal arthritis, systemic lupus erythematosus (SLE), and polymyalgia rheumatica (PMR) typically occur as polyarthritic disease. Gout, septic arthritis, and pseudogout most often occur as monoarthritis.

26. Answer: 4

Rationale: A patient who sustained a meniscal tear can usually recall a twisting injury of the knee followed by pain and effusion over the joint line. A strong force or injury that causes external rotation or hyperextension of the knee is a common mechanism of injury for collateral or cruciate ligament injuries. Valgus and varus are tests for stability of the knee joint, which involve applying medial and lateral pressure to the knee during full extension and flexion of 30 degrees.

27. Answer: 4

Rationale: As the soft tissue swells, pain onset is usually about 12–36 hours after injury.

28. Answer: 2

Rationale: Herniated intervertebral disc pain typically descends to the lower leg and foot. Lumbosacral strain causes pain in the back, buttock, and sometimes thigh. Osteomyelitis must be preceded by an event that permits an infectious agent to enter the bone. Osteoporosis occurs most often in postmenopausal women.

29. Answer: 4

Rationale: At the time a patellar subluxation occurs, a traumatic event causes the knee to "give out," and the patella is usually laterally displaced; severe pain and an effusion result. Subsequent to the injury, the patient will notice a locking sensation in the knee with pivoting or turning. Patellofemoral stress syndrome is a form of overuse syndrome. Pain of a dull, aching quality is present in the knee, sometimes with clicking. Long periods of sitting or activities that involve knee flexion as well as compression of the patella in the groove cause increased pain. Growing pains usually occur at night and resolve by morning. The pain is deep and does not involve the joints. In shin splints, inflammation of muscles along the medial shaft of the tibia due to overuse causes aching pain. Rest improves the pain.

30. Answer: 1

Rationale: In quadriceps setting, with the foot dorsiflexed, the thigh is pressed downward against the floor and held for 5 seconds. The straight leg raise involves lifting an extended leg while sitting on the floor and leaning back on the elbows with the opposite leg flexed to 90 degrees. A terminal arc extension requires that the patient lie on the floor supine with extended legs flexed to 20 degrees over a rolled towel. The patient then extends one leg and holds for 5 seconds. The exercise is repeated with the opposite leg. All of these exercises can be used to stretch and strengthen the quadriceps muscles in those with patellofemoral stress syndrome. Resistive exercises with an elastic band are general exercises that can be done with the extremities.

31. Answer: 3

Rationale: Gout generally affects men over age 30 and is associated with obesity, lead intoxication, starvation, and use of some medications, including salicylates, diuretics, pyrazinamide, and alcohol.

32. Answer: 4

Rationale: A third-degree sprain is a complete tear of a ligament resulting in marked edema, ecchymosis, pain, and an unstable joint.

33. Answer: 3

Rationale: Morning stiffness or activity and the length of time required for maximal improvement are American Rheumatism Association Classification criteria for rheumatoid arthritis (RA) and useful, measurable tools for effects of treatment. The other questions are good indicators of quality of activities of daily living but do not give a full, overall, measurable picture of the patient's joint discomfort.

34. Answer: 1

Rationale: This patient meets the classification criteria for fibromyalgia based on history of widespread pain and pain in 11 of 18 tender points. Myofascial syndrome symptoms are more focal, with no associated fatigue or sleep disorder. Rheumatoid arthritis (RA) would have abnormal serologic studies. Depression may cause musculoskeletal pain and fatigue but would not have reproducible tender points.

35. Answer: 2

Rationale: This is a subtherapeutic amount of calcium and vitamin D. The other choices are recommendations for prevention of osteoporosis.

36. Answer: 4

Rationale: Most whiplash injuries are associated with a cervical neck strain related to spasm of the cervical and upper back muscles from injury.

37. Answer: 2

Rationale: The patient's symptoms are indicative of septic arthritis, which is a medical emergency; if not treated promptly, the joint may be severely damaged or destroyed. Exam of the joint fluid is the most important diagnostic test. The other choices may provide some symptomatic relief, but the first goal of treatment is to determine whether the joint is septic.

38. Answer: 3

Rationale: When developing a differential diagnosis, the history and physical will help narrow the differentiation. Other procedures are important in completing the evaluation, but the most important information is the pattern of joints affected and whether it is inflammatory or noninflammatory disease.

39. Answer: 2

Rationale: Corticosteroids have limited value in treating ankylosing spondylitis (AS), and long-term use is associated with many serious side effects. Important treatment includes regular exercise to strengthen supporting muscles and use of nonsteroidal anti-inflammatory drugs (NSAIDs) for pain. Approximately one third of patients have recurrent attacks of acute iritis.

40. Answer: 1

Rationale: Trauma, increased alcohol intake on weekends, and physical stress have all been implicated in acute gout. Gout occurs primarily in adult men. Decreased circulation, ecchymosis, and bone deformity are not likely with acute gout.

41. Answer: 2

Rationale: The calcium intake is important in minimizing the development of osteoporosis. Both these foods contain calcium. The other options are not focused on the calcium intake.

42. Answer: 4

Rationale: Signs and symptoms of osteoarthritis include asymmetric joint pain exacerbated by movement and relieved by rest. Stiffness is of short duration (<15 minutes) after inactivity or in the morning. Pain may be described as aching and poorly localized. The other questions are indicative of rheumatoid arthritis (RA).

43. Answer: 3

Rationale: Low back pain is the number-one cause of disability and accounts for 25% of disabling work-related injuries.

44. Answer: 1

Rationale: The RICE principle is used for initial treatment: **R**est, **I**ce, **C**ompression, and **E**levation. All other treatments mentioned may be appropriate but not as the primary treatment.

45. Answer: 1

Rationale: Although all symptoms may be associated with cauda equina syndrome, urinary retention and loss of bowel or bladder control are important clues to the immediate need for surgery.

46. Answer: 2

Rationale: Annular tears are tears of the annulus fibrosus of the intervertebral disc and are the first step toward herniation. Early recognition can help avoid the need for surgical repair of a subsequent herniation.

47. Answer: 4

Rationale: Fibromyalgia is a poorly understood condition that can prolong the normal treatment course of an injury considerably and is very difficult to treat. Osteoarthritis may follow an injury, as can reflex sympathetic dystrophy and tendinitis, but they do not have specified tender points.

48. Answer: 2

Rationale: The five risk factors for osteoporosis include being female, Caucasian or Asian, over age 45, low body weight, postmenopausal, sedentary lifestyle, low calcium intake, and smoker.

49. Answer: 1

Rationale: The patient's occupation and symptoms both suggest carpal tunnel syndrome. Initial treatment would involve night splinting, ice, and anti-inflammatory medication.

50. Answer: 3

Rationale: Polymyalgia rheumatica (PMR) is an inflammatory disorder of the proximal muscles presenting as described. Polyarteritis nodosa, an inflammatory disorder affecting the small arteries, presents with muscle weakness, myalgias, headache, and subcutaneous nodules along leg and arm arteries. Wegener's disease presents with mild anemia, dyspnea, cough, chest pain, hemoptysis, and abnormal urinalysis.

51. Answer: 3

Rationale: Up to 40% of patients with temporal arteritis have a previous history of polymyalgia rheumatica (PMR). Presenting complaints include headache, low-grade fever, muscle aching and stiffness, fatigue, malaise, and anorexia.

52. Answer: 1, 2, 4

Rationale: The patient is presenting with the classic symptoms of nerve root compression secondary to pressure from a protruding lumbar disc. The sciatic stretch test (straight leg raise) maneuver will increase the radiation of pain down the hip. In piriformis syndrome, the piriformis muscle (a narrow muscle located in the buttocks) compresses or irritates the sciatic nerve. Spinal cord injury will result in focal pain or tenderness, bruising, hematoma, and palpable step-offs along the spine.

53. Answer: 2

Rationale: This patient is likely experiencing an acute exacerbation of his osteoarthritis because he is constantly rubbing his knees. Because 85% of the residents of long-term care facilities have uncontrolled pain, he probably has uncontrolled pain. Starting him on routine acetaminophen (Tylenol) would be an excellent start to pain management. It is unlikely that the patient's dementia is worsening because this is an acute problem. Although UTI is a good choice, the cues of rubbing the major joints would likely rule out a UTI as the problem. The patient is not exhibiting any neurologic symptoms, which would rule out an acute cerebral infarct.

Pharmacology

54. Answer: 2

Rationale: Patients on chronic steroid therapy should be evaluated for adrenal insufficiency during an acute illness, which increases stress. Signs and symptoms indicate subtle clinical manifestations of adrenal insufficiency. Recommended treatment is to treat empirically with stress-dose corticosteroid during acute illness. Stopping the medication or maintaining the same dose may precipitate acute adrenal insufficiency.

55. Answer: 2

Rationale: Aspirin is the first choice. Nonsteroidal anti-inflammatory drugs (NSAIDs) can be used, but the anti-inflammatory and antipyretic effects of aspirin, plus low cost, make it the initial drug of choice. Methotrexate is used for severe cases that do not respond to aspirin or NSAIDs. Steroids may be given but are not the drug of choice.

56. Answer: 2

Rationale: The patient needs to understand the importance of maintaining the prescribed steroid dose. When symptoms decrease, the medication is effective. It is not influenced by fluids and should be taken with food.

57. Answer: 3

Rationale: This is the only effective dose listed for the treatment of an acute episode of gout. The other doses are incorrect and insufficient as dosed. The maximum dose of colchicine for an acute gout attack is 1.8 mg.

58. Answer: 4

Rationale: Allopurinol works to keep the serum uric acid level lower. The goal of therapy is a serum uric acid level of <6.5 mg/dL. The other medications listed do not help lower serum uric acid levels, and aspirin can precipitate a gout attack.

59. Answer: 4

Rationale: These drugs modify the disease when nonsteroidal anti-inflammatory drugs (NSAIDs), such as ibuprofen, sulindac, and salicylates, have not worked. Corticosteroids can be used until the disease-modifying agents begin to work. Misoprostol is used to prevent ulcer development related to long-term medication use.

60. Answer: 3

Rationale: Gold is indicated for treatment of rheumatoid arthritis (RA) and is contraindicated in the presence of the other listed diseases.

61. Answer: 1

Rationale: Acetaminophen or nonsteroidal anti-inflammatory drugs (NSAIDs) are generally used for pain relief for patients with osteoarthritis. Systemic corticosteroids are not indicated in osteoarthritis. Gold salts may be one of several pharmacologic approaches to the treatment of rheumatoid arthritis. Misoprostol is used to minimize the development of NSAID-induced gastric ulcers.

62. Answer: 2

Rationale: Renal function may already be reduced in older adults, and ibuprofen can further impair renal function, which, in turn, can result in nephrosis, cirrhosis, and congestive heart failure.

63. Answer: 1

Rationale: The patient should be monitored for blood dyscrasias on a monthly basis, which would be a CBC with differential and platelet count. Women of childbearing age should avoid pregnancy.

64. Answer: 3

Rationale: Nonsteroidal anti-inflammatory drugs (NSAIDs) (naproxen) are recommended treatment for an acute gout attack in patients able to tolerate NSAID therapy. Allopurinol is contraindicated in an acute attack and can even precipitate an attack in the early stages of treatment. Low-calorie diets increase risks of gouty attacks. Joint injection would not be a first-line treatment choice, but for refractory cases in patients unable to take oral medication, it may be an option.

65. Answer: 4

Rationale: Gastritis and oral ulcers are common complications of alendronate (Fosamax). Alendronate is used to increase calcium absorption in patients with osteoporosis. If these effects occur, the medication should be discontinued. The medications in the other options do not cause this problem.

Neurology

Physical Exam & Diagnostic Tests

1. To evaluate the neurologic system for appropriate sensory system functioning in the geriatric patient, it is appropriate to determine the presence of stereognosis. This is done by having the patient:

   1. Rapidly touch the index finger and then the nose.
   2. Distinguish between a coin and a key by touch.
   3. Stand with heels together and eyes closed.
   4. Close eyes and identify familiar odors.

2. To determine cerebellar functioning in the geriatric patient, the family nurse practitioner would perform:

   1. The Get Up and Go test.
   2. The Romberg test.
   3. Kinesthesia assessments.
   4. The SPICES assessment.

3. What is considered a "soft" (or equivocal) neurologic sign?

   1. Positive Babinski's reflex in an adult.
   2. Mirroring hand movements of the extremities.
   3. Brudzinski's sign.
   4. Kernig's sign.

4. A patient is having difficulty controlling seizures and is referred for an electroencephalogram (EEG). The family nurse practitioner explains:

   1. This test will cause some discomfort and a sedative will be provided before the test.
   2. It will be important for her to take her regular dosages of paroxetine (Paxil) and phenytoin (Dilantin) before the test.

3. The procedure is painless and she will not experience discomfort or electrical shock.
4. After the test she will be on bed rest for 8 hours and will be given clear liquids for 12 hours.

5. Which cranial nerve is being tested when the family nurse practitioner asks the patient to raise the eyebrows, smile, frown, or puff out the cheeks?

   1. Hypoglossal nerve.
   2. Acoustic nerve.
   3. Glossopharyngeal nerve.
   4. Facial nerve.

6. The family nurse practitioner notes an absent patellar reflex in a healthy patient. What might the practitioner ask the patient to do?

   1. Lift both arms above the head and count to 5 slowly as the reflex is tested.
   2. Raise both legs slowly and then lower and immediately test for the reflex.
   3. Clench both hands together and pull while the reflex is tested.
   4. Close eyes and hold breath while examiner tests for the reflex.

7. With the patient in the supine position, the family nurse practitioner gently flexes the patient's neck in the direction of the chin touching the chest. If there is pain and resistance to the flexion, and if the hips and knees flex at the same time, the nurse accurately describes this finding as:

   1. Phalen's sign.
   2. Romberg's sign.
   3. Kernig's sign.
   4. Brudzinski's sign.

8. **QSEN** The family nurse practitioner is seeing an 82-year-old patient who lives in a townhome and routinely needs to climb two sets of stairs to get to the bedroom. Which two instruments would be appropriate to assess the patient's fall risk?

   1. The Tinetti Balance and Gait assessment.

   2. The Timed Get Up and Go test.

   3. The SPICES questionnaire.

   4. The Strength and Timing instrument.

   5. Trendelenburg test.

   6. Phalen's test.

9. The family nurse practitioner understands that dysdiadochokinesia refers to:

   1. Trouble with speech.

   2. Memory impairment.

   3. Impaired rapid alternating movements.

   4. Neurologic triad of gait, memory, and speech dysfunction.

Disorders

10. The family nurse practitioner understands that the most common form of facial paralysis in the adult patient is:

    1. Facial nerve fasciitis.

    2. Trigeminal neuralgia.

    3. Bell's palsy.

    4. Herpes zoster.

11. A patient has a history of injury at the fifth thoracic vertebra (T5), and his condition has stabilized. The family nurse practitioner understands that, with this level of injury, the patient most likely will not be able to:

    1. Perform coordinated movements with his hands, such as writing.

    2. Achieve lower body strength and coordination for walking.

    3. Have adequate upper body strength to drive a car.

    4. Maintain the upper body coordination required for eating.

12. An older patient is diagnosed with postpolio syndrome. The most common symptom is:

    1. Gastrointestinal upset, headache, and malaise.

    2. New onset of weakness, fatigue, and pain.

    3. Sudden onset of lower limb paralysis after an acute infection.

    4. Headache, fever, and elevated blood pressure and pulse.

13. The family nurse practitioner is discussing safety measures for the home environment of a patient with Parkinson's disease. It would be important for the family nurse practitioner to include what information?

    1. Sleep on a firm mattress that is high off the floor to facilitate getting into and out of bed.

    2. Pour hot liquids with the cup or container placed on the table to avoid spilling.

    3. Place a sheepskin pad on the bed to decrease the development of decubiti.

    4. Perform passive and active range of motion twice daily to prevent contracture.

14. A patient presents to a rural clinic after a diving accident. The family nurse practitioner suspects a spinal cord injury at the fifth cervical vertebra (C5). While awaiting emergency transport services, the family nurse practitioner assesses for the development of complications by:

    1. Checking for voluntary movement of extremities and sensation below the level of injury.

    2. Assessing breath sounds and evaluating movement of diaphragm with respiration.

    3. Maintaining cervical flexion to facilitate airway until cervical traction is initiated.

    4. Beginning neurologic checks with careful documentation of location of pain sensations.

15. Many patients who suffer from recurrent headaches have similar symptoms with each episode. Which is a sign that a headache may be from a more serious cause?

    1. It occurs on the right side.

    2. Rhinorrhea occurs with the headache.

    3. It becomes more and more painful.

    4. It increases when the patient bends over.

16. Epidemic meningococcal meningitis occurs rarely. This control is a result of:

    1. Live immunization recommendations on a national level.

    2. Lower community carrier rates.

    3. Improved socioeconomic conditions.

    4. Earlier detection and recognition of outbreaks.

17. The family nurse practitioner understands that benign paroxysmal positional vertigo:

    1. Is described as vertigo and nystagmus with positional change and occurs most often in older adults.

    2. Is more common in young persons and occurs suddenly and in episodes that include vertigo, tinnitus, hearing loss, feeling of fullness in the ears, and nausea and vomiting.

    3. Follows a viral syndrome (upper respiratory or gastrointestinal) with exacerbation of the vertigo with position change without hearing loss or tinnitus.

    4. Involves gradual hearing loss and tinnitus along with vertigo, eventually with facial numbness and weakness.

18. Which of the following three conditions are included in the differential diagnosis of a patient with facial paralysis?

    1. Herpes zoster.

    2. Bell's palsy.

    3. Trigeminal neuralgia.

    4. Otitis media.

    5. Myasthenia gravis.

19. What would be appropriate to include in the health promotion plan for a patient with a diagnosis of multiple sclerosis?

    1. Avoid aerobic exercise, due to muscle weakness.

    2. Keep warm (especially extremities) to improve neurologic function.

    3. Avoid antioxidants (vitamins C and E, beta-carotene); they contribute to loss of myelin sheath.

    4. Consume a low-fat, high-fiber diet with daily naps and multivitamin supplement.

20. A patient has had a stroke and is incontinent of urine. The family should be taught to:

    1. Restrict fluid intake.

    2. Insert a Foley catheter.

    3. Establish a scheduled voiding pattern.

    4. Reposition the patient often to reduce the discomfort of urgency.

21. What is the best approach to test the hearing of a patient with Bell's palsy?

    1. Stand out of sight of the patient and ask the patient to move or do something.

    2. Use a tuning fork to test for lateralization of sound.

    3. Stand in front of the patient and whisper, "Raise your hand."

    4. Snap your fingers next to the patient's ear and ask if the sound was heard.

22. Physical findings in a 50-year-old female patient who wears a left lower leg brace are weight of 100 lb, height of 65 inches, and vital signs within normal limits. She has developed postpolio symptoms. The family nurse practitioner suggests that the patient:

    1. Gain weight to prevent further disability.

    2. Exercise all muscle groups vigorously to prevent disuse syndrome.

    3. Avoid exposure to cold or chilling, which may cause a loss of strength in the affected muscle.

    4. Reduce the amount of time using the brace for joint support to prevent further loss of strength.

23. Inflammation and swelling of the seventh cranial nerve with resultant unilateral facial muscle paralysis is called:

    1. Bell's palsy.

    2. Temporal (giant cell) arteritis.

    3. Facial droop.

    4. Trigeminal neuralgia.

24. The family nurse practitioner understands that the following trigger helps differentiate a migraine from a tension headache:

    1. Alcohol.

    2. Bright lighting and noxious stimuli.

    3. Stressful situations.

    4. Sleep pattern disturbances.

25. The family nurse practitioner is teaching a patient about migraine headaches. Select three statements that are true about migraine headaches.

    1. Migraine is likely related to both vascular and chemical changes in the brain.

    2. Migraine and related headaches are disorders of an infectious response in the neurons.

    3. Genetic and environmental factors are influential in migraine.

    4. During migraine, the pain is described as pounding or throbbing and is aggravated by physical activity.

    5. Migraine headache feels like a tight band around the head.

    6. Migraine headache is unilateral, reaches maximum intensity in 15 minutes, and lasts 90 minutes.

26. Which symptom(s) can occur in a patient who has experienced a transient ischemic attack (TIA) in the anterior cerebral circulation?

    1. Bilateral vision disturbance and diplopia.

    2. Dysarthria (speech disturbance).

    3. Disorders of behavior and cognition.

    4. Bilateral motor and sensory dysfunction.

27. Many visits to emergency departments by adults are prompted by headaches. Which symptom may help the family nurse practitioner differentiate a migraine headache from a headache that may indicate severe problems?

    1. It is preceded by an "aura."

    2. It occurs mainly behind one eye and tends to be grouped.

    3. Onset is sudden and accompanied by nuchal rigidity.

    4. It occurs mainly on awakening.

28. An adult patient presents with a complaint of facial paralysis that started suddenly. In making a diagnosis, the family nurse practitioner considers which of the following symptoms of Bell's palsy?

    1. Concurrent paralysis of the opposite arm and leg.

    2. Pain in the (ipsilateral) ear that accompanied or preceded the paralysis.

    3. Loss of bowel control.

    4. Loss of hearing on the opposite side.

29. An older adult woman is present when her husband is admitted for a myocardial infarction. She complains that she is having numbness and tingling in her hands and face. Her heart rate is 98 beats/min, and her respiratory rate is 32 breaths/min. What is the best action for the family nurse practitioner to take?

    1. Administer oxygen per nasal cannula at 3 L/min.

    2. Schedule a magnetic resonance imaging (MRI) appointment.

    3. Provide calming interventions by explaining the probable reason for the symptoms.

    4. Administer amitriptyline (Elavil) 25 mg PO.

30. The family nurse practitioner is evaluating an older adult's tremor. Which assessment finding would be characteristic of an essential tremor rather than a parkinsonian tremor?

    1. The handwriting is not affected.

    2. The tremor occurs with purposeful movements.

    3. The tremor occurs at rest.

    4. The tremor worsens with beta blockers or alcohol.

31. Which assessment may be evaluated in a patient with Parkinson's disease?

    1. Macrographia.

    2. Micrographia.

    3. Exaggeration of rapid successive movements.

    4. Increased swinging of arms while walking.

32. A patient recently diagnosed with multiple sclerosis asks the family nurse practitioner about the disease process. The family nurse practitioner knows that:

    1. 90% of patients have a quickly progressive form of the disease.

    2. 90% of patients, after the first onset of symptoms, have relapses and remissions.

    3. 10% of patients will respond to corticosteroids.

    4. 10% of patients have problems with optic neuritis and sensory loss.

33. A 30-year-old female patient has had several episodes of incontinence, weakness, visual loss, and some ataxia. Physical exam reveals slight swelling of the optic disc on funduscopy, difficulty with heel-to-toe walking, lower extremity weakness, and 2+ deep tendon reflexes. Which condition does the family nurse practitioner suspect?

    1. Multiple sclerosis.

    2. Parkinson's disease.

    3. Amyotrophic lateral sclerosis.

    4. Myasthenia gravis

34. A patient has a 3-year history of recurrent headaches once or twice a month lasting 12–18 hours. When the patient presents at the clinic, she has taken 6 g of acetaminophen in the past 12 hours with no relief. The family nurse practitioner would:

    1. Recommend a parenteral narcotic analgesic as well as prescribe opioids for prn use.

    2. Consider an analgesic rebound relative to the dose of acetaminophen taken.

    3. Order naproxen (Anaprox) for prophylactic treatment of the headaches.

    4. Order an EEG and MRI to rule out pathology.

35. A patient presents to the emergency department, stating it is the "worst headache of my life." The patient reports that the headaches have not responded to the usual over-the-counter headache remedies. What is a priority differential?

    1. Brain tumor.

    2. Migraine.

    3. Onset of newly diagnosed seizure disorder.

    4. Subarachnoid hemorrhage.

36. A patient with a recent history of a left hemisphere stroke returns to the clinic for a checkup. What symptoms would the family nurse practitioner anticipate the patient to exhibit?

    1. Left-sided weakness.

    2. Bilateral weakness of lower extremities.

    3. Difficulty with speech.

    4. Left visual field deficit.

37. The family nurse practitioner is evaluating a group of older adult patients for risk factors of an embolic stroke. Which condition would be least likely to precipitate this type of stroke?

    1. Mitral valve disease.

    2. Atrial fibrillation.

    3. Endocarditis.

    4. Diabetes mellitus.

38. A patient returns to the clinic for a follow-up visit. She has a history of simple partial seizures. When questioning the patient, the family nurse practitioner would identify recurrence of this seizure activity if the patient reported:

    1. Short episodes when she loses consciousness but does not fall.

    2. No loss of consciousness but jerking and tingling of her right leg and then right hand.

    3. Auditory hallucinations, unconsciousness, and urinary incontinence.

    4. Short period of unconsciousness, followed by period of confusion.

39. An older adult woman comes to the clinic complaining of having difficulty when she tries to do her needlework. She walks straight, although somewhat slowly, and no rigidity is noted on movement. She states the shaking in her hands stops when she holds her hands in her lap. What tentative diagnosis would the family nurse practitioner make?

    1. Parkinson's disease.

    2. Transient ischemic attack.

    3. Benign essential tremor.

    4. Resting tremor.

40. A patient with a history of myasthenia gravis presents with ptosis, facial weakness, dysphagia, and generalized weakness. What is important for the family nurse practitioner to ask and establish initially?

    1. When did the symptoms first begin, and have they increased in severity?

    2. What medications is the patient taking, and when did he last take them?

    3. What activity was the patient participating in when the symptoms began?

    4. Has the patient experienced any seizure activity with the increase in symptoms?

41. A patient presents with miosis and ptosis with anhidrosis of the ipsilateral face and neck. The initial diagnosis would be:

    1. Horner's syndrome.

    2. Damage to cranial nerves III and IV.

    3. Ménière's syndrome.

    4. Mycotic aneurysm.

42. The family nurse practitioner is talking with a well-appearing, 42-year-old patient who mentions a concern over the past 3 months with swallowing. Which four differentials should be considered?

    1. Cranial nerve XI (glossopharyngeal nerve) dysfunction.

    2. Cranial nerve X (vagus nerve) dysfunction.

    3. Thyroidmegaly.

    4. Esophageal cancer.

    5. Epiglottitis.

    6. Multiple sclerosis.

43. The initial symptoms of amyotrophic lateral sclerosis are:

    1. Weakness in the lower extremities and urinary incontinence.

    2. Weakness in the upper extremities and dysfunction in fine motor skills.

    3. Spasticity and hyperreflexia.

    4. Loss of continence and drooling.

44. Which of the four findings below are associated with Guillain-Barré syndrome?

    1. A recent viral illness.

    2. Weakness more profound in the upper extremities.

    3. Headache and nuchal rigidity.

    4. Visual changes.

    5. Respiratory distress or failure.

    6. Protein in cerebral spinal fluid analysis.

45. The family nurse practitioner is seeing a patient for new onset headaches. Which statement by the patient would cause the most concern?

    1. "This headache makes me sick to my stomach."

    2. "This headache is behind my right eye and is giving me stabbing pain."

46.

    3. "This headache has awakened me from sleep for the past week."

    4. "I have needed to wear dark glasses for the past 3 days in a row."

46. The family nurse practitioner is treating a patient with Parkinson's disease. What finding should the family nurse practicitioner anticipate?

    1. Visual hallucinations and paranoia.

    2. Bowel and bladder dysfunction.

    3. Disorders in extraocular movements.

    4. Pulmonary hypertension associated with left ventricular failure.

47. Which of the following statements is correct concerning brain tumors?

    1. Meningiomas are the most frequent type of primary malignant tumors.

    2. A history of breast cancer has no associated risk for brain tumor.

    3. Seizures are a common clinical finding.

    4. Increased intracranial pressure is a classic early finding in meningioma.

48. The family nurse practitioner recognizes that cerebral edema usually presents within what time frame following a head trauma?

    1. 24 hours.

    2. 48 hours.

    3. 72 hours.

    4. One week.

49. What four symptoms are findings associated with post-concussion syndrome?

    1. Anxiety.

    2. Behavioral disturbances.

    3. Headaches.

    4. Fine tremors.

    5. Hallucinations.

    6. Sleep disturbances.

50. The family nurse practitioner recognizes which of the following two criteria as correct concerning multiple sclerosis (MS)?

    1. The onset is most likely between the ages of 20 and 50 years.

    2. It affects males and females equally.

    3. It is more commonly diagnosed in northern climates.

    4. Native Americans, Eskimos, and Asians are affected more than other ethnicities.

    5. MS is a result of exclusively an autoimmune disorder.

51. The family nurse practitioner is reviewing the records of a patient who is recovering from a stroke. The records indicate the patient is experiencing homonymous hemianopia. This is interpreted as:

    1. Partial loss of visual acuity in the peripheral area of the visual field.

    2. Diplopia in the eye contralateral to the cerebral lesion.

    3. Nystagmus in both eyes, but movements are dissimilar.

    4. Loss of vision in both eyes in either the right or the left half of the visual field.

Pharmacology

52. A patient is taking an antiepileptic medication. The family nurse practitioner understands that the antiepileptic medication:

    1. Must be taken indefinitely.

    2. Is usually discontinued after 4 years of no seizure activity, and EEG confirms lack of seizure activity.

    3. Is usually given in combination with other antiepileptics or sedatives to reduce the seizure threshold.

    4. Must be given to all patients who experience a seizure.

53. Pharmacologic management of patients with peripheral vestibulopathy includes:

    1. Meclizine (Antivert) 100 mg PO qid.

    2. Dimenhydrinate (Dramamine) 5 mg PO tid to qid.

    3. Scopolamine transdermal patch, 1 disc applied behind ear and left in place for 3 days.

    4. Prochlorperazine 25–50 mg PO q4h prn.

54. The family of a Parkinson's patient brings him to the clinic because he is experiencing increasing difficulty with ambulation. The family nurse practitioner increases the patient's dose of carbidopa (25 mg)/levodopa (100 mg) (Sinemet 25–100 mg) from three to four times daily. What is important for the family nurse practitioner to teach the family regarding the increase in the dose of this medication?

    1. Sleep disorders and hallucinations are common side effects of carbidopa/levodopa.

    2. Carbidopa/levodopa has shown efficacy in slowing disease progression.

    3. Orthostatic hypotension can be problematic at higher dosing ranges.

    4. The medication should be given on an empty stomach.

55. Which medication class is recognized for the treatment of moderate to severe dementia?

    1. Cholinesterase inhibitors.

    2. NMDA receptor antagonists.

    3. SSRIs.

    4. Central alpha$_2$ agonists.

56. Before prescribing an abortive agent for migraines, a priority question to ask the patient would be:

    1. "Do you have a history of gastric colic?"

    2. "Do you have a history of anxiety or panic episodes?"

    3. "Do you have a history of cardiac disease?"

    4. "Do you have a history of seizure disorder?"

57. **QSEN** What would be a priority teaching in a newly diagnosed patient initially using an anticonvulsant?

    1. Contact sports pose no risk to persons with epilepsy.

    2. The anticonvulsant medication will cause drowsiness.

    3. Avoid solitary activities.

    4. Medical alert bracelets are unhelpful.

58. Which factor is the greatest positive intervention for ischemic stroke?

    1. Cardiac rhythm control.

    2. Blood pressure control.

    3. Timely use of thrombolytics.

    4. Renal protection, including fluid support.

59. The family nurse practitioner recognizes that which antibiotic class can interfere with the metabolism of first-generation antiepilepsy drugs, such as carbamazepine?

    1. Cephalosporins.

    2. Quinolones.

    3. Sulfonamides.

    4. Macrolides.

60. The family nurse practitioner is discussing the worth of the herpes zoster vaccination with a 62-year-old patient. What would be an accurate statement in promoting the vaccine?

    1. Postherpetic neuralgia is not a reason to accept the vaccine.

    2. A severe case of zoster increases the risk of postherpetic neuralgia.

    3. Age is not correlated with risk for postherpetic neuralgia.

    4. Herpes zoster cannot affect the central or peripheral nervous systems.

61. What information is important for the family nurse practitioner to teach the patient regarding the use of medications to treat trigeminal neuralgia?

    1. Medications may cause seizure-like activity.

    2. Therapeutic levels of the drug may take up to a month to be reached.

    3. Relief of the symptoms should occur within 24 hours of starting the medication.

    4. Permanent side effects are not a concern of this condition.

11 Neurology Answers & Rationales

Physical Exam & Diagnostic Tests

1. Answer: 2

Rationale: Stereognosis is the ability to determine familiar objects by shape rather than visual identification. Rapidly touching the index finger and then the nose determines fine motor skills and coordination, standing with heels together and eyes closed determines proprioception (balance; posture), and closing the eyes and identifying familiar odors determines the functioning of the first cranial (olfactory) nerve.

2. Answer: 2

Rationale: The Romberg test assesses cerebellar function so would be a reasonable method to evaluate an elder's balance. The Get Up and Go test assesses gait and strength. Kinesthesia assessments determine proprioception ability. The SPICES assessment is an acronym of common older adult syndromes: **S** is for Sleep Disorders, **P** is for Problems with Eating or Feeding, **I** is for Incontinence, **C** is for Confusion, **E** is for Evidence of Falls, **S** is for Skin Breakdown.

3. Answer: 2

Rationale: Soft neurologic signs involve slight deviations of the central nervous system (CNS) that are present occasionally or inconsistently. Examples are short attention span; clumsiness; frequent falling (disturbances of gait); hyperkinesis; left-handed but right-footed; language disturbances; anisocoria; and mirroring movements of the extremities (when one hand performs a movement, the other is also in motion). The other three options indicate a CNS problem that occurs consistently; Brudzinski's and Kernig's signs indicate meningeal irritation, and a positive Babinski's reflex in an adult may indicate an upper motor lesion in the corticospinal tract.

4. Answer: 3

Rationale: The procedure is painless with no danger of electrical shock. All anticonvulsants, antidepressants, stimulants (caffeine, tobacco), and alcohol should be stopped. It would be concerning to see a selective serotonin reuptake inhibitor (SSRI) prescribed in a patient with seizures because SSRIs lower seizure threshold. There is no restriction on movement or diet after the procedure.

5. Answer: 4

Rationale: The facial nerve is tested by facial movement, taste, sensation, and corneal reflex. The hypoglossal nerve is tested by the patient sticking out the tongue. The acoustic nerve is tested by a hearing test. The glossopharyngeal nerve is tested by taste, gag reflex, and having the patient drink and swallow.

6. Answer: 3

Rationale: Augmentation of the patellar reflex can be obtained by having the patient isometrically tense muscles not directly involved with the reflex arc being tested, called Jendrassik's maneuver.

7. Answer: 4

Rationale: This describes Brudzinski's sign. Phalen's sign (maneuver) is elicited in carpal tunnel syndrome. The Romberg's sign test is done to assess gross swaying by asking the patient to stand with feet together and eyes closed for 5 seconds. Kernig's sign (inability to extend lower leg when leg is flexed at hip or when there is resistance or pain) along with Brudzinski's sign indicate meningeal irritation and should be evaluated further.

8. Answer: 1, 2

Rationale: Both the Tinetti and the Timed Get Up and Go tests assess functional ability and fall risk. The SPICES questionnaire assesses various geriatric syndromes. The Strength and Timing instrument is not a valid assessment tool. The Trendelenburg test measures competency of the leg vein valves in patients with varicosities. The Phalen's test is used to assess for carpal tunnel syndrome.

9. Answer: 3

Rationale: Dysdiadochokinesia is difficulty with attempts at rapidly alternating movements (e.g., finger to nose).

Disorders

10. Answer: 3

Rationale: The most common form of facial paralysis is Bell's palsy, a disorder affecting the facial nerve characterized by muscle flaccidity of the affected side of the face. Trigeminal neuralgia is a disorder of cranial nerve V that is characterized by an abrupt onset of pain in the lower and upper jaw, cheek, and lips. Herpes zoster affects the dermatomes and does not cause a paralysis but rather pain, herpetic grouped skin vesicles, and possibly postherpetic neuralgia.

11. Answer: 2

Rationale: Fifth thoracic vertebra (T5) injuries do not affect the coordination or capacity of the upper body, arms, and hands; the lower body is paralyzed. The patient should be able to do all activities listed except walk.

12. Answer: 2

Rationale: The cardinal signs of postpolio syndrome include onset of new weakness; fatigue; and pain along with hot or cold intolerance; and swallowing, speech, breathing, and sleep disturbances.

13. Answer: 2

Rationale: Pouring liquids is frequently a complicated task for this patient due to the tremors. If the cup or container to be filled is placed on the table, there is less chance of spilling the contents.

14. Answer: 2

Rationale: At this level of injury (C5), the intercostal muscles and diaphragm can be affected, and the patient may have respiratory compromise. Airway maintenance and avoiding flexion of the neck are critical.

15. Answer: 3

Rationale: If a headache becomes more and more severe, if there is new onset of severe headache in a patient over 35 years old, if the headache's character or progression is different from other headaches, or if there is vomiting, but no nausea, there could be a new and serious cause for the headache. The side on which the headache occurs, and accompanying rhinorrhea, may or may not be significant. Increasing pain when bending over is characteristic of sinus pressure or infection.

16. Answer: 3

Rationale: Improved sanitary and socioeconomic conditions have led to the marked reduction in the number of cases of epidemic meningitis. There is no research to support increased cases in communities with higher carrier numbers. Meningitis vaccine is not a live vaccination.

17. Answer: 1

Rationale: Benign paroxysmal positional vertigo usually occurs in older patients. Younger persons who experience a sudden episode of vertigo, tinnitus, hearing loss, sensation of fullness, and nausea and vomiting typically have Ménière's disease. Peripheral vestibulopathy usually follows upper respiratory or gastrointestinal viral illness and involves nearly incapacitating vertigo that increases with positional changes, but not hearing loss or tinnitus. The family nurse practitioner should suspect acoustic neuroma if gradual hearing loss, tinnitus, and vertigo occur before the development of facial numbness and weakness.

18. Answer: 1, 2, 4

Rationale: The differential diagnosis for facial paralysis includes bacterial ear infections, Bell's palsy, Lyme disease, herpes zoster, mumps, temporal bone fracture, acoustic neuroma, other tumors, and demyelinating diseases. Trigeminal neuralgia is associated with intense facial pain, not paralysis. Myasthenia gravis is characterized by fluctuating weakness and fatigability, often subtle, that worsens during the day and after prolonged use of affected muscles; may improve with rest; ptosis may be observed.

19. Answer: 4

Rationale: In addition to the factors listed, keeping cool, not warm, is associated with improvement of neurologic function. A regular exercise program is encouraged, along with daily intake of a multivitamin, antioxidants, and low-dose aspirin (81 mg). Maintaining ideal body weight, having rest periods or naps daily, and becoming informed about the disease process are important aspects of promoting health.

20. Answer: 3

Rationale: Reestablishing regularity will assist in maintaining bladder control. A catheter exposes the patient to infection. Fluids should not be restricted.

21. Answer: 1

Rationale: Bell's palsy involves a sensorineural hearing loss. In contrast to being able to read lips, this patient must be able to hear the direction of sound without any visual prompting. The tuning fork assists in differentiating between air and bone conduction of sound.

22. Answer: 3

Rationale: In addition to regular health maintenance visits, the patient should be advised to avoid gaining weight and exercising to the point of muscle pain. Cold temperatures can cause a loss of muscle strength in the affected muscle groups and should be avoided. Assistive or orthotic devices (canes, walkers, braces) should be used, along with periodic evaluation of muscle strength and function.

23. Answer: 1

Rationale: The symptoms describe Bell's palsy, which is thought to be caused by a virus. This sudden onset of unilateral facial paralysis usually resolves within 2 weeks but can endure for months. A few patients may have residual problems. Temporal or giant cell arteritis (GCA) is a generalized, large-vessel vasculitis commonly affecting the branches of the proximal aorta that supply the neck and the extracranial structures of the head. Facial droop occurs with Bell's palsy because of paralysis of the muscles innervated by the facial (seventh cranial) nerve. Trigeminal neuralgia is sudden pain along the fifth cranial nerve.

24. Answer: 4

Rationale: Sleep pattern disturbances, either too little or too much, may trigger a migraine headache. Lighting and noxious stimuli, along with alcohol use and stress, may trigger both tension and migraine headaches.

25. Answer: 1, 3, 4

Rationale: Headache disorders, including migraine, are disorders of neurovascular regulation and chemical changes in the brain and are not associated with an infectious response. Migraine headache pain is described as pounding or throbbing and is aggravated by physical activity. A tension headache is described as a feeling of a tight band around the head with no nausea and vomiting. A cluster headache is severe, unilateral, retro-orbital pain reaching intensity within 15 minutes and lasting 90 minutes.

26. Answer: 3

Rationale: A wide variety of changes can occur in behavior and cognition after a transient ischemic attack (TIA). Bilateral vision disturbance, diplopia, dysarthria (speech disturbance), and motor/sensory problems on both sides of the body are problems associated with TIA in the posterior cerebral circulation.

27. Answer: 3

Rationale: A sudden onset headache and nuchal rigidity may indicate a subarachnoid hemorrhage. Migraine headache without aura is the most common; however, migraine with aura occurs before the onset of pain. Cluster headaches occur behind one eye and are grouped. Headaches associated with hypertension occur mainly on awakening.

28. Answer: 2

Rationale: Bell's palsy is typically preceded or accompanied by pain in the ear on the paralyzed side often 1–2 days before the onset of facial paralysis. The paralysis is confined to the face, and there is no bowel involvement. Postauricular pain, tinnitus, and a mild hearing deficit may occur on the affected side.

29. Answer: 3

Rationale: Patients who are under stress have periods of hyperventilation in which they "blow off" more carbon dioxide (CO_2) than necessary. They experience numbness and tingling in their hands and faces and may experience syncope. Reassurance and calming intervention techniques by explaining the voluntary component of the rapid breathing will often have dramatic results of correcting the symptoms. In the past, breathing into a paper bag was recommended because it was supposed to increase CO_2 level and relieve the symptoms of respiratory alkalosis; however, this is not supported in evidenced-based literature and may be dangerous in patients with hypoxia or other physiologic/pathologic causes for the hyperventilation.

30. Answer: 2

Rationale: The differentiating feature between the two tremors is that the essential tremor occurs with purposeful movements. Handwriting may be affected with both tremors. The tremor with Parkinson's disease occurs at rest. Essential tremors improve with beta blockers as well as with alcohol.

31. Answer: 2

Rationale: Micrographia (small, cramped handwriting) is a classic manifestation of Parkinson's disease. The patient has impairment of rapid successive movements and loss of automatic movements, such as swinging the arms while walking.

32. Answer: 2

Rationale: Multiple sclerosis (MS) is characterized by exacerbations and remissions of the symptoms. Only 10% of MS patients have a progressive form of the disease from the onset. Many patients (35%–40%) have problems of optic neuritis, sensory loss, and weakness and do respond to corticosteroids.

33. Answer: 1

Rationale: Involvement of more than one CNS area, age 15–60 years, two or more separate episodes of symptoms involving different sites, or gradual progression over at least 6 months meet the criteria for multiple sclerosis.

34. Answer: 2

Rationale: The recommended dose for acetaminophen is no more than 4 g/day. This patient may be experiencing an analgesic rebound headache. Appropriate prophylactic medications for migraine include beta blockers (propranolol), tricyclic antidepressants (amitriptyline), selective serotonin reuptake inhibitors (paroxetine), anticonvulsants (topiramate), and calcium channel blockers (verapamil). It is not necessary to order expensive tests for patients with migraine or tension headache. Usually a careful, thorough history is sufficient.

35. Answer: 4

Rationale: This is a common patient complaint ("worst head-ache of my life") with a subarachnoid hemorrhage. This patient should have an emergent noncontrast CT scan of the brain and lumbar puncture with immediate referral to a neurologic surgeon, if either is positive.

36. Answer: 3

Rationale: The speech center (Broca's area) is most often located in the left cerebral hemisphere. The patient would experience weakness of the right side of the body and a right-sided visual deficit as well.

37. Answer: 4

Rationale: Mitral valve disease, atrial fibrillation, and endocarditis all precipitate the development of an embolus that can result in an embolic stroke. Diabetes will precipitate occlusive disease of the cerebral arteries and the possible development of a thrombotic stroke, not an embolic stroke.

38. Answer: 2

Rationale: A simple partial seizure is characterized by unilateral paresthesia, numbness and tingling, and spastic movement of the extremities. The patient has no loss of consciousness or incontinence of the bowel or bladder.

39. Answer: 3

Rationale: The characteristics of a benign tremor are fine-to-coarse rhythmic tremors of the hands and feet that increase with activity and may be absent at rest. Frequently the voice is also involved. An ingestion of a small amount of alcohol may decrease symptoms.

40. Answer: 2

Rationale: It is important to determine first whether the patient has stayed on the medication schedule. The symptoms may be the result of missed medication, especially with pyridostigmine (Mestinon). The symptoms may also be exacerbated by exercise and heat.

41. Answer: 1

Rationale: The clinical presentation is classic for Horner's syndrome, especially the lack of sweating (anhidrosis) on the ipsilateral (same) side of the face and neck as the eye symptoms. The patient needs to be referred for further neurologic workup.

42. Answer: 1, 3, 4, 6

Rationale: The glossopharyngeal nerve's motor function assists in swallowing. Thyromegaly can produce a feeling of fullness in the throat that is accompanied by dysphagia. Swallowing dysfunction is a late sign of esophageal cancer. Neuromuscular disorders, including multiple sclerosis, may be associated with dysphagia. Cranial nerve X (vagus) provides parasympathetic stimulation to secrete digestive enzymes in the gut, aid in peristalsis, as well as to provide the carotid reflex, involuntary actions of the heart, lung, and digestive systems. Its sensory innervation affects the area behind the ear and part of the external ear canal. Epiglottis is an airway-threatening, acute bacterial infection that is most commonly associated with *Haemophilus influenzae* type B. Patients with epiglottitis would not appear well.

43. Answer: 2

Rationale: The upper extremities are affected initially in 40–60% of cases. A frequent sign is low-amplitude fasciculations. Lower extremity weakness occurs in 20% of cases initially. Spasticity and hyperreflexia are other symptoms as the disorder progresses. Loss of continence is not a common concern. Drooling is one of the bulbar symptoms that can be present early in the disease. Additional bulbar symptoms include dysarthria and dysphagia.

44. Answer: 1, 4, 5, 6

Rationale: Recent viral illnesses, visual changes, respiratory dysfunction, and protein in cerebral fluid analysis are all findings in Guillain-Barré syndrome. Weakness is most profound in the lower extremities, progressing upward, leading to the risk of respiratory dysfunction. Headache and nuchal rigidity are associated with meningitis. Visual changes are also associated with multiple sclerosis.

45. Answer: 3

Rationale: Headaches that awaken the patient from sleep are associated with intracranial tumors. While nausea can also be present with increased intracranial pressure, intracranial tumors are associated with vomiting. Headache behind one eye is associated with cluster headaches, and photosensitivity is a common finding in migraine headaches.

46. Answer: 1

Rationale: Psychosis is a common comorbidity of Parkinson's disease (PD) with up to 40% of patients experiencing hallucinations. Bowel/bladder dysfunction, extraocular movement disorders, and cardiac complications, including left ventricular pathology, are not associated with PD.

47. Answer: 3

Rationale: Approximately one half of patients with brain tumors have a seizure. A history of breast, lung, melanoma, renal, and colon cancer increases risk for brain metastases. Gliomas are the most common type of primary malignant brain tumor. Increased intracranial pressure is a late finding in slow-growing tumors.

48. Answer: 3

Rationale: Peak occurrence for cerebral edema usually is up to 72 hours after a neurologic insult. It gradually resolves over a 2- to 3-week period. Cerebral edema may be caused by either the initial injury to the neuronal tissue or secondarily in response to the biochemical cellular injury cascade, hypoxia, hypercarbia, or cerebral ischemia.

49. Answer: 1, 2, 3, 6

Rationale: Anxiety, behavioral changes, headaches, and sleep disturbances are associated with postconcussion syndrome. Hallucinations/psychosis and fine tremors are not associated with postconcussion syndrome.

50. Answer: 1, 3

Rationale: Multiple sclerosis (MS) is most commonly diagnosed in northern Europe, North America, and Australia. It is uncommon around the equator. It affects Caucasians more than other ethnicities and females three times more often than males. MS is not a result of any one disorder but is felt to be due to environmental, genetic, and autoimmune interactions.

51. Answer: 4

Rationale: Homonymous hemianopia is the loss of the vision in one half of the visual field. Either the right or left field of vision may be affected. It is most often caused by a lesion or pathology in the optic tract or occipital lobe.

Pharmacology

52. Answer: 2

Rationale: Although most medication is discontinued after 4 years of no seizure activity, a confirmatory EEG should be obtained. Not all seizure patients require medication; referral to and monitoring by a neurologist are appropriate.

53. Answer: 3

Rationale: Scopolamine patches are placed behind the ear and provide medication for 3 days. The correct dose for meclizine (Antivert) is 12.5–25 mg PO tid to qid; for dimenhydrinate (Dramamine) 50 mg PO tid or qid; and for prochlorperazine 5–10 mg PO q4h prn.

54. Answer: 3

Rationale: Carbidopa/levodopa (Sinemet) induces a number of adverse reactions, including hypotension, gastrointestinal (GI) upset, psychosis, and motor complications. For best absorption, it should not be given around meals, despite GI side effects. It exerts no known effect on slowing disease progression.

55. Answer: 2

Rationale: NMDA receptor antagonists (e.g., memantine) are recognized as the class for management of moderate to severe Alzheimer's dementia. This group of medications control the effects of glutamate (the major excitatory transmitter in the CNS) at NMDA receptors, which are believed to play a critical role in learning and memory. The NMDA receptor regulates calcium entry into the neuron. Selective serotonin re-uptake inhibitors (SSRIs) are antidepressants used in the treatment of depression and anxiety. Central alpha$_2$ agonists are used in the treatment of hypertension.

56. Answer: 3

Rationale: Abortive medications for migraines cause cranial vasoconstriction, which will be generalized to all vessels, including cardiac. A history of cardiac disease, especially ischemia, increases risk for cardiac event.

57. Answer: 2

Rationale: Patients should be aware that all antiseizure medications can cause drowsiness, so driving, bathing, swimming, using machinery, climbing, etc., are all risky behaviors, especially when starting new medications. Contact sports would not be encouraged because the patient would be at risk of worsening seizure control should a head injury occur. Avoiding solitary activities is not discouraged, providing machinery and high areas are not involved. Medical alert bracelets or necklaces allow expedient information should the patient be injured and unconscious following a seizure.

58. Answer: 3

Rationale: Timely intervention with thrombolytics has the best evidence for patient outcomes. The goal from onset of symptoms to thrombolytics is 180 minutes. The risk of disability is greatly reduced with thrombolytic use, and the benefits outweigh the risk of a bleed.

59. Answer: 4

Rationale: Macrolide antibiotics, such as erythromycin and clarithromycin, can increase the plasma concentration of carbamazepine; therefore, when these medications are used together, carbamazepine levels must be closely monitored.

60. Answer: 2

Rationale: The risk for postherpetic neuralgia increases with age as well as zoster severity. Postherpetic neuralgia can be a chronic, life-altering condition and is associated with increased risks of suicide. Zoster targets the peripheral nervous system (individual dermatomes) but can also infect the central nervous system, causing myelitis and encephalitis.

61. Answer: 3

Rationale: Onset of drug action and relief of trigeminal neuralgia symptoms occur in 24 hours, usually in 4–6 hours. Laboratory tests are usually monitored based on the specific medication, not a peak and trough. These medications may be given to treat seizures.

Gastrointestinal & Liver

12

Physical Exam & Diagnostic Tests

1. The family nurse practitioner is preparing to examine the abdomen of a patient. What is the correct sequence in which to conduct the exam?

   1. Inspection, palpation, percussion, auscultation.

   2. Palpation, percussion, auscultation, inspection.

   3. Percussion, palpation, auscultation, inspection.

   4. Inspection, auscultation, percussion, palpation.

2. When obtaining a history from a young female adult patient with abdominal pain, which of the following should initially be assessed?

   1. Food effects on the pain.

   2. Location and onset of the pain.

   3. Change of pain with bowel movements.

   4. First day of last menstrual period.

3. To test for a positive obturator sign in a patient with abdominal pain, the family nurse practitioner:

   1. Passively flexes, and laterally and medially rotates the right leg from the 90-degree hip/knee flexion position.

   2. Asks the patient to take a deep breath while palpating in the abdominal right upper quadrant.

   3. Passively extends and elevates the right leg.

   4. Palpates the right abdomen one third the distance from the anterior superior iliac spine to the umbilicus.

4. The family nurse practitioner is performing the initial physical exam on a 51-year-old man. The history reveals that the patient's father died of colon cancer, but the patient is asymptomatic and has not had any screening for colon cancer. What is the best test to use to screen the patient?

   1. Barium enema and flexible sigmoidoscopy.

   2. CT colonography.

   3. Colonoscopy.

   4. Fecal occult blood and stool DNA testing.

5. Once a positive anti-HCV test is found, the next step for the family nurse practitioner to do is:

   1. Call the patient and explain that hepatitis C is active and treatment is needed.

   2. Repeat the anti-HCV test to assure it is positive.

   3. Test the hepatitis B panel.

   4. Test for an HCV RNA viral load.

6. Diagnosis of acute hepatitis B includes the following results:

   1. Positive HB surface antigen (HBsAg) and HBe antigen (HbeAg).

   2. Positive HB surface antigen (HbsAg) and HB surface antibody (anti-HBs).

   3. Positive HB core antibody (HbcAg) and negative HB surface antigen (HbsAg).

   4. HB core antibody (HbcAg) and HB surface antibody (anti-HBs).

7. The diagnosis of early acute pancreatitis would be considered by the family nurse practitioner based on history of severe acute upper abdominal pain and which of the following laboratory results?

   1. White blood cell (WBC) count of 10,300/mm³.

   2. Serum albumin of 6.2 g/dL.

   3. Serum amylase of 350 U/L.

   4. Serum lipase of 75 U/L.

8. An overweight, middle-aged woman has right upper quadrant pain that radiates to her right subscapular area and is severe and persistent. She is also experiencing anorexia, nausea, and a fever. Her most recent meal was a double quarter-pound hamburger with cheese, french fries, and a vanilla shake. Based on this information, the family nurse practitioner examines the abdomen and percusses for costovertebral angle tenderness. The abdomen is tender in the right upper quadrant. Which of the following signs, if positive, corresponds to the correct diagnosis?

   1. Obturator sign; patient has appendicitis.

   2. Costovertebral angle tenderness; patient has a urinary tract infection.

   3. Murphy's sign; patient has cholecystitis.

   4. McBurney's sign; patient has acute appendicitis.

9. The family nurse practitioner reviews laboratory results for a patient that reveal a positive *Helicobacter pylori* stool antigen test. The family nurse practitioner would want to treat this if the patient complained of:

   1. Upper abdominal pain.

   2. Altered bowel habits.

   3. Dysphagia.

   4. Nausea.

Disorders

10. A sudden onset of diarrhea that consists of 5–6 loose stools a day and awakens the patient at night with cramping, but without blood in the stools, would most likely be caused by:

    1. Infection.

    2. Irritable bowel syndrome.

    3. Ischemic colitis.

    4. Lactose intolerance.

11. An adult male presents with midsternal chest pain with radiation to the neck and left arm. He denies other symptoms. He was seen in the emergency room and had a negative cardiac workup. What might be the diagnosis?

    1. Pneumonia.

    2. Costochondritis.

    3. Gastroesophageal reflux.

    4. Esophageal spasm.

12. The family nurse practitioner suspects peritonitis in a patient. What assessment finding is most indicative of peritonitis?

    1. Palpate and watch for a positive Murphy's sign.

    2. Perform a rectal exam and test the stool for blood.

    3. Auscultate the abdomen for increased bowel sounds.

    4. Palpate for rebound tenderness.

13. An older adult woman is noted to have iron-deficiency anemia. She has no pain. What history would raise the suspicion of a gastric ulcer?

    1. Symptoms of acid reflux for the past 2 years, occurring at least 3 times a week.

    2. Postmenopausal with no recent history of vaginal bleeding.

    3. Weight loss of 10 lbs in the past 2 months.

    4. An ankle sprain requiring 800 mg of ibuprofen three times a day for the past 6 weeks.

14. A history of a patient with a chief complaint of diarrhea alternating with constipation, intermittent cramping, and bloating and relieved by a bowel movement is most likely:

    1. Drug-induced diarrhea.

    2. Inflammatory bowel disease.

    3. Gastroenteritis.

    4. Irritable bowel syndrome (IBS).

15. Which patient presentation would most likely suggest dysphagia caused by esophageal spasm?

    1. They usually have more difficulty swallowing solids than liquids.

    2. There is a long history of gastroesophageal reflux.

    3. They have difficulty swallowing both solids and liquids.

    4. They have marked weight loss.

16. Which problem would most likely worsen the symptoms of gastroesophageal reflux disease (GERD)?

    1. Small sliding hiatal hernia.

    2. An empty stomach when lying down.

    3. Gaining 30 pounds over a period of months.

    4. Gastroparesis.

17. A patient comes to the emergency department concerned about pain and swelling in his groin. He tells the family nurse practitioner that his doctor said he has an incarcerated hernia. Which assessment finding correlates with an incarcerated hernia?

    1. Hernia that easily moves back and forth across the abdominal wall.

    2. Hernia that protrudes from the groin area and cannot be reduced into the abdomen.

    3. Hernia that is very painful to palpation with significant abdominal swelling.

    4. Hernia that decreases in size when the patient increases intra-abdominal pressure.

18. Which finding most likely indicates a need for an endoscopy in patients with heartburn?

    1. All new cases of heartburn.

    2. Symptoms persisting after 8–12 weeks of empiric therapy.

    3. Negative *Helicobacter pylori (H. pylori)* test.

    4. Good response to empiric treatment after 7–10 days.

19. The family nurse practitioner knows that the following principle is most important in understanding the pathophysiology of gastroesophageal reflux disease (GERD):

    1. A hiatal hernia is always a coexisting and major contributing factor.

    2. The lower esophageal sphincter (LES) has become a poor antireflux barrier.

    3. The amount of acid reflux depends on a familial tendency for GERD.

    4. Overeating and use of caffeine and alcohol cause GERD.

20. Irritable bowel syndrome (IBS) affects:

    1. Men more than women.

    2. Children more than young adults.

    3. Women more than men.

    4. Older adults more than young adults.

21. The family nurse practitioner understands that hepatitis B can be transmitted through blood and blood products. Another mode of transmission of hepatitis B is:

    1. Respiratory contact.

    2. Arthropod vectors.

    3. Fecal-oral route.

    4. Perinatal exposure.

22. Which two forms of viral hepatitis are transmitted by the fecal-oral route?

    1. Hepatitis A.

    2. Hepatitis B.

    3. Hepatitis C.

    4. Hepatitis D.

    5. Hepatitis E.

23. An exam of the male genitalia that consists of inserting a finger into the lower scrotum and into the inguinal canal and asking the patient to cough that causes the family nurse practitioner to feel a sudden presence of a viscus that lies within the inguinal canal and comes through the external canal passing into the scrotum is most likely called:

    1. An indirect inguinal hernia.

    2. A direct inguinal hernia.

    3. A strangulated inguinal hernia.

    4. A femoral hernia.

24. Which is true about enterobiasis (pinworm infection)?

    1. The parasite is in the soil and enters the body through the feet. It can cause anemia.

    2. The parasite causes pruritus around the anus because the gravid females exit through the anus at night and lay eggs on the skin. The human is the only host of this parasite.

    3. The eggs of this parasite enter the body by ingestion of dirt (pica) or dirt on unwashed vegetables that contain the eggs, or through water containing the eggs.

    4. This parasite is a protozoan. The source is usually contaminated water, but it is spread from person to person by fecal-oral contamination.

25. Nonpharmacologic management of GERD includes which of the following?

    1. Weight reduction and sleep with head of bed elevated 4–6 inches with blocks.

    2. Lying down and resting after meals and weight reduction.

    3. Drinking large amounts of fluids with meals and avoiding alcohol.

    4. Avoiding mint, orange juice, and milk.

26. An organism associated with etiology of peptic ulcer disease (PUD) is:

    1. *Streptococcus pneumoniae.*

    2. *Helicobacter pylori.*

    3. *Moraxella catarrhalis.*

    4. *Staphylococcus aureus.*

27. All of the following are common causes of cirrhosis in the United States except:

    1. Hepatitis A.

    2. Nonalcoholic fatty liver disease.

    3. Chronic hepatitis C.

    4. Alcohol ingestion.

28. Prolapse of the anal cushion, made up of vascular, connective and muscular tissue, through the anal canal below the dentate line describes:

    1. Rectal prolapse.

    2. External hemorrhoid.

    3. Rectocele.

    4. Internal hemorrhoid.

29. An acute illness with jaundice, anorexia, malaise, arthralgias, an incubation period of 2–6 months, a chronic and acute form, and that is transmitted by parenteral, sexual, and perinatal routes describes:

    1. Hepatitis A.

    2. Hepatitis B.

    3. Hepatitis C.

    4. Hepatitis E.

30. A patient with a history of cholelithiasis presents to the office complaining of increased right upper quadrant abdominal pain. The family nurse practitioner would arrange immediate hospital admission for possible prompt intervention if the history also showed that the patient is:

    1. HIV positive.

    2. 75 years old and diabetic.

    3. 5 weeks pregnant.

    4. Vomiting with a slight fever.

31. An older adult male presents to the family nurse practitioner for evaluation of years of "heartburn" and recent significant weight loss (30 lb in 1 month). He has been taking antacids and an oral histamine (H_2) blocker for "years off and on" and has not had relief of his symptoms. He has a 60-pack-year history of cigarette smoking and drinks alcohol daily. What differential diagnosis must the family nurse practitioner consider first?

    1. Gastric ulcer.

    2. Gastroesophageal reflux disease (GERD).

    3. Esophageal cancer.

    4. Lung cancer.

32. An adult patient presents to the family nurse practitioner complaining of weakness and vomiting. He gives a history of "several" drinks per day for the past 22 years and cirrhosis, diagnosed 6 months ago. The family nurse practitioner questions the patient about excessive bleeding. The patient reports 2 episodes of hematemesis. What emergent condition is the family nurse practitioner most concerned about?

    1. Bleeding peptic ulcer (PUD).

    2. Excessive nosebleed.

    3. Hemoptysis.

    4. Esophageal varices.

33. A young adult female presents to the family nurse practitioner for evaluation of 2 days of increasing crampy abdominal pain. She states that she also has some mild nausea, anorexia, and a low-grade fever. The patient states that the pain is periumbilical. Her STAT complete CBC reveals a slightly elevated WBC but is otherwise normal. What is the family nurse practitioner's next step in the care of this patient?

    1. Refer to a gynecologist for evaluation of possible ectopic pregnancy.

    2. Order a CT of the abdomen and refer to surgeon for evaluation of possible appendicitis.

    3. Observe overnight and reassess the next day.

    4. Place on a clear liquid diet and have patient watch for increasing symptoms.

34. An adult patient has early alcoholic cirrhosis diagnosed by a liver biopsy. While teaching the patient to manage her symptoms, the family nurse practitioner instructs that it is most important that the patient:

    1. Take a daily vitamin E supplement.

    2. Decrease her alcohol intake to less than 2 drinks a day.

    3. Abstain from alcohol.

    4. Maintain a nutritious diet.

35. An older adult patient presents with fever, leukocytosis, and a sudden onset of lower left quadrant pain for the past 12 hours. She has not had a bowel movement since the pain began. The family nurse practitioner's top differential diagnosis would be:

    1. Appendicitis.

    2. Diverticulitis.

    3. Irritable bowel syndrome.

    4. Ruptured ovarian cyst.

36. Which patient would be at lowest risk for developing diverticular disease?

    1. A vegetarian on a high-fiber diet.

    2. A patient with chronic constipation for 10 years.

    3. An older adult on a small-meal diet.

    4. A fad dieter on a fiber diet.

37. The family nurse practitioner knows that colon cancer screening with colonoscopy is definitely warranted in a patient with:

    1. Anemia.

    2. Diarrhea.

    3. Bright-red rectal bleeding.

    4. Change in bowel habits.

38. The family nurse practitioner knows that in patients with ulcerative colitis that involve the entire colon, careful surveillance of the colon is required because of an increased risk of:

    1. Colon cancer.

    2. Diverticulosis.

    3. Ischemic colitis.

    4. Irritable bowel syndrome.

39. Which is true of peptic ulcer disease (PUD) in older adult patients?

    1. Smoking does not increase the risk of PUD.

    2. Duodenal ulcers are more common in older adults.

    3. Perforation is a common complication.

    4. Weight loss and anorexia are often the only symptoms.

40. Which is true of early cancer of the esophagus in the older adult patient?

    1. Alcoholism and smoking increase the risk for adenocarcinoma of the esophagus.

    2. It is associated with high caffeine use.

    3. Dysphagia for solids and cough may be the first symptoms.

    4. Boring-type midchest pain indicates mediastinal involvement and requires immediate surgery.

41. A patient has a history of colon polyps. The family nurse practitioner knows:

    1. A history of polyps increases the risk of colon cancer, and more frequent screening is required.

    2. Hyperplastic polyps are a concern for malignancy.

    3. Small polyps <1 cm are not a concern.

    4. A colonoscopy is 99% accurate for finding colon polyps and cancer.

42. A young adult patient presents with a complaint of intermittent diarrhea and cramping for the past 2 years. Screening blood tests reveal iron-deficiency anemia and elevated liver transaminases. The family nurse practitioner suspects:

    1. Hepatitis B.

    2. Celiac sprue.

    3. *Salmonella* infection.

    4. Bleeding peptic ulcer.

43. A middle-aged male patient with elevated liver enzymes and no other symptoms has a history of type 2 diabetes and hypercholesterolemia. The family nurse practitioner would first consider:

    1. Nonalcoholic fatty liver disease (NAFLD).

    2. Autoimmune hepatitis.

    3. Celiac sprue.

    4. Drug-induced liver disease.

44. In patients suspected of having celiac sprue with elevated antibodies, but negative biopsy, the family nurse practitioner knows:

    1. The patient may have a negative biopsy because she has been gluten free for 3 weeks.

    2. The positive antibodies are likely a laboratory error.

    3. The patient may have a gluten sensitivity.

    4. The biopsy may be a false negative result.

45. A young female adult reports she had the flu and recovered 2 weeks ago. She reports resolution of her symptoms, except she continues to have nausea, decreased appetite, and early satiety. The family nurse practitioner suspects:

    1. A relapse of the influenza infection.

    2. Post-viral gastroparesis.

    3. Vertigo, causing nausea related to a possible ear infection.

    4. Peptic ulcer from taking ibuprofen.

46. Irritable bowel syndrome (IBS) can produce which of the following symptoms?

    1. Abdominal cramping, rectal bleeding, and diarrhea.

    2. Diarrhea alternating with constipation but no pain.

    3. Abdominal cramping, diarrhea, and fecal incontinence.

    4. Abdominal cramping, diarrhea, and bloating.

47. When discussing diet with a patient with irritable bowel syndrome (IBS), the family nurse practitioner tells the patient to avoid:

    1. Simple sugars.

    2. Dairy products.

    3. Red meat.

    4. Vegetables.

48. Patient education for a patient with nonalcoholic fatty liver disease (NAFLD) should include:

    1. Lowering cholesterol intake.

    2. To not take a statin medication.

    3. Exercise and weight loss.

    4. To take vitamin A.

Pharmacology

49. The family nurse practitioner is examining a 30-year-old obese man with a body mass index (BMI) of 35 who complains of almost daily indigestion and heartburn for the past year with a strong acid taste in the mouth about an hour after meals, and frequent belching and awakening at night with choking. The history is negative for chronic illnesses and alarm symptoms. A diagnosis of gastroesophageal reflux disease (GERD) is made. What is the best initial treatment for the patient?

    1. Omeprazole (Prilosec) 20 mg after breakfast daily.

    2. Hyoscyamine (Levsin) 0.125 mg tid 15 minutes before eating.

    3. Ranitidine (Zantac) 150 mg bid.

    4. Omeprazole (Prilosec) 20 mg every morning 30 minutes before breakfast.

50. Which of the following would be prescribed as initial treatment for uncomplicated peptic ulcer disease (PUD) with negative *Helicobacter pylori*?

    1. Clarithromycin 500 mg bid.

    2. Famotidine (Pepcid) 25 mg daily.

    3. Omeprazole (Prilosec) 20 mg qd.

    4. Bismuth (Pepto-Bismol) 2 tablets twice a day.

51. Which drug would be most useful for the family nurse practitioner to prescribe for an adult patient's arthritis pain to reduce the risk of ulcers?

    1. Celecoxib (Celebrex).

    2. Cimetidine (Tagamet).

    3. Misoprostol (Cytotec).

    4. Omeprazole (Prilosec).

52. After percutaneous or permucosal exposure to a hepatitis B source, what is the appropriate treatment for the patient?

    1. In an unvaccinated patient, begin the hepatitis B series.

    2. In a person with a positive hepatitis B surface antibody, no treatment is necessary.

    3. In a vaccinated person with a negative antihepatitis B surface antigen, give hepatitis B immune globulin (HBIG), and initiate a new hepatitis B vaccine series.

    4. In a patient with a positive antihepatitis B surface antibody who completed the entire hepatitis B vaccine series, give a hepatitis B booster.

53. Successful treatment for an adult patient with *Helicobacter pylori (H. pylori)*-induced peptic ulcer disease requires therapy with which regimen?

    1. Clarithromycin, amoxicillin, and omeprazole (Prilosec).

    2. Bismuth (Pepto-Bismol), cephalexin (Keflex), and metronidazole (Flagyl).

    3. Amoxicillin, bismuth (Pepto-Bismol), metronidazole (Flagyl), and cimetidine (Tagamet).

    4. Clarithromycin, cephalexin (Keflex), and lansoprazole.

54. A primary therapy for patients with mild ulcerative colitis is:

    1. Metronidazole (Flagyl).

    2. Mesalamine (Pentasa).

    3. Ciprofloxacin (Cipro).

    4. Prednisone (Deltasone).

55. For a patient exposed to household or sexual contacts with hepatitis A, the family nurse practitioner would:

    1. Give immunoglobulin 0.02 mL/kg as soon as possible but no later than 2 weeks after exposure.

    2. Give one dose of HBIG and immunoglobulin 0.02 mL/kg as soon as possible.

    3. Give immunoglobulin 0.02 mL/kg and two doses of HBIG.

    4. Understand that no injections are needed.

56. A young woman presents with a history of recent unprotected sexual activity (in the past 2 weeks) with a partner now diagnosed with hepatitis B. She is currently asymptomatic and does not recall having a vaccine in the past. What is the best action for the family nurse practitioner?

    1. Obtain a hepatitis B e antibody test (anti-HBe).

    2. Administer one dose of HBIG.

    3. Obtain a viral load for hepatitis B.

    4. Administer one dose of HBIG and initiate vaccination.

57. What condition is a contraindication for the administration of the hepatitis B vaccine?

    1. Pregnancy.

    2. Lactation.

    3. Severe hypersensitivity.

    4. Age >60 years.

58. A 78-year-old patient is diagnosed with *Clostridium difficile* infection, and the physician prescribes vancomycin (Vancocin) 125 mg PO qid. In following the patient's progress, the family nurse practitioner would monitor which of the following in regard to medication tolerance?

    1. CBC, platelet count, clotting studies.

    2. Serum creatinine, BUN, hearing changes.

    3. Serum electrolytes, urinalysis, ataxia.

    4. Changes in bowel habits, diarrhea, ECG changes.

59. A patient with PUD is treated with a regimen that includes bismuth subsalicylate (Pepto-Bismol), tetracycline, and metronidazole (Flagyl). The patient calls the family nurse practitioner to report that his stools are unusually dark. He is not experiencing any gastric discomfort, orthostatic hypotension, or increased lethargy. How would the family nurse practitioner interpret the information?

    1. He is probably bleeding and should come in immediately.

    2. He ate something to affect the color of his stool.

    3. His stools are dark, secondary to Pepto-Bismol.

    4. The stool discoloration is caused by metronidazole.

12 | Gastrointestinal & Liver Answers and Rationales

Physical Exam & Diagnostic Tests

1. Answer: 4

Rationale: Inspection and auscultation should be conducted first to prevent eliciting pain and undue guarding. The family nurse practitioner should auscultate and listen to the abdomen before percussing and palpating it, because palpation may alter the frequency of bowel sounds. If the exam is painful initially, the patient will be uncomfortable, which will not allow the examiner to continue.

2. Answer: 4

Rationale: Although all the information is important in determining the cause of abdominal pain, for a young female patient of childbearing age, ascertaining whether the patient is pregnant is a priority. A possibility of pregnancy would alter the testing that might need to be ordered, so a pregnancy test should be ordered. Additionally, abdominal pain may be from pelvic inflammatory disease or related gynecologic disorders. The family nurse practitioner should obtain a gynecologic, pregnancy, and recent sexual history, including dates of last two normal menstrual periods, condom use and other birth control use, and timing of last sexual intercourse. Food effects are important to ascertain because it may lead to a diagnosis of dietary intolerances. Location and associated symptoms are valuable to narrow down the differential diagnoses of the pain. Abrupt onset of pain has differential diagnoses that are different from pain that is recurrent or has occurred for weeks or longer (chronic). Acute pain can be visceral (internal), somatic (superficial), or referred, which arises from the viscera and terminates in the spinal cord where there are fibers in the skin. These sensations produce the perception of pain at the referred site. Change in bowel habits may indicate an intestinal origin if there is relief, even if only temporary. Pain not affected by a bowel movement or passing gas is not likely intestinal/colonic pain and may be related to other sources, such as kidney/bladder or the musculoskeletal system.

3. Answer: 1

Rationale: If abdominal pain results from passive flexion to 90 degrees and lateral and medial rotation of the right leg causes right hypogastric pain, then inflammation of the obturator internus muscle, a positive obturator sign, suggests a ruptured appendix or pelvic abscess. A positive Murphy's sign, severe pain, and a brief inspiratory arrest result when a patient takes a deep breath while the examiner applies pressure over the right upper quadrant suggestive of cholecystitis. McBurney's point and sign, eliciting pain in the right lower quadrant, is associated with acute appendicitis. The psoas sign, extension and

elevation of the right leg that causes pain, is a sign of inflammation of the psoas muscle, which is a sign of appendicitis.

4. Answer: 3

Rationale: A colonoscopy is the most accurate and best test to use to screen for colon cancer. The improved equipment and medication for sedation and colon preparation have made this test safe and effective. Finding and removing colon polyps increase the prevention of colon cancer. A barium enema has poor sensitivity and specificity for locating polyps and cancer. The test requires a bowel preparation and is uncomfortable for the patient. A flexible sigmoidoscopy is a test with a limited exam of the lower portion of the colon. The "virtual colonoscopy" is performed by a CT scan. It requires a bowel preparation and can be uncomfortable. It does not examine the rectum and can miss smaller polyps. Fecal occult blood testing has low sensitivity and specificity and has limited use for screening. Stool DNA is new technology and will likely have an increasing role, but it detects early cancer, not polyps.

5. Answer: 4

Rationale: Hepatitis C exposure will produce a positive anti-HCV. However, it is not necessarily indicative of active infection. Twenty percent of patients exposed to hepatitis C will clear the virus without treatment but will continue to have a positive antibody. The best approach is to confirm that hepatitis C is present is with the viral load test. Repeating the antibody is not useful. Without confirmation, it is not appropriate to inform the patient of an active infection, but it should be explained that it is possible there is infection.

6. Answer: 1

Rationale: Hepatitis B surface antigen (HBsAg) indicates active infection. HBe antigen (HbeAg) is present in early and active disease with high infectivity and can predict chronic infection. HB core antibody (HbcAg) can indicate chronic infection or exposure without having acquired infection. HB surface antibody (anti-HBs) indicates the end of acute infection and can also indicate immunity.

7. Answer: 3

Rationale: In acute pancreatitis, the serum amylase increases within 3–6 hours of onset. A level 3 times normal is more diagnostic. The serum lipase elevates after the increase in amylase. In adults, the normal level for serum amylase is 30–110 IU/L and for serum lipase 13–141 IU/L. An elevated serum albumin occurs with dehydration and high-protein diets.

8. Answer: 3

Rationale: The history, right upper quadrant pain that radiates to the right subscapular area, especially after a fatty meal, and positive Murphy's sign are all associated with cholecystitis. A positive Murphy's sign is noted with severe pain with inspiratory arrest on palpation of the right upper quadrant.

9. Answer: 1

Rationale: *Helicobacter pylori* is a bacteria that is responsible for most duodenal and gastric ulcers. The most accurate non-invasive test for active infection is the stool antigen test. Serum IgG and IgM antibody testing may not indicate a current infection. The bacteria cause ulcers and gastric inflammation, which can present as upper abdominal pain. Altered bowel habits may be indicative of irritable bowel syndrome, which has no relation to the bacteria. Nausea is a nonspecific symptom with no strong correlation to the bacteria.

Disorders

10. Answer: 1

Rationale: Diarrhea is a common symptom with a wide differential. Clues include awakening at night and cramping without blood. A sudden onset that awakens a patient suggests pathology, which could be inflammation or infection. Obtaining a travel history, exposure to infection, and medication history will suggest infection. Irritable bowel syndrome is a functional disorder that does not awaken the patient. Ischemic colitis presents with rectal bleeding, as well as pain and diarrhea. Lactose intolerance and other dietary triggers cause functional diarrhea and cramping.

11. Answer: 3

Rationale: A negative workup for cardiac disease leads to other considerations for chest pain. Gastroesophageal reflux can cause chest pain, and patients do not always have classic symptoms of reflux. This would be the most likely diagnosis to consider. Pneumonia is very unlikely without any respiratory symptoms. Costochondritis is a common musculoskeletal symptom that is noted on palpation of the rib cage. Esophageal spasm can cause pain but is usually accompanied by dysphagia.

12. Answer: 4

Rationale: Rebound tenderness is found with palpation of the abdomen and quickly lifting the hand. Patients will complain of more pain with releasing the pressure on the abdomen. This suggests peritoneal irritation and inflammation. Stool for occult blood is not a test for peritonitis. Increased bowel sounds would not be present with peritonitis. Decreased bowel sounds may be present.

13. Answer: 4

Rationale: Nonsteroidal anti-inflammatory drugs (NSAIDs), such as ibuprofen, cause a high risk of gastrointestinal erosion and ulcers. There may be no symptoms until anemia is noted. Gastroesophageal reflux does not contribute to anemia, unless there is gastritis with erosions or other signs of bleeding. Postmenopausal history is significant because it rules out a cause of anemia but not a concern for ulcer development. Weight loss of 5 lb a month is a nonspecific symptom that needs further exploration.

14. Answer: 4

Rationale: Irritable bowel syndrome (IBS) presents with abdominal pain and altered bowel habits that can be erratic and unpredictable. These symptoms can be aggravated by stress and food triggers. Diarrhea does not occur during sleep, but abdominal pain can occur at any time. Drug-induced diarrhea occurs in association with certain medications, usually taken within the previous few months. Prime offending medications include antibiotics (may cause *Clostridium difficile* colitis) and metformin, for example. Bacterial or viral gastroenteritis presents with a sudden onset of diarrhea and does not alternate with constipation. Inflammatory bowel disease presents with more consistent symptoms of diarrhea and pain and possibly rectal bleeding. In fact, the symptoms can be present for months to years before diagnosis. Extraintestinal manifestations, such as arthritis and skin lesions, may be present, and nocturnal diarrhea and fecal incontinence can be present if rectal inflammation is present.

15. Answer: 3

Rationale: Patients with dysphagia due to an esophageal spasm may report difficulty with both liquids and solids, as the spasm has closed the esophagus temporarily. Relaxation of the esophagus usually occurs within a minute, and the food will pass down. This can cause choking with liquids as well. Spasm can occur for many reasons, one of which can be acid reflux. It is episodic, nonprogressive, and unpredictable. Difficulty swallowing solids and feeling that food is sticking is most likely because of an esophageal stricture or obstruction. Marked weight loss is not usually a symptom of dysphagia, unless is it related to esophageal cancer.

16. Answer: 4

Rationale: Gastroparesis can be a significant complication for patients with reflux. The lingering contents in the stomach will contain acid and the frequency of reflux will be increased. Persons with a small sliding hiatal hernia are not likely to have a significant change in their symptoms. Reflux is less likely to occur after lying down with an empty stomach.

17. Answer: 2

Rationale: The most common hernia is an inguinal hernia, protruding at the inguinal canal. Incarcerated means the hernia cannot be reduced or returned to the abdominal cavity. A reducible hernia easily moves across the abdominal wall. There should be no abdominal swelling, and if the hernia is particularly painful and associated with nausea and vomiting, strangulation/incarceration should be considered as a surgical emergency.

18. Answer: 2

Rationale: An endoscopy is needed for patients with no/minimal response to therapy, indicated by persistent symptoms after 8–12 weeks of therapy. Heartburn may be characterized by burning substernal chest pain and may have gastroesophageal reflux. The factors that would raise a red flag would be long-term history of reflux, dysphagia, or weight loss.

19. Answer: 2

Rationale: The factor contributing most to reflux is an incompetent lower esophageal sphincter (LES), the antireflux barrier. A hiatal hernia is frequently present with reflux but is not a significant factor in the pathophysiology, unless it is large, but may be associated with greater reflux and delayed esophageal acid clearance in patients with reflux. Gastroesophageal reflux disease (GERD) can be familial but is not always a factor. Overeating, alcohol, and caffeine all affect the LES pressure and increase stomach acid production, affecting symptoms, but are not the main cause.

20. Answer: 3

Rationale: The female/male ratio for irritable bowel syndrome (IBS) is thought to be 3:1. It is a functional disorder, not a disease that can affect any age, children to older adults, but IBS frequently has an onset in young adults.

21. Answer: 4

Rationale: A means of hepatitis B (HBV) transmission is from mother to baby, perinatally. Before the hepatitis B vaccine, it was estimated that 30–40% of chronic HBV infections were transmitted perinatally. Since the widespread use of the vaccine and guidelines of vaccinating newborns, this rate has dropped dramatically. The main routes of transmission are percutaneous or mucosal contact with infectious blood or body fluids, such as semen and saliva. The exposure can occur with sexual contact, intravenous drug use with shared needles and other equipment, contact with blood or open sores, needle sticks, and sharing razors or toothbrushes with an infected person. HBV is not spread by food, water, sharing eating utensils, breastfeeding, hugging, kissing, coughing, or sneezing.

22. Answer: 1, 5

Rationale: Hepatitis A and E are transmitted by the fecal-oral route. Hepatitis A spreads rapidly in households and daycare centers for children. Risk is higher in daycare centers with young children who wear diapers. Outbreaks can also occur from contaminated food and water infected with human sewage. Hepatitis C and hepatitis D are transmitted by blood transfusion, needle sharing, sexual contact, and vertical (perinatal) transmission. Hepatitis D occurs as a coinfection with hepatitis B.

23. Answer: 1

Rationale: When there is a defect in the abdominal wall, a hernia can develop. The hernia is a protrusion of a peritoneal-lined sac (i.e., bowel or omentum) through the weakness in the abdominal wall. An indirect hernia protrusion occurs directly through the floor of the inguinal canal and exits through the external inguinal ring. A direct hernia is less common and occurs more in those over 40 years of age. It may be felt medial to the external canal and rarely passes into the scrotum. A femoral hernia is noted when the femoral artery exits the abdomen and is the least common of pelvic hernias. It occurs more in females. A strangulated hernia is nonreducible and can be a surgical emergency.

24. Answer: 2

Rationale: The pinworm parasites reside in the intestine. Females lay eggs on the skin outside the anus, resulting in extreme pruritus. The only host is humans, and it is transmitted by the fecal-oral route, easily spreading among households, daycares and schools. Hookwoom larvae reside in the soil, enter the body through the feet, and can cause anemia. When dirt containing roundworm eggs is ingested through pica or unwashed vegetables, or if contaminated water is consumed, an intestinal infestation occurs. Giardiasis results from ingestion of the protozoan *Giardia lamblia* through contaminated water or oral-fecal transmission.

25. Answer: 1

Rationale: An important nonpharmacologic intervention for gastroesophageal reflux disease (GERD) is to advise the patient not to lie down within 2–3 hours after meals to allow the stomach to empty. Patients with GERD also should reduce weight, avoid large meals and exercise after meals, and elevate the head of the bed. Certain drinks (alcohol, mint, and orange juice) should be avoided because they can increase acid production and can relax the lower esophageal sphincter (LES). Acidic foods (tomato products; spicy foods) may worsen symptoms of reflux and should be avoided. The patient should be taught to avoid bending after meals. Drinking large amounts of fluid with meals may affect GERD, depending on the volume of the fluids.

26. Answer: 2

Rationale: *Helicobacter pylori* has been shown to be responsible for most duodenal and gastric ulcers. The other common cause of ulcers is from use of nonsteroidal anti-inflammatory drugs (NSAIDs) at regular and/or high doses. The other organisms listed are implicated in other types of infections (e.g., acute otitis media; skin infections). *Streptococcus pneumoniae* and *Moraxella catarrhalis* have been implicated as causative agents in pneumonia.

27. Answer: 1

Rationale: Hepatitis A never becomes chronic and is not a cause of cirrhosis. Nonalcoholic fatty liver disease (NAFLD) is common, affects 20% of the general population, and is related to metabolic syndrome. There are excess fat deposits in the liver in persons who drink little or no alcohol, which can cause inflammation and scarring (cirrhosis). NAFLD has become a common cause of cirrhosis. Chronic hepatitis C is a major cause of cirrhosis and need for liver transplantation. It is estimated that 3 million people in the United States are infected. Alcohol is the most common cause of cirrhosis worldwide. Daily drinking and recent alcohol consumption have an increased risk of liver disease and cirrhosis.

28. Answer: 2

Rationale: A hemorrhoid is a vascular anal cushion and can be internal (above the dentate line) or external (below the dentate line), which can enlarge and bleed. Everyone has internal hemorrhoids even without any symptoms. In a rectal mucosa prolapse, the wall of the rectum prolapses through the anal canal on straining. A rectocele is a herniation into the vaginal wall and can cause constipation.

29. Answer: 2

Rationale: These characteristics describe hepatitis B, which affects less than 1% of the U.S. population and is a much less common cause of cirrhosis. Hepatitis A has common causes of fever and up to 50% jaundice. Transmission is by the fecal-oral route or sexual contact and has an incubation period of 15–50 days (average 30 days) and no chronic form. Hepatitis C infection causes jaundice up to 25% of the time and can cause arthralgias, but there is no fever. It is transmitted parenterally, sexually, and perinatally and has an incubation period of 14–18 days (average 42–49 days). Up to 75% of those infected with hepatitis C will develop chronic infection. Hepatitis E is characterized by oral-fecal transmission that is associated with contaminated food and water and has an incubation period of 14–60 days and no chronic disease state.

30. Answer: 2

Rationale: Although most patients need eventual intervention, those who are older adults and diabetic are at increased risk and should be hospitalized for prompt diagnosis, which could include a right upper quadrant (RUQ) abdominal ultrasound, and/or a magnetic resonance cholangiopancreatography (MRCP). The MRCP is very sensitive at documenting a gallstone lodged in the bile duct. Abnormally elevated transaminases and possibly pancreatic enzymes would be present with bile duct blockage, and the patient may have secondary pancreatitis. Intravenous fluids, pain control, and surgical consultation would also be warranted.

31. Answer: 3

Rationale: Long-term GERD ("heartburn for years") without effective treatment carries a risk of Barrett's esophagus, a precursor to esophageal adenocarcinoma, especially in a non-Hispanic white male smokers over the age of 50 years. Rapid weight loss is a concerning clinical finding that may indicate esophageal cancer or other cancer. Squamous cell carcinoma of the esophagus is associated with cigarette smoking and alcohol use and is less common than adenocarcinoma (ratio 1:2). Adenocarcinoma of the esophagus most commonly develops in men (men/women ratio 6:1) age 65 years and older. The symptoms of heartburn caused by either gastric ulcer or long-term GERD will not likely be controlled with an H2 blocker/antacid and would require a proton pump inhibitor daily. A patient with a gastric ulcer would be tested for *Helicobacter pylori* and would be questioned about a history of nonsteroidal anti-inflammatory drug (NSAID) use and then treated appropriately. Clinical manifestations of lung cancer include cough, hemoptysis, dyspnea, chest pain, and weight loss, and the substantial pack-year history does place the patient at risk.

32. Answer: 4

Rationale: Esophageal varices are dilated submucosal veins that are a late sign and complication of cirrhosis because of scarring of the liver and portal hypertension. The cirrhosis would likely be advanced for varices to develop, usually in the esophagus, but can also occur in the stomach. As these varices are under high pressure, the patient can have anything from a slow leak of blood to a major, life-threatening bleed. The patient is diagnosed by endoscopy and treated with beta blockers to lower the blood pressure. Of patients with cirrhosis, approximately 50% will develop gastroesophageal varices and will have a yearly rate of bleeding from 5–15%. A history of heavy alcohol intake may be the cause of this patient's cirrhosis. These patients can present clinically with bleeding, spontaneous "coffee ground" or bright-red blood, hypotension, and eventual shock. The other choices could all be associated with this patient. A bleeding peptic ulcer is possible but is not the first concern. An excessive nosebleed is possible because of thrombocytopenia from cirrhosis and would need to be explored. Hemoptysis implies lung disease.

33. Answer: 2

Rationale: Increasing crampy abdominal pain that starts as periumbilical pain, anorexia, and fever are classic symptoms of appendicitis. A surgeon should evaluate the patient to decrease the risk of rupture. An abdominal CT scan has a high sensitivity to document appendicitis. Although ectopic pregnancy should always be a consideration in young females with abdominal pain, the characteristics of the pain and other symptoms are not typical of an ectopic pregnancy. However, a good gynecologic history would be needed. The patient should not be sent home unless the CT scan is negative, and then follow-up within 24 hours would be warranted.

34. Answer: 3

Rationale: Abstinence from alcohol, the most important treatment for cirrhosis, can halt progression of cirrhosis and reverse the damage, if the liver is minimally scarred. Continuing to drink even occasionally can be detrimental and rapidly increase the disease process. It is known that 1–2 drinks a day for a woman raises her risk of cirrhosis up to 4 times the risk of the general population. Recent research shows that current drinking may be more of a factor than a lifetime amount. The patient's diet should be nutritious, and she should avoid herbal and other supplements because some have been known to cause liver toxicity. Vitamin E supplementation is controversial and may be recommended by the patient's hepatologist. It is not a routine part of care.

35. Answer: 2

Rationale: Diverticulitis usually presents with a sudden onset of abdominal pain in the left lower quadrant. The patient may have a low-grade fever and leukocytosis. Patients with diverticulitis have a range of mild to severe disease. Severe pain may be accompanied by nausea and vomiting. Appendicitis may present with pain in the periumbilicus that eventually travels to the right lower quadrant and may not be severe for several hours after onset. Other signs, including nausea and vomiting, leukocytosis, and fever, may or may not be present. Irritable bowel syndrome (IBS) may present with aching or cramping periumbilical or lower abdominal pain, often precipitated by meals and relieved by defecation. The pain can be severe occasionally, and there is an altered frequency and consistency of the stools. Fever, leukocytosis, and awakening at night are not indicative of IBS. A ruptured ovarian cyst would not be a differential in an older adult woman because the ovaries shrink and stop functioning with menopause.

36. Answer: 1

Rationale: A high-fiber diet is the treatment for diverticular disease, and vegetarians who eat increased amounts of fruits, vegetables, grains, and cereals are in the lowest risk category. Chronic constipation causes chronic increased pressure in the sigmoid colon, which increases the likelihood of bowel wall weakening and diverticula (outpouches) developing. Small meals and low-fiber diets would also increase the risk of constipation.

37. Answer: 3

Rationale: The risk of colorectal cancer increases in patients over age 50 years. The most frequent ages that colon cancer is found are in the 6th and 7th decades of life. Almost all colon cancers begin as polyps, which can be slow growing, taking 8–15 years to begin to grow and eventually turn into cancer. Therefore, colon screening is recommended beginning at age 50 to find and remove polyps before cancer can develop. Frequently, there are no symptoms, even with left-sided colon cancers, and because of the bright red rectal bleeding always should be explored. Although hemorrhoidal bleeding would be most common, without a colonoscopy one cannot be sure. Anyone over the age of 45 years, if African American, or 50 years, for all other races, needs regular screening. Colonoscopy is the most accurate and the only test where polyps can be removed at the time of testing. Symptoms such as weight loss, pain, and change in bowel habits are usually a late sign and do not frequently occur. Anemia can be present, but it may not necessarily indicate a need for a colonoscopy, although blood loss would be in the differential. Diarrhea is not typically a sign of cancer.

38. Answer: 1

Rationale: Colon cancer risk in patients with universal ulcerative colitis increases by 0.5%–1% per year after the 10th year of diagnosis. Ulcerative colitis limited to the left colon carries less of a risk. Colonoscopy with random biopsies every 1–2 years is recommended 8–10 years after diagnosis. Diverticulosis is common in the general population but is less common in ulcerative colitis. Ischemic colitis occurs when a mesenteric artery is temporarily blocked and the colon at the splenic flexure develops ischemia from lack of blood flow, which is usually temporary. There is not a higher risk for patients with ulcerative colitis. Irritable bowel syndrome is common in patients with ulcerative colitis, but it is a functional disorder and does not require surveillance.

39. Answer: 4

Rationale: Patients with a gastric ulcer may not have any symptoms, especially in the older adult. Weight loss and anorexia may be present. The patient may not realize an ulcer is present until it bleeds and causes significant anemia. Smoking does increase the risk, and perforation can occur. Gastric ulcers are more common in older adult patients.

40. Answer: 3

Rationale: Dysphagia and cough with solid and liquid intake may be the first indication that the patient has cancer, but this is usually late in development. Alcoholism and smoking are the primary risk factors for squamous cell esophageal cancer, which is not as common as adenocarcinoma. Midchest pain indicates late disease, which does not usually respond to treatment, including surgery.

41. Answer: 1

Rationale: A history of polyps does increase the risk of colon cancer and on average patients will need a repeat colonoscopy in 3–5 years rather than the recommended 10 years if there are no polyps and no family history. Hyperplastic polyps, in general, are not a concern and do not turn into cancer. Adenomatous polyps can turn into cancer. Small polyps may or may not be cancerous. A colonoscopy is sensitive and specific for polyps and cancer, but there is a miss rate that can vary with the endoscopist. It is not as high as 99%.

42. Answer: 2

Rationale: Celiac sprue is a genetic disease of the small bowel that is caused by gluten intolerance. The diarrhea and cramping are related to the gluten effects. Because of malabsorption, many patients have iron-deficiency anemia and can have elevated liver enzymes. Hepatitis B would produce elevated liver enzymes but not the other symptoms. *Salmonella* infection could produce diarrhea and cramping. A bleeding ulcer could produce anemia but not the other symptoms.

43. Answer: 1

Rationale: Nonalcoholic fatty liver disease (NAFLD) is associated with diabetes, hyperlipidemia, and obesity. The liver is storing excessive amounts of fat, which can, over time, cause inflammation of the liver. If the inflammation continues, the liver can become scarred, which can lead to cirrhosis. Autoimmune hepatitis is not common and affects women more than men. Celiac sprue is not associated with obesity or diabetes. Drug-induced liver disease is related to certain medications that can cause acute injury to the liver. Depending on the medications he is taking and the elevation of the enzymes, this diagnosis would be considered.

44. Answer: 3

Rationale: Abnormal villi found on the small bowel biopsy are the gold standard for diagnosis. A negative biopsy is sufficient for diagnosis. The antibody panel is a blood test and the tissue transglutaminase (TTG) antibody is the most sensitive test for celiac sprue. The patient likely has gluten sensitivity, meaning the genetic abnormality of celiac sprue is not present, but removing gluten may improve the patient's symptoms. A gluten-free diet will reverse the abnormal findings on biopsy and convert the antibodies to negative, but both tests would be affected and it could 2–3 months or longer to have normal results.

45. Answer: 2

Rationale: A common sequela of a viral infection is gastroparesis. The virus can affect the gastric pacer, causing it to malfunction and result in slow gastric emptying. Typical symptoms of nausea, decreased appetite, and early satiety occur because of the lingering of solid food in the stomach, which can be more than 4 hours. Accumulation throughout the day can result in a full stomach that does not empty. These are not typical symptoms of an influenza infection. Vertigo causes nausea, but not the other symptoms. Although the patient may have taken ibuprofen for several days, it is less likely that an ulcer would have developed with a short course, but it should be in the differential.

46. Answer: 4

Rationale: The symptoms of cramping, diarrhea, and bloating are classic for irritable bowel syndrome (IBS) with diarrhea predominant. Abdominal pain is a hallmark symptom of IBS but is not associated with rectal bleeding or fecal incontinence.

47. Answer: 1

Rationale: People with irritable bowel syndrome (IBS) can have many food triggers. The challenge is to identify the foods without having them avoid entire food groups. Simple sugars, specifically fermentable oligo-, di-, and monosaccharides and polyols (FODMAPS), can cause symptoms of cramping, gas, bloating, and diarrhea. Rather than avoiding all fruits and vegetables, patients need to be aware of the most offending foods and carefully avoid those that cause a problem. Dairy products have lactose, which is not able to be broken down when someone is lacking some or all lactase, the enzyme needed for digestion of lactose. Although people have IBS and lactose intolerance, it should not be assumed the patient has both. Red meat and saturated fat can cause some problems but are not the prime offenders.

48. Answer: 3

Rationale: One of the ways patients can decrease the fat in the liver is to lose weight with exercise. It is important to treat hyperlipidemia because this is associated with fatty liver, and statins should not be discontinued. Lowering cholesterol is not as effective as lowering saturated fats in the diet. Excessive doses over 10,000 mg of vitamin A daily can cause liver damage.

Pharmacology

49. Answer: 4

Rationale: Omeprazole is a proton pump inhibitor (PPI) that blocks acid production for up to 24 hours. It is recommended for patients with frequent symptoms, at least several times a week. It is important to take the PPI on an empty stomach, and then eat 20–30 minutes after for maximum efficacy. PPIs need food to work, and, if a second dose is required, it should be taken before the evening dose. Anticholinergics (hyoscyamine) will likely increase his symptoms by lowering the lower esophageal sphincter (LES) pressure. Anticholinergics are effective for the cramping of IBS. Ranitidine is a histamine blocker (H2-Bl). This blocks one pathway for acid secretion, but there are two other pathways that continue to secrete. H2-Bl is effective for occasional symptoms, a few times a week or less, or as a short trial for new onset of symptoms.

50. Answer: 3

Rationale: Goals of peptic ulcer disease (PUD) treatment include relief of pain, healing of ulcer, and cost-effectiveness. Proton pump inhibitors (PPIs) heal 90% of duodenal ulcers after 4 weeks and 90% of gastric ulcers after 8 weeks, if *Helicobacter pylori (H. pylori)* is negative. PPIs, such as omeprazole, are recommended for ulcers because these drugs provide faster pain relief and more rapid healing than H2 antagonists, because of their ability to decrease acid production. Clarithromycin and bismuth (Pepto-Bismol) are some of the accepted treatment therapies against active *H. pylori*–associated ulcers, but not as single agents. Eradication of *H. pylori* requires a combination regimen.

51. Answer: 1

Rationale: Treating a patient who has arthritis pain with a nonsteroidal anti-inflammatory drug (NSAID) that is a cyclooxygenase (COX-2) selective agent (celecoxib, rofecoxib) is recommended for the majority of patients at high risk of NSAID-induced complications. Prostaglandins help protect the gastrointestinal (GI) mucosa and are blocked by COX-1 agents, such as ibuprofen and other NSAIDs that make the class of drugs risky. Misoprostol is used to prevent stomach ulcers when patients take NSAIDs by protecting the stomach lining by decreasing the amount of acid that comes in contact with it. Additionally, there are risks because it is a prostaglandin analog and should not be taken by pregnant women. Cimetidine would not be suggested because it is an H2-blocker and carries side effects. Omeprazole can help protect the mucosa if the patient is taking an NSAID, but, ideally, not using a COX-1 inhibitor may be the best solution.

52. Answer: 2

Rationale: If a person exposed to a patient known to be positive for hepatitis B has sufficient immunity to hepatitis B, no treatment is necessary. If this same person had not been vaccinated, in addition to initiation of the hepatitis B vaccine series, HBIG 0.06 mL/kg IM is also administered. If an exposed person has had an inadequate immune response to the hepatitis B vaccine series (negative antihepatitis surface antibody), a hepatitis B booster should be given.

53. Answer: 1

Rationale: Patients with gastric or duodenal ulcers due to *Helicobacter pylori (H. pylori)* are successfully treated with the triple-drug therapy of omeprazole, amoxicillin, and clarithromycin. Other FDA-approved regimens include proton pump inhibitor (PPI), clarithromycin, and metronidazole or bismuth, metronidazole, tetracycline, and ranitidine. Treatment should be given for 10–14 days. After completion of *H. pylori* eradication therapy, treatment should continue with a proton pump inhibitor for 4–8 weeks to promote healing of the ulcer. Cephalosporins are not recommended.

54. Answer: 2

Rationale: Mesalamine (5-aminosalicylic acid) therapy for patients with mild ulcerative colitis has been shown to improve symptoms and induce and maintain remission. There are several mesalamine products available, including rectal suspension and suppositories that can be very helpful for left-sided colitis. If no response is seen after 2–4 weeks, the addition of corticosteroids (prednisone) can be helpful, but they are not first-line therapy. Ciprofloxacin and metronidazole are typically used for gastrointestinal infections.

55. Answer: 1

Rationale: To minimize the risk of a contact developing hepatitis A, immunoglobulin 0.02 mL/kg should be given as soon as possible after exposure. It has not been shown to be effective if administered more than 2 weeks after exposure. Hepatitis B immune globulin (HBIG) is for hepatitis B.

56. Answer: 4

Rationale: For unvaccinated patients with exposure to hepatitis B, one dose of hepatitis B immune globulin (HBIG) is administered and the HBV series initiated. HBIG may be protective or may attenuate the severity of the illness if given within 7 days of exposure (adult dose of 0.06 mL/kg). If the patient thinks the individual may have been vaccinated, but does not know whether there was a response, the family nurse practitioner can test antihepatitis B surface antibody. Neither the HBe antibody nor the viral load would be a first-line test. Because of the timing of appearance of the antibodies to hepatitis B, testing would need to be delayed.

57. Answer: 3

Rationale: The only contraindication to the hepatitis B vaccine is prior anaphylaxis or severe hypersensitivity to the vaccine or components of the vaccine.

58. Answer: 2

Rationale: Vancomycin causes problems with nephrotoxicity and ototoxicity (eighth cranial nerve). Renal function should be monitored regularly with laboratory tests (serum creatinine and BUN) and the patient evaluated frequently for hearing loss. The geriatric patient is particularly susceptible.

59. Answer: 3

Rationale: This is a common observation for a patient taking Pepto-Bismol. The patient may also experience a problem with discoloration of his tongue. The stool discoloration is not related to bleeding or metronidazole. Certain foods can affect the stool color, but bismuth is more likely the cause.

Hematology

13

Physical Exam & Diagnostic Tests

1. On physical exam, a palpable, firm, nontender supraclavicular lymph node is noted on the left side of the body. The finding is consistent with a diagnosis of:

   1. Bacterial infection draining from the internal jugular vein.
   2. Thoracic or abdominal malignancy.
   3. Inflammation of the tonsils and adenoids.
   4. Non-Hodgkin's lymphoma.

2. Which test is most important for diagnosing iron-deficiency anemia?

   1. Direct Coombs.
   2. Serum folate level.
   3. Serum ferritin.
   4. RBC count.

3. The term "shotty" is often used to describe lymph nodes that are:

   1. Tender, mobile, and >5 mm.
   2. Small and pellet-like.
   3. Discrete and cystic.
   4. Irregular, soft, and fixed to surrounding tissue.

4. A macrocytic, normochromic anemia is diagnosed in an older adult male patient. What should be the next test(s) ordered?

   1. Serum iron and TIBC levels.
   2. Bone marrow biopsy.
   3. Colonoscopy.
   4. Vitamin B_{12} and RBC/folate levels.

5. The family nurse practitioner would suspect disseminated intravascular coagulation (DIC) if the patient's laboratory results, including prothrombin time (PT), indicated:

   1. Increased PT, decreased platelet count, and decreased fibrinogen.
   2. Decreased PT, increased hematocrit, and increased fibrinogen.
   3. Increased platelet count, decreased hematocrit, and increased PT.
   4. Increased platelet count, increased hematocrit, and decreased PT.

6. When examining lymph nodes, the family nurse practitioner understands:

   1. Children are more likely to develop generalized lymphadenopathy than adults in response to a mild infection.
   2. Older adults frequently have enlarged, nontender supraclavicular and epitrochlear lymph nodes due to aging.
   3. Lymphadenopathy in an adult indicates acute or chronic infection and rarely malignancy.
   4. Enlarged neck lymph nodes in children with no other physical findings are highly suspicious of Burkitt's lymphoma.

7. After confirming the diagnosis of iron-deficiency anemia in an older adult male patient based on CBC, peripheral smear, serum iron, TIBC, and serum ferritin, what would be the next essential test for the family nurse practitioner to order?

   1. Stool guaiac × 3.
   2. Prothrombin time/partial thromboplastin time (PT/PTT).
   3. Liver function tests.
   4. Endoscopy.

8. Evaluation of an older adult male patient reveals a macrocytic, normochromic anemia. Subsequent testing shows normal folate level and decreased vitamin B_{12} level. Further evaluation could include:

   1. Referral to a hematologist for a bone marrow biopsy.

   2. Assay for anti-IF antibodies.

   3. Upper gastrointestinal (GI) series.

   4. No tests are indicated at this time.

9. The most sensitive test for the diagnosis of sickle cell anemia is:

   1. CBC with a peripheral smear.

   2. Bone marrow biopsy and aspiration.

   3. Hemoglobin electrophoresis.

   4. Hemoglobin and hematocrit.

10. An older adult male patient presents to the office with complaints of fatigue, dizziness, decreased activity tolerance, and occasional bounding heart rate. Physical exam reveals pallor (including mucous membranes), tachycardia, and general appearance of lethargy. The family nurse practitioner orders CBC with differential, peripheral smear, serum iron, TIBC, and serum ferritin because there is a high index of suspicion for:

    1. Sideroblastic anemia.

    2. Pernicious anemia.

    3. Folic-acid-deficiency anemia.

    4. Iron-deficiency anemia.

11. Anemia of chronic disease would reveal which of the following laboratory findings?

    1. Decreased iron, decreased TIBC, and decreased serum ferritin.

    2. Decreased iron, decreased TIBC, and increased serum ferritin.

    3. Decreased iron, increased TIBC, and decreased serum ferritin.

    4. Decreased iron, increased TIBC, and increased serum ferritin.

12. Which of the following statements is true concerning the leukemias?

    1. Liver function studies are decreased in the later stages of the disease process.

    2. Initial white blood cell (WBC) count is the most important predictor of prognosis.

3. Thrombocytopenia is rarely present.

4. The prognosis is better if a child is younger than 2 years.

Disorders

13. Sickle cell anemia is caused by:

    1. Exposure to ionizing radiation.

    2. Genetically induced production of abnormal hemoglobin S.

    3. Deficiency of dietary folic acid.

    4. Long-term use of thiazide diuretics.

14. An adult patient presents to the family nurse practitioner with a history of erythrocytosis. One common complaint that could cause a serious complication for the patient is:

    1. A laceration.

    2. Vomiting and diarrhea.

    3. Coughing.

    4. Dizziness.

15. A patient has a folic-acid-deficiency anemia. The family nurse practitioner teaches the patient to eat foods rich in folic acid, such as:

    1. Green leafy vegetables, nuts, and liver.

    2. Carrots, salmon, and avocados.

    3. Cottage cheese, yogurt, and skim milk.

    4. Lima beans, Brussels sprouts, and potatoes.

16. Which of the changes occurs in the RBC indices for pernicious anemia?

    1. Microcytic, normochromic.

    2. Microcytic, hypochromic.

    3. Normocytic, normochromic.

    4. Macrocytic, normochromic.

17. Which statement is true concerning thalassemia?

    1. It is characterized by defective lymphocyte synthesis.

    2. Thalassemia minor does not require pharmacologic treatment.

    3. Thalassemia major is associated with high RBC counts and elevated serum iron.

    4. It is characterized with an acute onset of symptoms leading to leukocytosis.

18. Iron-deficiency anemia is an example of:

    1. Macrocytic, normochromic anemia.

    2. Macrocytic, hypochromic anemia.

    3. Microcytic, hypochromic anemia.

    4. Normocytic, normochromic anemia.

19. An adult patient with pernicious anemia may present with which signs and symptoms?

    1. Peripheral neuropathy, ataxia, lethargy, and fatigue.

    2. Hepatomegaly, jaundice, and right upper quadrant pain.

    3. Hypertension, angina, and peripheral edema.

    4. Blurred vision, diplopia, and decreased vibratory sensation.

20. Anemia of chronic disease is a:

    1. Normochromic, normocytic anemia.

    2. Normochromic, microcytic anemia.

    3. Hypochromic, microcytic anemia.

    4. Hypochromic, macrocytic anemia.

21. A young adult presents to the clinic for a routine checkup. History is unremarkable, but on physical exam, the family nurse practitioner palpates an enlarged (2 cm), mobile, nontender, rubbery lymph node on the left posterior cervical chain. What is the family nurse practitioner's next step?

    1. Order a throat culture and monospot test.

    2. Refer to a surgeon for a lymph node biopsy.

    3. Order a STAT chest x-ray.

    4. No intervention is necessary at this time.

22. The family nurse practitioner understands that "B" symptoms associated with non-Hodgkin's lymphoma (NHL) include:

    1. Bruising and bleeding.

    2. Peripheral edema, shortness of breath, and ascites.

    3. Fever, night sweats, and unexplained weight loss.

    4. Headache, fatigue, and weakness.

23. In teaching a patient with anemia to include foods rich in iron in the diet, the family nurse practitioner encourages the patient to eat:

    1. Cheese, milk, and yogurt.

    2. Red beans, whole-grain bread, and bran cereal.

    3. Tomatoes, cabbage, and citrus fruits.

    4. Beef, spinach, and peanut butter.

24. Anemia of chronic disease is associated with:

    1. Malnutrition and vitamin B_{12} deficiency.

    2. Infections, inflammation, and neoplasms.

    3. Traumatic injuries and folate deficiency.

    4. Excessive menstrual flow, trauma, and heredity.

25. The family nurse practitioner understands that most adult patients with Hodgkin's lymphoma present with:

    1. Nausea, vomiting, and diarrhea.

    2. Night sweats, weight loss, and fever.

    3. Painless, movable mass in the neck, axilla, or groin.

    4. Hepatosplenomegaly with a painful mass in the mediastinum.

26. What is the most common leukemia found in the older adult, typically asymptomatic and characterized by median survival of about 10 years?

    1. Acute myelogenous.

    2. Chronic myelogenous.

    3. Acute lymphocytic.

    4. Chronic lymphocytic.

27. A female patient tells the family nurse practitioner her family has a diagnosis of hemophilia A. What is the family nurse practitioner's understanding of the condition?

    1. Her mother was a carrier for the disease and her father had the disease.

    2. Both mother and father have the disease.

    3. Her mother was a carrier.

    4. Both grandparents were carriers of the disease.

28. Folic-acid deficiency most often results from:

    1. Lead exposure.

    2. Poor dietary habits.

    3. Gastrointestinal bleeding.

    4. Genetic defect.

Pharmacology

29. The family nurse practitioner determines that an adult male patient has an iron deficiency anemia and has ruled out gastrointestinal (GI) bleeding as the cause. The family nurse practitioner:

    1. Refers the patient to a hematologist.

    2. Orders iron dextran 50 mg IM weekly for 4 weeks and schedules the patient for weekly office visits for the injection.

    3. Prescribes ferrous sulfate 325 mg PO tid and schedules the patient to return in 1 month for a repeat CBC, serum iron, and TIBC.

    4. Schedules the patient to return in 6 months for additional stool guaiac testing.

30. What information would the family nurse practitioner include in teaching a patient about the treatment of vitamin B_{12} deficiency following a total gastrectomy?

    1. The patient will be taking vitamin B_{12} tablets twice daily for 1 year.

    2. The patient will be taking oral folic acid supplements daily for life.

    3. The patient will receive monthly cyanocobalamin (vitamin B_{12}) injections for life (after being given daily weekly injections for the first month).

    4. The patient will require iron supplementation and monthly blood transfusions until the deficiency is corrected.

31. Treatment of anemia of chronic disease should include:

    1. Folic acid supplement 1 mg PO qd.

    2. Iron sulfate ($FeSO_4$) supplement 300 mg PO tid.

    3. Treatment of the underlying condition.

    4. Weekly epoetin alfa (Epogen) injections.

32. The family nurse practitioner has prescribed elemental iron 6 mg/kg/day in three divided doses for a toddler diagnosed with iron-deficiency anemia. What instructions would the family nurse practitioner include for the parents?

    1. Give the iron with food to increase the absorption of the medication.

    2. Give the medication through a straw to decrease the staining of the teeth.

    3. Avoid foods containing ascorbic acid, which decreases absorption of the medication.

    4. If a dose is missed, double up on the next two doses.

33. After initiating vitamin B_{12} therapy, the family nurse practitioner would expect which of the following at a 4-week follow-up visit to the clinic?

    1. Ferritin level of 40 ng/mL.

    2. Reduced RBCs, WBCs, and platelets.

    3. Increased macrocytosis and anisocytosis.

    4. Increased hemoglobin/hematocrit and reticulocyte count.

34. It is recommended to administer a 0.5 mL (25 mg) test dose of which medication?

    1. Nascobol (intranasal B_{12} gel).

    2. Folic acid.

    3. Iron dextran.

    4. Ferrous sulfate (Feosol).

13 | Hematology Answers and Rationale

Physical Exam & Diagnostic Tests

1. Answer: 2

Rationale: A Virchow's node in the left supraclavicular region is of concern because of the high correlation with abdominal or thoracic malignancy. Infections and inflammatory conditions produce tender, inflamed lymph nodes.

2. Answer: 3

Rationale: The serum ferritin correlates with total body iron stores because it is the major iron storage protein. Its value is reduced in iron-deficiency anemia. Direct Coombs measures in vivo red blood cell (RBC) coating by immunoglobulins and is positive in autoimmune hemolytic anemia, blood transfusion reactions, and drug-induced hemolysis. Serum folate measures the folic acid level in the blood.

3. Answer: 2

Rationale: "Shotty," or small and pellet-like, lymph nodes that are movable, cool, nontender, discrete, and less than 1 cm in diameter are usually considered normal and often represent enlargement of the lymph nodes following a viral infection. They feel like BBs or buckshot under the skin and move under the examiner's fingers when palpated. If shotty nodes are found in the epitrochlear or supraclavicular regions, they require additional evaluation. A fixed, or nonmovable, lymph node is cause for concern.

4. Answer: 4

Rationale: It is important to determine the type of macrocytic anemia so that the appropriate therapy can be ordered. Therefore, the vitamin B_{12} and RBC/folate levels would be ordered. These tests would determine whether the patient has a pernicious anemia (the most common type) or a folate deficiency (also common in older adult patients). Serum iron and total iron-binding capacity (TIBC) would be ordered if an iron-deficiency anemia was suspected (not in this case because this is a microcytic anemia). There is no indication for a colonoscopy. It would be premature to order a bone marrow biopsy without performing initial testing and potentially overlooking an easily treated condition (e.g., pernicious anemia, folate-deficiency anemia). Measurement of certain metabolites of vitamin B_{12}, methylmalonic acid and homocysteine, provide additional information to help identify the cause of the anemia.

5. Answer: 1

Rationale: Disseminated intravascular coagulation (DIC) is a complication of infection, malignancy, blood transfusions, liver disease, complications of pregnancy, and sometimes trauma. DIC is the inappropriate accelerated systemic activation of the coagulation cascade, resulting in simultaneous hemorrhage and thrombosis. Laboratory results would show increased PT and decreased platelet count and fibrinogen in response to the hemorrhage and clotting.

6. Answer: 1

Rationale: Children often have generalized lymphadenopathy in response to mild infections of the skin or respiratory tract. Palpable lymph nodes are generally not present in healthy individuals, but some may have small, discrete, nontender nodes that are not clinically significant. Enlarged lymph nodes may indicate infection, inflammation, and malignancy in both children and adults. Tender lymph nodes are noted with inflammatory processes. Hard, fixed, and painless lymph nodes may indicate a malignant process. A painless, firm supraclavicular or cervical lymph node is a common sign of Hodgkin's disease in children, not Burkitt's lymphoma, in which the child has other associated symptoms depending on the system affected.

7. Answer: 1

Rationale: Stool guaiac testing would identify blood loss from the gastrointestinal tract—the most common cause of iron-deficiency anemia, along with menorrhagia in females. The other tests should be done if the stool guaiac results are positive. Finding the cause of the iron deficiency is paramount, and the stool guaiac test is an easy, noninvasive method of ruling out gastrointestinal bleeding as the cause.

8. Answer: 2

Rationale: The anti-intrinsic factor (anti-IF) or antiparietal cell antibody (APCA) assay test is the currently accepted method to verify the diagnosis of pernicious anemia. The presence of anti-IF antibodies is highly specific for pernicious anemia. In the past, the Schilling's test was used to determine the cause of the vitamin B_{12} deficiency. In pernicious anemia, it will be important to distinguish between inadequate intake (an intrinsic-factor deficiency) or a malabsorption problem. This will allow the practitioner to prescribe the most appropriate therapy for the patient. A bone marrow biopsy and an upper gastrointestinal (GI) series are not indicated at this time.

9. Answer: 3

Rationale: Normal and abnormal hemoglobin can be detected by electrophoresis, which matches hemolyzed RBC material against standard bands for the various known hemoglobins, including hemoglobin S, the abnormal hemoglobin associated with sickle cell anemia. CBC with peripheral smear and hemoglobin/hematocrit would not yield enough information to diagnose sickle cell anemia. Low hemoglobin, normal to increased MCV, increased MCHC, chronic reticulocytosis, mild to moderate anisocytosis, and poikilocytosis with numerous sickle cells and Howell-Jolly bodies would be noted on the CBC and differential. A bone marrow biopsy would not be necessary and would not indicate the presence of hemoglobin S.

10. Answer: 4

Rationale: This patient's clinical picture is a classic presentation for anemia. Further testing is needed to determine the type of anemia involved. The most common cause in older adult men is GI bleeding, which would cause an iron-deficiency anemia. The tests that were ordered would confirm or rule out this diagnosis. The peripheral smear is especially important in diagnosing the specific type of anemia, i.e., hypochromic and microcytic. TIBC would be increased, and serum ferritin and serum iron are decreased. If the smear ruled out the diagnosis of iron-deficiency anemia, it would lead the practitioner to other diagnoses (including the remaining choices) and the appropriate laboratory tests required for confirmation.

11. Answer: 2

Rationale: Normal to increased iron stores (serum ferritin) with concurrent low-serum iron is the hallmark finding of anemia of chronic disease. Serum iron is decreased along with total iron-binding capacity (TIBC). Decreased iron, increased TIBC, and decreased serum ferritin contain the findings for iron-deficiency anemia.

12. Answer: 2

Rationale: The patient is at higher risk if initial WBC count is >50,000 cells/mm³. Liver function studies and uric acid levels are increased. Approximately 75% of patients have marked thrombocytopenia with platelets <100,000 cells/mm³. Prognosis is poor for children <2 years and >10 years of age. The most likely diagnosis in children is acute lymphocytic leukemia (ALL). For adults, the most likely diagnosis is chronic lymphocytic leukemia (CLL), with the second most common type being acute myelogenous leukemia (AML).

Disorders

13. Answer: 2

Rationale: Sickle cell anemia is a genetic disorder characterized by the production of hemoglobin S, an anemia secondary to shortened erythrocyte survival, microvascular occlusion by sickle-shaped erythrocytes, and increased susceptibility to certain infections. Exposure to ionizing radiation has been associated with the development of certain malignancies, especially leukemia. A deficiency of dietary folic acid does not cause sickle cell anemia, although folic acid is used in the treatment of these patients to help increase hematopoiesis and aid in recovery from aplastic events. Long-term use of thiazide diuretics has been implicated in the development of hemolytic or aplastic anemias in rare cases.

14. Answer: 2

Rationale: Erythrocytosis (or polycythemia) can be worsened by dehydration from any cause, i.e., vomiting and diarrhea. Coughing and dizziness will have no effect on the condition, and a laceration may actually improve the symptoms because of the blood loss.

15. Answer: 1

Rationale: Green leafy vegetables, oranges and orange juice, and nuts are excellent sources of folic acid. Also, cereals and breads are now fortified with folic acid. Be sure to stress that folate is heat labile and rapidly destroyed by prolonged cooking or food processing. The other foods are not significant sources of folic acid.

16. Answer: 4

Rationale: A macrocytic (MCV >100 fL), normochromic anemia resulting from atrophic gastric mucosa not secreting intrinsic factor is the definition of pernicious anemia. These indices could also include folic-acid-deficiency anemia. Microcytic normochromic or hypochromic could include iron-deficiency anemia or anemia of chronic disease. Normocytic and normochromic could also include anemia of chronic disease.

17. Answer: 2

Rationale: Thalassemias are chronic, inherited anemias characterized by defective hemoglobin synthesis leading to a decreased RBC count, hypochromia (MCH <20 pg), microcytosis (MCV <70 fL), normal serum iron, and normal RBC distribution width (RDW) in thalassemia minor, which does not require pharmacologic treatment. This should be noted that although the RDW is usually normal, it can be elevated in about 50% of patients with thalassemia trait, which is in contrast to iron-deficiency anemia, where the RDW is almost always elevated (90%). Patients with thalassemia minor should not be given iron supplements to resolve anemia. Patients with thalassemia major are usually managed by a hematologist.

18. Answer: 3

Rationale: Iron-deficiency anemia is a microcytic, hypochromic anemia. The RBCs are smaller (microcytic) because of the decrease in hemoglobin production caused by inadequate amounts of iron, which also makes the cell appear pale (hypochromic). The other selections describe other types of anemias, which would be determined by the peripheral smear.

19. Answer: 1

Rationale: Vitamin B_{12} deficiency may result in neurologic signs and symptoms, including peripheral neuropathy, paresthesias, unsteady gait (ataxia), loss of proprioception, decreased vibratory sensation, lethargy, and fatigue. In the later stages of severe B_{12} deficiency, spasticity, hyperactive reflexes, and presence of Romberg's sign is noted because of the formation of a demyelinating lesion of the neurons of the spinal cord and cerebral cortex. These findings are specific to pernicious anemia and must be assessed in all patients who present with anemia. The other signs and symptoms are not characteristic of pernicious anemia.

20. Answer: 1

Rationale: Anemia of chronic disease is a chronic normochromic, normocytic, and hypoproliferative anemia. There is normal production of hemoglobin, along with normal maturation of RBCs. The serum iron is low; ferritin level and TIBC are elevated.

21. Answer: 2

Rationale: Lymphadenopathy as described, without evidence of infection, should always be referred to a surgeon for biopsy, the only definitive test to rule out a malignancy (a frequent cause of lymphadenopathy not caused by infectious processes). No signs or symptoms suggest the need for a throat culture, monospot test, or chest x-ray. Not intervening is inappropriate because the cause of lymphadenopathy needs to be determined.

22. Answer: 3

Rationale: This constellation of symptoms (fever, night sweats, and weight loss) is used in the staging of non-Hodgkin's lymphoma (NHL), the presence of which is considered to be a poor prognostic indicator. The other symptoms may occur depending on the amount of disease involvement, but they are not considered "B" symptoms, also known as constitutional symptoms.

23. Answer: 4

Rationale: Beef, spinach, and peanut butter are iron-rich foods. The other options are examples of foods rich in calcium, fiber, and vitamin C, respectively.

24. Answer: 2

Rationale: Anemia or chronic disease is associated with infections (e.g., tuberculosis), chronic inflammatory conditions (e.g., systemic lupus erythematosus; rheumatoid arthritis), and malignancies. Excessive blood loss from menstrual flow or traumatic injuries would more likely cause an iron-deficiency anemia. Malnutrition can contribute to iron, vitamin B_{12}, and folate deficiencies.

25. Answer: 3

Rationale: Most patients with Hodgkin's lymphoma present with a painless, movable mass in the neck, axilla, or groin. Constitutional symptoms may also occur, which include weight loss, persistent fever, and night sweats. Often the patient may experience pruritus and pain in the lymph node area after consuming alcohol (an unexplained finding). Hepatosplenomegaly presents with advanced disease.

26. Answer: 4

Rationale: Chronic lymphocytic leukemia (CLL) is found primarily in middle-aged and older adults (<10% of patients under age 50). Median age of diagnosis of CLL is 70 years, affecting more males than females. Acute myelogenous leukemia (AML) incidence increases with age, with median age greater than 70 years. Chronic myelogenous leukemia (CML) occurs between 50 and 60 years. Acute lymphocytic leukemia (ALL) is most common in children and gradually increases in frequency in later life with the median age of 35–40 years.

27. Answer: 1

Rationale: Hemophilia A is characterized by a deficiency of factor VIII and is due to an X-linked chromosome recessive inheritance disorder. This means that males are almost exclusively affected with hemophilia and females are carriers. When a female has hemophilia, they are the offspring of a father with hemophilia and a mother who is a carrier. In the past, this rarely occurred because males with hemophilia rarely lived to adult reproductive age. Now with the availability of replacement factor VIII, male patients with hemophilia can live to reproductive age.

28. Answer: 2

Rationale: Folic-acid deficiency most often results from dietary deficits and frequently affects the older adult, chronically ill, alcoholic patients, and food faddists (poor food selections). Pregnancy requires an increase in folic acid, as do disease states such as cancer, chronic inflammation, Crohn's disease, rheumatoid arthritis, and malabsorption syndromes.

Pharmacology

29. Answer: 3

Rationale: Treatment with iron orally for at least 6 months is necessary to correct both the anemia and the depleted body iron stores. Ferrous sulfate should be taken on an empty stomach 1 hour before meals. If the patient experiences GI symptoms, the dose can be reduced or the patient can take the iron with the meal; however, taking it with meals will reduce the delivery and absorption of the iron by 50%. Iron dextran (parenteral) may be used if the patient is unable to take PO medications or if the hemoglobin is less than 6 g/dL. The patient should have hemoglobin/hematocrit, iron, and total iron-binding capacity (TIBC) rechecked after 1 month on iron supplementation. If there is no improvement in all parameters, most notably a rise in the hemoglobin by 1 g/dL, the patient should be referred to a hematologist. Referral to a GI specialist or repeat of stool guaiac testing is unnecessary because there is no indication that this patient's condition is caused by bleeding.

30. Answer: 3

Rationale: If the deficiency is not caused by inadequate intake, the patient will require lifetime supplementation of vitamin B_{12} (1000 μg of cyanocobalamin) by intramuscular injection to ensure absorption. In patients with irreversible malabsorption (total gastrectomy) and severe neurologic symptoms, parenteral therapy is indicated: 1000 μg/day for 7 days, and then 1000 μg weekly for 4 weeks, followed by 1000 μg monthly for life. The family nurse practitioner should keep in mind that high-dose, daily oral cyanocobalamin (1000–2000 μg) are as effective as monthly intramuscular injection and is the preferred route of initial therapy in most circumstances because it is cost-effective and convenient. Oral folic acid, iron, and blood transfusions would not treat the cause of the deficiency, and, therefore, the resulting anemia would not be corrected.

31. Answer: 3

Rationale: Treatment of the underlying condition leads to resolution of the anemia of chronic disease. Folic acid and iron supplements are indicated for folate and iron-deficiency anemias, respectively. Epoetin alfa injections are indicated for conditions that affect erythropoiesis, including chronic renal failure, chemotherapy-induced anemia, and acquired immunodeficiency syndrome (AIDS). Patients with underlying iron-deficiency anemia and anemia of chronic disease may benefit from a trial of iron therapy.

32. Answer: 2

Rationale: Iron medications can cause staining of the teeth, so it is a good practice to give the medication through a straw. It is best to give iron on an empty stomach (if tolerable) to increase absorption. Ascorbic acid increases absorption of iron. If a dose is missed, it is best to give the dose when it is remembered as long as it is not too close to the next dose. The next two doses would not be increased.

33. Answer: 4

Rationale: In addition to a sense of well-being, improved appetite, and decreased neurologic symptoms (gait disturbances, peripheral neuropathy, paresthesias (numbness/tingling in fingers), and extreme weakness), the hemoglobin/hematocrit and reticulocyte count should increase with vitamin B_{12} therapy.

34. Answer: 3

Rationale: The use of IM or IV iron dextran is for patients who cannot tolerate oral supplementation or who have GI disease that limits oral absorption. Therapy should be initiated with an IV test dose of 0.5 mL (25 mg) to observe for anaphylaxis. If the test dose appears safe, slowly administer a larger dose (500 mg over a 10- to 15-minute interval), and if the 500-mg dose is uneventful, additional doses may be given as needed.

Urinary

14

Physical Exam & Diagnostic Tests

1. A basic urinary continence evaluation done by the family nurse practitioner should include:

    1. History, physical exam, postvoid residual volume, and urinalysis (UA).

    2. Postvoid residual volume, blood urea nitrogen (BUN), serum creatinine, and UA.

    3. History, physical exam, serum glucose, BUN, serum creatinine, and UA.

    4. Urodynamic/endoscopic/imaging tests, UA, and serum creatinine.

2. Which one of the following is the most useful tool in diagnosing congenital anomalies, stone formation, and foreign bodies in the urinary tract?

    1. Intravenous urography (IVU).

    2. Voiding cystourethrography.

    3. Intravenous pyelogram (IVP).

    4. Computed tomography urography (CTU).

3. Which of the following patients would be a good candidate for urodynamic studies (UDS)?

    1. Patient with history of stress incontinence and urge incontinence.

    2. Patient with recent surgery for bladder suspension.

    3. Patient with initial incontinence episode after total knee replacement.

    4. Older adult male with residual volume of 45 mL after 250-mL voiding.

4. The family nurse practitioner is evaluating blood chemistries on a patient who is experiencing a slight increase in blood pressure (BP). She has no previous history of high BP or other chronic disease. Which serum laboratory value would be of most concern to the practitioner?

    1. Serum creatinine 4.2 mg/dL.

    2. Blood urea nitrogen (BUN) 30 mg/dL.

    3. Serum potassium 4.5 mEq/L.

    4. Serum osmolarity 290 mOsm/kg.

5. When taking a history on voiding patterns in adults, the family nurse practitioner knows:

    1. Adults normally void q2–3h in a 24-hour period (8–12 times a day).

    2. First sensation to void occurs when the bladder fills to 200–300 mL.

    3. Normally, 15–20 minutes pass between first urge to void and reaching functional capacity.

    4. Adults typically reach functional (comfortable) capacity at 200–300 mL and normally experience some leakage if voiding is delayed.

6. The family nurse practitioner expects which findings on exam of an older adult patient with dehydration?

    1. Tongue furrows and skin tenting over the clavicle.

    2. Specific gravity of urine 1.004.

    3. Pulse rate 58 beats/min (strong, regular) and BP 100/62 mm Hg.

    4. Geographic tongue and reduced saliva pool.

7. Which diagnostic test is considered essential in the preliminary workup of a patient with incontinence?

    1. UA with C&S.

    2. Bedside urodynamic studies.

    3. Intravenous and retrograde pyelography.

    4. Renal sonography.

Disorders

8. A young woman explains to the family nurse practitioner that she has been having frequent and painful urination. The family nurse practitioner orders a clean-catch urine specimen for routine UA with C&S. Laboratory results show 10^5/mL of *Escherichia coli (E. coli)* and 10^4/mL of *Staphylococcus epidermidis (S. epidermidis).* The family nurse practitioner would:

    1. Treat the *E. coli.*

    2. Order amoxicillin.

    3. Treat the *S. epidermidis.*

    4. Encourage citric fruit juices.

9. An older adult woman is incontinent of urine. Her perineal area is red and excoriated. What would the family nurse practitioner advise the family caregiver to **avoid** using on the skin in the perineal area?

    1. Petrolatum.

    2. Moisture-barrier films.

    3. Mild soap and water.

    4. Zinc oxide ointment.

10. A young adult comes to the student health clinic complaining of severe abdominal discomfort and bloody urine. An initial priority in the diagnostic workup would include:

    1. Intravenous pyelography to rule out a kidney stone.

    2. Straining all urine.

    3. Microscopic urine exam.

    4. 24-hour urine culture.

11. Which plan would be most appropriate for an older patient with functional incontinence?

    1. Evaluate need for incontinence pads.

    2. Limit fluid intake in the evenings.

    3. Perform Credé's maneuver.

    4. Provide a bedside commode.

12. A 60-year-old man presents with recurrent urinary tract infections (UTIs). What is the most likely cause?

    1. Balanitis.

    2. Epididymitis.

    3. Chronic bacterial prostatitis.

    4. Benign prostatic hypertrophy.

13. What is a possible cause of transient and reversible urinary incontinence?

    1. Poor pelvic support causing hypermobility of the base of the female bladder.

    2. Lower urinary tract problems, such as carcinoma.

    3. Cystocele or uterine prolapse in women.

    4. Ingestion of certain medications, such as sedatives, diuretics, anticholinergics, and α-adrenergic agents.

14. Which statement best characterizes functional incontinence?

    1. Leakage of urine during activities that increase abdominal pressure, such as coughing, sneezing, and laughing.

    2. Mainly caused by factors outside the urinary tract, especially immobility, that prohibit proper toileting habits.

    3. Characterized by the inability to delay urination, with an abrupt and strong desire to void.

    4. Occurrence of incontinence with overdistention of bladder.

15. What are the two most common pathogens in community-acquired UTIs?

    1. *Klebsiella pneumoniae.*

    2. *Proteus mirabilis.*

    3. *Staphylococcus saprophyticus.*

    4. *Escherichia coli.*

    5. *Staphylococcus aureus.*

    6. *Streptococcus pyogenes.*

16. What is the usual clinical presentation of an adult patient with cystitis?

    1. No symptoms noted.

    2. Acute onset of chills, fever, flank pain, headache, malaise, and costovertebral angle tenderness.

    3. Complaints of dysuria, urgency, frequency, nocturia, and suprapubic heaviness.

    4. Signs and symptoms of fever, irritability, decreased appetite, vomiting, diarrhea, constipation, dehydration, and jaundice.

17. Recurrent UTIs in women are caused by relapse or reinfection. The family nurse practitioner understands which of the following about relapse?

    1. Is less common than reinfection and occurs within 2 weeks of completing drug therapy for the infection.

    2. Is responsible for most recurrent UTIs in women.

    3. May result from residual urine after voiding due to prolapsed uterus or bladder or lack of estrogen.

    4. Can be treated with the same medication regimen used for the original infection.

18. The family nurse practitioner understands that the treatment of pyelonephritis:

    1. Suggests a structural problem in female patients.

    2. Requires hospitalization, parenteral antibiotic therapy, and intravenous voiding pyelography in male patients.

    3. Requires hospitalization, parenteral antibiotic therapy, and intravenous voiding pyelography in female patients.

    4. Requires no follow-up.

19. What is the term given to the type of urinary incontinence associated with conditions such as Parkinson's disease or Alzheimer's disease?

    1. Stress incontinence.

    2. Urge incontinence.

    3. Functional incontinence.

    4. Overflow incontinence.

20. A 40-year-old white man presents to the clinic with a history of uric acid renal calculi. Knowing that the alkaline-ash, low-purine diet is difficult for patients to adhere to, which other option should the family nurse practitioner consider?

    1. Monitor the patient for another episode.

    2. Discuss the alkaline-ash, low-purine diet in detail with the patient.

    3. Start the patient on allopurinol (Zyloprim) and monitor serum uric acid level.

    4. Refer the patient to a urologist.

21. A male patient presents with complaints of blood in his urine; it is painless and he has no difficulty with urination. The family nurse practitioner obtains UA to confirm the presence of blood, and no bacteria are present. What is the priority diagnosis that must be ruled out on the patient?

    1. Cancer of the prostate.

    2. Prerenal failure.

    3. Renal calculi.

    4. Cancer of the bladder.

22. The family nurse practitioner is taking the history of a patient who has been diagnosed with renal calculi. What information in the history would the family nurse practitioner identify as a precipitating factor in the development of renal calculi?

    1. Increased incidence of UTIs over the past 3 years.

    2. Drinking 6–8 oz of milk daily.

    3. History of fractured femur and prolonged bed rest.

    4. High intake of citrus fruit and high-fiber carbohydrates.

23. A patient is diagnosed with renal failure, thought to be post renal in origin. What would the family nurse practitioner identify as a possible precipitating cause of the patient's renal failure?

    1. History of MI with severe hypotensive episode.

    2. Advanced prostatic hypertrophy with hematuria.

    3. Renal vascular changes secondary to long history of diabetes.

    4. Exposure to carbon tetrachloride at the job site.

24. A family nurse practitioner recognizes which factor as contributing to the development of prerenal failure?

    1. History of an anaphylactic reaction that rendered the patient unconscious.

    2. Extended treatment of an infection with gentamicin (Garamycin).

    3. Acute pyelonephritis with subsequent glomerulonephritis.

    4. Renal vascular changes secondary to atherosclerotic disease.

25. The family nurse practitioner teaching a female patient about bladder health would include which of the following three guidelines:

    1. Drink at least six to eight glasses of water per day.

    2. Avoid doing Kegel's exercises.

    3. Avoid constipation.

    4. Consider weight loss, if incontinence occurs.

    5. Have at least one cup of coffee or tea daily.

26. Which one of the following objective findings on a 56-year-old male is consistent with a diagnosis of benign prostatic hyperplasia (BPH)?

    1. Elevated PSA.

    2. Gross hematuria.

    3. A nodular firm prostate palpated on DRE.

    4. A smooth enlarged prostate palpated on DRE.

27. Which two situations should the family nurse practitioner refer to a urologist?

    1. Patient with a smooth enlarged prostate palpated on DRE.

    2. Patient with a nodular firm prostate palpated on DRE.

    3. If initial treatment for BPH is not effective.

    4. When the patient with BPH develops a UTI.

28. Which of the following three findings are characteristics of nephrotic syndrome?

    1. Hematuria.

    2. Peripheral edema.

    3. Proteinuria.

    4. Hypoalbuminemia.

    5. Hypolipidemia.

    6. Decreased coagulation.

29. Signs of renal damage in patients with diabetes mellitus and hypertension include which two of the following?

    1. Increased BUN.

    2. Increase in serum creatinine.

    3. Presence of proteinuria.

    4. Decrease in GFR.

    5. Hematuria.

    6. Elevated A1C.

30. A 75-year-old Caucasian female patient presents to the clinic with her husband, her primary caregiver. She has a history of multi-infarct dementia (MID), likely from a long history of untreated hypertension. Her husband reports that for the past 2 days she has been agitated and increasingly confused, and he has not been able to redirect her. He denies the addition of new medications or over-the-counter herbal supplements. What would the family nurse practitioner suspect?

    1. New infarct.

    2. Worsening of dementia.

    3. Urinary tract infection.

    4. Underlying stress to caregiver.

Pharmacology

31. A patient is diagnosed with benign prostate hypertrophy. Which medication should be recognized by the family nurse practitioner as likely to aggravate this condition?

    1. Glyburide (DiaBeta).

    2. Oral buspirone (Buspar).

    3. Inhaled ipratropium (Atrovent).

    4. Ophthalmic timolol (Timoptic).

32. Which of the following agents can be useful for stress incontinence in the female patient?

    1. Propantheline (Pro-Banthine) 7.5–30 mg three to five times a day.

    2. Oxybutynin (Ditropan) 2.5–5 mg tid to qid.

    3. Doxepin (Sinequan) 10–25 mg qd/bid/tid initially to maximum total daily dose of 25–100 mg.

    4. Conjugated estrogen (Premarin) 0.3–1.25 mg/day orally or vaginally and medroxyprogesterone (progestin) 2.5–10 mg/day continuously or intermittently.

33. To decrease the production of uric acid stones, the family nurse practitioner orders which medication?

    1. Allopurinol (Zyloprim).

    2. Indomethacin (Indocin).

    3. Bethanechol (Urecholine).

    4. Phenazopyridine (Pyridium).

34. A 70-year-old woman is treated with oxybutynin (Ditropan) for her urinary frequency and urgency. The family nurse practitioner would explain to the patient she will probably experience:

    1. Increased sensitivity to sunlight.

    2. Dizziness on standing.

    3. Dry mouth and increased thirst.

    4. Increased bruising.

35. Which of the three medications listed can cause urinary incontinence in the older adult?

    1. Hypnotics.

    2. Antibiotics.

    3. Sedatives.

    4. Bulk-forming laxatives.

    5. Antidepressants.

    6. Opioids.

36. The family nurse practitioner has selected nitrofurantoin (Macrodantin) for treatment of a chronic UTI in a female patient. Which parameter should the nurse evaluate before administration of this medication?

    1. Creatinine clearance (>50 mL/min).

    2. Levels of serum alanine aminotransferase (ALT).

    3. Current medications that include anticoagulants.

    4. History of allergic reactions to sulfa-based medications.

37. A 46-year-old man with a history of renal calculi presents with complaints of severe flank pain radiating to his groin area. He is also experiencing nausea and vomiting, and his temperature is 99°F (37.2°C). What is the best initial therapy that the family nurse practitioner can provide?

    1. Ketorolac 20 mg IM.

    2. Ibuprofen (Advil) 600 mg PO q6h.

    3. Increase fluid intake and strain all urine.

    4. Trimethobenzamide (Tigan) 250 mg PO.

38. The family nurse practitioner is prescribing nitrofurantoin (Macrodantin) for a woman who is experiencing problems with UTIs. What specific directions should the nurse give the patient regarding administration of nitrofurantoin?

    1. Take with food and expect brownish discoloration of urine.

    2. Do not take with milk products; take on empty stomach for better absorption.

    3. Take four times a day until symptoms have subsided for at least 24 hours.

    4. Do not take acetaminophen (Tylenol) or ibuprofen (Advil) with nitrofurantoin.

39. A young woman presents with complaints of burning on urination, frequency, and urgency. Phenazopyridine (Pyridium) is prescribed. What specific directions should the family nurse practitioner provide for the patient regarding phenazopyridine?

    1. May discolor contact lenses; if sclerae begin to turn yellow, return to the office.

    2. Always take on an empty stomach to increase absorption.

    3. Do not take any medication containing aspirin or salicylate.

    4. May interfere with effectiveness of mini-pill for birth control.

40. When prescribing oxybutynin (Ditropan) for the patient with overactive bladder symptoms, which disorder in the patient's medical history must the family nurse practitioner consider before prescribing?

    1. Diabetes.

    2. Cough.

    3. Narrow-angle glaucoma.

    4. Gallstones.

41. Angiotensin-converting enzyme (ACE) inhibitors are recommended for slowing the progression of chronic renal disease but are contraindicated in the following disorder:

    1. Cardiovascular disease.

    2. Hypertension.

    3. Diabetes.

    4. Renal artery stenosis.

14 | Urinary Answers and Rationale

Physical Exam & Diagnostic Tests

1. Answer: 1

Rationale: A basic evaluation of urinary incontinence should include a history and physical, measurement of postvoid residual volume, and urinalysis (UA). The other tests may be performed based on the findings from the initial evaluation.

2. Answer: 4

Rationale: Computed tomography urography (CTU) has become the most useful diagnostic tool in different urinary tract abnormalities, such as complex congenital anomalies, trauma, infection, and tumors. The use of CTU in different anomalies including vascular, parenchymal, and urothelial evaluation has a great impact in management of patients. CTU has many disadvantages over intravenous urography (IVU), including its high cost and the higher radiation dose, but it is more effective than IVU at visualizing the structures of the kidney.

3. Answer: 1

Rationale: The optimal patients for urodynamic studies (UDS) include those who have not had prior incontinence surgery or who have clear symptoms of stress or urge incontinence. Postvoid residual volume may be seen in an older adult male patient.

4. Answer: 1

Rationale: The primary concern in the patient is the greatly elevated serum creatinine level of 4.2 mg/dL. All the other blood chemistry values are within normal limits. The patient should be referred to a nephrologist immediately because of the elevated creatinine level. The family nurse practitioner should order whole parathyroid hormone level, liver function tests, lipid and renal panels, and magnesium/calcium levels. Having these laboratory tests completed will assist the nephrologist in determining the cause of the patient's renal failure. A complete review of the patient's medications should be initiated to determine whether she is taking any medication that may cause renal failure, including angiotensin-converting enzyme (ACE) inhibitors (e.g., captopril). The patient's family history may be reviewed to rule out familial kidney disorders (e.g., Alport's syndrome).

5. Answer: 2

Rationale: Adults normally void four to six times in a 24-hour period (q4–6h). Most adults usually do not awaken to void at night unless they have a medical problem (e.g., benign prostatic hypertrophy, urge incontinence, or diuretic therapy). The feeling of the bladder filling occurs at about 90–150 mL, with the first urge at 200–300 mL. Normally, 1–2 hours pass between the first urge to void and reaching functional capacity. Adults typically reach functional (comfortable) capacity at 300–600 mL and should never experience leakage if voiding is delayed.

6. Answer: 1

Rationale: Signs of dehydration in the older adult are skin tenting over the clavicle, concentrated urine (specific gravity >1.025), oliguria, sunken eyes, lack of axillary moisture, orthostatic blood pressure (BP) changes, tachycardia, dry mucous membranes of mouth and nose, and absent or small saliva pool. In the obese older adult patient who has lost weight, tenting of the forehead is not always a reliable clinical sign because of excessive loss of subcutaneous fat. As the older patient becomes dehydrated, aqueous humor of the eye also decreases. Gentle palpation of the eyeball will reveal a boggy versus a firm eyeball, a useful assessment tool in these patients. It is important to examine the mouth because it reveals reliable assessment data in the older adult suspected of dehydration. A geographic tongue (patchy papillary loss that causes a maplike appearance) should not be confused with tongue furrows and tongue coating.

7. Answer: 1

Rationale: Urinalysis (UA) with culture and sensitivity (C&S) is essential to an incontinence workup and can be done in the primary care office before more discriminating tests to evaluate bladder storage and emptying. A symptomatic or asymptomatic urinary tract infection (UTI) can cause symptoms of urgency and frequency, which are associated with incontinence.

Disorders

8. Answer: 1

Rationale: *Escherichia coli (E. coli)* is the most common organism causing urinary tract infections (UTIs) in young women, and counts of 10^5 are diagnostic. *E. coli* will likely respond to trimethoprim-sulfamethoxazole (Septra DS) or any suitable, sensitive anti-infective agent, and the patient should also be treated for the UTI. *Staphylococcus epidermidis (S. epidermidis)* is normal skin flora and is likely a contaminant because of an inappropriate clean-catch specimen collection technique.

9. Answer: 2

Rationale: Although effective in protecting healthy skin from urine, moisture-barrier films contain alcohol and can burn and irritate denuded skin and, therefore, should be used sparingly. If the perineal area is already red and excoriated, using a moisture-barrier film is contraindicated. Each time the patient is changed, the caregiver should cleanse the perineal area with mild soap and water, and then apply a thin layer of petrolatum or zinc oxide to treat the irritant dermatitis. The addition of vitamin C 250mg and zinc 220mg daily will aid the healing process. Once the perineal area is healed, vitamin C and zinc should be discontinued.

10. Answer: 3

Rationale: The family nurse practitioner suspects UTI and needs to confirm the diagnosis with microscopic urine exam to identify white blood cells (WBCs) and bacteria. If no WBCs or bacteria are seen, an abdominal radiograph should be ordered to rule out a kidney stone, which is also part of the differential diagnosis.

11. Answer: 4

Rationale: Functional incontinence is the inability to toilet appropriately because of impaired mobility. Ensuring that the patient has the appropriate equipment in the home (bedside commode, walker, wheelchair, accessible bathroom, and clothing that is easily removed) will assist the patient in maintaining independence. The patient may also benefit from scheduled toileting every 2 hours to reduce "accidents." Often these patients become socially isolated and depressed because of their concern about an accident in public. The family nurse practitioner should explore all options available. Evaluating the need for incontinence pads is effective with stress incontinence. Limiting fluid intake in the evenings to reduce nocturnal incontinence is appropriate for urge incontinence. Performing Credé's maneuver is appropriate for overflow incontinence.

12. Answer: 3

Rationale: The patient likely has chronic bacterial prostatitis, which is difficult to treat because the bacteria reside in prostatic calculi and corpora amylacea. Chronic bacterial prostatitis requires 3–4 months of therapy with trimethoprim-sulfamethoxazole (Septra DS), or a quinolone (e.g., ciprofloxacin) may be necessary to prevent urinary symptoms, although care should be taken when prescribing quinolones in patients 60 years and older because of risks of Achilles tendon rupture and other potential side effects.

13. Answer: 4

Rationale: Sedative-hypnotics, diuretics, anticholinergics, α-adrenergic agents, and calcium channel blockers can cause reversible transient urinary incontinence. Poor pelvic support is a possible cause of stress incontinence. Urge incontinence, or the inability to delay urination with a sudden and powerful urge to void, is a possible result of lower urinary tract problems. A prolapsed uterus or bladder can cause overflow incontinence with overdistention of the bladder.

14. Answer: 2

Rationale: Functional incontinence is the inability to toilet appropriately because of impaired mobility. Stress incontinence is leakage from the bladder during activities that increase intra-abdominal pressure and, therefore, pressure on the bladder, forcing urine leakage. Urge incontinence is an inability to delay urination, with a strong, abrupt urge to void, caused by bladder hyperactivity or hypersensitive bladder. The patient often has little warning before urine passes out of the bladder. Incontinence with overdistention of the bladder is called overflow incontinence, caused by an underactive or noncontracting detrusor muscle or by bladder outlet or urethral obstruction. It is characterized by frequent urination in small amounts.

15. Answer: 3, 4

Rationale: *E. coli* is the pathogen in 80%–90% of community-acquired UTIs. Gram-positive *Staphylococcus saprophyticus (S. saprophyticus)* is the second most common pathogen. *Klebsiella pneumoniae (K. pneumoniae)* and *Proteus mirabilis (P. mirabilis)* are also possible pathogens. In hospital settings, *E. coli* is less prevalent. *Streptococcus pyogenes,* also known as the flesh-eating bacteria, usually begins as a skin infection or in the throat and then spreads to deeper areas of the skin, which ultimately leads to potentially life-threatening diseases. *Staphylococcus aureus* infections typically are not associated with UTIs but are found more often with skin (impetigo; mastitis), lung (pneumonia), bone (osteomyelitis), and blood vessel (thrombophlebitis) infections.

16. Answer: 3

Rationale: Cystitis in adults usually presents with dysuria, urgency, frequency, nocturia, and suprapubic heaviness. Acute onset of chills, fever, flank pain, headache, malaise, and costovertebral angle tenderness are common in pyelonephritis in adults. Infants with cystitis may exhibit fever, irritability, decreased appetite, vomiting, diarrhea, constipation, dehydration, and jaundice.

17. Answer: 1

Rationale: Relapse is an uncommon cause of recurrent UTIs in women and occurs within 2 weeks of completion of antibiotic therapy. It may need to be treated for 2–12 weeks. Reinfection is the cause of most UTIs in women and may be caused by residual urine resulting from a prolapsed uterus or bladder or by lack of estrogen in perimenopausal women. If the patient has up to two UTIs a year, single-dose or 3-day antibiotic therapy may be used.

18. Answer: 2

Rationale: Pyelonephritis in men suggests a structural abnormality and is usually an indication for hospitalization, parenteral antibiotics, and an intravenous voiding pyelogram. Pyelonephritis in women is usually a result of invasion of the urinary tract by bacteria that have ascended the urethra from the introitus of the urethra. If bacteremia is suspected, women need to be hospitalized as well. Suggested follow-up is by telephone contact within 12–24 hours of initiation of antibiotic therapy and at 2 weeks and 3 months for posttreatment urine cultures.

19. Answer: 2

Rationale: Urge incontinence is associated with conditions such as Parkinson's disease or Alzheimer's disease and involves the central nervous system causing detrusor motor and/or sensory instability. Urge incontinence is the involuntary leakage accompanied by or immediately preceded by urgency.

20. Answer: 3

Rationale: Although discussing the alkaline-ash, low-purine diet with the patient is appropriate, most patients, when they learn how difficult the diet is to follow, will be noncompliant with the diet even though they realize they risk developing another uric acid renal calculi. Starting the patient on allopurinol (Zyloprim) 100mg qd PO and monitoring to ensure that the serum uric acid level remains at normal levels will control the incidence of uric acid stones while allowing the patient freedom without such strict dietary restrictions. Monitoring the patient for another episode is inappropriate because the serum uric acid is likely elevated and a repeat incident is likely imminent. Referral to a urologist is inappropriate at this time because there is no acute episode.

21. Answer: 4

Rationale: Painless hematuria is the most common presenting symptom in the patient with bladder cancer. Painless hematuria often occurs early in the course of bladder cancer and is often the only symptom the patient will exhibit. There is

no evidence of renal failure (oliguria; edema). Renal calculi would be characterized by both hematuria and flank pain. Prostate cancer often presents with the other symptoms of benign prostatic hypertrophy.

22. Answer: 3

Rationale: A sedentary lifestyle or episodes of immobilization can predispose a patient to the development of renal calculi. UTIs usually do not precipitate problems with renal calculi; however, the presence of renal calculi will predispose the patient to UTIs. Milk intake of 6–8 oz daily is not excessive and will not predispose a patient to renal calculi, and increased intake of citrus and high-fiber carbohydrates is good for the patient's dietary needs.

23. Answer: 2

Rationale: Postrenal failure results from development of an obstructive problem distal to the kidney, as seen in advanced prostatic hypertrophy with hematuria. A severe hypotensive episode, often seen after acute myocardial infarction (MI), is considered prerenal. The vascular changes resulting from diabetes and the exposure to nephrotoxic chemicals are considered intrarenal.

24. Answer: 1

Rationale: The precipitating factor in prerenal failure is most often an incident that precipitated renal ischemia, such as a shock situation (anaphylactic reaction). Treatment with nephrotoxic medications such as gentamicin (Garamycin), pyelonephritis, and renal vascular changes are causes of intrarenal failure.

25. Answer: 1, 3, 4

Rationale: Routinely performing Kegel's (pelvic floor) exercises should be taught because they assist in maintaining strong pelvic floor musculature. Weak pelvic floor musculature may contribute to urinary incontinence, especially with activity. The family nurse practitioner should include teaching about avoiding dietary substances that can irritate the bladder, such as caffeine, alcohol, and spicy foods.

26. Answer: 3

Rationale: A smooth enlarged prostate palpated on DRE is found with BPH. An elevation in prostate specific antigen (PSA) can be found in prostate cancer as well as benign prostatic hyperplasia (BPH), but is not diagnostic for either. Gross hematuria may be found in men over the age of 60 with BPH because of the chronicity of the disorder that leads to chronic cystitis. A nodular firm prostate is indicative of prostate cancer.

27. Answers: 2, 3

Rationale: Subsequent testing by a urologist is done if cancer is a concern, which is suspected when the prostate is nodular and firm, or if the patient does not improve with medication management. The subsequent testing may include uroflow to help diagnose obstruction, a cystometrogram that measures bladder compliance for patients with suspected neurologic disease, and a cystoscopy to determine whether surgical intervention is required for obstruction or cancer. Oftentimes, one of the symptoms that accompany initial diagnosis of BPH is a urinary tract infection (UTI). Unless the patient develops chronic UTIs, the family nurse practitioner can treat UTI with routine antibiotics.

28. Answers: 2, 3, 4

Rationale: Nephrotic syndrome is damage to the kidneys that is caused by disorders that lead to increased protein in the urine and to a subsequent decrease in serum albumin, which leads to peripheral edema (third spacing). Other objective findings include an increase in lipids because of an increase in synthesis of very low-density lipoproteins (VLDL) as well as cholesterol and triglycerides. This leads to lipiduria, which is the sloughing of tubular cells containing fat. Increased coagulation occurs, along with reduced kidney function.

29. Answers: 3, 4

Rationale: The National Kidney Foundation recommends screening patients with diabetes mellitus and hypertension for proteinuria as well as a decrease in GFR. Chronic renal failure is diagnosed when there is evidence of persistent kidney damage noted to be over a period of 6 months, which is proteinuria, but other markers of damage may include persistent glomerulonephritis or structural damage from polycystic kidney disease and a GFR of less than 60. Hematuria is not usually found. Elevated A1C is related to diabetic control and not specifically indicative of renal damage, although consistently high levels do correlate with the long-term complication of nephropathy.

30. Answer: 3

Rationale: Acute onset of increased confusion, inability to redirect, and increased agitation indicate an infection, likely a UTI, in the older adult patient with dementia. The family nurse practitioner should obtain a UA and empirically treat for UTI until the UA results are received. Because the patient has no neurologic symptoms (e.g., weakness; flaccidity), a new infarct is unlikely. Acute confusion is not a sign of worsening dementia because dementia is a gradual process. The caregiver bringing the patient with this acute problem would not indicate underlying caregiver stress, which usually presents when persons complain of stress to their own primary care provider.

Pharmacology

31. Answer: 3

Rationale: Benign prostatic hypertrophy is a common cause of urinary retention in older men. Inhaled ipratropium is an atropine-like bronchodilator used to treat chronic bronchitis, and its anticholinergic agent may aggravate urinary retention. Neither glyburide (oral antihyperglycemic) nor buspirone (oral antianxiety agent) has an effect on the urinary system. Timolol is a topical agent used to treat glaucoma and does not have a systemic effect.

32. Answer: 4

Rationale: Combination hormone replacement therapy using conjugated estrogen (Premarin) 0.3–1.25 mg/day orally or vaginally and medroxyprogesterone (progestin) 2.5–10 mg/day continuously or intermittently can be useful for management of stress incontinence. Propantheline and oxybutynin may be useful in urge incontinence; research is limited on their use for urge incontinence. Doxepin (Sinequan) is a tricyclic antidepressant and is used infrequently.

33. Answer: 1

Rationale: To decrease the formation of uric acid stones, a urinary alkylating agent, such as allopurinol, is frequently used. As standard practice, the family nurse practitioner should check the patient's serum uric acid level monthly for 3 months to ensure the levels are decreasing to normal ranges, and then annually once serum uric acid levels are normalized. Indomethacin is used for its anti-inflammatory properties in the treatment of gout. Urecholine is a cholinergic agent that stimulates the bladder to contract, which improves urine flow. Phenazopyridine is a urinary tract analgesic.

34. Answer: 3

Rationale: Oxybutynin produces anticholinergic effects, and dry mouth is a common side effect. Because this patient is an older adult, the family nurse practitioner should review the patient's list of medications to verify that no other medications will exacerbate dry mouth. If another medication will increase this side effect (e.g., diuretic), the family nurse practitioner should advise the patient of methods to relieve the dry mouth, such as hard candy or chewing gum. The patient may also be taking other medications with anticholinergic side effects, which could be increased with the addition of oxybutynin to the point the patient could be at risk for falls. Careful review of the patient's medication list is essential before adding a new drug. The other reactions are not consistent with oxybutynin administration.

35. Answer: 1, 3, 5

Rationale: Sedatives and hypnotics lead to sedation and muscle relaxation in all groups, but particularly in the older adult population; central nervous system (CNS) changes from aging may lead to increased muscle relaxation, with the addition of a sedative-hypnotic leading to urinary incontinence. Antidepressants have anticholinergic effects and lead to sedation. CNS changes and the addition of antidepressants with anticholinergic side effects will increase muscle relaxation in the older adult patient and contribute to urinary incontinence. Antibiotics and bulk-forming laxatives have not been implicated in the development of urinary incontinence in older patients. Opioids increase the tone in the urinary bladder sphincter, leading to urinary retention.

36. Answer: 1

Rationale: Nitrofurantoin is contraindicated if renal function is impaired, antibacterial concentration in the urine is inadequate, or risk of toxicity is increased. To treat chronic UTI, the family nurse practitioner would consider nitrofurantoin 100 mg PO hs as prophylactic treatment. Using this dose in the adult patient should not cause serum or tissue accumulation of the drug. Liver function studies may be indicated if the patient experiences adverse reactions to the medication. Anticoagulants and sulfa-based drugs are not reported to cause significant drug interactions.

37. Answer: 1

Rationale: The severe pain of renal calculi should be addressed before other treatments or diagnostics. Narcotics and now nonsteroidal anti-inflammatory drugs (NSAIDs) are commonly used for pain relief. In most randomized, blinded studies of NSAIDs versus narcotics, NSAIDs have shown equal or greater efficacy for pain relief, shorter duration to pain relief, with equal or fewer side effects. Ketorolac works at the peripheral site of pain production rather than on the CNS and, based on clinical findings, has been proven to be as effective as opioid analgesics, with fewer adverse effects.

38. Answer: 1

Rationale: The most important side effects of nitrofurantoin are gastrointestinal upset, which can be decreased if the medication is taken with food or milk, and discoloration of the urine. The patient should continue taking nitrofurantoin for at least 3 days after sterile urine is obtained. If applicable to the patient, the drug may interfere with the efficacy of oral contraceptives.

39. Answer: 1

Rationale: The family nurse practitioner should advise the patient that if she experiences yellow discoloration of the sclerae while taking phenazopyridine, she is to return to the office immediately. This may indicate poor renal excretion and requires a renal workup (renal panel, parathyroid and thyroid-stimulating hormone, serum magnesium/calcium, and a 24-hour urine for creatinine clearance) and possible referral to a nephrologist. Phenazopyridine should be administered with food, and no drug interactions occur with aspirin or oral contraceptives.

40. Answer: 3

Rationale: Oxybutynin is contraindicated in patients with narrow-angle glaucoma. Patients with open-angle glaucoma may take this medication. Anticholinergics may increase the pressure within the eye, which puts the patient at risk for progression of the glaucoma, which is blindness.

41. Answer: 4

Rationale: Angiotensin-converting enzyme (ACE) inhibitors increase pressure within the kidney in renal artery stenosis, causing an increase in serum creatinine and potassium. ACE inhibitors have protective properties for patients with cardiovascular disease, hypertension, and diabetes.

15

Male Reproductive

Physical Exam & Diagnostic Tests

1. Which organ is not palpable on physical exam of a male patient?
   1. Vas deferens.
   2. Testes.
   3. Epididymis.
   4. Cowper's glands.

2. Review of a lab report indicating elevated serum gonadotropin would raise suspicion of which disorder?
   1. Seminal vesiculitis.
   2. Vas deferens disease.
   3. Testicular disease.
   4. BPH.

3. Which of the following structures can be palpated during an external exam of a male patient?
   1. Epididymis.
   2. Cowper's ducts.
   3. Seminal vesicles.
   4. Ejaculatory ducts.

4. What would be most helpful in diagnosing gynecomastia?
   1. History and physical.
   2. Liver function test.
   3. Thyroid function test.
   4. Mammogram.

5. The correct position in which to place a healthy adult male patient to examine the rectum and prostate is:

   1. Left lateral Sims' position with right knee flexed and left leg extended.
   2. Supine position with hips and legs flexed and feet positioned on the examining table.
   3. Modified knee-chest position with patient prone and knees flexed under hips.
   4. Leaning over the exam table with chest and shoulders resting on the table.

6. How is prostate cancer appropriately diagnosed?
   1. An elevated PSA.
   2. Upon palpating a nodule during a DRE.
   3. Biopsy via transrectal ultrasonography.
   4. An elevated prostatic acid phosphatase.

7. Which statement is correct about the PSA test?
   1. PSA can be elevated in patients with BPH.
   2. PSA is not elevated in patients with prostatitis.
   3. Prostatic massage will not elevate PSA levels.
   4. PSA does not increase in recurrence of prostate cancer.

8. The United States Preventive Services Task Force recommends against routine screening for prostate cancer screening because:
   1. There is a high mortality rate from prostate cancer regardless of screening.
   2. There is harm associated with a high number of false positives.
   3. Digital rectal exam is shown to be superior to serological testing.
   4. Ultrasonography is now the screening of choice.

9. When examining the scrotum of a dark complexion male, a normal finding is:

   1. Symmetric scrotal sac with two movable testes.

   2. Smooth, rubbery, saclike surface that is sensitive to gentle compression.

   3. Asymmetric sac with left side lower than right side.

   4. Reddish color that is darker than body skin with sebaceous cysts.

Disorders

10. A 49-year-old male smoker presents to the clinic with complaints of painless gross hematuria. What is the most serious problem that needs to be considered by the family nurse practitioner?

    1. Bladder cancer.

    2. Benign prostatic hypertrophy.

    3. Erectile dysfunction.

    4. Urinary tract infection.

11. What finding is indicative of testicular torsion?

    1. Scrotal swelling with tenderness that occurs only after age 40.

    2. Sudden onset of pain with a firm, tender mass in the scrotum.

    3. A scrotum that transilluminates.

    4. Cremasteric reflex.

12. On a routine physical exam, a patient expresses concern over the observation that one side of his scrotum is larger than the other side. He states that it has been getting larger for the past few months and that the scrotum is smaller in the morning and enlarges through the day. He has felt a heaviness in the scrotum, denies any acute pain, but does confirm some discomfort in his lower back. He reports no history of trauma to the scrotal area. On exam, the family nurse practitioner confirms the enlargement. Further exam reveals that the scrotum will transilluminate and that manual manipulation of the scrotum does not cause pain. What is the initial diagnosis for the patient?

    1. Hydrocele.

    2. Orchitis.

    3. Epididymitis.

    4. Traumatic injury.

13. Which statement is correct concerning circumcision?

    1. Circumcision is helpful in preventing phimosis.

    2. Circumcision is a cause of paraphimosis.

    3. Balanoposthitis is the direct result of circumcision in older men.

    4. Circumcision increases the incidence of cancer of the penis.

14. Acute epididymitis is characterized by:

    1. Absence of dysuria.

    2. Nonenlarged scrotum.

    3. Tenderness over epididymis.

    4. Lack of abdominal pain.

15. In a 70-year-old man, which of the following bacteria is likely responsible for epididymitis?

    1. *Escherichia coli.*

    2. *Treponema pallidum.*

    3. *Neisseria gonorrhoeae.*

    4. *Chlamydia trachomatis.*

16. Which of the following is true about hypogonadism?

    1. Usually presents with decreased libido.

    2. May cause an increase in muscle mass.

    3. Is not associated with gynecomastia.

    4. Does not contribute to infertility.

17. Which of the following is a common cause of impotence?

    1. The use of antihypertensives.

    2. Dietary supplements.

    3. Masturbation.

    4. It is a natural part of aging.

18. Which action is true about the prostate?

    1. Secretes fluid that is acidic.

    2. Secretes fluid that is alkaline.

    3. Secretes androgens.

    4. Produces sperm.

19. An older adult man presents to the clinic with complaints of difficulty voiding and hematuria. The digital rectal exam reveals a firm prostate about 5 cm in diameter, asymmetric, with firm nodules. The PSA level is 14. The next action is to:

    1. Medicate with finasteride (Proscar) 5 mg PO daily and reevaluate in 3 months.

    2. Advise patient to avoid caffeine, alcohol, and over-the-counter decongestants.

    3. Obtain a urinalysis to determine presence of infection and amount of hematuria.

    4. Refer to urologist for biopsy and diagnostic evaluation for prostatic cancer.

20. A 20-year-old male patient presents with scrotal pain. A suspected diagnosis that requires immediate referral is:

    1. Testicular torsion.

    2. Hydrocele.

    3. Epididymitis.

    4. Inguinal hernia.

21. An adult male patient is being evaluated for dysuria, fever, and perineal pain. The physical exam by the family nurse practitioner reveals a distended bladder. Which of the following should be avoided?

    1. Urine culture.

    2. Prostate massage.

    3. Cultures for gonorrhea and chlamydia.

    4. CBC.

22. An older adult male presents with a history of burning on urination and difficulty urinating that has been increasing over the past few days. He often has to void a short time later to fully empty his bladder. A digital rectal exam reveals an enlarged prostate. What is the primary diagnosis considered by the family nurse practitioner?

    1. Bladder cancer.

    2. Testicular torsion.

    3. Benign prostatic hypertrophy.

    4. Renal failure.

23. The patient with localized prostate cancer will exhibit which symptoms?

    1. Hesitancy, frequency, and dysuria.

    2. Fatigue, severe constipation, and dysuria.

    3. Hematuria, nocturia, and weight loss.

    4. Myalgia, confusion, and lethargy.

24. A young patient presents with a complaint of a feeling of fullness in the scrotum. Physical exam reveals a round, soft, nontender, nonadherent, bluish testicular mass resembling a "bag of worms." No variation in size occurs with respiration or Valsalva maneuver. The mass transilluminates and is located anterior to the testes. The most likely diagnosis is:

    1. Varicocele.

    2. Hernia.

    3. Tumor.

    4. Spermatocele.

25. An uncircumcised patient presents with a complaint of not being able to retract the foreskin over the glans penis. What is the most likely diagnosis?

    1. Lateral phimosis.

    2. Phimosis.

    3. Peyronie's disease.

    4. Paraphimosis.

26. A middle-aged patient complains of a tight band causing a dorsal curvature of the penis and shortening of the penis both with and without an erection. What is the most likely diagnosis?

    1. Phimosis.

    2. Lateral phimosis.

    3. Lateral paraphimosis.

    4. Peyronie's disease.

27. A middle-aged, uncircumcised patient presents with tender or pruritic red pinpoint pustules and papules on the prepuce and glans. The most likely diagnosis is:

    1. Peyronie's disease.

    2. Balanitis.

    3. Phimosis.

    4. Paraphimosis.

28. A male patient is diagnosed with balanitis. The most likely cause is:

    1. Candidiasis.

    2. Herpes genitalis.

    3. Lichen planus.

    4. Psoriasis.

29. A male patient presents with a complaint of sexual dysfunction. The family nurse practitioner understands that sexual dysfunction is impairment of:

    1. Erection only.

    2. Emission only.

    3. Ejaculation only.

    4. Erection, emission, or ejaculation.

30. A man presents with a complaint of dysuria, enlarged scrotal tenderness over the epididymis, and abdominal pain. What is the most likely diagnosis for the patient?

    1. Testicular torsion.

    2. Vas deferens inflammation.

    3. Epididymitis.

    4. Balanitis.

31. The family nurse practitioner knows that erectile dysfunction is:

    1. Primarily psychological in origin.

    2. Unusual in older men.

    3. The persistent inability to achieve and maintain an erection adequate for sexual intercourse.

    4. The physiologic dysfunction when smooth muscle contracts, causing a lack of adequate amount of blood in the penis to render a rigid, larger penis.

32. Priapism is classified as which type of sexual dysfunction?

    1. Erection.

    2. Emission.

    3. Ejaculation.

    4. Priapic.

33. Which of the following is correct in response to a patient's question concerning a possible cause of testicular cancer?

    1. Syphilis.

    2. Gonorrhea.

    3. Cryptorchidism.

    4. Balanitis.

34. A male patient complains of impotence. Which of the following may be a contributing factor?

    1. Antihypertensive drugs.

    2. Sexual intercourse.

    3. Rheumatoid arthritis.

    4. Frequent masturbation.

35. A 16-year-old boy presents with gynecomastia. The family nurse practitioner knows that it is likely:

    1. A result of hypogonadism.

    2. Caused by medication.

    3. Due to the hormonal imbalances of adolescence.

    4. An aggressive form of breast cancer.

36. Which is true of prostate cancer?

    1. Rarely diagnosed in men >50 years of age.

    2. Soft, indiscrete, symmetric nodules of the prostate.

    3. Obstructive symptoms rarely present.

    4. Firm prostate, often with hard nodules.

37. Which symptoms would be most concerning about a possible diagnosis of prostate cancer in a male over 50 years of age?

    1. Hesitancy, dribbling, and urgency.

    2. Decreased force of urine stream.

    3. Pain and feeling of a full bladder.

    4. Urinary symptoms coupled with pain in the hips or back.

38. Which statement is correct concerning testicular cancer?

    1. It is a common problem in men over age 50.

    2. It is directly related to testicular trauma.

    3. It presents suddenly with pain.

    4. It is primarily found in young men.

39. Which of the following is true about acute bacterial prostatitis?

    1. Characterized by recurrent urinary tract infections.

    2. Involves an ascending infection of the urinary tract.

    3. Always occurs in men under age 30.

    4. Usually treated with one month of antibiotics.

40. Which of the following is true of orchitis?

    1. Is rarely viral.

    2. The lesion transilluminates.

    3. Is relatively painless.

    4. Can be associated with a worsening epididymitis.

41. A patient has nongonococcal urethritis (NGU). The family nurse practitioner understands that:

    1. No related problems occur if NGU is untreated.

    2. Patients with NGU are often asymptomatic.

    3. NGU is easily differentiated from gonococcal urethritis on physical exam.

    4. There is a very purulent discharge with a foul odor.

42. What organism is the most common cause of nongonococcal urethritis (NGU) in men?

    1. *Chlamydia trachomatis.*

    2. *Neisseria gonorrhoeae.*

    3. *Escherichia coli.*

    4. *Streptococcus faecalis.*

43. Which test is a useful tumor marker for testicular cancer?

    1. Alpha-fetoprotein (AFP).

    2. Prostate-specific antigen (PSA).

    3. Prostatic acid phosphatase (PAP).

    4. Alkaline phosphatase (ALP).

44. The most common causative agent of orchitis is:

    1. Arbovirus.

    2. Echovirus.

    3. Mumps.

    4. Rubeola.

45. What are common symptoms of benign prostatic hypertrophy (BPH)?

    1. Dribbling, hesitancy, loss of stream volume and force, and recurrent urinary tract infections.

    2. Dysuria, urgency, frequency, nocturia, and suprapubic heaviness or discomfort.

    3. Obstructive symptoms, such as a weak urine stream, abdominal straining to void, hesitancy, incomplete bladder emptying, and terminal dribbling.

    4. Acute onset of fever, chills, flank pain, headache, malaise, costovertebral angle tenderness, and possibly hematuria.

46. A 25-year-old patient with a history of sickle cell disease complains of a sudden problem with erections that are not sexually oriented. He is currently experiencing a painful erection and he is unable to void. The family nurse practitioner determines the treatment of choice is:

    1. Morphine sulfate and bed rest.

    2. Immediate referral to a urologist.

    3. Increased hydration for sickle cell crisis.

    4. Determination of PSA level.

47. The family nurse practitioner is speaking with a group of male teenagers who are most concerned about symptoms associated with gonorrhea. Which of the following would the family nurse practitioner include in the discussion?

    1. Reddish lesions may appear on the palms of the hands and soles of the feet.

    2. Men may observe a rash over the body of the penis.

    3. Urinary dribbling may result from irritation of the urinary tract.

    4. Painful urination results from inflammation of the urethra.

48. A 65-year-old uncircumcised man presents to the clinic with complaints of a painless "bump" on his penis, difficulty retracting the foreskin, and serosanguineous drainage from beneath the foreskin. The family nurse practitioner must first consider a possible diagnosis of:

    1. Balanitis.

    2. Penile cancer.

    3. Herpes.

    4. Penile trauma.

49. What is considered a major contributing factor in erectile dysfunction?

    1. Diet high in vitamin C.

    2. Diabetes mellitus.

    3. Allergies.

    4. Low-sodium diet.

50. A 30-year-old male presents with a maculopapular rash on his body, including the soles of his feet and his palms. He is also complaining of fatigue, fever, malaise, and swollen lymph nodes. On further questioning, it is revealed that the illness began several weeks ago with several papules on his penis. The family nurse practitioner suspects:

    1. Herpes simplex.

    2. Granuloma inguinale.

    3. Gonorrhea.

    4. Syphilis.

51. Which of the following sexually transmitted infections often begins with a prodrome of headaches, fever, malaise, and myalgia?

    1. Genital herpes.

    2. Granuloma inguinale.

    3. Gonorrhea.

    4. Syphilis.

52. Which of the following clinical presentations are commonly associated with genital herpes?

    1. Vesicular lesions on an erythematous base.

    2. Chancres on the penis.

    3. Purulent urethral discharge.

    4. Small, flattened papules and larger verrucous lesions.

53. Which of the following is true of testicular cancer?

    1. It affects hundreds of thousands of adolescent boys each year.

    2. It has a high mortality rate.

    3. Early detection via testicular self-exam improves morbidity and mortality.

    4. Cryptorchidism is a risk factor for testicular cancer.

Pharmacology

54. A patient has been taking doxazosin (Cardura) 2 mg PO daily for 3 weeks for treatment of BPH. He returns to the clinic and is complaining of feeling dizzy when he stands up. Which action would the family nurse practitioner take?

    1. Determine blood pressure (BP) with patient lying down, standing, and sitting.

    2. Order urinalysis (UA) to determine hematuria and presence of bacteria.

3. Review with patient his symptoms over the past 3 weeks.

4. Perform digital rectal exam to determine if prostate is smaller than previously noted.

55. In planning treatment for a patient with balanitis, the family nurse practitioner orders:

    1. Rest, ice, and elevation.

    2. Massage therapy.

    3. Antifungal agents.

    4. Emergency circumcision.

56. A 28-year-old man presents with complaints of fever, low back pain, perineal pain, and intense pain on voiding. Rectal exam reveals a tender, swollen, firm, warm prostate. Based on the patient's symptoms, the treatment of choice is:

    1. Ceftriaxone (Rocephin) 250 mg IM × 1, followed by doxycycline 100 mg PO bid × 10 days.

    2. Tetracycline (Achromycin) 250 mg PO qid × 10 days.

    3. Amoxicillin (Amoxil) 500 mg PO tid × 14 days.

    4. Erythromycin (Ilosone) 250 mg PO q6h × 24 days.

57. A 70-year-old man complains of scrotal pain with dysuria and frequency that has been increasing over the past 2 weeks. Physical exam reveals extreme scrotal tenderness and swelling, urethral discharge, and testes normal in size and position. UA reveals pyuria. What is the treatment of choice for the patient?

    1. Nitrofurantoin (Macrodantin) 100 mg PO qid × 14 days.

    2. Levofloxacin (Levaquin) 500 mg PO qd × 10 days.

    3. Doxazosin (Cardura) 1 mg PO qd × 10 days.

    4. Oxybutynin (Ditropan) 5 mg PO tid × 10 days.

58. Finasteride (Proscar) is prescribed for a 50-year-old man who is experiencing a problem with urination secondary to an enlarged prostate. The family nurse practitioner would teach the patient that while he is taking this medication, it is important to:

    1. Increase his fluid intake.

    2. Restrain from sexual activity.

    3. Take special precautions around women of childbearing age.

    4. Increase intake of folic acid.

59. A 75-year-old patient is diagnosed with chronic bacterial prostatitis, and the family nurse practitioner selects ciprofloxacin (Cipro) as the treatment. How should the ciprofloxacin be prescribed for this patient?

    1. 500 mg PO bid × 10 days.

    2. 500 mg PO tid × 3 days, then 500 mg PO bid × 10 days.

    3. 500 mg PO bid × 21 days.

    4. 500 mg PO bid × 30–45 days.

60. Which of the following would be considered an initial treatment for Peyronie's disease?

    1. Surgery.

    2. Trial of vitamin E 400 IU bid.

    3. Circumcision.

    4. Oxybutynin (Ditropan).

15 | Male Reproductive Answers and Rationales

Physical Exam & Diagnostic Tests

1. Answer: 4

Rationale: Cowper's glands (bulbourethral glands) are located near the prostate and beside the urethra near the base of the penis. These internal glands are nonpalpable. The testes, vas deferens, and epididymis are all palpable on exam.

2. Answer: 3

Rationale: Gonadotropin is often elevated in testicular disease, whereas prostate specific antigen (PSA) is elevated in disease of the prostate, such as benign prostatic hypertrophy (BPH).

3. Answer: 1

Rationale: The epididymis is palpable, whereas the ducts and glands are not. The comma-shaped epididymis is palpated on the posterolateral surface of each testis. The seminal vesicles (pair of glands) lie behind the urinary bladder in front of the rectum. These vesicles join the ampulla of the vas deferens to form the ejaculatory duct.

4. Answer: 1

Rationale: A complete history and physical usually provide the cause of gynecomastia without further testing, since it can be caused by medication, starving and refeeding, or lack of androgen production (atrophying testes), which changes the estrogen/androgen ratio. Serologic tests are considered only when history and physical suggest an underlying endocrine disorder.

5. Answer: 4

Rationale: For patient comfort and ease of exam, the healthy ambulatory adult is asked to lean over the exam table with his chest and upper body resting on the table. Although left lateral Sim's position is correct, it is the position used for examining a patient who is confined to bed or requests an alternative to standing.

6. Answer: 3

Rationale: The standard for diagnosing prostate cancer is a biopsy obtained by a urologist via transrectal ultrasonography. An elevated PSA is usually present during prostate cancer but can also be present in noncancerous disorders, such as benign prostatic hyperplasia. A nodule palpated on exam is suggestive of prostate cancer but is not diagnostic. Prostatic acid phosphatase is an enzyme present in prostate cancer that is an older test for prostate cancer and is also present in other diseases and when taking some medications.

7. Answer: 1

Rationale: PSA can be elevated in patients with benign prostatic hypertrophy (BPH) and those with prostatitis, as well as after prostate gland massage. PSA does increase with the increasing burden of the tumor, as in recurrent prostate cancer.

8. Answer: 2

Rationale: Prostate cancer has a low mortality regardless of screening, as only 2.8% of men will die of the disease. Over 80% of PSAs are false positives and not attributed to prostate cancer. Biopsies to rule out prostate cancer can cause anxiety, pain, bleeding, and urinary dysfunction. Digital rectal exam (DRE) and ultrasonography have not been proven to be effective methods of detecting prostate cancer.

9. Answer: 3

Rationale: The scrotal sac is asymmetric. In darker complexion men, the scrotal skin is often darker than the body. On all men, the scrotal surface may be coarse with small lumps on the skin, which are sebaceous or epidermoid cysts that may have an oily discharge.

Disorders

10. Answer: 1

Rationale: Gross hematuria in a patient over 40 years old should be considered as possible bladder cancer until proven otherwise. Smoking increases the patient's risk of bladder cancer.

11. Answer: 2

Rationale: The sudden pain in testicular torsion is not relieved when the involved testicle is elevated to relieve pressure. Transillumination is associated with cystic masses, such as a hydrocele. The cremasteric reflex is absent. Testicular torsion is most common among neonates and adolescents, with the highest incidence during puberty.

12. Answer: 1

Rationale: The lack of pain, increase in size of scrotal contents, and transillumination are characteristic of a hydrocele. Orchitis and epididymitis are usually characterized by pain; orchitis is most often associated with parotitis or mumps. There is no history of injury, and the scrotum would be tender to palpation.

13. Answer: 1

Rationale: Circumcision can be helpful in preventing chronic or severe phimosis and paraphimosis because both are a retraction dysfunction of the prepuce. In phimosis, the foreskin is too tight to be retracted backward over the glans penis. In paraphimosis, once the foreskin has been retracted behind the glans penis, it is too constricted to return to a position of covering the glans penis. Balanoposthitis is inflammation of the foreskin and glans in an uncircumcised male.

14. Answer: 3

Rationale: Acute epididymitis is characterized by an acute scrotal pain, dysuria, and enlarged unilateral scrotum with abdominal pain. Scrotal pain is relieved when the involved testicle is elevated.

15. Answer: 1

Rationale: In men over age 35, the most likely cause of epididymitis is *Escherichia coli (E. coli)*. These men usually have BPH or urinary tract disorders that make them more susceptible to *E. coli*. Sexually active men under age 35 are more likely to have epididymitis because of a sexually transmitted disease, such as *Neisseria gonorrhoeae* or *Chlamydia trachomatis*. *Treponema pallidum* is the causative agent of syphilis.

16. Answer: 1

Rationale: A man with primary hypogonadism will often present with low energy and decreased libido. These same men will often have gynecomastia because of the low or absent production of gonadotropin. Males with Klinefelter's syndrome (chromosomal abnormality with karyotype of 47,XXY–47,XXXXY) is the most common genetic cause of male hypogonadism, with failure of both spermatic function and virilization.

17. Answer: 1

Rationale: Impotence can be commonly caused by antihypertensives, particularly beta blockers and diuretics. Other causes of impotence are diabetes, trauma, and vascular and psychological disorders.

18. Answer: 2

Rationale: The prostate secretes an alkaline fluid that helps sperm survive in the acidic environment of the female reproductive tract. Androgens are produced by Leydig's cells of the testes. Sperm are produced in the seminiferous tubules of the testes.

19. Answer: 4

Rationale: The digital rectal exam (DRE) and levels of PSA are the primary indicators of prostatic cancer and should be thoroughly evaluated by a urologist. The other options are directed toward treatment of BPH and should be considered only after prostatic cancer has been ruled out.

20. Answer: 1

Rationale: Testicular torsion and testicular cancer are considerations that may be curable but must be treated early. Hydrocele, epididymitis, and inguinal hernias also require referral but do not require immediate attention.

21. Answer: 2

Rationale: In suspected acute prostatitis, only a rectal exam should be performed, if at all. Vigorous massage must be avoided because of the risk of inducing bacteremia. Although diagnostically helpful, palpation of the prostate in acute disease can be quite painful. Urine culture, urethral cultures for gonorrhea and chlamydia, and an elevated white blood cell count may be helpful in making the diagnosis.

22. Answer: 3

Rationale: BPH is often seen in men over age 50. Bladder cancer should be ruled out as a diagnosis in any patient presenting with microscopic or gross hematuria.

23. Answer: 1

Rationale: All the symptoms listed can be found in the patient with prostate cancer, but only the symptoms of hesitancy, frequency, and dysuria are localized. The patient often is asymptomatic.

24. Answer: 1

Rationale: A varicocele presents as described, whereas a hernia may transilluminate, and bowel sounds sometimes can be auscultated in the scrotum. Hernias vary in size with Valsalva maneuver. Tumors are solid and, therefore, do not transilluminate.

25. Answer: 2

Rationale: Phimosis is a retraction disorder of the penile foreskin or prepuce. It can occur at any age and is usually the result of poor hygiene and chronic infection (the foreskin cannot be retracted back over the glans penis). Paraphimosis is the inability to retract the foreskin from behind the glans penis.

26. Answer: 4

Rationale: Peyronie's disease is a fibrotic condition that causes a lateral curvature of the penis during erection. Most patients simply require reassurance. Some patients with more severe symptoms may require surgical intervention.

27. Answer: 2

Rationale: Inflammation of the glans penis and prepuce (balanitis) can be associated with poor hygiene and is often found in men with poorly controlled diabetes.

28. Answer: 1

Rationale: Candidiasis is the usual cause of balanitis and is often found in men with poorly controlled diabetes.

29. Answer: 4

Rationale: In sexual dysfunction, erection, emission, or ejaculation may not be functioning because of multifactorial causes, such as medications, vascular disorders, neuropathy, and trauma. Peyronie's disease and priapism are examples of erection dysfunction.

30. Answer: 3

Rationale: Epididymitis presents as described. Testicular torsion does not usually present with dysuria, although if there is any doubt, an ultrasound should be immediately performed.

31. Answer: 3

Rationale: This is the correct definition of erectile dysfunction (ED). The incidence of erectile dysfunction increases significantly in men as they age, particularly at age 60 and over. It involves a dysfunction in the hemodynamic mechanism of smooth muscle relaxation that increases blood flow in the penis and ultimately causes venous trapping (compression of subtunical venules) and rigidity. Patients who present with vascular ED are at a higher risk for cardiovascular events.

32. Answer: 1

Rationale: Priapism is a condition of prolonged penile erection related to venous obstruction and unrelated to sexual arousal. Erections lasting longer than 4 hours should be evaluated immediately by a urologist.

33. Answer: 3

Rationale: Patients with undescended testicles are more prone to developing testicular cancer. The other conditions listed are not causes of testicular cancer.

34. Answer: 1

Rationale: Antihypertensive drugs, such as propranolol (Inderal LA), can cause impotence. Other common causes include cardiovascular disease, diabetes, smoking, prostate surgeries, antidepressants, and depression.

35. Answer: 3

Rationale: Gynecomastia in adolescent boys is most likely a result of hormonal imbalances experienced during puberty. In older men, it is frequently caused by medications, such as spironolactone and H2 blockers. In adolescents, the condition requires reassurance that it rarely persists beyond the age of 17.

36. Answer: 4

Rationale: Prostate cancer is usually found in men over age 65 and causes rapid onset of urinary obstructive symptoms. Palpation reveals a firm prostate, often with discrete, hard nodule(s). Advanced stages may include complaints of bone pain.

37. Answer: 4

Rationale: Urinary symptoms coupled with pain in the hips or back are concerning for metastatic prostate cancer. It is difficult to differentiate between BPH and prostate cancer based on symptoms alone. Prostate cancer usually has no symptoms in early stages.

38. Answer: 4

Rationale: Although rare, testicular cancer is primarily found in men under age 40 and presents as nonpainful nodules of the involved testicle. It is second to leukemia as the most common cause of cancer in adolescent boys and is the most common cancer in men age 20–40. Trauma is not a causal factor.

39. Answer: 2

Rationale: Acute bacterial prostatitis is caused by an infection in the urinary tract moving up the urethra into the prostate. The most common organisms are *Escherichia coli, Pseudomonas,* and *Enterococcus.* The condition tends to occur in men ages 30 to 50 but can be associated with BPH in older men. Chronic bacterial prostatitis is characterized by recurrent urinary tract infections. The usual antibiotic course is 2 weeks in acute prostatitis and is 1 to 3 months for chronic prostatitis.

40. Answer: 4

Rationale: Orchitis can be either bacterial or viral in nature. The viral form is often caused by mumps, and the bacterial form of the disease is often a result of *Escherichia coli,* spread from a worsening epididymitis. The disorder can range from being uncomfortable to painful and often with constitutional symptoms.

41. Answer: 2

Rationale: Nongonococcal urethritis (NGU) is often asymptomatic and is difficult to diagnose. NGU typically has a clear discharge and usually is caused by chlamydiae. Gonococcal urethritis produces a yellow, purulent discharge. If there is a discharge, NGU is difficult to differentiate from gonorrhea without a culture. Epididymitis and reactive arthritis are also associated with untreated chlamydial infection of the urogenital tract.

42. Answer: 1

Rationale: *Chlamydia trachomatis* is the most common organism in male patients with NGU.

43. Answer: 1

Rationale: Alpha-fetoprotein (AFP), lactate dehydrogenase (LDH), and human chorionic gonadotropin (hCG) are all useful tumor markers for testicular cancer.

44. Answer: 3

Rationale: The mumps virus is responsible for causing orchitis. Arbovirus and echovirus are implicated in meningitis and encephalitis. Rubeola is associated with complications of otitis media, pneumonia, croup, and encephalitis.

45. Answer: 3

Rationale: Obstructive symptoms are common in BPH. Dribbling, hesitancy, loss of normal urine stream, and recurrent urinary tract infections are present in chronic bacterial prostatitis. Dysuria, urgency, frequency, nocturia, and suprapubic heaviness are common symptoms of cystitis. Fever, chills, flank pain, headache, malaise, and costovertebral angle tenderness of acute onset with or without hematuria are indications of pyelonephritis.

46. Answer: 2

Rationale: This is considered a urologic emergency because of the inability to void and because the circulation to the penis may be compromised. The patient should be referred immediately to a urologist.

47. Answer: 4

Rationale: Dysuria is one of the most common complaints of young men with gonorrhea. No lesions, rash, or urinary dribbling accompanies the yellow discharge.

48. Answer: 2

Rationale: The patient's age, presentation, and uncircumcised state put him at risk for the relatively rare condition of penile cancer. Balanitis does not present with a serosanguineous drainage. Human papillomavirus (HPV) is frequently associated with this type of cancer.

49. Answer: 2

Rationale: Diabetes is a common contributor to erectile dysfunction because of the impaired circulation.

50. Answer: 4

Rationale: This patient has classic symptoms of secondary syphilis. Granuloma inguinale also presents with ulcerative lesions on the penis and lymphadenopathy but lacks the maculopapular rash and the systemic symptoms associated with syphilis. In this stage, syphilis is particularly infectious.

51. Answer: 1

Rationale: Many patients with genital herpes experience a prodrome of constitutional symptoms with their primary infection. In syphilis, systemic symptoms appear weeks to months after the genital lesions. Gonorrhea and granuloma inguinale are not typically associated with constitutional symptoms.

52. Answer: 1

Rationale: Vesicular lesions on an erythematous base are typical of genital herpes. Later in the course of the outbreak, the blisters break and leave a painful sore. Chancres on the penis are associated with syphilis. Purulent urethral discharge is found in those with gonorrhea or chlamydia infection. Small, flattened papules are associated with genital warts.

53. Answer: 4

Rationale: Testicular cancer affects around 8500 men per year in the United States. Treatment is effective and there are fewer than 400 who will die of the disease. The United States Preventive Services Task Force recommends against screening for testicular cancer because it is unreliable, is of low incidence, and false positives cause anxiety. A major risk factor for testicular cancer is cryptorchidism (undescended testicles).

Pharmacology

54. Answer: 1

Rationale: Doxazosin is also used as an antihypertensive agent; the patient may be experiencing orthostatic hypotension. The other options are directed toward evaluating his BPH, which has already been diagnosed.

55. Answer: 3

Rationale: Topical antifungals, such as clotrimazole, are appropriate for mild to moderate disease. Oral agents, such as metronidazole or fluconazole, can also be used to treat this disorder.

56. Answer: 1

Rationale: The patient is presenting with classic symptoms of acute bacterial prostatitis. The treatment of choice is IM ceftriaxone plus oral tetracycline.

57. Answer: 2

Rationale: The patient is presenting with classic symptoms of epididymitis. The treatment of choice is a fluoroquinolone, such as levofloxacin or ciprofloxacin. Nitrofurantoin is a urinary antiseptic, doxazosin is given for BPH, and oxybutynin is indicated for incontinence or enuresis.

58. Answer: 3

Rationale: Finasteride has some risk to women of childbearing age. It is important that women of childbearing age not be exposed to the sperm of a patient taking finasteride. These women and pregnant women should avoid handling crushed tablets. Exposure can cause fetal abnormalities.

59. Answer: 4

Rationale: The recommended treatment is for at least 30–45 days to prevent recurrence. Patients may require continued suppression therapy for an extended period.

60. Answer: 2

Rationale: Vitamin E promotes softening of fibrous tissue, which forms the plaques in Peyronie's disease. Pentoxifylline (TRENtal) is also commonly used.

Female Reproductive

Physical Exam & Diagnostic Tests

1. When obtaining a cervical specimen for a conventional Pap smear, the family nurse practitioner:

   1. Lubricates the speculum with a non-water-soluble lubricant to assist in the insertion of the instrument.

   2. Uses a cotton-tipped applicator when obtaining the cervical cells from a prenatal patient.

   3. Uses warm water to lubricate the speculum to assist in the insertion of the instrument.

   4. Completes the bimanual portion of the exam first in order to determine the relative position of the cervix to assist in the comfortable insertion of the speculum.

2. To promote patient comfort before performing a pelvic exam, the family nurse practitioner:

   1. Asks the patient to bear down slightly as the speculum is inserted.

   2. Has the patient empty her bladder.

   3. Explains each step of the procedure in a calm manner.

   4. Carefully reassures the patient that the exam will only take a few minutes.

3. What finding is considered a normal surface characteristic of the cervix?

   1. Small, yellow, raised round area on cervix.

   2. Red patches with occasional white spots.

   3. Friable, bleeding tissue at opening of cervical os.

   4. Irregular granular surface with red patches.

4. The primary role of a breast ultrasound is to:

   1. Screen for breast cancer.

   2. Definitively diagnose breast cancer.

   3. Determine if a breast lesion is cystic or solid.

   4. Locate small lesions before surgery.

5. The screening bone mineral density (DEXA) report ordered for a 60-year-old postmenopausal woman shows a result of –1.5 SD (standard deviation) at the hip. She gives a past history of myocardial infarction (MI) 1 year ago and wrist fracture at age 32. What option would **not** be considered for this patient?

   1. Counsel on smoking cessation and alcohol consumption.

   2. Initiate therapy with continuous conjugated estrogen 0.625 mg and medroxyprogesterone acetate (MPA) 2.5 mg.

   3. Initiate therapy with raloxifene (Evista).

   4. Encourage weight-bearing exercises and increased calcium intake.

6. When is the optimal time to perform a hysterosalpingogram (HSG)?

   1. During menses.

   2. Immediately after ovulation.

   3. After menses but before ovulation.

   4. 3–4 days before menses.

7. Which statement about mammography is false?

   1. Mammography detects all breast cancers.

   2. Mammography should be accompanied by a breast exam.

   3. Negative mammography should not delay biopsy of a clinically suspicious mass.

   4. Mammography is a cost-effective method to screen for breast cancer.

8. The use of potassium hydroxide (KOH) when doing a wet mount assists in the diagnosis of:

   1. Bacterial vaginosis and candida vaginitis.

   2. Trichomoniasis and chlamydia cervicitis.

   3. Syphilis and gonorrhea.

   4. Herpes simplex and condyloma.

9. The family nurse practitioner is reviewing the laboratory results of an 18-year-old patient seen recently for a Pap smear: Classification—high-grade squamous intraepithelial lesion; endocervical cells seen; adequate smear. The family nurse practitioner phones the patient and tells her which of the following?

   1. "Your Pap smear was normal. Follow up in 1 year or sooner if problems arise."

   2. "Your Pap smear shows invasive cancer. I would like you to see a gynecologic oncologist for treatment."

   3. "Your Pap smear shows abnormal tissue that needs to be evaluated. Please schedule an appointment for a colposcopy."

   4. "Your Pap smear shows a minor abnormality. Sometimes this can signify a disease process just beginning. Please schedule another Pap smear in 4 months for follow-up."

10. A 27-year-old patient reports the desire to become pregnant. She and her husband have had regular, unprotected intercourse for more than 1 year. The family nurse practitioner completes a thorough history and gynecologic exam, which appear normal. What diagnostic test might be ordered early in the workup?

    1. Hysterosalpingogram.

    2. Tests for antisperm antibodies.

    3. Semen analysis.

    4. Endometrial biopsy.

11. For which of the following women does the National Osteoporosis Foundation (NOF) recommend a screening bone DEXA scan? Select two responses.

    1. A 48-year-old Caucasian woman who smokes and has excessive alcohol intake.

    2. A 50-year-old woman having irregular menstrual cycles.

    3. A 51-year-old woman on long-term corticosteroid therapy.

    4. A 54-year-old woman receiving hormone replacement therapy (HRT).

    5. A 45-year-old woman who plays tennis regularly and recently fractured her ulna while playing.

12. When describing the findings from a normal breast exam, what would the family nurse practitioner document on the patient record?

    1. Left nipple everted, several coarse black hairs arising from areola, enlarged axillary lymph nodes palpated bilaterally, tender nodes in supraclavicular area.

    2. No dimpling or retraction; 1-cm hard, fixed, stellate mass noted next to nipple with scant nipple discharge; no pain or tenderness on palpation.

    3. Right breast slightly larger and denser than left with no nipple discharge, right areola dark pink in color and inverted, left areola dark brown in color and everted, breasts tender to palpation with no axillary nodes noted.

    4. Pendulous breasts with no dimpling, retraction, nipple discharge, or areas of discoloration; numerous small nevi near areola with Montgomery's tubercles noted, no supraclavicular or axillary lymph nodes palpated.

13. In an infertility workup, what is the best way to evaluate ovulation?

    1. Hysterosalpingogram.

    2. Postcoital test.

    3. Endometrial biopsy.

    4. Basal body temperature (BBT) chart.

14. The family nurse practitioner is reviewing the laboratory results of a 61-year-old patient seen recently for a Pap smear: atrophic changes, scant endocervical cells, and adequate smear. She has been treated for breast cancer with mastectomy and tamoxifen (Nolvadex). She has never received hormone replacement therapy (HRT). What is appropriate for the family nurse practitioner to tell the patient when she phones her with her results?

    1. "Your Pap smear is slightly abnormal. I would recommend the use of some estrogen vaginal cream nightly for 3 weeks, and then return to the office to have the Pap smear repeated."

    2. "Your Pap smear is normal but shows a mild thinning of the tissue. This is to be expected in someone who is postmenopausal and not on hormones, and it does not pose a threat to your health. Please return to the office in 1 year for your annual exam or sooner if needed."

3. "Your Pap smear shows that you don't have enough endocervical cells. Please make an appointment for endocervical curettage."

4. "Your Pap smear is abnormal. This could signify a disease state of the cervix. Please schedule a colposcopy at your earliest convenience."

15. Which test is the "gold standard" for the diagnosis of chlamydial infection?

   1. KOH wet mount "whiff" test.

   2. Nucleic acid amplification test (NAAT).

   3. Direct fluorescent antibody (DFA) test.

   4. Culture with special media and collection technique.

16. The family nurse practitioner is discussing mammography with a group of women and providing the recommendation from the American Cancer Society. What important information should the family nurse practitioner include in the discussion?

   1. A mammogram should be done annually for all women of childbearing age.

   2. All women age 40 years and older should have a mammogram annually.

   3. A mammogram should be done annually after pregnancy if the woman does not breast-feed.

   4. A mammogram should be done only if the woman has breast pain or nipple retraction.

17. Which is the **most** accurate statement regarding a reactive serologic test for syphilis?

   1. All reactive serologic tests require confirmation with a treponemal test.

   2. Reactive serologic tests are highly suspicious for active syphilis.

   3. A false-positive serologic test, although rare, can be unnecessarily traumatizing to a patient.

   4. A reactive serologic test most likely implies the need for re-treatment.

18. In the workup for a patient with secondary amenorrhea, the prolactin serum assay results show a level of 24 ng/mL. Appropriate management includes:

   1. Administering medroxyprogesterone acetate (MPA; Provera) 10 mg PO bid × 5 days.

   2. Referral to a specialist.

3. Recording the results as WNL (within normal limits).

4. Assessment for nipple discharge.

19. In the evaluation of a young adult with amenorrhea and normal secondary sex characteristics, the purpose of the progesterone challenge is to determine the presence of:

   1. Endogenous estrogen.

   2. Thyroxine.

   3. Prolactin.

   4. Adequate body fat.

20. A patient comes to the office complaining of fatigue, breast tenderness, abdominal bloating, fluid retention, and irritability about a week before onset of her menses. This has been occurring for the past 4 months. What is the most important information for the family nurse practitioner to obtain to assist in determining the diagnosis of premenstrual syndrome (PMS)?

   1. Point in menstrual cycle when symptoms occur.

   2. Severity of symptoms.

   3. Number and frequency of symptoms over past 4 months.

   4. Presence or absence of anxiety or depression.

21. A 65-year-old woman reports to the clinic stating she has been experiencing intermittent vaginal bleeding over the past 2 months. Her last menstrual period was more than 10 years ago. Her last Pap smear at the clinic 9 months ago was within normal limits (WNL). She is not taking any hormonal products. She is sexually active with occasional complaints of dyspareunia. What is the **most** appropriate response of the family nurse practitioner at this time?

   1. Order CBC and TSH and repeat Pap smear.

   2. Schedule laparoscopy.

   3. Schedule endometrial biopsy.

   4. Schedule pelvic/transvaginal ultrasonography.

Normal Gynecology

22. The endometrial cycle is often described in three phases. Select the correct phases:

   1. Follicular, menstrual, and luteal.

   2. Proliferative, luteal, and menstrual.

   3. Follicular, secretory, and menstrual.

   4. Proliferative, secretory, and menstrual.

23. The family nurse practitioner understands that PMS occurs with greatest frequency and severity in the:

    1. Late luteal phase.

    2. Follicular phase.

    3. Proliferative phase.

    4. Ovulatory phase.

24. Which hormones are released from the anterior pituitary gland? Select three hormones.

    1. Follicle-stimulating hormone (FSH).

    2. Luteinizing hormone (LH).

    3. Oxytocin.

    4. Prolactin.

    5. Antidiuretic hormone (ADH).

25. What is the primary function of FSH?

    1. Stimulation of maturation of ovarian follicles.

    2. Milk secretion.

    3. Triggering ovulation.

    4. Inhibiting release of luteinizing hormone (LH) from the pituitary gland.

26. How is the term *menopause* best defined?

    1. Cessation of ability for natural reproduction.

    2. Completion of 12 months of amenorrhea after last menstrual period.

    3. FSH level of 30 and estradiol level of 30.

    4. Last menstrual period.

27. In the ovarian cycle, what phase begins with ovulation and ends with the onset of menses?

    1. Follicular phase.

    2. Ovulation.

    3. Proliferative phase.

    4. Luteal phase.

28. Which is not a risk factor for heart disease in the postmenopausal female?

    1. Regular exercise.

    2. Cigarette smoking.

    3. Hormone replacement therapy.

    4. Diabetes mellitus.

29. An adult patient's last menstrual period (LMP) was 2 months ago. She has had an intrauterine device (IUD) in place for the past 4 months. She is complaining of nausea, fatigue, breast tenderness, and abdominal bloating. Physical exam reveals the following:

    - Abdomen: WNL.

    - Pelvic: Cervix—positive Chadwick's sign, IUD strings protruding from cervical os.

    - Uterus: Enlarged and nontender.

    - Adnexae: Nontender, without mass and no cervical motion tenderness.

    What is the most likely diagnosis?

    1. Uterine fibroid.

    2. Ovarian cancer.

    3. Dislodged IUD.

    4. Pregnancy.

30. What function do the Bartholin's glands have in reproduction?

    1. Prevent vaginitis by maintaining adequate pH.

    2. Prepare the mucous plug that occurs during early pregnancy.

    3. Produce an alkaline secretion that enhances sperm viability.

    4. Produce small amounts of hormones necessary for ovulation.

31. Which is not a risk factor for osteoporosis?

    1. Cigarette smoking.

    2. Caucasian.

    3. Alcohol consumption.

    4. Obesity.

32. A young woman complains to the family nurse practitioner that she is experiencing headaches, irritability, decreased appetite, and fatigue about 1 week before menses. Appropriate management includes which of the following?

    1. Treat PMS with increased protein and salt in the diet.

    2. Incorporate daily aerobic exercise and dietary changes into her lifestyle.

    3. Order CBC, comprehensive metabolic panel, and urinalysis.

    4. Supplement her diet with an additional 1–2 g of vitamin C.

33. A middle-aged female presents with abnormal uterine bleeding. A hormonal profile reveals increased FSH and LH levels. What is the most likely cause for these findings?

    1. Hypothalamic disorder.
    2. Onset of climacteric.
    3. Premature ovarian failure.
    4. Anterior pituitary disorder.

34. A 29-year-old patient presents to the family planning clinic for her annual exam. She had a tubal ligation postpartum 6 months ago. She has been feeling tired, is nauseated, and is slowly gaining weight. She had one menses postpartum, 4 months ago. The family nurse practitioner notes the following on physical exam:

    - Abdomen: Bowel sounds × 4, soft, no hepatosplenomegaly, palpable mass in lower abdomen measures 14 cm, no tenderness.
    - Pelvic: Bartholin's/urethral/Skene's glands (BUS) normal; cervix—os closed, smooth pink mucosa.
    - Bimanual: Uterus enlarged, nontender, smooth contours, no cervical motion tenderness.
    - Adnexae: Not palpable.

    What is the likely diagnosis?

    1. Pregnancy.
    2. Uterine fibroid.
    3. Premature menopause.
    4. Colon cancer.

35. Menopause occurs at a mean age of 51 years. Which of the following factors has been linked to influencing the age at which menopause occurs?

    1. Use of oral contraceptives.
    2. Socioeconomic status.
    3. Age at menarche.
    4. Smoking.

Gynecologic Disorders

36. During a yearly physical exam, a family nurse practitioner asks a woman if she has any problems or questions about sexual function or activity. Initially the patient hesitates, but with further questioning and discussion, she states that she is unsure if she has ever experienced an orgasm. The family nurse practitioner suspects:

    1. Vaginismus.
    2. Primary orgasmic dysfunction.
    3. Secondary orgasmic dysfunction.
    4. Dyspareunia.

37. The family nurse practitioner is talking with a young woman who has been diagnosed with herpes simplex type 2. In discussing her care, it would be important for the family nurse practitioner to include what information?

    1. The initial lesions are usually worse than lesions that occur with outbreaks at a later time.
    2. Her sexual partner will not contract it if she does not have sex when the lesions are present.
    3. This condition can be treated and cured if she takes all of the antibiotics for 2 weeks.
    4. If she becomes pregnant in the future, she will need to have a cesarean delivery.

38. The definition of bacterial vaginosis is:

    1. A syndrome resulting from homeostatic disruption in the vagina.
    2. Vaginitis caused by a flagellated protozoan.
    3. A bacterial sexually transmitted infection that can be symptomatic or asymptomatic.
    4. A virus characterized by recurrent outbreaks and remissions.

39. A 22-year-old married patient complains of severe dysmenorrhea. Her gynecologic exam is normal. Which management protocol is preferred?

    1. Assess for contraceptive interest and, if interested, suggest use of oral contraceptives (OCs).
    2. Suggest use of a prostaglandin synthetase inhibitor.
    3. Suggest use of over-the-counter ibuprofen.
    4. Assess exercise patterns and use of relaxation techniques.

40. Which is not a criterion for the diagnosis of bacterial vaginosis?

    1. Positive amine test (whiff test).
    2. Presence of clue cells.
    3. Vaginal pH >4.5.
    4. Presence of pseudohyphae.

41. A patient with a history of dilation and curettage (D&C) after a first-trimester spontaneous abortion and subsequent amenorrhea would lead the family nurse practitioner to a working diagnosis of which of the following?

    1. Polycystic ovarian syndrome.

    2. Asherman's syndrome.

    3. Hypogonadism.

    4. Premature ovarian failure.

42. The LH/FSH ratio in polycystic ovarian syndrome (Stein-Leventhal syndrome) is:

    1. 1.5:1

    2. 3:1

    3. 6:1

    4. 1:3

43. What are common findings in a patient with polycystic ovarian syndrome?

    1. Weight loss, dental caries, and amenorrhea.

    2. Hyperprolactinemia and galactorrhea.

    3. Dysmenorrhea, nodules palpated on bimanual exam, and infertility.

    4. Chronic irregular menses, hirsutism, and increased abdominal girth.

44. What is the most common cause of dysfunctional uterine bleeding?

    1. Thyroid disorder.

    2. Blood dyscrasia.

    3. Anovulation.

    4. Uterine tumor.

45. A 30-year-old patient presents with scant pubic hair, minimal breast development, absent cervix, and uterus with a 46,XY karyotype. Which diagnosis would the family nurse practitioner suspect?

    1. Turner's syndrome.

    2. Müllerian agenesis.

    3. Testicular feminization.

    4. Gonadal dysgenesis.

46. The most common cause of a breast mass in patients ages 15–25 is:

    1. Fibroadenoma.

    2. Intraductal papilloma.

    3. Infiltrating lobular carcinoma.

    4. Fibrocystic breast syndrome.

47. An effective treatment for primary dysmenorrhea is:

    1. NSAIDs.

    2. Tranquilizers.

    3. Progestins.

    4. Steroids.

48. What is a cause of secondary amenorrhea?

    1. Testicular feminization.

    2. Hypogonadotropic hypogonadism.

    3. Congenital absence of uterus.

    4. Extreme exercise.

49. A young woman comes into the clinic for a well-woman checkup. She states that, about 3 weeks ago, she had a sore on her labia that went away. It was not particularly painful, did not itch, and apparently caused no residual problems. The family nurse practitioner would treat this patient by:

    1. Ordering the treponemal-specific test (FTA-ABS).

    2. Swabbing the area of the lesion for a viral culture.

    3. Advising her to notify her sexual contacts to determine if they have had any symptoms.

    4. Ordering nystatin (Mycostatin) cream to be applied to the area three or four times a day.

50. Which is not a risk factor for the development of cervical cancer?

    1. Human papillomavirus (HPV).

    2. Virginal status.

    3. Multiple sexual partners.

    4. Previous high-grade squamous intraepithelial lesion (HSIL).

51. A young woman is complaining of tenderness and burning of her vulva. On exam, the vulva is edematous and excoriated. The family nurse practitioner performs a wet mount preparation of the vaginal secretions. It reveals pseudohyphae and spores. The diagnosis for this patient is:

    1. Vulvovaginal candidiasis.

2. Chlamydial infection.

3. Bacterial vaginosis.

4. Gonorrhea.

52. The leading cause of mortality in women with genital cancer, excluding breast cancer, is:

1. Ovarian cancer.

2. Endometrial cancer.

3. Cervical cancer.

4. Vulvar/vaginal cancer.

53. A young woman presents with complaints of an irritation in the vaginal area. This is the first time it has occurred. On vaginal exam, the cervix is inflamed and friable. Flagellated protozoa are seen on the wet mount. The most likely diagnosis is:

1. Trichomoniasis.

2. Cervicitis.

3. Chlamydial infection.

4. Bacterial vaginosis.

54. A 26-year-old female patient presents to the emergency department complaining of gradual onset of abdominal pain. The pain started in the periumbilical region and is now in the right lower quadrant, accompanied by nausea, anorexia, constipation, and low-grade fever. Physical exam confirms the diagnosis of acute appendicitis. What diagnostic studies are least useful in confirming this diagnosis?

1. CBC with differential.

2. Flat plate of abdomen, KUB.

3. Pelvic ultrasound.

4. Pregnancy test.

55. Which is not a risk factor for endometrial cancer?

1. Obesity.

2. Oral contraceptive use.

3. Unopposed estrogen use.

4. Advancing age, >50 years.

56. Which statement is true regarding the diaphragm?

1. May be inserted up to 24 hours before intercourse.

2. May be inserted any time up to 6 hours before intercourse.

3. Should be removed within 1 hour after intercourse.

4. May be left in place up to 24 hours following intercourse.

57. A contraceptive method associated with an increase in UTI is the:

1. Intrauterine device.

2. Diaphragm.

3. Norplant.

4. Oral contraceptive.

58. Which is not a risk factor for ovarian cancer?

1. Family history of ovarian cancer.

2. Advancing age, >50 years.

3. Oral contraceptive use.

4. Positive BRCA-2 gene.

59. What is the most common female genital malignancy, excluding the breast?

1. Ovary.

2. Endometrium.

3. Cervix.

4. Vulva/vagina.

60. A 20-year-old college student presents to urgent care with new onset of painful sores in the vulva. These erupted yesterday and are associated with exquisite pain, fever, and flulike symptoms of headache, general body aches, and mild dysuria. She has a new sexual partner. The exam reveals vesicular lesions covering the labia, extreme tenderness of external genitalia to palpation, normal BUS, normal vaginal inspection with mild leukorrhea, normal cervical mucosa, and slightly tender, minimally enlarged inguinal lymph nodes bilaterally. What is the likely diagnosis?

1. Gonorrhea.

2. Chlamydial infection.

3. Herpes simplex virus.

4. Lymphogranuloma venereum.

61. A 21-year-old patient is seen for her annual gynecologic exam. She is sexually active, rarely uses condoms for STD (STI) prevention, and has multiple sexual partners. She smokes one pack of cigarettes per day, admits to a sedentary lifestyle, and eats two meals per day, most often at fast-food restaurants. Her exam is negative for any abnormalities. Her family history and personal medical history are negative for major disease. She has no menstrual abnormalities; her last menstrual period (LMP) was 1 week ago. The family nurse practitioner has done her Pap smear. Which would not be appropriate for this patient?

    1. Cultures for gonorrhea and Chlamydia.

    2. Laboratory testing of glucose, cardiac risk profile, and TSH.

    3. HIV titer and RPR.

    4. Counseling on safe sex practice and contraceptive information.

62. Which are considered to be risk factors in the development of breast cancer? Select three responses.

    1. Early menopause.

    2. High-fat diet.

    3. Advancing age.

    4. Early menarche.

    5. Nonproliferative fibroadenomas.

63. A 32-year-old female patient, G2 T1 P1 A0 L2, is seen in the clinic by the family nurse practitioner for her annual exam and is requesting information on preconception counseling. She has been taking oral contraceptives (OCs) for 3 years without complications. During the past year she has started an exercise program at a health club 5 days a week and is eating three nutritionally sound meals daily. She has lost 33 lb and is now at her ideal body weight. She quit her job as a postal worker and now stays home with her children. As part of her preconception care, what should the family nurse practitioner recommend?

    1. Start prenatal vitamins with folic acid.

    2. Discontinue exercise.

    3. Update measles-mumps-rubella (MMR) vaccine.

    4. Start genetic counseling due to advanced maternal age.

64. The initial workup for abnormal uterine bleeding should include:

    1. Referral for diagnostic D&C.

    2. Referral for endometrial biopsy to rule out cancer.

    3. CBC, pregnancy test, and endocrine studies.

    4. Coagulation studies and STD cultures.

65. Which is not a risk factor for breast cancer?

    1. History of maternal breast cancer, premenopausal onset.

    2. First pregnancy after age 35.

    3. Late menopause, after age 54.

    4. Fibrocystic breast disease.

66. A 21-year-old female patient presents for her first well-woman exam. She never has been sexually active. Her family history and past medical history are negative for any gynecologic diseases. Her menses occur every 28 days and last 5 days, with a relatively moderate flow and no significant abdominal cramps. Her physical exam/visit today should include which tests?

    1. Pap smear.

    2. Cultures for gonorrhea and Chlamydia.

    3. Stool hemoccult.

    4. Baseline mammogram.

67. What is the leading cause of death for women in the United States?

    1. Breast cancer.

    2. Colon cancer.

    3. Heart disease.

    4. Stroke.

68. Reactive cellular changes noted on a Pap smear are most often associated with:

    1. Inflammation.

    2. Use of estrogen vaginal cream.

    3. Drying artifact.

    4. Use of OCs.

69. Risk factors for cervical cancer include:

    1. Pregnancy after age 35.

    2. Viral exposure.

    3. Low parity.

    4. Prolonged contraceptive use.

70. What is the most common cancer in women in the United States?

    1. Breast cancer.

    2. Colon cancer.

    3. Malignant melanoma.

    4. Lung cancer.

71. A 48-year-old patient presents to the clinic complaining of hot flashes, no menses for 14 months, insomnia, crying spells, irritability, decreased libido, and fatigue. At the end of her history and physical, she begins to cry and tells the family nurse practitioner that she "thinks she's going crazy." She then begs the family nurse practitioner to tell her what is wrong. Which action is inappropriate for the family nurse practitioner to do at this point?

    1. Obtain laboratory tests, including FSH and LH.

    2. Discuss HRT, including risks and benefits and short- and long-term treatment strategies.

    3. Provide antidepressant therapy and a referral for counseling sessions for depression.

    4. Provide written information regarding menopause and options for treatment of symptoms.

72. Care for a patient with chancroid should include:

    1. Screening for HIV as well as syphilis.

    2. Mandatory notification and treatment of all sexual partners.

    3. Screening for lymphogranuloma venereum.

    4. Culture for gonorrhea.

73. During her annual exam, a 35-year-old patient complains of recent breast changes. She states that her breasts are painful and frequently feel "lumpy." Because of this, she has stopped doing monthly breast self-exam (BSE), believing BSE is a "waste of time." What would be the most appropriate advice for the family nurse practitioner to give to this patient?

    1. Stress the importance of the woman knowing the normal look and feel of her breasts and to report any changes.

    2. Suggest she do BSE at least every 2 months.

    3. Suggest she start having mammograms to establish some baseline data about her breasts.

    4. Determine when her breasts are nontender and least "lumpy," and change her BSE schedule.

74. During a breast exam on a young woman, palpation reveals a painless, 2-cm lobular mass in the right breast that is firm and freely mobile. Appropriate management includes:

    1. Continued observation and rechecking in 3 months.

    2. Referral for a mammogram.

    3. Referral for probable surgical excision.

    4. Detailed family history to determine breast cancer risk.

75. A woman with bilateral breast implants asks if it is really necessary to do monthly breast self-exam (BSE) because she "does not know what to feel for." The most appropriate response would be:

    1. Suggest she involve her sexual partner in assessing her breasts on a regular basis.

    2. Review the steps in BSE until she feels comfortable with the process.

    3. Acknowledge the difficulty of doing BSE after implant surgery.

    4. Explain the usefulness of regular mammograms for implant patients.

76. An adult patient comes to the clinic complaining of abnormal vaginal discharge (dark watery brown) along with postcoital bleeding. The family nurse practitioner suspects the possibility of cancer of the cervix. During the vaginal exam, suspicious physical results would be:

    1. Soft, cylindrical-shaped cervix.

    2. Very firm cervix with an ulcer.

    3. Vague lower abdominal discomfort.

    4. Tender, enlarged lymph nodes.

77. A postmenopausal patient is worried about pain in the upper outer quadrant of her left breast. The family nurse practitioner should:

    1. Do a breast exam and order a mammogram.

    2. Explain that the pain is related to hormone fluctuations, and order laboratory studies.

    3. Reassure the patient that pain is not a presenting symptom of breast cancer, and check for proper fit of the brassiere.

    4. Teach the patient breast self-exam (BSE).

78. A 22-year-old female patient comes to the family nurse practitioner's office with a complaint of 1 day of fever of 102°F (38.9°C), a diffuse macular rash, vomiting, headache, and decreased urine output. The history obtained by the family nurse practitioner must include:

    1. Whether the patient's immunizations are up-to-date.

    2. If the patient is currently menstruating.

    3. If the patient has a history of tuberculosis.

    4. What type of contraception the patient uses.

79. A young female patient presents to the family nurse practitioner's office with a complaint of abdominal pain. In the United States which of the following diagnoses results in about 1 death per 1000 and, therefore, must be considered early in the decision process?

    1. Irritable bowel syndrome.

    2. Appendicitis.

    3. Pyelonephritis.

    4. Ectopic pregnancy.

80. A young adult patient presents with a history of vaginal itching and heavy white discharge. The patient gives a history of no sexual activity. On exam, the family nurse practitioner finds a red, edematous vulva and white patches on the vaginal walls. The discharge has no odor. The family nurse practitioner expects which factors in the patient's history?

    1. Vegetarian diet.

    2. Recent diarrhea.

    3. Early menopause.

    4. Recent antibiotic use.

81. A young patient comes to the office complaining of vaginal bleeding. The patient states that she has used 5 tampons in the past 3 hours. She admits to sexual activity and takes OCs. On further questioning, the patient states that she started her last pack of OCs "about 2 weeks late." The family nurse practitioner should:

    1. Perform a STAT urine pregnancy test.

    2. Perform a STAT CBC.

    3. Discuss proper use of OCs.

    4. Send the patient for a pelvic sonogram.

82. The family nurse practitioner knows that the majority of breast cancers occur in which area of the breast?

    1. Upper inner quadrant.

    2. Upper outer quadrant.

    3. Beneath the nipple and areola.

    4. Lower outer quadrant.

83. The patient presents with abnormal uterine bleeding and has been found to have endometrial cancer. She returned to the family nurse practitioner because she does not understand how this is possible when the Pap smear 6 months ago was negative. What is the family nurse practitioner's best response?

    1. "Uterine cancer develops quickly."

    2. "Pap smears are difficult to read, and mistakes can happen."

    3. "Pap smears are not useful in detecting uterine cancers in most cases."

    4. "The previous Pap smear did not have an adequate sample."

84. A postmenopausal woman is seen in the office with complaints of frequent urination, stress incontinence, vaginal dryness, and dyspareunia. Her last menstrual cycle was 6 years ago, and she elected not to take HRT. She has increased her intake of soy products. What is the most common cause of her symptoms?

    1. Urinary tract infection.

    2. Cystocele.

    3. Bacterial vaginitis.

    4. Atrophic vaginitis.

Pharmacology

85. A 42-year-old female patient presents to the office with complaints of dysuria, urinary frequency, and urgency. These symptoms began early this morning. She leaves a clean-catch midstream urine specimen, which shows white blood cells (WBCs) too numerous to count (TNTC)/high-power field (HPF), 4–5 red blood cells (RBCs)/HPF, and positive nitrites. A urine culture will be ready in 3 days. Which of the following three medications might be prescribed for an uncomplicated lower urinary tract infection (UTI)?

    1. Phenazopyridine (Pyridium) 200 mg 1 tab PO tid × 2 days.

    2. Trimethoprim-sulfamethoxazole (TMP-SMX; Septra DS) 1 tab PO bid × 5 days.

    3. Ceftriaxone (Rocephin) 1 g IM.

    4. Nitrofurantoin (Macrobid) 1 tab PO bid × 5 days.

    5. Neomycin 1 g PO q6h × 5 days.

86. The results of the Women's Health Initiative (WHI) provided evidence-based data that have led to new guidelines in assessing the risk/benefit ratio for initiation of HRT in postmenopausal women. Which statement is not correct?

    1. HRT is indicated for the treatment of menopausal symptoms, such as vasomotor and urogenital symptoms.

    2. HRT should be continued for primary prevention of coronary heart disease.

    3. HRT can be continued for the prevention of postmenopausal fractures due to osteoporosis.

    4. HRT should be limited to the shortest duration consistent with treatment goals and benefits in consideration with risks in the individual woman.

87. A 46-year-old female patient is being seen in the clinic by the family nurse practitioner. She was last seen 2 weeks ago for an upper respiratory tract infection and was treated with amoxicillin (Amoxil) 250 mg PO tid × 10 days. She completed her medication last week but now is aware of vaginal itching and has cottage cheese-like vaginal discharge. She states that she has never experienced such intense itching. She is in a mutually monogamous relationship. Her LMP was 2 weeks ago. Her partner had a vasectomy 2 years ago. Wet mount with KOH shows negative whiff test, rare clue cells, positive lactobacilli, positive hyphae and spores, few WBCs, and no trichomonads. She is leaving tomorrow for a week-long cruise. She is not taking any medications and has no known drug allergies. The family nurse practitioner knows that the best treatment for this problem is:

    1. Metronidazole (Flagyl) 500 mg PO bid × 7 days.

    2. Clindamycin (Cleocin) vaginal cream one applicator full vaginally hs × 7 days.

    3. Fluconazole (Diflucan) 150 mg 1 tab PO one time.

    4. Hydrocortisone (Cortaid) 1% cream sparingly bid × 7 days.

88. A 25-year-old patient presents with complaints of a malodorous vaginal discharge, which is described as white and watery. She douches with vinegar and water every 2 weeks. She uses a diaphragm for contraception. She and her boyfriend have been sexually active for 2 years, using condoms for STD prevention with every act of coitus. She denies any dyspareunia. Her LMP was 1 week ago, and there are no noted changes in her normal menstrual pattern. Her wet mount with KOH results show a positive whiff test, TNTC clue cells/HPF, no lactobacilli, no hyphae or spores, no trichomonads, and few WBCs. What is the diagnosis and treatment for this patient?

    1. *Chlamydia trachomatis*; doxycycline (Vibratabs) 100 mg PO bid × 10 days.

    2. *Candida albicans;* terconazole (Terazol 7) vaginal cream 1 applicator hs × 7 days.

    3. Herpes simplex type 2; acyclovir (Zovirax) 200 mg PO q4h × 5 days.

    4. Bacterial vaginosis; metronidazole (Metrogel) vaginal gel 1 applicator hs × 5 days.

89. A 55-year-old patient, G2 T2 P0 A0 L2, is being seen in the clinic for her annual exam. She went through a natural menopause 5 years ago and has never been interested in HRT. She smokes one pack per day and does no formal exercise. Her family history is positive for osteoporosis in her mother, positive for MI in her father, and negative for cancer. She has a normal physical exam today and had a negative mammogram yesterday. She is now interested in HRT but wants to know her alternatives. Which choice has not been clinically proven for prevention of osteoporosis?

    1. Estradiol (Estrace) 0.5 mg 1 tab PO qd and micronized progesterone (Prometrium) 100 mg 1 tablet PO qd.

    2. Weight-bearing exercise three times weekly.

    3. Discontinue cigarette smoking.

    4. Wild Mexican yam cream applied to skin tid.

90. A young woman is seen in the STD clinic. She noticed some itchy bumps in the vulvar area and is concerned that they could be cancer. On careful inspection, the family nurse practitioner notes five cauliflower-like, warty, pinkish lesions in the lower introitus. Two smaller lesions nestled anterior to the hymeneal ring of the vagina and cervix fail to reveal any abnormalities. Wet mount with KOH is negative. Culture for gonorrhea and *Chlamydia trachomatis* was obtained, Pap smear done, and HIV titer and RPR drawn. Which is not an appropriate treatment for this patient?

    1. Podophyllin (Podoben) application; wash off in 6 hours with soap and water.

    2. Trichloroacetic acid application; do not wash off.

    3. Cryotherapy with liquid nitrogen to lesions.

    4. Benzathine penicillin 2.4 million units IM weekly × 3 weeks.

91. A young adult complaining of vaginal itching, thick yellow mucous discharge, and urinary discomfort is seen in the urgent care unit by the family nurse practitioner. She is sexually active and uses condoms with only one of her two partners. On physical exam, the abdomen is negative; pelvic exam reveals the BUS WNL, cervix with mucopurulent discharge from the os, and mucosa friable to palpation; bimanual exam is negative. Cultures were taken, but are not yet available. Wet mount with KOH reveals a negative whiff test, few clue cells, TNTC WBCs/HPF, no yeast, and no trichomonads. What is the likely diagnosis and appropriate treatment?

    1. Chlamydia; azithromycin (Zithromax) 1 g PO single dose.

    2. Chlamydia; ceftriaxone (Rocephin) 125 mg IM.

    3. Herpes simplex virus; acyclovir (Zovirax) 200 mg 1 cap PO q4h × 5 days.

    4. Trichomoniasis; metronidazole (Flagyl) 2 g PO single dose.

92. A 52-year-old woman presents for her annual gynecologic exam from her primary care provider. She received a hysterectomy with ovarian conservation at age 40 for uterine fibroids and dysfunctional uterine bleeding. She has been taking oral estrogen (conjugated equine estrogen 0.625 mg) replacement therapy (HRT) for 1 year. Although HRT has definitely reduced the discomfort of hot flashes, vaginal dryness, and mood swings from insomnia, she still experiences flushes and some night sweats. Her diagnostic lipid panel shows total cholesterol 180, LDL 112, HDL 52, and triglycerides 325. What, if any, change might be considered in her medication regimen?

    1. No change should be considered at this time.

    2. Decrease estrogen dosage to 0.3 mg daily.

    3. Recommend stopping estrogen therapy.

    4. Suggest changing route of administration to transdermal.

93. An adult female patient is seen in the family planning clinic for a consultation on contraception. She is using OCs but forgets to take them because her work schedule changes every week; she is looking for an effective method that will be easy to remember. She has been married for 14 years, is G2 T2 P0 A0 L2, and is a nonsmoker. She has a negative past history for major diseases and a negative gynecologic history for abnormalities. She has never been treated for an STD and is in a mutually monogamous relationship. She is needle phobic and faints when she has to have blood drawn. What contraceptive method would be a good choice for the patient?

    1. Depo-Provera injection every 3 months.

    2. Implantation system for 5 years.

    3. Intrauterine device (IUD).

    4. Diaphragm.

94. A young woman is seen at the family planning clinic by the family nurse practitioner. The patient wants birth control pills but has heard that oral contraceptives (OCs) are "dangerous to one's health." When asked for clarification, she lists weight gain, ovarian cancer, heavy or irregular periods, and infertility. After saying, "I can see that you are concerned about your health," what would be appropriate for the family nurse practitioner to tell the patient?

    1. "There are a lot of fallacies about birth control pills. They actually are thought to reduce the risk of ovarian cancers and to help regulate the bleeding, and they are not associated with causing infertility. There can be a minor increase in body weight of 3 to 5 pounds."

    2. "Perhaps you would be better off trying the implantation system or Depo-Provera."

    3. "What you have heard is true. They can be dangerous to your health, and many women experience these problems."

    4. "There are a lot of fallacies about birth control pills. Ovarian cancer and infertility are risks when taking the pills, but they do not cause weight gain or bleeding changes during periods. Pap smears done every year will detect such problems as ovarian cancer."

95. An adult female patient is taking OCs. She calls into the clinic with complaints of bleeding through the first 2 weeks of every package of pills. She has been taking this pill for 4 months at the same time every day. Her present OC is a low-dose monophasic pill. She is not taking any other medications and denies any adverse effects from the OCs. She would prefer to keep taking the OCs if possible. The family nurse practitioner's advice should include:

    1. Discontinue the pills and do not restart them. Use an alternative contraceptive method.

    2. Change to a higher dosage, and higher progestational agent.

    3. Try taking the pills early in the morning on an empty stomach to improve their metabolism.

    4. There is no cause for concern; breakthrough bleeding is a normal side effect of OCs.

96. An adult female patient is seen by the family nurse practitioner at the family planning clinic. The patient notes heavy, irregular menses and an increase in facial acne and facial/abdominal hair growth over the past few years. She is G1 T1 P0 A0 L1 and is not planning future

pregnancies. After a normal pelvic exam, she decides she wants oral contraceptives (OCs). What is a good choice for this patient?

1. Loestrin 1/20.

2. Triphasil.

3. Demulen 1/35.

4. OCs are inappropriate for this patient.

97. A 41-year-old patient is seen for her 6-week postpartum exam by the family nurse practitioner. She is breast-feeding without difficulty and plans to continue for a year. She wants to begin using a contraceptive and plans no further pregnancies. Which is an inappropriate choice for this patient?

1. Depo-Provera 150 mg IM every 3 months.

2. Intrauterine device.

3. Progestin-only OC.

4. Combination OC.

98. A 38-year-old patient is seen for her 6-week postpartum exam by the family nurse practitioner. The patient was breast-feeding for a short time but discontinued 4 weeks ago. Her menses have resumed. She is contemplating another pregnancy in about a year, but if she became pregnant before then, she "wouldn't mind." She is seeking contraception. She smokes one pack per day. Her exam is normal, with the uterus well involuted. Which of the following is contraindicated in this patient?

1. Progestasert intrauterine device (IUD).

2. Oral contraception.

3. Depo-Provera injection.

4. Condoms and spermicide.

99. A 22-year-old female patient presents to the urgent care department and is seen by the family nurse practitioner. She is complaining of abdominal pain, low-grade fever, and mucopurulent vaginal discharge. Her symptoms began 3 days ago and are worsening. She has a new sexual partner and has not yet used condoms with him. Her menses just ended; she is taking OCs. She denies nausea, vomiting, or anorexia. Her exam reveals findings consistent with pelvic inflammatory disease (PID). Cultures are taken for gonorrhea and chlamydia. Which of the following represents an inappropriate treatment plan for the family nurse practitioner to follow?

1. Ceftriaxone (Rocephin) 250 mg IM.

2. Doxycycline (Vibratabs) 100 mg PO bid × 10 days.

3. CBC, erythrocyte sedimentation rate (ESR).

4. Hospitalization.

100. What is the primary role of progestins in prescribing postmenopausal HRT?

1. Reduce side effects of estrogen-related breast tenderness.

2. Provide endometrial protection against hyperplasia.

3. Stabilize mood swings and reduce hot flashes.

4. Reduce occurrence of breakthrough bleeding.

101. An older female patient is seen by the family nurse practitioner for her annual exam. She has been on HRT for 6 months, having started herself on the pills left over by her deceased mother. She brings the pills, which she wants to keep taking, and requests a prescription for Estrace 1 mg daily. She has an intact uterus, is in excellent health, and denies any complaints. She does not have any contraindications to the use of HRT. Her exam is normal. Which represents an incorrect and potentially dangerous plan for the family nurse practitioner to follow?

1. Endometrial biopsy.

2. Prescription for Estrace 1 mg daily plus medroxy-progesterone acetate (Provera) 2.5 mg daily.

3. Prescription for Estrace 1 mg daily.

4. Instruct patient on the risks and benefits of HRT.

102. An older adult patient is seen for follow-up to discuss her HRT that she began 3 months ago. She needs a refill on her HRT but is not sure "if it is working right." She continues to feel hot flashes, moodiness, and decreased libido and has many sleep disturbances. She is taking Premarin 0.625 mg daily and Provera 2.5 mg daily. She denies any vaginal bleeding. Which is not an acceptable choice for the patient?

1. Premarin 0.9 mg 1 tab PO qd and Provera 5 mg 1 tab PO qd days 1–12.

2. Premarin 0.9 mg 1 tab PO qd and Provera 5 mg 1 tab PO qd days 16–25.

3. Premarin 0.3 mg 1 tab PO qd and Provera 2.5 mg 1 tab PO qd.

4. Premarin 1.25 mg 1 tab PO qd and Provera 10 mg 1 tab PO qd days 1–12.

103. Which is not a contraindication to the use of HRT in the postmenopausal woman?

    1. Recent deep vein thrombosis.

    2. Chronic active hepatitis.

    3. Controlled hypertension.

    4. Undiagnosed abnormal genital bleeding.

104. A young adult patient presents to the clinic with complaints of a malodorous, yellowish vaginal discharge and vulvovaginal itching. She has never had a gynecologic exam and is extremely apprehensive. She is sexually active and has had a new sexual partner for 2 months. She states that they use condoms "most of the time" and are not interested in alternate forms of contraception at this time. Her LMP was 1 week ago. Her wet mount with KOH shows few clue cells, moderate lactobacilli, few WBCs, no yeast, and TNTC mobile trichomonads. Appropriate treatment for this patient would include:

    1. Metronidazole (Flagyl) 2 g PO single dose.

    2. Metronidazole (Metrogel) vaginal cream 1 applicator hs × 5 days.

    3. Fluconazole (Diflucan) 150 mg PO single dose.

    4. Terconazole (Terazol) vaginal cream 1 applicator hs × 7 days.

105. Which dose of conjugated equine estrogen (Premarin) is the minimal effective dose to prevent osteoporosis?

    1. 0.3 mg.

    2. 0.625 mg.

    3. 0.9 mg.

    4. Premarin is inappropriate.

106. A single woman presents for contraceptive counseling, expressing preference for a diaphragm. Which factor in her history would make a diaphragm a poor choice?

    1. Three urinary tract infections (UTIs) in the past year.

    2. Strong desire to avoid pregnancy.

    3. Last two Pap smears showing atypical cells.

    4. Nulliparous cervix.

107. Combination OCs prevent pregnancy primarily by:

    1. Decreasing fallopian tube motility.

    2. Thinning of cervical mucus.

    3. Suppressing ovulation.

    4. Causing inflammation of the endometrium.

108. A young adult patient is hesitant to be fitted for an IUD because of strong antiabortion views and asks for the family nurse practitioner's opinion. Which explanation least accurately describes an IUD's probable action?

    1. Slows transport of ovum through the fallopian tube, causing it to age and die in transit.

    2. Prevents effective implantation of a fertilized ovum.

    3. Action is no different from that of a spermicide.

    4. Slows transport of sperm.

109. What is a unique advantage of a Progesterone T IUD?

    1. Lowest failure rate of IUDs.

    2. May be left in place for up to 10 years.

    3. Decreases menstrual blood loss and dysmenorrhea.

    4. Must be replaced annually.

110. An older female patient is seen by the family nurse practitioner for her annual exam and needs a refill on her HRT. She is feeling well and has not voiced concerns. The patient had a total abdominal hysterectomy and bilateral salpingo-oophorectomy 2 years ago for benign fibroids. Her exam is normal. She takes conjugated estrogen (Premarin) 0.625 mg days 1–25 and medroxyprogesterone acetate (Provera) 10 mg from days 16–25. What changes would be appropriate for the family nurse practitioner to make in the HRT regimen?

    1. No changes needed; the patient is doing well on the present regimen.

    2. Premarin 0.625 mg daily and discontinue the Provera.

    3. Premarin 0.625 mg daily and Provera 2.5 mg daily.

    4. Premarin 0.625 mg days 1–25 and Provera 5 mg days 16–25.

111. Which statement about progestin-only pills is true?

    1. Women who are breast-feeding should not use progestin-only pills.

    2. Ovulation suppression is as effective with progestin-only pills as with combination OCs.

3. There is an increased incidence of functional ovarian cysts.

4. The risk of ectopic pregnancy is lower for women using progestin-only pills.

112. Before prescribing HRT, which clinical approach should have the highest priority?

1. The decision about use should rest primarily with the patient after providing appropriate education and counseling.

2. For most women the benefits of HRT far outweigh any possible side effects, so HRT should be actively encouraged.

3. Involving the sexual partner in the counseling session is likely to lead to a higher compliance rate for HRT.

4. Education regarding HRT should include a thorough review of risk factors and possible side effects to avoid liability issues.

113. The most common side effect associated with depomedroxyprogesterone (DMPA; Depo-Provera) is:

1. Nausea.

2. Acne.

3. Menstrual cycle changes.

4. Increased menstrual cramps.

114. What information should the family nurse practitioner include when teaching a patient about taking alendronate (Fosamax)?

1. Take it midmorning.

2. Take with food.

3. Take with a full glass of orange juice.

4. Remain upright after taking medication.

115. The addition of a progesterone to an estrogen regimen in a postmenopausal woman with a uterus reduces the risk of:

1. Endometrial cancer.

2. Cervical cancer.

3. Gallbladder disease.

4. Breast cancer.

116. The single-dose treatment of choice for trichomoniasis is:

1. Azithromycin (Zithromax) 1 g PO.

2. Ofloxacin (Floxin) 500 mg PO.

3. Metronidazole (Flagyl) 2 g PO.

4. Clindamycin (Cleocin) 300 mg PO.

117. A 25-year-old woman comes into the office with complaints of profuse malodorous discharge. The family nurse practitioner makes a diagnosis of bacterial vaginosis and then would:

1. Advise the patient to notify her sexual contacts regarding the diagnosis.

2. Treat the problem with metronidazole (Flagyl) 500 mg PO bid x 7 days.

3. Initiate treatment with doxycycline (Vibramycin) 100 mg PO bid × 7 days.

4. Determine the presence of pregnancy before initiating a course of treatment.

118. A young woman who is taking a low-dose OC calls the clinic in a panic, stating that she forgot her pill 2 days ago. She is taking phenytoin (Dilantin) for seizure activity and has been seizure free for over a year. She asks, "What should I do about my pills?" What would be the family nurse practitioner's most appropriate response?

1. "Take the forgotten dose today along with the regular dose."

2. "See your physician for advice about the Dilantin."

3. "Continue the pills, but use another contraceptive through the rest of this cycle."

4. "Come to the clinic for a 'morning-after' pill."

119. A vaginal culture has confirmed the presence of a chancroid in a homeless woman who presented with a painful genital ulcer. The treatment regimen of choice should be:

1. Ceftriaxone (Rocephin) 250 mg IM single dose.

2. Erythromycin (E-Mycin) 500 mg PO qid × 7 days.

3. Metronidazole (Flagyl) 2 mg PO single dose.

4. Clindamycin (Cleocin) 2% vaginal cream 1 applicator × 5 days.

120. You are counseling a 49-year-old woman who had her LMP 10 months ago. She is experiencing some hot flashes and night sweats and is not sleeping well. These symptoms are affecting her ability to work effectively because she finds herself tired and "cranky." She does not want HRT. Which of the following evidence-based alternative measures is most accurately described?

    1. Venlafaxine (Effexor SR) has been effective in reducing hot flashes in randomized controlled trials.

    2. Raloxifene (Evista) has demonstrated a significant reduction in hot flashes compared with placebo in clinical trials.

    3. Black cohosh (*Cimicifuga racemosa*) has been reported as efficacious in treating menopausal symptoms in many large controlled trials.

    4. Isoflavones, specifically soy, have been shown in studies to be significantly more effective than placebo in reducing hot flashes.

121. A young woman presents to the office for evaluation of abdominal pain. The patient admits to recent sexual activity and states that she does not have her partner use condoms. On exam, the family nurse practitioner finds vaginal discharge and cervical motion tenderness. Besides sending cultures to the laboratory, the family nurse practitioner's treatment plan for the patient would also include which two medications?

    1. Penicillin G 2.4 million units IM.

    2. Metronidazole (Flagyl) 500 mg PO bid × 7 days.

    3. Ceftriaxone (Rocephin) 250 mg IM.

    4. Azithromycin (Zithromax) 1 g PO.

    5. Acyclovir (Zovirax) 400 mg PO bid × 7 days.

122. Which information about HRT should the family nurse practitioner understand when discussing HRT with patients?

    1. Estrogen replacement delays the onset of menopause.

    2. Estrogen and progesterone cause vasomotor symptoms.

    3. Estrogen decreases the risk of osteoporosis.

    4. Estrogen replacement with progesterone increases the risk of ovarian cancer.

16 | Female Reproductive Answers and Rationale

Physical Exam & Diagnostic Tests

1. Answer: 3

Rationale: Lubricants, other than water, should not be used if a cervical specimen is being obtained for conventional Papanicolaou (Pap) smear analysis; some can alter the appearance of the cells and affect cytologic accuracy. For a liquid-based Pap test, in addition to the use of water, the posterior blade of the speculum may also be lubricated with a small amount of water-based lubricant before insertion. The endocervical cell retrieval is diminished with use of a cotton-tipped applicator and is not recommended in any female patient regardless of pregnancy status. The bimanual exam is performed after the internal vaginal exam.

2. Answer: 2

Rationale: To aid in the exam, an empty bladder provides comfort for the patient and assists the family nurse practitioner in making a more accurate assessment during the bimanual portion of the exam. Asking the patient to bear down slightly while the speculum is inserted and explaining each step of the procedure helps reduce the patient's anxiety, which ultimately may help achieve comfort.

3. Answer: 1

Rationale: A nabothian cyst (nabothian follicle) is a small, white or yellow, raised, round area on the cervix and is considered to be a normal variant. The surface of the cervix should be smooth and may have a symmetric, reddened circle around the os (squamocolumnar epithelium or ectropion). The other options are all unexpected, abnormal findings.

4. Answer: 3

Rationale: A breast ultrasound is used to determine whether a lesion is solid or cystic. Ultrasound misses 50% of lesions <2 cm. The test is not sensitive enough to be used for routine screening and cannot replace mammography. The definitive diagnosis of breast cancer is the breast biopsy.

5. Answer: 2

Rationale: The World Health Organization defines osteoporosis as a bone mineral density T-score below –2.5 SD and osteopenia as a T-score between –1 and –2.5. The woman has early signs of osteopenia. She is not a candidate for HRT (estrogen + MPA) because of her past cardiovascular history. Raloxifene has been shown to prevent the progression of osteoporosis and, as a selective estrogen-receptor modulator (SERM), may be a good alternative to HRT. The other two lifestyle modifications are important counseling issues to reduce the risk of developing osteoporosis.

6. Answer: 3

Rationale: The hysterosalpingogram (HSG) is used to document the presence of a normal uterine cavity and the patency of the fallopian tubes. A contrast dye is injected into the uterus and radiographs are taken to assess anatomy. The best time to do this test is 2–5 days after menses but before ovulation.

7. Answer: 1

Rationale: Approximately 10% of breast cancers are not seen mammographically.

8. Answer: 1

Rationale: KOH lyses epithelial and white blood cells, making it easier to visualize *Candida albicans* (yeast). *C. albicans* cells are resistant and remain intact. KOH also assists with diagnosing bacterial vaginosis by alkalinizing vaginal discharge, causing a distinct fishy odor. This is a positive amine or whiff test.

9. Answer: 3

Rationale: The Pap smear is a screening test for cervical cancer and precancerous states. The diagnostic test needed to confirm the diagnosis of a high-grade lesion is the colposcopy with guided biopsies. The results of this test are clearly abnormal and must be addressed. Waiting a year could be deleterious to the patient's health. This is not a Pap smear report that one would choose to redo in 4 months; the patient needs a diagnostic test, not another screening test. Because this is not a diagnosis of cervical cancer on this Pap smear, referral to a gynecologic oncologist is premature at this time.

10. Answer: 3

Rationale: All the tests listed may be included in the workup for infertility. Because male factors account for 35%–40% of infertility, a semen analysis should be done early in the workup. HSG and endometrial biopsy require scheduling at specific times of the menstrual cycle. Tests for antisperm antibodies would be done if the postcoital test revealed abnormalities.

11. Answer: 1, 3

Rationale: The National Osteoporosis Foundation (NOF) has conducted cost analyses on the value of screening bone DEXA scans for evaluation of bone mineral density (BMD). The NOF reports that BMD testing is cost-effective for postmenopausal women ages 50–60 who have other risk factors for development of osteoporosis, including lifestyle factors of minimal exercise, smoking, excessive alcohol intake, and low calcium intake. Other risk factors include genetic history of disease, slender physical frame, premature menopause, hyperthyroidism, multiple myeloma, rheumatoid arthritis, chronic renal disease, corticosteroid use, and long-term anticonvulsant therapy. The woman with the history of long-term corticosteroid therapy would meet the NOF criteria.

12. Answer: 4

Rationale: Longstanding nevi and Montgomery's tubercles are normal findings; pendulous breasts is only a description of size, which is important to note. Enlarged lymph nodes and tender supraclavicular nodes are potential cause for concern. A fixed stellate mass with nipple discharge is not normal, and although asymmetry might be normal, the different colors of the areolae and unilateral nipple inversion could represent a problem.

13. Answer: 4

Rationale: The basal body temperature (BBT) chart is an easy and inexpensive tool to evaluate for ovulation. Patients should be instructed on the first visit how to use a BBT thermometer and record the findings on a BBT chart. The remaining answers are usually included in an infertility workup but do not evaluate the presence of ovulation.

14. Answer: 2

Rationale: Atrophic changes on the cervix of a postmenopausal woman are to be expected, as is the paucity of endocervical cells. Because of her past medical history of breast cancer, she is not a candidate for the use of estrogen vaginal cream, and the Pap smear interpretation is not abnormal. Endocervical curettage is used as a biopsy technique for sampling tissue from the endocervical canal; however, it is not appropriate to recommend this invasive procedure for someone with scant endocervical cells but rather for one with abnormal endocervical cells. Because this Pap smear report really is not classified as abnormal, there is no need to recommend a diagnostic procedure for the patient.

15. Answer: 2

Rationale: Nucleic acid amplification test (NAAT) is the preferred screening test and is generally more sensitive and specific than other tests for chlamydia infections and provides results faster than culturing. Patients can be given a vaginal swab to collect the specimen themselves or it can be collected during a vaginal exam by the family nurse practitioner. The other chlamydia tests include culture, which grows the bacteria, direct fluorescent antibody stain (DFA), and DNA probe, but these are used less commonly since they are less sensitive.

16. Answer: 2

Rationale: Mammography is recommended annually by the American Cancer Society for all women 40 years of age and older. Currently, the U.S. Preventive Services Task Force has a draft recommendation of screening mammography every 2 years for women ages 50 to 74. At the time of writing this test item, the American Cancer Society still recommends annual mammography for all healthy women beginning at age 40. There is no place for annual mammographic testing for all women of childbearing age. Breast-feeding does not preclude the use of mammography, and screening is not done only for breast symptoms.

17. Answer: 1

Rationale: Serologic tests are good screening tests, but positive results require follow-up with a treponemal test to detect specific antibodies.

18. Answer: 2

Rationale: Serum prolactin assay levels >20 ng/mL indicate the need for medical referral, usually to an endocrinologist. The most common cause of hyperprolactinemia and galactorrhea is a pituitary tumor or lesion of the hypothalamus. Other causes include hypothyroidism, medications (narcotics, tranquilizers, and antihypertensives), and oral contraceptives.

19. Answer: 1

Rationale: A positive withdrawal bleed after a progesterone challenge indicates adequate levels of endogenous estrogen. A serum prolactin level should be obtained as part of the amenorrhea workup in addition to a serum pregnancy test. A diagnosis of anovulation can be made on the basis of the successful withdrawal bleed and normal prolactin levels. Low body fat and abnormal thyroxine levels can also lead to amenorrhea but do not affect the progesterone challenge test.

20. Answer: 1

Rationale: The occurrence of the symptoms during the luteal phase of the cycle (following ovulation) will assist the family nurse practitioner in making the diagnosis of premenstrual syndrome (PMS). Having the patient keep a calendar to track her symptoms for three cycles is helpful in making the diagnosis and measuring successful treatment. Severity of symptoms, although important, is not the most important information.

21. Answer: 3

Rationale: If bleeding resumes after 1 year of amenorrhea in a postmenopausal woman or persists longer than 6 months after HRT initiation, further evaluation is necessary. The most common cause of this abnormal finding is endometrial atrophy, but more serious pathology must be definitively ruled out. An endometrial biopsy should be scheduled to further evaluate the cause of bleeding.

Normal Gynecology

22. Answer: 4

Rationale: The uterine lining first *proliferates* and then prepares for implantation. During the *secretory* phase, glandular epithelium develops, further enhancing the lining. If no fertilized egg arrives for implantation, the lining sloughs off; this is the *menstrual* phase.

23. Answer: 1

Rationale: Premenstrual syndrome (PMS) occurs approximately 5–11 days before onset of menses (late luteal phase) and subsides within 1–2 days of menses onset. This phase is progesterone dominant. The follicular phase is estrogen dominant.

24. Answer: 1, 2, 4

Rationale: Oxytocin and antidiuretic hormone (ADH) are released from the posterior pituitary. FSH, LH, and prolactin are all released from the anterior pituitary gland. The other hormones released from the anterior pituitary are thyroid-stimulating hormone (TSH), adrenocorticotropic hormone (ACTH), and growth hormone.

25. Answer: 1

Rationale: FSH stimulates the maturation of ovarian follicles, resulting in a dominant follicle. Milk secretion depends on prolactin. The production and release of LH is regulated by estrogen. LH is responsible for ovulation.

26. Answer: 2

Rationale: Menopause is one point in time and is defined after 12 months of amenorrhea, following the final menstrual period. In postmenopause, FSH levels rise 10-fold to 15-fold with marked reductions in estradiol, but other menstrual irregularities can create a variation in these levels. Therefore, these levels are not considered the best definition for menopause.

27. Answer: 4

Rationale: The ovarian cycle is divided into three phases. The follicular phase begins on the first day of menses and continues until day 14, when ovulation usually occurs. Immediately after ovulation, the empty follicle begins to enlarge and develops into a corpus luteum, which releases increasing amounts of progesterone. If implantation does not occur, the corpus luteum regresses, causing the onset of menses. This phase, from ovulation to menses, is the luteal phase.

28. Answer: 1

Rationale: Regular exercise and a healthy diet reduce the risk for heart disease in postmenopausal women. As many as 30% of all coronary events are associated with tobacco use. HRT increases the risk of cardiovascular disease. Diabetes increases the mortality from cardiovascular disease two to four times compared with nondiabetic patients.

29. Answer: 4

Rationale: Pregnancy is the most likely diagnosis in this patient, given the list of symptoms and physical findings. She could have a uterine fibroid, but it is not contributing to the symptoms listed. Ovarian cancer could present with nausea, fatigue, and abdominal bloating but would not cause the enlarged uterus or the positive Chadwick's sign. A dislodged IUD will usually change the position of the IUD, decreasing visibility of the strings or causing the IUD itself to be expelled into the vagina or endocervical canal.

30. Answer: 3

Rationale: Maintaining an alkaline pH is important to promote viability of sperm that are deposited into the vaginal vault.

31. Answer: 4

Rationale: Obesity is not a risk factor for osteoporosis. Cigarette use, Caucasian race, and alcohol consumption, among others, are considered risk factors for osteoporosis.

32. Answer: 2

Rationale: Conservative management for PMS includes daily exercise, stress reduction, dietary changes, and reassurance that her symptoms are valid should help the patient gain more control. A low-salt diet is encouraged; when necessary, a diuretic may be used for fluid retention. The use of vitamins B$_6$, A, and E may be helpful as well. Laboratory studies are not indicated here but might be helpful if the symptoms were sustained throughout the menstrual cycle.

33. Answer: 2

Rationale: As the function of the ovaries declines and the amount of circulating estrogen begins to fall, the middle-aged woman may begin to experience the symptoms typically associated with menopause. The body's feedback system will attempt to stimulate the ovaries and increase estrogen level. FSH and LH levels rise in response to these efforts.

34. Answer: 1

Rationale: Pregnancy is the most likely diagnosis, requiring a pregnancy test and pelvic ultrasound to confirm it. Even though the patient has had a tubal ligation, failure rates of 1 in 300 have been reported. This patient could have uterine fibroids, but these do not generally present with this symptom complex and are not associated with amenorrhea, although they do cause uterine enlargement. Premature menopause could cause all these symptoms, including amenorrhea, but not the enlarged uterus. Colon cancer can present with these symptoms and could be responsible for an abdominal mass but not for uterine enlargement or amenorrhea.

35. Answer: 4

Rationale: The age of menopause has fluctuated little over the past several centuries, even though life expectancy has increased. Of the options, only smoking has been found to cause an earlier menopause (average 1.5 years). Research shows a direct correlation among number of cigarettes smoked, number of years of smoking, and age at menopause. Nulliparity and epilepsy have also been associated with an earlier age at menopause.

Gynecologic Disorders

36. Answer: 2

Rationale: Dyspareunia is painful intercourse, and vaginismus is painful vaginal spasms on penetration. Primary orgasmic disorder is when an individual has never achieved orgasm, usually a lifelong problem. Secondary orgasmic dysfunction refers to an acquired problem of loss of orgasmic function after an individual has experienced orgasm.

37. Answer: 1

Rationale: The initial outbreak is usually the worst. It can be transmitted even when there is no lesion present, and it cannot be cured. Vaginal delivery is allowed if there are no genital lesions at the time of labor.

38. Answer: 1

Rationale: Bacterial vaginosis results when the normal environment in the vagina is disrupted. The normal vaginal lactobacilli are decreased or absent, and there is an overgrowth of many different types of anaerobic bacteria. Trichomoniasis is caused by a flagellated protozoan, and gonorrhea is caused by a bacterium and may be asymptomatic. The virus that causes recurrent outbreaks of genital lesions is herpes simplex type 2 (HSV-2).

39. Answer: 1

Rationale: Oral contraceptives (OCs) will reduce prostaglandin production, which is thought to be the primary cause of dysmenorrhea.

40. Answer: 4

Rationale: The criteria for the diagnosis of bacterial vaginosis are characteristic milky homogeneous discharge, pH >4.5, amine odor (positive whiff test) with addition of potassium hydroxide (KOH), and presence of epithelial cells studded with coccobacilli that obscure the borders (clue cells). Pseudohyphae are present in candidiasis.

41. Answer: 2

Rationale: In Asherman's syndrome, a normally functioning uterus has been damaged and scarred secondary to instrumentation, usually a dilation and curettage (D&C). Ovulation may be occurring normally, but no endometrium is built up and, therefore, no endometrium is shed (menstruation does not occur). Pregnancy, as well as the other diseases listed, should be ruled out in this patient.

42. Answer: 2

Rationale: The LH/FSH ratio in polycystic ovarian syndrome is 3:1. The normal LH/FSH ratio is 1.5:1.

43. Answer: 4

Rationale: The criteria for the diagnosis of polycystic ovarian syndrome include menstrual irregularity, increased body weight, hirsutism, androgen excess evidenced by laboratory studies and physical findings, chronic anovulation, and multiple bilateral ovarian cysts. Weight loss, dental caries, and amenorrhea would be more common in anorexia nervosa/bulimia. Hyperprolactinemia and galactorrhea are found with a prolactin-secreting pituitary tumor. Dysmenorrhea, nodules palpated on bimanual exam, and infertility are associated with endometriosis.

44. Answer: 3

Rationale: Anovulation causes 90% of dysfunctional uterine bleeding. The lack of progesterone allows for asynchronous, excessive proliferation of the endometrium to take place. This tissue is fragile, and the normal hemostatic mechanism is altered. Thyroid disease, blood dyscrasias, and uterine tumors can mimic dysfunctional uterine bleeding and must be excluded.

45. Answer: 3

Rationale: A female-appearing person with a 46,XY karyotype has androgen insensitivity syndrome, or testicular feminization. This maternal X-linked recessive disorder accounts for approximately 10% of all cases of amenorrhea, and these persons appear normal until puberty. These patients present with amenorrhea, scant or absent pubic hair, and abnormal or no breast development. Persons with müllerian agenesis have a normal XX karyotype with congenital absence of the vagina, uterus, or both. In Turner's syndrome, congenital absence of ovaries results from loss of one X chromosome.

46. Answer: 1

Rationale: The most common breast mass in young women <30 years old is the fibroadenoma. This benign breast mass is the third most common breast mass after fibrocystic changes and carcinoma. Fibrocystic breast changes are seen most commonly in women 30–50 years old. Intraductal papilloma is a wartlike growth located in the mammary duct and occurs in women 40–50 years old. Malignant breast neoplasms occur most frequently in women over 40 and are rarely seen in women 15–25 years old.

47. Answer: 1

Rationale: Nonsteroidal anti-inflammatory drugs (NSAIDs) inhibit prostaglandin synthesis and are effective agents in primary dysmenorrhea. The other agents listed have not demonstrated effectiveness in primary dysmenorrhea. Other measures to decrease discomfort are exercise, relaxation techniques, heat application, and low-dose OCs.

48. Answer: 4

Rationale: Secondary amenorrhea is defined as no menses for three-cycle lengths or 6 months in a woman with previously established menses. Exercise can cause an increase in estrogen and endorphin levels, which influences the release of gonadotropin-releasing hormone (GnRH). Without appropriate GnRH release, FSH and LH are not released adequately, resulting in anovulation, which may lead to amenorrhea. The other conditions listed are causes of primary amenorrhea.

49. Answer: 1

Rationale: This has the characteristics of a syphilitic lesion and needs to be evaluated. Only after determining the presence or type of STD (sexually transmitted infection [STI]) can it be treated effectively. The herpes viral culture should be done while the lesion is present and the fluid from the vesicles can be obtained.

50. Answer: 2

Rationale: A person who has never engaged in coital activity is not considered at risk for cervical cancer because exposure to human papillomavirus (HPV) is unlikely. In addition to other factors not listed, the presence of HPV, multiple sexual partners, and previous high-grade squamous intraepithelial lesion (HSIL) are considered to be risk factors in the development of cervical cancer.

51. Answer: 1

Rationale: The pseudohyphae and spores on the wet mount with KOH are diagnostic for *Candida* infection. *Chlamydia trachomatis* is diagnosed by nucleic acid amplification test (NAAT). Gonorrhea is diagnosed by NAAT or cervical culture, and bacterial vaginosis has microscopic findings of clue cells and positive amine odor (Whiff test).

52. Answer: 1

Rationale: Cancer of the ovary is the leading cause of death from female genital cancer, excluding the breast, in the United States.

53. Answer: 1

Rationale: Flagellated protozoan confirms the diagnosis of trichomoniasis. Chlamydial infection is best diagnosed by nucleic acid amplification test (NAAT). Bacterial vaginosis is diagnosed by wet mount revealing clue cells and positive amine test. Inflammatory cervicitis is generally asymptomatic and will not cause vaginal irritation.

54. Answer: 3

Rationale: The pelvic ultrasound is not a useful test for appendicitis because it does not allow for adequate exam of the appendix. The CBC with differential is useful because of the expected rise in WBCs seen in this inflammatory state. The flat plate of the abdomen and kidney–ureters–bladder (KUB) are helpful to determine the extent of the problem and to rule out other diagnoses. Because pregnancy can cause these symptoms if complicated by an ectopic state, the family nurse practitioner should consider it as part of the differential diagnosis.

55. Answer: 2

Rationale: Oral contraceptives (OCs) have been shown to reduce the risk of endometrial cancer. Obesity, unopposed estrogen use, and advanced age, in addition to others not listed here, are considered to be risk factors for developing endometrial cancer.

56. Answer: 4

Rationale: The diaphragm may be inserted up to 2 hours before intercourse and should be removed no sooner than 6 hours after intercourse has ended. It should not be left in place longer than 24 hours.

57. Answer: 2

Rationale: Urethral discomfort and recurrent urinary tract infections (UTIs) are associated with diaphragm use and are the most common reasons for discontinuing use and changing birth control methods.

58. Answer: 3

Rationale: OC use has been shown to reduce the risk of ovarian cancer. Family history of ovarian cancer, advancing age, and positive BRCA-2 gene are considered risk factors for developing ovarian cancer.

59. Answer: 2

Rationale: Endometrial cancer is the most common female genital cancer, with ovarian cancer causing the most deaths annually. Endometrial cancer is more common than ovarian cancer and is easier to cure with just surgery alone. Because ovarian cancer is usually diagnosed in a later stage, the condition is more difficult to cure.

60. Answer: 3

Rationale: Herpes simplex virus type 2 (HSV-2) typically presents dramatically in the newly infected primary outbreak. Gonorrhea generally is associated with a mucopurulent vaginal discharge and is not accompanied by vesicular lesions. Chlamydial infection may be associated with dysuria and, unless accompanied by pelvic inflammatory disease (PID), is not generally accompanied by fever or body aches and is not associated with vesicular lesions. Lymphogranuloma venereum is a rare disease classically accompanied by pustular enlargement of the lymph nodes, particularly the inguinal nodes. It is associated not with vesicles, but buboes.

61. Answer: 2

Rationale: Screening blood studies for glucose, cardiac risk profile, and TSH in this age group without any stated risk factors is not cost-effective and is of little value. The patient can be better served with a discussion regarding diet and exercise. Because this patient is at risk for STDs, counseling and testing for these are reasonable approaches. Contraceptive information educates the patient and allows her to make wiser choices in her family planning.

62. Answer: 2, 3, 4

Rationale: High-fat diet, advancing age, and early menarche have been identified as risk factors in the development of breast cancer. Early menopause and nonproliferative fibroadenomas have not been associated with the development of breast cancer.

63. Answer: 1

Rationale: The use of prenatal vitamins with folic acid before conception has been found to reduce the risk of neural tube defects in the fetus. It is important for the patient to continue her exercise program, although some discussion about the type of exercise and any limitations are important once pregnancy is achieved. Because the patient has had two previous pregnancies, it is likely that her rubella immune status has been determined; if she is found to not be immune to rubella, an MMR vaccination should be recommended. This patient is not of advanced maternal age and, therefore, does not require genetic counseling for this reason.

64. Answer: 3

Rationale: Baseline laboratory work should be obtained to determine the presence of anemia, possible pregnancy, and endocrine dysfunction.

65. Answer: 4

Rationale: Fibrocystic breast disease is not a risk factor for breast cancer. In addition to others, those listed in the other options are considered to be risk factors for breast cancer.

66. Answer: 1

Rationale: The recommended age for a female to begin screening Pap smears is at the onset of sexual activity or at 21 years of age. Because this patient is 21 years old and has not yet had her first Pap smear, this would be the most appropriate test to perform. It is not necessary to perform STD screening on patients who have not been sexually active. Stool guaiac (hemoccult) testing and mammography are not recommended as screening procedures in the young adult.

67. Answer: 3

Rationale: Heart disease remains the leading cause of death for women in the United States.

68. Answer: 1

Rationale: Reactive cellular changes are most often associated with inflammation, including typical repair. Other causes include atrophy with inflammation (atrophic vaginitis), IUD use, radiation, and diethylstilbestrol exposure in utero. OCs do not cause reactive changes, and estrogen vaginal cream may be used to improve atrophy.

69. Answer: 2

Rationale: Cervical cancer has been directly linked with high-risk types of human papillomavirus (HPV). Pregnancy after age 35, low parity, and prolonged contraceptive use are not risk factors for cervical cancer.

70. Answer: 1

Rationale: Breast cancer is the most common cancer in women in the United States. Lung cancer mortality is higher than that for breast cancer.

71. Answer: 3

Rationale: These symptoms are classic for menopausal syndrome, although some depressive symptoms are listed. Antidepressant therapy and counseling for depression at this stage of treatment is not appropriate. Testing, teaching, and treatment in this case should be aimed at the menopause. The depressive symptoms will undoubtedly improve with greater understanding and treatment of the menopausal symptoms.

72. Answer: 1

Rationale: Chancroid is well established as a cofactor for HIV transmission. Chancroid is a sexually transmitted infection (STI) of the genitals that is caused by the bacteria *Haemophilus ducreyi*. It is characterized by an open sore or ulcer and can be transmitted from skin-to-skin contact with an infected person. It should be noted that is rarely seen in the United States but occurs more in third-world countries.

73. Answer: 1

Rationale: According to the American Cancer Society, women should be advised of the benefits and limitations of monthly breast self-exam (BSE), should be aware of how their breasts normally look and feel, and should report any new breast changes.

74. Answer: 2

Rationale: Symptoms are most likely indicative of benign fibroadenoma. Mammography is indicated. Surgical excision is unlikely for a young woman.

75. Answer: 2

Rationale: This patient needs to become more knowledgeable about the normal feel of implants as well as her own breast tissue. Mammography is not a substitute for breast self-exam (BSE).

76. Answer: 2

Rationale: A very firm cervix along with a cervical lesion/ulcer is suspicious for cancer of the cervix, which can be confirmed with a Pap smear.

77. Answer: 1

Rationale: This complaint is an indication for clinical breast exam and mammography. Although uncommon, breast pain can be a presenting symptom for breast cancer. Teaching breast self-exam (BSE) is important but not the most important action at this point. Hormonal fluctuations can explain breast pain, as can excessive caffeine intake, but should be a diagnosis of exclusion after ruling out malignancy.

78. Answer: 2

Rationale: Toxic shock syndrome occurs primarily in menstruating women ages 12–24 who use tampons. The diagnosis is made with the presence of fever over 102°F (38.9°C), macular rash, hypotension, and involvement of three or more organ systems.

79. Answer: 4

Rationale: More than 16% of ectopic pregnancies present as surgical emergencies. In the United States blood loss causes 1 death in 1000 ectopic pregnancies.

80. Answer: 4

Rationale: Almost half of all vaginal infections are caused by candidiasis. The majority of women who develop the infection have recently taken antibiotics. It is not a sexually transmitted infection (STI).

81. Answer: 1

Rationale: It is important to evaluate the patient for threatened abortion as soon as possible. It is most likely too soon for the CBC to reflect blood loss. A pelvic sonogram takes longer than a urine pregnancy test, and the patient must be immediately referred for a D&C if her pregnancy test is positive.

82. Answer: 2

Rationale: The most common site for breast cancer occurrence is the upper outer quadrant (tail of Spence), followed by the area beneath the nipple.

83. Answer: 3

Rationale: Pap smears are crucial for the detection of cervical cancer but do not diagnose uterine cancer. In the early stages, uterine cancer can be asymptomatic and would not be detectable even on bimanual exam.

84. Answer: 4

Rationale: Vulvovaginal changes, such as atrophic vaginitis, often become apparent and bothersome several years after the LMP in women not receiving estrogen therapy. Insufficient data are available to demonstrate that isoflavones in soy products have a positive effect on vaginal symptoms. Vaginal lubricants are therapeutic in relieving symptoms of vaginal dryness. If nonprescription remedies do not provide relief and no contraindications exist, estrogen (often topical) is the treatment of choice.

Pharmacology

85. Answer: 1, 2, 4

Rationale: TMP-SMX and nitrofurantoin are both effective against UTI. Phenazopyridine helps make the patient more comfortable until the antibiotic reaches effective levels for treatment. Ceftriaxone is an effective drug for complicated UTI but is unnecessary in an uncomplicated lower UTI. Neomycin is an aminoglycoside and would not be used for an uncomplicated UTI but rather for severe systemic infections and preoperatively to sterilize the bowel for intestinal surgery.

86. Answer: 2

Rationale: The Women's Health Initiative (WHI) study was stopped early because after 5.2 years, in the opinion of the Safety/Data Monitoring Board, the health risks for the women on the study (mean age 63) taking estrogen plus progestin exceeded the benefits. Women taking estrogen/progestin were at higher risk for developing MIs, strokes, and thromboemboli as well as developing breast cancer than women taking placebo. However, women taking HRT were less likely to have a fracture caused by osteoporosis and less likely to develop colorectal cancer. The study did not address the shorter term use of HRT for treatment of menopausal symptoms, the primary indication for initiating the therapy. This landmark study stresses the need for providers to discuss the risks/benefits of initiating or continuing HRT with postmenopausal women.

87. Answer: 3

Rationale: Fluconazole is now approved for a single-dose oral treatment of uncomplicated vulvovaginal candidiasis. It is the most convenient approach for this patient, who is unlikely to be compliant with vaginal creams, given the upcoming travel. She does not have contraindications to its use. Metronidazole and clindamycin are for bacterial vaginosis, not *Candida albicans* infections. Hydrocortisone is a topical steroid used for inflammatory dermatologic conditions, and although it may help the itching, it would not treat the candidiasis.

88. Answer: 4

Rationale: Metronidazole vaginal gel is the treatment of choice for bacterial vaginosis in the nonpregnant female. The presence of clue cells and the associated malodorous discharge and absence of lactobacilli are markers for the diagnosis of bacterial vaginosis.

89. Answer: 4

Rationale: Although some authors may recommend herbal treatments for menopausal symptoms, no controlled studies have been done on disease prevention. Traditional allopathic Western medicine supports the use of HRT for the prevention of osteoporosis. Weight-bearing exercise and increased calcium intake have been shown to help maintain bone health. Cigarette smoking increases the risk for bone loss. This patient can reduce her risk by quitting smoking.

90. Answer: 4

Rationale: Benzathine penicillin 2.4 million units IM is the treatment of choice for syphilis, but this patient has condyloma acuminatum, not condyloma latum. Topical use of podophyllin, trichloroacetic acid, and cryotherapy are all accepted treatment modalities for condyloma acuminatum.

91. Answer: 1

Rationale: Chlamydia often presents this way (dysuria, mucopurulent discharge, and cervical friability). The treatment of choice in ambulatory care settings is single-dose azithromycin 1 g PO. The treatment dose should be 250 mg IM for a chlamydial infection, not 125 mg. Herpes simplex virus will present with painful vesicles in the vulvovaginal region and is treated with acyclovir 200 mg 1 cap PO q4h × 5 days for recurrences. Trichomoniasis can present this way, but trichomonads on the wet mount are absent. Therapy for trichomoniasis is single-dose metronidazole 2 g PO.

92. Answer: 4

Rationale: A hepatic effect due to the first-pass metabolism in the liver occurs with oral estrogen products. A 25% increase in triglycerides has been associated with this route of administration. Because transdermal estrogen is not dependent on gastrointestinal absorption or affected by the first-pass metabolic effect, this option should be considered. A discussion regarding risks/benefits of continuing HRT is appropriate from the primary provider. Because the patient is only 52 years old and is still experiencing menopausal symptoms, reducing the most common dosage or stopping the medication, unless significant risks are apparent, is probably not the most therapeutic option.

93. Answer: 3

Rationale: The IUD would be a good choice for this patient because it is extremely effective (>99%). Maintenance is minimal, and no injections are involved for insertion or removal. The Depo-Provera injections, although extremely effective as well (>99%), require an injection every 3 months, which could lead to decreased patient compliance. The system of implants is also very effective (>99%) but also requires injections for insertion and removal, which this patient is trying to avoid. The diaphragm is a noninvasive contraceptive that is effective (88%) but requires her to be more active in its use. None of these methods is contraindicated for this patient, but an attempt should be made to help her choose one with which she is likely to be comfortable.

94. Answer: 1

Rationale: The family nurse practitioner should try to determine what the patient has heard and dispel the fallacies if possible. Recent research supports the protective benefit of OCs against ovarian cancer as well as endometrial cancer. Amount of menstrual bleeding usually is decreased and the cycle regulated. Minimal weight fluctuations are reported. Infertility is not associated with OC use. To suggest either implantation system or Depo-Provera injections to someone who voices concerns about irregular menses or weight gain is sure to lead to an unhappy patient because these are common side effects of both methods. Pap smears do not screen for ovarian cancer.

95. Answer: 2

Rationale: Changing to a pill with a stronger progestational agent or changing to a different progestational agent often will resolve the problem of bleeding irregularities with OCs. Many choices are available regarding the dose or strength of an OC, and her problem likely can be resolved with a different pill. Taking the pills at a different time of day or on an empty stomach will do nothing to resolve the stated problem, which is not breakthrough bleeding but rather prolonged bleeding, probably secondary to poor endometrial support. If a change is not made in the pills, the patient will continue to bleed and may eventually develop anemia.

96. Answer: 3

Rationale: An OC such as Demulen 1/35 is a good choice for women with more androgenic characteristics because of its strong estrogenic effect with moderate progestational effect. Loestrin 1/20 is a poor choice; the weaker dose of estrogen and progestin may not adequately support her endometrium and will not have a positive effect on this patient's androgenic characteristics. Triphasil is a triphasic pill and does have a positive progestational effect that should support the endometrium, but the progestin in this OC tends to be slightly more androgenic, which is undesirable in this patient.

97. Answer: 4

Rationale: Combination OCs are not recommended for breast-feeding mothers because of the potential effect on decreasing milk quantity and quality. Progestin-only OCs are approved for nursing mothers because no deleterious effect on milk quantity or quality have been shown. Depo-Provera and the IUD are also accepted contraceptive methods for lactating females.

98. Answer: 2

Rationale: OCs are contraindicated in a cigarette smoker age 35 years or older. No contraindication exists to the use of Depo-Provera injection in the cigarette smoker. The IUD would probably be a good IUD choice for this patient because it is only approved for 1 year's use and is safe in a cigarette smoker. The only contraindication to condoms and spermicide is allergy to either substance.

99. Answer: 4

Rationale: It is not necessary to hospitalize the patient with acute pelvic inflammatory disease (PID) who is not vomiting or pregnant. If she does not respond well to outpatient treatment, hospitalization may be recommended. The medications listed are the accepted treatment of choice for outpatient management of PID and should be started before lab results are available, based on the patient's clinical presentation. The CBC and ESR are helpful to track the WBC count and inflammatory response of the body.

100. Answer: 2

Rationale: Unopposed estrogen in a woman with an intact uterus increases her risk of endometrial hyperplasia and progression to endometrial cancer. Women who have taken unopposed estrogen for more than 3 years have a five-fold increased risk of endometrial cancer compared with women not on this regimen. The addition of progesterone to the regimen provides uterine protection. However, the progestin component of HRT is responsible for the breakthrough bleeding, a chief complaint at the initiation of therapy that may lead to discontinuance of the drug. Some women also are intolerant of progestins, which have been linked to irritability.

101. Answer: 3

Rationale: The use of unopposed estrogen in the patient with an intact uterus could put her at risk for endometrial hyperplasia or cancer. The addition of a progestin protects the endometrium adequately. The patient is an excellent candidate for endometrial biopsy to document the status of the endometrium. This patient also needs to be educated on the risks and benefits of HRT.

102. Answer: 3

Rationale: Lowering the dose of the estrogen would not help this patient's symptoms. The other dosage regimens listed are all acceptable choices for this patient, proving that there are many effective ways to utilize HRT, allowing for individualization of the regimen to the patient.

103. Answer: 3

Rationale: Well-controlled hypertension is not a contraindication to the use of HRT.

104. Answer: 1

Rationale: Metronidazole 2g PO in a single dose is the treatment of choice for trichomoniasis. Metronidazole vaginal cream does not effectively treat vaginal trichomoniasis. Fluconazole and terconazole are treatments for vaginal candidiasis.

105. Answer: 1

Rationale: A dose of 0.3 mg of conjugated equine estrogen (Premarin) is the minimal effective dose to prevent osteoporosis. HRT helps maintain bones, but this effect only lasts as long as HRT is taken. Because of the risks for cardiovascular disease from using HRT, it is no longer recommended for osteoporosis prevention. Other methods of osteoporosis prevention include regular exercise, smoking cessation, and sufficient calcium (1200–1500 mg of elemental calcium) and vitamin D (400–800 IU) daily.

106. Answer: 1

Rationale: The diaphragm predisposes many women to UTIs. Some women are sensitive to the contraceptive cream or jelly. The diaphragm has been associated with toxic shock syndrome, so its use should be avoided during menses, and it should not be left in place longer than 24 hours.

107. Answer: 3

Rationale: The primary mechanism of action of OCs is suppression of ovulation. Ovulation is suppressed in 95%–98% of patients. Should ovulation occur, the other mechanisms of action likely to prevent conception are thickening of cervical mucus, causing the endometrium to become atrophic and making the uterine environment unfavorable for implantation.

108. Answer: 3

Rationale: Although still unproven conclusively, mechanisms of action for IUDs include prevention of blastocyst implantation by inducing low-grade endometritis, the copper's effects on enzymes, progesterone's actions on the endometrium, and inhibition of sperm/ovum migration.

109. Answer: 3

Rationale: A progesterone-releasing IUD acts to decrease blood loss and cramping. Progesterone-releasing IUDs thicken the cervical mucus, thicken the endometrium, and inhibit ovulation. Copper-containing IUDs can increase bleeding and dysmenorrhea. There are two hormonal IUDs available; one works for 3 years (Skyla) and the other for 5 years (Mirena). The copper IUD can stay in place for up to 10 years.

110. Answer: 2

Rationale: The patient no longer requires Provera to protect the endometrium from the potential effects of estrogen; therefore, the progestin can be discontinued and the patient given continuous estrogen therapy without concern. The other dosage regimens listed are appropriate for an HRT patient with an intact uterus.

111. Answer: 3

Rationale: The progestin-only pill does not consistently suppress ovulation. This suppression only occurs in 40%–60% of cycles, which makes the progestin-only pill less effective than combination OCs. Mechanisms of action that contribute to the progestin-only pill's effectiveness include creating an atrophic endometrium and possibly altering tubal physiology by decreasing ovum transport. Progestin-only pills contain no estrogen and are a good choice for the breastfeeding woman. There is an increased incidence of functional ovarian cyst.

112. Answer: 1

Rationale: Informed consent is essential. The pros and cons of HRT should be explained, but the choice is up to the patient.

113. Answer: 3

Rationale: Depo-Provera is frequently associated with menstrual cycle changes. In fact, this irregular bleeding is the most frequently cited reason for discontinuation. These menstrual changes range from heavy, irregular bleeding to spotting and even amenorrhea. Nausea and acne are usually effects of estrogen and are not seen with Depo-Provera.

114. Answer: 4

Rationale: Patients taking alendronate are instructed to take the medication on awakening, 30 minutes before eating, and with a full glass of water. Patients should be instructed to remain upright to prevent esophageal irritation. Taking medication with food (reduces bioavailability by 40%), coffee or orange juice (decreases bioavailability by 60%), or after eating significantly reduces absorption.

115. Answer: 1

Rationale: Women with a uterus taking unopposed exogenous estrogen have an increased risk of endometrial cancer. The addition of progesterone decreases this risk. The addition of progesterone may prompt bleeding, which many women view unfavorably. Progesterone does not affect cervical cancer, breast cancer, or gallbladder disease.

116. Answer: 3

Rationale: Metronidazole in a single 2g dose is the treatment of choice for trichomoniasis. An alternative is giving the 2 g in divided doses the same day to reduce nausea and improve compliance.

117. Answer: 4

Rationale: Metronidazole is the treatment of choice for bacterial vaginosis. Data suggest that metronidazole therapy poses low risk in pregnancy and according to the CDC (2015), "multiple studies and meta-analyses have failed to demonstrate an association between metronidazole use during pregnancy and teratogenic or mutagenic effects in newborns." The sexual partners do not require treatment, and doxycycline is not the drug of choice.

118. Answer: 3

Rationale: This patient requires added protection through this cycle because of the low-dose oral contraceptive (OC). Phenytoin may also decrease the effectiveness of OCs, especially low-dose forms.

119. Answer: 1

Rationale: Because of the patient's homeless status, the family nurse practitioner needs to use a single-dose treatment. Erythromycin, although a correct second line medication, is a poor dosing choice for this patient.

120. Answer: 1

Rationale: The most accurate answer is venlafaxine. This combination serotonin and norepinephrine reuptake inhibitor has been found to reduce hot flashes at doses of 25–150 mg/day in several clinical trials. Although many individuals consider the "natural" over-the-counter products to be safer than prescription drugs, these products can have pharmacologic effects and side effects. Use of these drugs by patients should be questioned at the time of the exam. Critics argue that the trials studying black cohosh (*Cimicifuga racemosa*) have been too small, uncontrolled, and not randomized to provide evidence-based information on the herb's efficacy and safety. Soy has been found to be moderately effective in reducing hot flashes, but comparable results have been seen in the placebo groups as well. A side effect of raloxifene used to prevent postmenopausal osteoporosis, is hot flashes.

121. Answer: 3, 4

Rationale: The most common cause of PID in sexually active women is gonococcal infections. These infections are often accompanied by *Chlamydia trachomatis*, and usually both are treated.

122. Answer: 3

Rationale: HRT may be considered for short-term use (3–4 years) to alleviate menopausal symptoms and the risk of osteoporosis in high-risk patients. The ovarian cancer risk may increase for women using estrogen alone for 10 years or longer. Current data are insufficient to know if combination HRT has the same risk. HRT reduces colorectal cancer risk.

Maternity

17

Physiology of Pregnancy

1. Normal cardiovascular physiologic responses to pregnancy include:

    1. Increased heart rate, increased cardiac output, decreased blood volume, and systolic murmur.

    2. Increased heart rate, decreased cardiac output, increased blood volume, and systolic murmur.

    3. Increased heart rate, increased cardiac output, increased blood volume, and systolic murmur.

    4. Decreased heart rate, increased cardiac output, increased blood volume, and diastolic murmur.

2. How does progesterone affect the gastrointestinal (GI) system during pregnancy?

    1. Causes nausea and vomiting early in pregnancy.

    2. Causes hypertrophy and bleeding of gums.

    3. Delays gastric emptying time and decreases intestinal peristalsis.

    4. Causes diarrhea due to increased intestinal peristalsis.

3. A pregnant patient has a hemoglobin value of 11.7 g/dL. Which factor explains this finding?

    1. Presence of iron-deficiency anemia.

    2. Nausea and vomiting.

    3. Physiologic anemia of pregnancy.

    4. Anemia of chronic disease.

4. Several physiologic changes in pregnancy may mimic heart disease. Which of the following is an abnormal finding in pregnancy?

    1. Third heart sound.

    2. Leg edema.

    3. Systolic murmur.

    4. Diastolic murmur.

5. What are three common urinary system findings during pregnancy?

    1. Physiologic hydronephrosis.

    2. Increased glomerular filtration rate.

    3. Increased urinary frequency.

    4. Proteinuria.

    5. Decreased renal plasma blood flow.

6. Which laboratory finding remains unchanged during pregnancy?

    1. White blood cell (WBC) count.

    2. Red blood cell (RBC) volume.

    3. Fibrinogen level.

    4. Prothrombin level.

7. During pregnancy, estrogen is responsible for:

    1. Hyperpigmentation.

    2. Facilitating implantation.

    3. Reducing smooth muscle tone.

    4. Decreased uterine contractility.

8. Which is not a placental hormone?

    1. Human chorionic gonadotropin (hCG).

    2. Estrogen.

    3. Relaxin.

    4. Cortisol.

9. What is the function of the placental hormone relaxin?

   1. Causes changes in endometrium and relaxes smooth muscle.

   2. Stimulates development of the ductal system of the breasts and causes hypertrophy and hyperplasia of the uterus.

   3. Aids in softening smooth muscle and connective tissue.

   4. Involved with metabolizing certain nutrients and aids in the growth of breasts and other maternal tissues.

10. The family nurse practitioner understands that at 12 weeks of fetal development:

    1. Quickening is felt.

    2. Fetal heart rate should be heard with Doppler ultrasound.

    3. Fetal heart rate is heard with the stethoscope.

    4. Respiratory movements occur.

11. A positive sign of pregnancy is:

    1. Softening of the cervix.

    2. Fetal heartbeat.

    3. Enlargement of uterus and abdomen.

    4. Mother's perception of fetal movement.

12. The bluish discoloration of the cervix and vagina is known as:

    1. Goodell's sign.

    2. Chadwick's sign.

    3. Hegar's sign.

    4. Braxton Hicks sign.

13. What is MacDonald's method of abdominal measurement in the pregnant woman?

    1. With woman on her back and knees slightly flexed, top of fundus is palpated, and measuring tape is stretched from top of symphysis pubis over the abdomen to top of fundus.

    2. Midline of abdomen is determined, and measuring tape is placed around abdomen and measured at the point where fundus is determined to be at midline.

    3. Distance from xiphoid process to symphysis pubis is measured, and dimensions of abdominal curve or fundus is calculated.

    4. With woman on her back and knees flexed, bony pelvis is determined, ischial tuberosities are identified, and distance from tuberosities to top of fundus is measured.

14. During the regular prenatal visits, what assessment data other than vital signs and weight are determined with each visit?

    1. Fundal height, fetal heart rate, urine dip for protein and glucose, and presence of edema.

    2. Urinalysis, glucose screen, fundal height, and fetal heart rate.

    3. Presence of/changes in Chadwick's sign, complete blood count, and blood glucose screening.

    4. Pelvic measurements, fundal height, urinalysis, and complete blood count.

Perinatal Care & Newborn

15. A patient is pregnant for the fifth time and is in her 7th month. She had two spontaneous abortions in the first trimester. She has a son and daughter, both full-term pregnancies. What is her calculation of gravida and para using the TPAL acronym?

    1. Gravida 2, para 5, T1, P1, A2, L4.

    2. Gravida 5, para 2, T2, P0, A2, L2.

    3. Gravida 2, para 4, T0, P2, A0, L2.

    4. Gravida 5, para 2, T0, P2, A2, L2.

16. A patient comes in for her first prenatal visit. Her last menstrual period (LMP) was on June 15, 2016. Using Nägele's rule, the family nurse practitioner computes the estimated date of delivery (EDD) as:

    1. March 22, 2017.

    2. April 20, 2017.

    3. February 15, 2017.

    4. April 3, 2017.

17. Dietary changes to reduce nausea and vomiting in pregnancy include:

    1. Consuming small, frequent, low-fat meals and avoiding spicy foods.

    2. Avoiding carbonated beverages.

    3. Avoiding eating when awakening in the morning.

    4. Increasing iron and prenatal vitamins to twice daily.

18. The pregnant woman requires an average of how many extra calories per day?

    1. 100.

    2. 300.

    3. 500.

    4. 800.

19. A pregnant patient at 22 weeks' gestation is planning a prolonged car trip. The family nurse practitioner's recommendations would not include:

    1. Support stockings.

    2. Frequent (every 1–2 hours) walking.

    3. Wearing a seat belt.

    4. Knee-high stockings.

20. The recommended office visit interval for a low-risk patient at 28 weeks of pregnancy is every:

    1. 4 weeks.

    2. Week.

    3. 2 weeks.

    4. 6 weeks.

21. At 20 weeks' gestation, the family nurse practitioner would expect to palpate the fundus at:

    1. The symphysis pubis.

    2. The umbilicus.

    3. Halfway between symphysis pubis and umbilicus.

    4. The xiphoid.

22. Which is not an expected complication of the pregnant patient age 35 years or older?

    1. Spontaneous abortion (SAB).

    2. Preeclampsia.

    3. Gestational diabetes mellitus (GDM).

    4. Anemia.

23. At an initial prenatal visit occurring in the first trimester, which blood test is not recommended?

    1. Antibody screen.

    2. Rubella.

    3. Maternal serum alpha-fetoprotein (MSAFP).

    4. Hepatitis B surface antigen.

24. The most common indication for genetic counseling is:

    1. Maternal age.

    2. Drug exposure during the first trimester.

    3. Increased maternal alpha-fetoprotein.

    4. History of previous stillbirth.

25. Patients at highest risk for having a child with Tay-Sachs disease are:

    1. Black.

    2. Jewish.

    3. Asian.

    4. 35 years or older at conception.

26. The family nurse practitioner teaches a prenatal patient that a significant source of toxoplasmosis is:

    1. Rare hamburger.

    2. Fresh fruits.

    3. Raw oysters.

    4. Raw vegetables.

27. Which finding would the family nurse practitioner assess in a patient with a ruptured tubal pregnancy?

    1. Sharp, stabbing pain localized to left lower quadrant with BP of 90/58 mm Hg.

    2. Boardlike rigidity of the uterus with abdominal distention.

    3. Dilation of the cervix and rapidly falling BP and pulse.

    4. Serosanguineous vaginal fluid with grapelike vesicles.

28. A pregnant patient at 20 weeks' gestation comes into the clinic with complaints of vaginal bleeding for the past 6 hours as well as abdominal cramping before the bleeding started. Vaginal exam reveals a decrease in the uterine size, loss of pregnancy symptoms, and a closed, firm cervix. The most likely diagnosis for this patient is:

    1. Threatened abortion.

    2. Braxton Hicks contractions.

    3. Placenta previa.

    4. Missed abortion.

29. The family nurse practitioner schedules a 38-year-old primigravida for an amniocentesis at 16 weeks' gestation. The family nurse practitioner would explain that the purpose of this procedure is to:

    1. Assess for the possibility of twins.

    2. Determine the bilirubin level.

    3. Perform genetic studies.

    4. Assess lecithin/sphingomyelin (L/S) ratio.

30. Management of a patient after an amniocentesis includes assessing for:

    1. Increased fetal activity.

    2. Elevated temperature.

    3. Spontaneous rupture of the membranes.

    4. Abnormal lung sounds.

31. What would be appropriate management for a primigravida at term who experiences rupture of the membranes?

    1. Begin timing contractions.

    2. Begin pushing.

    3. Take a warm bath.

    4. Immediately go to the emergency department (ED).

32. The family nurse practitioner would note which finding as a possible sign associated with preeclampsia?

    1. Urgency to urinate at night.

    2. Edema in extremities and puffy face.

    3. Stomach cramps.

    4. Clear fluid discharge from nipple.

33. The family nurse practitioner is discussing the monitoring of the growth of twins during the pregnancy with a patient in the first trimester. Which test would the family nurse practitioner explain to the patient?

    1. Nonstress test (NST).

    2. Sonogram.

    3. Lecithin/sphingomyelin (L/S) ratio.

    4. Amniocentesis.

34. A woman who has missed her period for 5 weeks states that she has been having nausea with some vomiting in the morning hours. The woman also states that she may have a urinary tract infection due to frequency and fatigue. The family nurse practitioner would recognize these symptoms to be:

    1. A possible systemic infection.

    2. Positive signs of pregnancy.

    3. Presumptive signs of pregnancy.

    4. Probable signs of pregnancy.

35. The family nurse practitioner managing a pregnant patient with sickle cell trait would include which information in the plan?

    1. CBC each trimester.

    2. Weekly nonstress test.

    3. Urine cultures each trimester.

    4. Frequent ultrasounds for growth.

36. Screening based on American College of Obstetricians and Gynecologists (ACOG) guidelines for gestational diabetes mellitus (GDM) during pregnancy includes:

    1. 1-hour postprandial 100g glucose screen for all women at 24–28 weeks' gestation.

    2. 3-hour, 150g glucose tolerance test (GTT) at initial visit for all women with GDM history.

    3. 1-hour postprandial 50g glucose screen at initial visit for women at risk.

    4. Glycosylated hemoglobin A1C (A1C) for all women at 24–28 weeks' gestation.

37. A 23-year-old (G3 P0) has a 50g glucose load with a 1-hour postprandial glucose screen result of 210 mg/dL. What is the next appropriate step for the family nurse practitioner to take?

    1. Order 3-hour 100g GTT.

    2. Order FBS.

    3. Order A1C.

    4. Refer immediately for diabetic treatment.

38. A teenager returns to the clinic for contraceptive follow-up after being on a low-dose oral contraceptive (OC) for 3 months. She complains of amenorrhea for 2 months, urinary frequency, and leukorrhea. Vaginal exam reveals the uterus to be about 6 cm and presence of Chadwick's sign. The first diagnostic test indicated should be:

    1. Pregnancy test.

    2. Complete blood count.

    3. Microscopic urinalysis.

    4. Culture for gonorrhea and Chlamydia.

39. An adult patient presents with her spouse for a prenatal visit. During the exam, the family nurse practitioner notices bruises on her abdomen and back. The spouse does most of talking during the history. What is the best approach for the family nurse practitioner to take in this situation?

    1. Ask the spouse to leave the room so the nurse can do a pelvic exam.

    2. Ask the woman to accompany the nurse to the lab for blood work, and ask about bruises.

    3. Ask the woman about the bruises during the exam.

    4. Do nothing; domestic violence is beyond the scope of the nurse's practice.

40. A pregnant employee who works at a daycare center is concerned about a recent outbreak of "fifth disease." The family nurse practitioner understands that:

    1. Most parvovirus B19 infections in utero are associated with an increased number of congenital anomalies.

    2. There are no isoimmunization-associated problems for the mother exposed to a young child with fifth disease.

    3. Parvovirus B19 has caused hydrops fetalis and death in some fetuses infected in utero.

    4. Mortality risk for a fetus is extremely high, especially if the mother has never had fifth disease.

41. Which is an abnormal complaint in the second trimester of pregnancy?

    1. Frequent uterine contractions.

    2. Frequent fetal movement.

    3. Calf cramps.

    4. Heartburn.

42. Which statement is true about smoking during pregnancy?

    1. The rate of spontaneous abortion among smokers is the same as in nonsmokers.

    2. Risks of complications increase with the number of cigarettes smoked.

    3. Discontinuation of smoking during pregnancy has no effect on pregnancy outcome.

    4. No relationship exists between smoking and sudden infant death syndrome (SIDS).

43. Chlamydial infections during pregnancy may be associated with:

    1. Transplacental transmission to fetus.

    2. Congenital anomalies of the eyes.

    3. Premature rupture of membranes.

    4. Fetal hydrops.

44. Cocaine use during pregnancy is associated with:

    1. Abruptio placentae.

    2. Postdate pregnancy.

    3. Macrosomatia infant.

    4. Maternal hypotension.

45. Which is not a normal cervical finding in the second trimester?

    1. Cervix firm.

    2. Cervical dilation.

    3. Cervix 2 cm long.

    4. Cervix posterior.

46. During pregnancy, sexual relations are contraindicated:

    1. During the first trimester when patient has a history of spontaneous abortion.

    2. After 36 weeks' gestation.

    3. With the diagnosis of placenta previa.

    4. With excessive maternal weight gain.

47. Which is an abnormal complaint in the first trimester of pregnancy?

    1. Nausea and vomiting.

    2. Fatigue.

    3. Vaginal bleeding.

    4. Low backache.

48. The recommended screening test for gestational diabetes mellitus (GDM) is:

    1. 3-hour GTT.

    2. 1-hour postprandial 50g glucose screen.

    3. 2-hour postprandial blood sugar measurement.

    4. Random blood sugar measurement.

49. Which is an abnormal complaint of the third trimester of pregnancy?

    1. Leukorrhea.

    2. Headache with blurred vision.

    3. Urinary frequency.

    4. Uterine contractions.

50. Which would be incorrect for the treatment of preeclampsia without severe features?

    1. Modified bed rest.

    2. Monitor BP, weight, and urinary protein.

    3. Methyldopa (Aldomet) 250 mg PO tid.

    4. Daily urine dipstick for protein.

51. What would be incorrect advice to a nonlaboring pregnant patient with a second-trimester diagnosis of marginal placenta previa?

    1. Pelvic rest.

    2. Report any bright-red bleeding.

    3. Planned cesarean section.

    4. Follow-up ultrasound at 32 weeks' gestation.

52. A pregnant patient requests further information regarding exercise guidelines. She runs on the treadmill 4 mph for 30 minutes daily and then does 30 additional minutes of free weight and lower leg exercises at the gym. General guidelines should include all except:

    1. Keep the heart rate <140 beats/min.

    2. Limit free weight for upper body to <10 lb each.

    3. Limit exercise time to 30 minutes total.

    4. Avoid breathlessness and excessive heat.

53. Testing for gestational diabetes mellitus (GDM) should be done in which of the following patients?

    1. Patient with previous macrosomatia infant.

    2. Obese patients.

    3. All pregnant patients.

    4. Patient with glycosuria.

54. Which is not a predisposing factor of preeclampsia?

    1. Primigravida.

    2. Age >35.

3. Multiple gestations.

4. Hyperthyroidism.

55. For a pregnant patient at 32 weeks' gestation with a BP of 140/92 mm Hg, weight gain the past 2 weeks of 4 lb, trace protein on urine dip, 1+ pitting edema in the feet, and 2+ reflexes, the probable diagnosis would be:

    1. Preeclampsia without severe features.

    2. Preeclampsia with severe features.

    3. Eclampsia.

    4. HELLP syndrome.

56. The family nurse practitioner is assessing a patient who has a positive pregnancy test. Laboratory data indicate that the mother's blood group is O positive and the father's AB negative. What risk is associated with this pregnancy?

    1. The mother may build up antibodies to the infant's blood if the infant is type B positive, which will be significant in future pregnancies.

    2. The mother is Rh positive; if the infant is Rh negative, there is an increased incidence of the infant building up Rh antibodies.

    3. Since the mother is O and the father is AB, there is an increased risk for the development of an ABO incompatibility.

    4. Type O blood is the dominant characteristic; the infant's blood will be in the O group, with no complications.

57. A young adult patient, G2 P1 A0 L1, 10 weeks' gestation with intrauterine pregnancy (IUP), is seen for her first obstetric intake history and physical. She knows when she conceived and denies any vaginal bleeding or abdominal pain. The patient has a soft, nontender fundus that measures 14 cm; adnexal exam negative for mass or tenderness; no fetal heart rate (FHR) audible with doptone. What is the most likely diagnosis seen on ultrasound?

    1. Multiple gestations.

    2. Fibroid uterus.

    3. Ectopic pregnancy.

    4. 14-week viable IUP.

58. A healthy patient is at 36 weeks' gestation. On her regular clinical visit, the fundus is measured at the level of the xiphoid process. At the 40-week gestational visit, the fundus is measured at just below the xiphoid

process. What is the most likely interpretation of this observation?

1. Fetus has stopped growing.

2. Fetal head has descended into pelvic cavity.

3. Labor will probably begin within 24 hours.

4. Amount of amniotic fluid is decreased.

59. On her first prenatal visit, a patient's blood work indicates that she is Rh negative. This is her first pregnancy, and she has no history of abortions. What will the family nurse practitioner explain to the patient regarding this information?

    1. To prevent complications of future pregnancies, the patient will receive an injection of RhoGAM at about 28 weeks' gestation and after the birth of an Rh-positive infant.

    2. Her husband needs to be tested to determine if his blood type is Rh positive and if there is a problem.

    3. The patient needs to receive RhoGAM at about 20 weeks' gestation and after the birth of the first child to prevent hemolytic disease.

    4. There could be a problem with the mother's blood sensitizing the infant's blood to the Rh factor; the mother will receive RhoGAM after the birth of each child.

60. During a postpartum assessment, the family nurse practitioner notes a cluster of external hemorrhoids. Which statement made by the patient indicates a need for additional teaching?

    1. "I can give myself an enema every other day to reduce constipation."

    2. "I can take sitz baths for pain."

    3. "I can decrease the swelling by using a topical hydrocortisone cream."

    4. "I can take a stool softener to decrease the pain of a bowel movement."

61. A 28-year-old female patient is seen by the family nurse practitioner for an office visit. Her LMP was 8 weeks ago; she is complaining of left lower quadrant (LLQ) abdominal pain, spotting, and fatigue. Her pelvic exam reveals cervical os closed, minimal blood in vaginal vault, uterus minimally enlarged, mild cervical motion tenderness (CMT), left adnexal fullness and tenderness, and right adnexa within normal limits (WNL). Vital signs are stable. The serum pregnancy test is positive. What is the most cost-effective and useful test for the family nurse practitioner to order?

1. Abdominopelvic CT scan.

2. Barium enema.

3. Pelvic ultrasound.

4. Flat plate of abdomen.

62. Ten days after delivery, a patient is diagnosed with mastitis. Which of the following would the family nurse practitioner expect to find on physical exam?

    1. Tender, hard, hot, and reddened area on breast.

    2. Dimpled skin on breasts and firm nodules around areola.

    3. Decreased milk production, inverted nipple, and firm, inflamed breast tissue.

    4. Soft, tender palpable masses with cracked, bleeding nipples.

63. In discussing the timing of contractions with a patient, the family nurse practitioner explains "frequency" as the interval from the:

    1. Beginning of one contraction to the beginning of the next.

    2. Beginning of one contraction to the end of that contraction.

    3. End of one contraction to the start of the next.

    4. End of one contraction to the end of the next.

64. Which is not an expected complication of the pregnant adolescent age 17 years or younger?

    1. Premature labor and birth.

    2. Anemia.

    3. Gestational diabetes mellitus (GDM).

    4. Gestational hypertension.

65. The biophysical profile includes which of the following parameters?

    1. Fetal breathing movements, fetal muscle tone, and amniotic fluid volume.

    2. Ultrasonography, alpha-fetoprotein screening, and fetal heart reactivity.

    3. Amniocentesis, amniotic fluid volume, and nonstress test.

    4. Contraction stress test, nonstress test, and gross fetal movement.

66. The most common reason for a nonreactive nonstress test (NST) is:

    1. Fetal hypoxia.

    2. Maternal drug use.

    3. Fetal inactivity or sleep.

    4. Congenital heart defect.

67. Which is least likely to be found in a patient presenting with an ectopic pregnancy?

    1. Pain.

    2. Missed menses.

    3. Vaginal bleeding.

    4. Abdominal mass.

68. Which is not true about an ectopic pregnancy?

    1. 90% occur in the fallopian tube.

    2. Ectopic pregnancies account for approximately 5% of maternal deaths.

    3. Prior history of pelvic inflammatory disease (PID) is reported in 50% of patients.

    4. Previous ectopic pregnancy does not increase risk of another ectopic pregnancy.

69. A patient presents to the clinic with a diagnosis of threatened abortion. The family nurse practitioner describes this as:

    1. Vaginal bleeding with or without cramping and no cervical change.

    2. Vaginal bleeding with cramping and cervical change.

    3. Loss of pregnancy symptoms, decrease in uterine size, and cervix closed and firm.

    4. Cramping, bleeding, and incomplete expulsion of products of conception.

70. A predisposing factor in preterm labor is:

    1. Obesity.

    2. Previous spontaneous abortions.

    3. Prior preterm delivery.

    4. Caucasian race.

71. The ability of amniotic fluid to produce a ferning pattern when dried may be altered by:

    1. Meconium.

    2. Changes in vaginal pH.

    3. Presence of cervical mucus.

    4. Heavy contamination with blood.

72. Ten weeks into her pregnancy, a patient begins to experience light vaginal bleeding. Her human chorionic gonadotropin (hCG) levels remain elevated. The family nurse practitioner would instruct the patient to report which of the following symptoms?

    1. Nausea and vomiting.

    2. Abdominal pain or severe cramping.

    3. Urinary frequency.

    4. Fatigue.

73. Which statement is true regarding the course of pruritic urticarial papules and plaques of pregnancy (PUPPP)?

    1. Perinatal mortality is increased.

    2. Pruritus is increased postpartum.

    3. Lesions first appear on abdomen.

    4. Onset is usually in the first trimester.

74. Why does an infant have increased loss of scalp hair 2–4 months after delivery?

    1. Increased number of hairs in telogen.

    2. Hyperthyroidism.

    3. Fatigue.

    4. Sudden postpartum cardiovascular changes.

75. In a breast-feeding patient having difficulty with milk production, the family nurse practitioner understands that milk production will be increased by:

    1. More frequent suckling of infant.

    2. Longer duration of suckling.

    3. Cessation of suckling for 24 hours.

    4. Cold compresses to the breast.

76. During a breast exam on a lactating woman, which finding is cause for concern?

    1. Leaking of "watery" fluid from left breast.

    2. Cracked nipples that are tender to touch.

    3. Warm breasts that are distended.

    4. Inverted left nipple and flat right nipple.

77. A new first-time mother is being evaluated for a complaint of breast pain. Her infant is 3 weeks old, and she is breast-feeding. The infant is gaining weight and seems satisfied after feeding. On exam, the family nurse practitioner finds red, irritated nipples on both breasts, but no masses or tenderness to the breasts themselves. What is an important part of the family nurse practitioner's evaluation?

    1. Mammogram of the breast.

    2. Exam of the infant's mouth.

    3. STAT CBC.

    4. Analysis of the milk.

78. A patient delivers a healthy newborn with a cleft lip and cleft palate. Which action by the family nurse practitioner would promote maternal-infant bonding?

    1. Point out the newborn's normal characteristics.

    2. Explain to the mother how the problem is not significant.

    3. Have the mother begin taking care of the newborn immediately after delivery.

    4. Explain to the mother that orofacial surgery will completely correct the defect.

79. When do most nonnursing mothers resume menstruation after childbirth?

    1. 30 days.

    2. 7–9 weeks.

    3. 45 days.

    4. 2–4 weeks.

80. What risk factor is often associated with puerperal infection?

    1. Rupture of membranes 36 hours before delivery.

    2. Excessive weight gain during pregnancy.

    3. 10 hours in the labor process.

    4. Premature labor and delivery.

Pharmacology

81. Which immunization is contraindicated in pregnancy?

    1. Polio vaccine.

    2. Hepatitis B vaccine.

    3. MMR.

    4. Tetanus.

82. If studies in animals or pregnant women demonstrate evidence of fetal abnormality or risk, or if the potential for fetal risk clearly outweigh the possible benefit of a drug, the U.S. Food and Drug Administration (FDA) category for this drug is:

    1. B.

    2. C.

    3. D.

    4. X.

83. The family nurse practitioner is aware that fetal exposure to tetracycline causes:

    1. Blindness.

    2. Hearing loss.

    3. Tooth discoloration.

    4. Limb deformities.

84. Which of the following may reduce the risk of neural tube defects when taken before conception?

    1. Vitamin A.

    2. Pyridoxine.

    3. Folic acid.

    4. Vitamin C.

85. The current recommendation for antepartum treatment of Rh-negative pregnant women with $Rh_o(D)$ immune globulin (RhoGAM) includes:

    1. Administration of 300 μg at 28 and 36 weeks' gestation.

    2. Administration of 300 μg at 28 weeks' gestation.

    3. Administration of 300 μg in each trimester.

    4. No administration is needed until postpartum.

86. The patient comes in for her first prenatal visit. She is healthy and has no history that would contribute to complications during the pregnancy. She asks the family nurse practitioner what she can take for her occasional headaches caused by eyestrain and allergies. Which of the following would the family nurse practitioner recommend for the patient?

    1. Ibuprofen (Advil) 200 mg q4–6h, not to exceed 600 mg over 24 hours.

    2. Naproxen (Aleve) 220 mg q8–12h.

    3. Aspirin (ASA) 60 mg q6h, not to exceed 300 mg over 24 hours.

    4. Acetaminophen (Tylenol) 650 mg q4–6h, not to exceed 650 mg over 24 hours.

87. Which medication would be considered safe to use in all trimesters of pregnancy?

    1. Metronidazole (Flagyl).

    2. Tetracycline (Achromycin).

    3. Isotretinoin (Accutane).

    4. Angiotensin-converting enzyme (ACE) inhibitors.

88. For the patient who wants to breast-feed and take oral contraceptives, the pill of choice is:

    1. 1/35 preparation.

    2. Triphasic preparation.

    3. Progestin-only preparation.

    4. 1/50 preparation.

89. A pregnant patient in the last trimester complains of a constant backache aggravated by walking, moving, and bending. The pain does not radiate to either leg. In addition to rest, massage, and physiotherapy, which of the following medications is appropriate?

    1. Acetaminophen.

    2. Codeine.

    3. Naproxen.

    4. Aspirin.

90. The family nurse practitioner has diagnosed mastitis in a 6-week postpartum patient. The patient has no known drug allergies. Which medication is appropriate for treatment?

    1. Doxycycline (Vibramycin) 100 mg PO bid × 10 days.

    2. Dicloxacillin (Dynapen) 250 mg PO qid × 10 days.

    3. Metronidazole (Flagyl) 500 mg PO bid × 10 days.

    4. Ciprofloxacin (Cipro) 500 mg PO bid × 7 days.

17 Maternity Answers and Rationales

Physiology of Pregnancy

1. Answer: 3

Rationale: During pregnancy, a hyperdynamic state is caused by an increase in blood volume, which results in a slightly increased heart rate and increased cardiac output. Systolic ejection murmurs are common and caused by increased flow across the pulmonic and aortic valves. Diastolic murmurs are abnormal and require referral.

2. Answer: 3

Rationale: Progesterone affects the GI system by decreasing smooth muscle tone, delaying gastric emptying, and decreasing intestinal peristalsis. Human chorionic gonadotropin (hCG) is associated with nausea and vomiting early in pregnancy. Estrogen causes the gums to become hyperemic, soft, and swollen with a tendency to bleed.

3. Answer: 3

Rationale: The increase in plasma volume combined with a slower rise in RBC production produces a dilutional anemia. Hemoglobin and hematocrit decrease in relation to plasma volume, reaching the lowest levels during the second trimester. True anemia occurs with hemoglobin <11 g/dL and hematocrit <35%, although some providers will allow the hemoglobin to drop to 10 g/dL and hematocrit to drop to 33% before treating. Nausea and vomiting will increase hemoglobin and hematocrit.

4. Answer: 4

Rationale: Leg edema is caused by increased venous pressure in the legs. Both components of the first heart sound become louder, with exaggerated splitting, and a third heart sound gallop is common after midpregnancy. Systolic ejection murmurs are common and result from the increased flow across the aortic and pulmonic valves. Diastolic murmurs are an abnormal finding and should always be referred.

5. Answer: 1, 2, 3

Rationale: Changes in renal structure are influenced by estrogen, progesterone, increased blood volume, and uterine pressure. Changes in the collection system, such as dilation of the renal pelvis and ureters, cause a physiologic hydronephrosis. The glomerular filtration rate does increase during pregnancy, along with renal plasma flow. Increased urinary frequency is related to increasing size of uterus and its pressure on the bladder. Proteinuria is abnormal when the amount exceeds 300 mg/24 hours or albuminuria is greater than 30 mg/24 hours, except in very concentrated urine or in the first voided specimen on arising. Proteinuria is a warning of impaired kidney function or preeclampsia.

6. Answer: 4

Rationale: RBC volume increases approximately 30%, and WBCs increase 5000–12,000/mm³. Fibrin, fibrinogen, and plasma levels of factors VII, IX, and X are also increased. Prothrombin levels remain unchanged.

7. Answer: 1

Rationale: During pregnancy, estrogen is responsible for stimulation of melanin-stimulating hormone, resulting in hyperpigmentation. Progesterone from the corpus luteum and later the placenta is responsible for facilitating implantation, decreasing uterine contractility, and reducing smooth muscle tone.

8. Answer: 4

Rationale: There are five placental hormones: human chorionic gonadotropin (hCG), estrogen, progesterone, human placental lactogen, and relaxin. Cortisol is produced in the adrenal glands.

9. Answer: 3

Rationale: Relaxin helps soften smooth muscle and connective tissue in preparation for labor and delivery. Progesterone relaxes smooth muscle and causes changes in the endometrium. Estrogen stimulates the development of the ductal system of the breasts and causes hypertrophy and hyperplasia of the uterus. Human placental lactogen is involved with metabolism of glucose, fatty acids, and amino acids. It also aids in the growth of the breasts and other maternal tissues.

10. Answer: 2

Rationale: Fetal heart rate should be heard by 12 weeks' gestation and may be heard as early as 10 weeks, dependent on the maternal adipose tissue and amniotic fluid. Quickening is felt at 16–22 weeks. Fetal heart rate can be heard by stethoscope at 20 weeks. Respiratory movements occur later in fetal development, at about 24 weeks.

11. Answer: 2

Rationale: Positive evidence of pregnancy includes fetal heartbeat, palpation of fetal movement by examiner, and visualization of fetus by ultrasonography. Amenorrhea, nausea, emesis, urinary frequency, fatigue, skin changes, and mother's perception of fetal movement are presumptive evidence of pregnancy. Probable evidence of pregnancy includes softening of cervix, softening of lower uterine segment, cyanosis of cervix and vagina, Braxton Hicks contractions, ballottement, palpation of fetal outline by examiner, and pregnancy tests.

12. Answer: 2

Rationale: Chadwick's sign occurs at 6–8 weeks' gestation and is the bluish discoloration of the cervix and vagina. Goodell's sign is the softening of the cervix that is seen as early as 4 weeks' gestation. Hegar's sign is the softening of the lower uterine segment. Braxton Hicks sign consists of contractions of the uterus that can occur as early as 16 weeks' gestation.

13. Answer: 1

Rationale: MacDonald's measurement is taken at each prenatal visit to estimate uterine size. Fundal height is measured with a tape that is stretched from the top of the fundus to the symphysis pubis. If the fundal height is less or more than expected based on the gestational age, the estimated date of delivery (EDD) should be reevaluated and confirmed. Further fetal assessment may be necessary.

14. Answer: 1

Rationale: Fundal height, fetal heart rate, urine dip for protein and glucose, and assessment for edema are determined with each prenatal visit. Urinalysis and CBC are done as part of initial exam and are repeated as necessary. Chadwick's sign is an early indication of pregnancy, and pelvic measurements are done to determine adequacy of the pelvic outlet for delivery.

Perinatal Care & Newborn

15. Answer: 2

Rationale: *Gravida* is the number of pregnancies, including the present pregnancy, gravida 5 for this patient. *Para* is the number of pregnancies that have progressed past 20 weeks, para 2. *T* is the number of pregnancies that have progressed to term, T2. *P* is the number of pregnancies with delivery preterm, P0. *A* is abortions, A2. *L* is living children, L2.

16. Answer: 1

Rationale: The family nurse practitioner counts back 3 months to March 15 and adds 7 days. This brings the date to March 22 of the next year.

17. Answer: 1

Rationale: Patients should eat frequent small meals to keep some food in the stomach at all times and to avoid stomach distention. Sipping on carbonated beverages may be helpful. Having crackers at the bedside to take before rising in the morning may be a successful preventive measure.

18. Answer: 2

Rationale: The pregnant woman requires about 15% more calories per day than the nonpregnant woman. This is approximately 300 calories per day and depends on the patient's weight and activity level.

19. Answer: 4

Rationale: Venous stasis occurs with prolonged sitting and may be a risk factor for thrombophlebitis. Support stockings and frequent walking should be encouraged. Knee-high stockings have elastic around the calf that may act as a tourniquet. They should be avoided during pregnancy. Seat belts are recommended.

20. Answer: 3

Rationale: The American College of Obstetricians and Gynecologists (ACOG) recommends visits every 2 weeks starting at 28 weeks until 36 weeks of pregnancy. At 36 weeks of pregnancy, visits are weekly until delivery.

21. Answer: 2

Rationale: The expected fundal height at 20 weeks' gestation is at the umbilicus. At 12 weeks' gestation, the fundus can be palpated just above the symphysis pubis, and at 16 weeks' gestation, between the symphysis and umbilicus. The fundus is palpated at the xiphoid process at approximately 36 weeks' gestation.

22. Answer: 4

Rationale: The risk for anemia in pregnancy does not increase with age. The risks for spontaneous abortion, preeclampsia, and gestational diabetes mellitus (GDM) do increase with maternal age.

23. Answer: 3

Rationale: Routine prenatal laboratory studies include CBC, blood type and Rh, antibody screen, hepatitis B surface antigen, syphilis screen, and rubella immune status. The MSAFP is done between 15 and 20 weeks. Before this time the fetus produces little alpha-fetoprotein, and results would be inaccurate.

24. Answer: 1

Rationale: The largest group of women who potentially benefit from genetic counseling are those age 35 and older. The number of births to women between age 35 and 40 years old has increased by approximately 35% in the 1990s. The primary cause of congenital abnormalities in women older than age 35 years is chromosomal abnormalities. The other answers are all reasons for genetic counseling, but to a much lesser degree.

25. Answer: 2

Rationale: The incidence of the Tay-Sachs gene in the Jewish population is 1 in 30, compared with 1 in 300 for the non-Jewish population.

26. Answer: 1

Rationale: Undercooked red meat is a major source of toxoplasmosis. Pregnant women should be cautioned against eating undercooked meats. Cats are also shown to be hosts. Toxoplasmosis is spread through cat feces. Pregnant women should be warned about cleaning the litter box and about contaminated soil.

27. Answer: 1

Rationale: The ruptured fallopian tube causes a sharp, sudden, stabbing pain. Symptoms of shock (decreased BP, increased pulse, and increased respiration) occur, and the patient quickly becomes a surgical emergency. The cervix does not dilate. Boardlike abdominal rigidity is often noted with abruptio placentae. Grapelike vesicles are associated with hydatidiform mole, a gestational trophoblastic disease.

28. Answer: 4

Rationale: A missed abortion is characterized by a loss of pregnancy symptoms, vaginal bleeding, and a closed cervix. A threatened abortion has vaginal bleeding and cramping, but the symptoms of pregnancy are still present. Placenta previa is bleeding without pain, and symptoms of pregnancy are present. Braxton Hicks contractions can occur as early as the second trimester but are more commonly experienced in the third trimester. The uterine muscles tighten for 30–60 seconds and then relax.

29. Answer: 3

Rationale: The woman's age places her at risk for a Down syndrome baby. Amniocentesis for lecithin/sphingomyelin (L/S) ratio is performed in the third trimester for fetal lung maturity, and amniocentesis for bilirubin level (delta optical density) is performed for a pregnancy complicated by isoimmunization.

30. Answer: 3

Rationale: Damage to the membranes is a possibility and a high-priority situation. Fever would not be an immediate problem. Fetal heart rate is monitored, not activity.

31. Answer: 1

Rationale: The patient should begin to count the contractions to determine the progress of beginning labor. Because she is a primagravida, delivery probably is not imminent, so going to the emergency department (ED) is not appropriate. She should not try to "push" this early in labor. Without the protective barrier of the amniotic membrane, the mother and fetus are susceptible to infection. Bathing would be a hazard because of the possibility of contracting an infection from the bath water. The patient should count the contractions and call the physician.

32. Answer: 2

Rationale: Classic signs of preeclampsia are hypertension and proteinuria. Generalized edema of the extremities and face occurs, as a result of increased permeability and capillary leakage. Stomach cramps could be an indication of early labor or gastrointestinal (GI) upset. Clear nipple fluid would be an early sign of colostrum.

33. Answer: 2

Rationale: The ultrasound test (sonogram) is used to assess growth of the fetus and position of the placenta and fetus. The nonstress test (NST) is used to observe the response of the fetal heart rate to activity. The lecithin/sphingomyelin (L/S) ratio determines whether there is sufficient surfactant. An amniocentesis is performed to obtain amniotic fluid for analysis later in the pregnancy, if indicated.

34. Answer: 3

Rationale: Missed menstrual periods, nausea, vomiting, frequency, and fatigue are presumptive signs (subjective) of pregnancy. Probable signs of pregnancy are objective, such as Chadwick's sign, ballottement, and a positive pregnancy test. Positive signs of pregnancy are fetal heart rate, fetal movement felt by a health care provider, and sonographic evidence.

35. Answer: 3

Rationale: Sickle cell trait occurs in 8% of African Americans. These women are asymptomatic, not anemic, and usually have no problems except under conditions of hypoxia. There is no difference in perinatal outcome, and these women do not require frequent ultrasounds or nonstress testing. They are at increased risk for asymptomatic bacteriuria and require a urine culture each trimester.

36. Answer: 3

Rationale: This is standard screening for women at risk of gestational diabetes mellitus (GDM). The American College of Obstetricians and Gynecologists (ACOG) recommends a two-step screening method that has been used for many years. The first step is a screen consisting of a 50g oral glucose load, followed by a plasma glucose measurement 1 hour later. An initial positive screening result is followed by step 2, a 3-hour (100g) oral glucose tolerance test (OGTT) on another day. The ACOG recommends use of the two-step screening procedure because there is no evidence that the one-step method leads to clinically significant improvement in maternal or newborn outcomes. This glucose screen should also be done for all other pregnant women between 24 and 28 weeks of gestation.

37. Answer: 4

Rationale: An extremely elevated result on the glucose challenge is considered diagnostic, alleviating the need for an oral glucose tolerance test (GTT) or fasting blood sugar (FBS).

38. Answer: 1

Rationale: This clinical picture is highly indicative of pregnancy, especially the presence of Chadwick's sign.

39. Answer: 2

Rationale: Although asking the spouse to leave the room during a pelvic exam may work, it may also arouse the spouse's suspicion and create a situation. Asking the woman to accompany the nurse to the lab and asking about the bruising is best because it gives a legitimate reason to move the woman quickly from the room, offers privacy to inquire about the bruises, and provides an opportunity to move the woman to a safe place, if needed, without creating confrontation.

40. Answer: 3

Rationale: Most fetuses are not affected; however, some undergo isoimmunization, which leads to hydrops fetalis and death. The mortality risk is actually low, and there are usually no associated congenital anomalies.

41. Answer: 1

Rationale: Contractions could represent early premature labor and should be monitored to rule out early cervical change. Not all contractions are Braxton Hicks, and contractions require serious consideration. The other symptoms listed are important to discuss and to rule out other associated symptomatology.

42. Answer: 2

Rationale: The risk of complications and perinatal loss increases with the number of cigarettes smoked. Discontinuation of or decrease in the amount of cigarettes smoked during pregnancy can reduce the risk of complications, especially for high-risk women.

43. Answer: 3

Rationale: Premature rupture of membranes may be associated with chlamydial infections. Intrauterine transmission of *Chlamydia trachomatis* to the fetus has not been demonstrated. There is no evidence of fetal eye anomalies; without prophylaxis, however, conjunctivitis will develop in 30%–50% of infants 7 days after birth.

44. Answer: 1

Rationale: Use of cocaine during pregnancy is associated with placental abruption, spontaneous abortion, and preterm labor. Maternal blood pressure and heart rate are increased. The fetus is at risk for intrauterine growth retardation, fetal distress, seizures, and death.

45. Answer: 2

Rationale: It is not considered normal or expected for a woman to have a dilated cervix at any time in the second trimester of pregnancy. The cervix will typically be firm, 2 cm long, and posterior, as well as closed.

46. Answer: 3

Rationale: In placenta previa, the placenta is improperly positioned in the lower uterine segment, covering all or part of the cervical os. There is an increased risk of bleeding. Management includes bed rest, no intercourse, no vaginal exams, instruction on managing bleeding, and close fetal surveillance.

47. Answer: 3

Rationale: Vaginal bleeding could represent a potential problem in the pregnancy during the first trimester. The other symptoms listed are important as well and warrant further discussion to rule out a problem.

48. Answer: 2

Rationale: The recommended screening test for gestational diabetes is a blood sugar measurement 1 hour after 50 g of glucose at 24–28 weeks' gestation. If the result of this test is 140 or above, a 3-hour glucose tolerance test (GTT) is done.

49. Answer: 2

Rationale: Headache associated with blurred vision could represent early symptoms of preeclampsia and warrants further workup to rule out a problem. The other symptoms are not of concern if not associated with other symptoms.

50. Answer: 3

Rationale: The use of medication is no longer thought to be useful in the treatment of preeclampsia without severe features and could be hazardous. The patient is best treated conservatively with modified bed rest on the left side and dietary counseling, along with close monitoring of BP, weight, and urinary protein. Close follow-up with exam for edema or symptomatic change and monitoring of the fetus are also performed.

51. Answer: 3

Rationale: There is no reason to plan a cesarean section on diagnosis of the placenta previa at this stage of the pregnancy because the lower segment of the uterus goes through its final maturation between 28 and 32 weeks of gestation. The placenta could likely migrate by the third trimester, thus allowing for vaginal birth, barring any other unforeseen factors.

52. Answer: 3

Rationale: No reason exists to limit the amount of time for exercise, provided the patient is feeling well. Keeping the heart rate below 140 beats/min reduces the risk of internal overheating and exhaustion. The American College of Obstetricians and Gynecologists (ACOG) suggests limiting free weights to <10 lb to avoid undue stress and strain on muscles and ligaments. Avoidance of breathlessness and excessive heat allows for better circulation to the fetus.

53. Answer: 3

Rationale: More than one half of pregnant women who exhibit gestational diabetes mellitus (GDM) lack the classic risk factors of family history of diabetes, unexpected stillbirth, prior macrosomatia infant, obesity, and advanced maternal age. Glycosuria in pregnancy is not necessarily an indication of diabetes. The best answer is that all women should be screened for gestational diabetes.

54. Answer: 4

Rationale: Predisposing factors in preeclampsia include primigravida, <20 years or >35 years, women with vascular diseases (hypertension, systemic lupus erythematosus, diabetes mellitus, and renal disease), family history, previous history of preeclampsia, and multiple gestations. Hyperthyroidism does not predispose to preeclampsia.

55. Answer: 1

Rationale: Preeclampsia without severe features is consistent with systolic BP >140 mm Hg or systolic rise >30 mm Hg, diastolic >90 or diastolic rise >15 mm Hg, weight gain >2 lb/wk, and nondependent edema >1+ with normal reflexes. Severe features of preeclampsia include BP >160/110 mm Hg, proteinuria > 2 g/24 hours, serum creatinine >1.2 mg/dL, platelets < 100,000, ↑ LDH, ↑ ALT, persistent headache or cerebral/visual disturbances, and persistent epigastric pain. Eclampsia includes the above plus seizures. The hemolysis, elevated liver enzymes, low platelets (HELLP) syndrome includes signs and symptoms of severe preeclampsia, an enlarged and firm liver, and epigastric or right upper quadrant pain.

56. Answer: 3

Rationale: There is an increased incidence of ABO incompatibility if the mother is blood group O and the infant is either blood group A or B. Rh incompatibility occurs only when the mother is Rh negative and is carrying an Rh-positive infant. In the most common cases of ABO incompatibility, there is production of maternal antibodies against the A or B cells.

57. Answer: 1

Rationale: Multiple gestations will cause the uterus to enlarge faster than normal. Fetal heart rate (FHR) may be inaudible with the doptone at 10 weeks' gestation. A fibroid could cause the uterus to enlarge, but it is generally accompanied by firmness to palpation of the uterus. Ectopic pregnancy could be the cause of an inaudible FHR but is usually accompanied by adnexal tenderness, a mass, or vaginal bleeding. A 14-week viable intrauterine pregnancy (IUP) should have an audible FHR with the doptone.

58. Answer: 2

Rationale: "Lightening" often occurs at about 40 weeks' gestation when the infant's head descends into the pelvic cavity and becomes "engaged." At any other time during pregnancy, a decrease in fundal height would cause concern for the infant's growth. There has been no decrease in amniotic fluid, and it does not indicate that labor is imminent.

59. Answer: 1

Rationale: The unsensitized Rh-negative pregnant woman is given RhoGAM at 28 weeks' gestation as a preventive measure. It effectively prevents the formation of active antibodies if there is accidental transport of fetal Rh-positive blood cells into the circulation during the remainder of the pregnancy. At delivery, the infant's blood type is determined. If the infant is Rh positive, the mother will receive another dose of RhoGAM within 72 hours of delivery. If the infant is Rh negative, there is no antibody formation and RhoGAM is unnecessary.

60. Answer: 1

Rationale: An enema every other day to reduce constipation would negatively affect the normal bowel movement pattern and deplete the patient's natural intestinal flora. Sitz baths, anti-inflammatory and analgesic topical ointments and sprays, stool softeners, and increased bulk in the diet would be indicated in the management of the external hemorrhoids.

61. Answer: 3

Rationale: This easy, inexpensive, and relatively noninvasive test assists the family nurse practitioner with confirming the diagnosis of ectopic pregnancy. It can be obtained quickly and is often available rapidly. Abdominopelvic CT will also show an ectopic pregnancy but is neither cost-effective nor noninvasive. Barium enema and flat plate of the abdomen are not useful in this patient.

62. Answer: 1

Rationale: A tender, hard, hot, and reddened area on the breast over the affected area is typically found with mastitis. The patient with mastitis will also typically be febrile. Dimpled skin (peau d'orange or orange-peel appearance) is a potential sign of breast cancer. Decreased milk production, inverted nipple, and firm breast tissue may be complications of engorgement. Cracked nipples may result from improper positioning or oversuckling. Soft, tender breast masses may be engorged milk ducts.

63. Answer: 1

Rationale: Frequency of contractions should be timed from the beginning of one contraction to the beginning of the next contraction.

64. Answer: 3

Rationale: The pregnant adolescent is at increased risk for premature labor, anemia, and preeclampsia. There is no documentation that the pregnant teen is at greater risk of gestational diabetes.

65. Answer: 1

Rationale: The biophysical profile includes observation of fetal respiratory movement, fetal tone, gross fetal movement, measurement of amniotic fluid volume, and fetal heart reactivity. Each parameter is given a score of 0 or 2; the scores from all parameters are then added together, the normal is 8 to 10. Ultrasonography, alpha-fetoprotein screening, nonstress testing, and stress test are not part of this profile.

66. Answer: 3

Rationale: The most common reason for a nonreactive nonstress test (NST) is fetal sleep or inactivity. The fetal sleep–wake cycle

ranges from 20–40 minutes. If reactivity is not demonstrated in 20 minutes, continuing to 40 minutes usually accommodates the sleep–wake cycles. Fetal hypoxia and maternal smoking and drug use certainly affect fetal heart rate but are not the most common causes. Infants with a congenital heart defect do not exhibit a significant incidence of nonreactive NSTs.

67. Answer: 4

Rationale: Greater than 90% of patients presenting with ectopic pregnancies will complain of pain and report a missed period. Approximately 80% will describe vaginal bleeding. Only 50% will have a palpable abdominal mass.

68. Answer: 4

Rationale: It is true that 90% of ectopic pregnancies are found in the fallopian tubes. Patients with pelvic inflammatory disease (PID) have a sevenfold increase in the rate of ectopic pregnancy. Maternal deaths from ectopic pregnancy have decreased markedly over the past few years as a result of improved diagnostic procedures. A previous ectopic pregnancy is a risk factor and does increase the risk of a subsequent ectopic pregnancy.

69. Answer: 1

Rationale: A threatened abortion progresses to complete spontaneous abortion in 50% of cases. Clinical findings are vaginal bleeding with or without cramping and no cervical change. Vaginal bleeding with cramping and cervical change is an inevitable abortion. An incomplete abortion is demonstrated by vaginal bleeding, cramping, and incomplete expulsion of the products of conception. A missed abortion is diagnosed when products of conception are retained after fetal death. There is a decrease in uterine size, loss of pregnancy symptoms, and often a closed and firm cervix.

70. Answer: 3

Rationale: History of preterm birth is associated with a 20%–40% recurrence risk. Low prepregnancy weight and inadequate weight gain, not obesity, are associated with preterm labor. Maternal smoking, drug use (especially cocaine), low socioeconomic status, maternal age <17 and >35 years, and non-Caucasian race are all predisposing factors for preterm labor. Previous spontaneous and elective abortions are not risk factors.

71. Answer: 4

Rationale: Ferning is due to high levels of estrogen and when air-dried, amniotic fluid produces a fern pattern. This microscopic arborization is accurate in confirming rupture of membranes in 90%–95% of cases. Samples heavily contaminated with blood may not fern.

72. Answer: 2

Rationale: Contractions, cramping, or abdominal pain along with continued bleeding could signify a spontaneous abortion. The other symptoms are common during the first trimester.

73. Answer: 3

Rationale: Pruritic urticarial papules and plaques of pregnancy (PUPPP) skin rash typically start on the abdomen and spread to the thighs and possibly the buttocks. Onset of lesions is usually in the third trimester and usually resolves postpartum. It is thought to be related to the stretching of the skin. There is no associated adverse perinatal outcome.

74. Answer: 1

Rationale: Normally, 15%–20% of hairs are in telogen (resting phase of hair cycle). In late pregnancy, this is reduced to <10%. After delivery the percentage increases, and by 2 months postpartum, 20% of hairs are in telogen. Therefore, a marked increase occurs in hair loss at 2–4 months after delivery.

75. Answer: 1

Rationale: More frequent suckling will increase production of milk more effectively than increasing the duration of suckling. Stopping or decreasing breast-feeding or applying cold compresses to the breasts will decrease milk production.

76. Answer: 2

Rationale: Cracked nipples are a sign of irritation and may eventually cause skin breakdown with severe pain and possible infection.

77. Answer: 2

Rationale: Breast irritation in nursing mothers is often caused by *Candida albicans*. The source of infection is most likely the infant's mouth (thrush).

78. Answer: 1

Rationale: Initially after delivery, the mother needs an opportunity to accept that her newborn has a congenital defect. Pointing out normal characteristics of the newborn will allow her to put the problem in perspective. Often the mother will focus on the defect. Orofacial surgery will provide closure of the defect but will not completely correct it because scarring will undoubtedly occur.

79. Answer: 2

Rationale: Most nonnursing mothers will resume menstruation 7–9 weeks after birth. About one half of them will ovulate during the first cycle. Most lactating women will resume menstruation in 12 weeks, although some do not menstruate during the entire lactation period.

80. Answer: 1

Rationale: Prolonged rupture of the membranes is defined as membrane rupture >24 hours before delivery. The rupture provides an increased opportunity for bacterial growth. Excessive weight gain and premature delivery are not associated with postpartum infection. Ten hours in labor is well within the normal time for labor.

Pharmacology

81. Answer: 3

Rationale: The measles-mumps-rubella (MMR) is a live virus vaccination and is contraindicated in pregnancy. Polio, tetanus, and hepatitis B vaccine are inactivated bacterial or DNA-based vaccines and are safe when indicated.

82. Answer: 4

Rationale: The FDA has five pregnancy risk categories for drugs. Category X indicates that fetal risk outweighs any benefit, and use in pregnancy is contraindicated. Category B drugs show no evidence of fetal abnormalities, and risk to the fetus is relatively unlikely. Category C drugs have potential for animal fetal abnormalities and/or no adequate well-controlled studies in pregnant women, but benefits of drugs are thought to justify risks to the fetus. Drugs classified as Category D demonstrate positive evidence of human fetal risk and should be used only in serious disease or life-threatening situations when safer drugs are ineffective.

83. Answer: 3

Rationale: Tetracycline binds with developing enamel and discolors the deciduous teeth between 26 weeks of gestation and 6 months of infancy.

84. Answer: 3

Rationale: Recent studies have confirmed that folic acid taken before conception can reduce the risk of neural tube defect.

85. Answer: 2

Rationale: Current recommendations for RhoGAM is administration of 300 μg to all Rh-negative women at 28 weeks of pregnancy. This is considered protective for the remainder of the pregnancy.

86. Answer: 4

Rationale: Acetaminophen is a risk category B drug, but problems have not been documented; it should be used with caution. Aspirin is risk category D and may cause bleeding disorders. Nonsteroidal anti-inflammatory drugs (NSAIDs) (ibuprofen; naproxen) are risk category B but have been associated with prolonging pregnancy and prematurely closing the fetal ductus arteriosus because of antiprostaglandin effects.

87. Answer: 1

Rationale: Metronidazole is safe to use in all trimesters of pregnancy. The other medications are known teratogens and contraindicated in pregnancy.

88. Answer: 3

Rationale: Estrogen inhibits milk production. Progestin-only preparations are ideal for the breast-feeding patient because they do not contain estrogen and, therefore, do not inhibit milk production. The other oral contraceptives (OCs) listed contain estrogen in varying amounts.

89. Answer: 1

Rationale: Acetaminophen can be safely prescribed to the pregnant patient. Aspirin and nonsteroidal anti-inflammatory drugs (NSAIDs) are contraindicated in the third trimester. The use of narcotics for the patient is inappropriate.

90. Answer: 2

Rationale: Dicloxacillin will treat *Staphylococcus aureus,* which is the most common organism associated with mastitis. None of the other medications is appropriate for treatment of mastitis, and both doxycycline and ciprofloxacin are contraindicated when breast-feeding.

18

Pediatrics

Endocrine

1. A common cause of poor control of type 1 diabetes during the adolescent period is:

   1. Too frequent evaluation of blood sugar.

   2. Increased intake of protein.

   3. Too much exercise.

   4. Denial of the severity of the condition.

2. An infant with congenital hypothyroidism is being discharged home. The family nurse practitioner would instruct the parents to:

   1. Watch for constipation and slow pulse as signs of toxicity.

   2. Reduce the medication as symptoms decrease.

   3. Give the medication as a single dose in the early morning.

   4. Expect weight loss until the child adjusts to the dose.

3. A goal in the management of a child with diabetes would be to maintain blood sugar level in a target range according to what?

   1. The target blood sugar level must be individualized based on the child's age and ability to recognize the symptoms of hypoglycemia.

   2. The target range for blood sugar level depends on the provider's judgment, the health care team, and the goals set with the child and parents.

   3. The overall goal is to maintain the child's blood sugar level in the range that allows the lowest A1C without significant hypoglycemia.

   4. All the above.

4. A mother presents her school-age child to the family nurse practitioner and expresses her concern that her son is the shortest child in his class and asks if something is wrong with him. Initial differentiation of cause by the family nurse practitioner of the child's short stature would include:

   1. History with familial height patterns, physical exam with Tanner stage, and radiography to assess skeletal maturation, if indicated.

   2. History with familial height patterns, physical exam, and trial treatment with growth hormone.

   3. Immediate referral to an endocrinologist.

   4. Physical exam and complete blood count (CBC), thyroid function panel, urinalysis, karyotyping, chemistry profile, and insulin sensitivity tests.

5. Which of the following findings would the family nurse practitioner expect to find in a child with pubertal gynecomastia?

   1. Tanner stage II with testes ≤4 cm in length.

   2. Breasts and nipples nontender and equal in size.

   3. Breast tissue enlargement mainly glandular, movable, and nonadherent to skin or underlying tissue.

   4. Lymphadenopathy, goiter, asymmetrical testes, and repaired hypospadias.

6. Which of the following is true regarding hyperthyroidism in children?

   1. Boys have a higher incidence of Graves' disease.

   2. Autoimmune response is most often triggered by the body's reaction to a bacterial or viral infection.

   3. Decreased production and secretion of thyroid hormone and presence of goiter.

   4. Common, endemic congenital disorder caused by iodine deficiency.

7. On physical examination of a 14-year-old girl complaining of amenorrhea, the family nurse practitioner notes BP 138/90 mm Hg; pulse of 98 beats/min; broad chest with widely spaced nipples; Tanner stage I; webbing of neck; low hairline; and prominent, anomalous ears. The family nurse practitioner suspects:

   1. Klinefelter's syndrome.
   2. Marfan's syndrome.
   3. Fragile X syndrome.
   4. Turner's syndrome.

8. The family nurse practitioner understands that growth retardation that appears after age 12 in boys is usually caused by:

   1. Chromosomal abnormalities.
   2. Hyperthyroidism.
   3. Hyperpituitarism.
   4. Hypogonadism.

9. The family nurse practitioner understands that the blood glucose level in diabetic children 7–12 years of age who can recognize the symptoms of hypoglycemia need to be maintained in which range?

   1. 60–75 mg/dL.
   2. 100–175 mg/dL.
   3. 80–140 mg/dL.
   4. >180 mg/dL.

10. An adolescent male patient presenting with recent-onset nocturia, polydipsia, polyphagia, weight loss, and blurred vision is most likely experiencing the symptoms of:

    1. Type 1 diabetes.
    2. Type 2 diabetes.
    3. Urinary tract infection (UTI).
    4. Mononucleosis.

11. In which of the following groups of patients is tight glycemic control contraindicated?

    1. Adolescent males.
    2. Middle-aged females.
    3. Middle-aged males.
    4. Children under age 6.

12. An infant with an abnormally pitched cry may demonstrate a genetic disorder or other problems, such as:

    1. Hypothyroidism.
    2. Hypertelorism.
    3. Cleft palate.
    4. Pyloric stenosis.

13. A 6-year-old child with hypothyroidism diagnosed shortly after birth is seen by the family nurse practitioner for a routine physical exam. Temperature is 96.8°F (36°C) and pulse is 68 beats/min. The mother states that the child has been constipated and seems to be more tired than usual. Based on this history, what should the family nurse practitioner suspect?

    1. The child has been taking too much levothyroxine and is exhibiting symptoms of toxicity.
    2. The child needs to add more fluids to his diet to correct the constipation.
    3. The child needs to have the dose of levothyroxine (Synthroid) increased because he is exhibiting signs of hypothyroidism.
    4. The child has "outgrown" the hypothyroidism and no longer needs levothyroxine.

Hematology

14. A mother brings her school-age child to the clinic and reports a recent history of easy fatigability ("he can't keep up with his brother anymore"), unexplained bruising, and multiple courses of antibiotics for symptoms of upper respiratory infection (URI) during the past 6 months. Physical examination reveals scattered bruising in no apparent pattern, pallor, and cervical lymphadenopathy. What should be the first step of the diagnostic workup for this child?

    1. Chest x-ray and ECG.
    2. Liver function tests and abdominal ultrasound.
    3. PT/PTT.
    4. CBC with differential and platelet count.

15. In evaluating the laboratory findings for a child with iron-deficiency anemia, the family nurse practitioner expects:

    1. Low MCV and low reticulocyte count.
    2. High MCV and hemoglobin 12 g/dL.
    3. Normal MCV and hematocrit 34%.
    4. High MCV and normal reticulocyte count.

16. The family nurse practitioner explains a bone marrow aspiration procedure to a 4-year-old child. Which behavior of the child would reflect effective teaching?

    1. Appears calm as the nurse takes her for the procedure.

    2. Asks if she can have ice cream after the procedure.

    3. States that her blood is bad and "the doctor will make it better."

    4. Points at her doll and says, "They have to put a needle here to look at my blood."

17. Which of the following signs and symptoms are associated with a diagnosis of childhood acute lymphocytic leukemia (ALL)?

    1. Splenomegaly, facial rash, and cough.

    2. Expiratory wheezing, bleeding, and hepatomegaly.

    3. Bleeding, fever, and pain.

    4. Bone pain, fever, and night sweats.

18. The family nurse practitioner is concerned about the development of which complication in a young child with a diagnosis of iron-deficiency anemia?

    1. Crohn's disease.

    2. Pernicious anemia.

    3. Impaired cognitive development.

    4. Hepatic and spleen dysfunction.

19. The family nurse practitioner is counseling a parent who has a child with sickle cell disease. The parent asks, "If my child has sickle cell disease, does that mean that I'm at an increased risk for developing the same problems?" The family nurse practitioner's response would be based on which principle of sickle cell disease?

    1. The mother is at an increased risk because the condition is inherited; she probably has the condition and has not had an active episode.

    2. The mother is not at risk for developing the condition because males are carriers of the trait.

    3. The mother has a 25% chance of being affected by the disease, especially during times of stress.

    4. Both parents are carriers of the trait but do not have active disease; each child has a 25% chance of having the condition.

20. During a clinic visit, the family nurse practitioner notes that an 11-month-old infant is pale. The physical examination reveals a pulse of 170 beats/min, height at the 25th percentile, and weight at the 95th percentile. The nurse questions the mother about the infant's diet. The mother states that the infant eats mostly puréed fruits and whole milk. The family nurse practitioner expects which diagnostic finding?

    1. Normal hemoglobin.

    2. Elevated MCV.

    3. Low serum ferritin level.

    4. Macrocytic, hyperchromic anemia.

21. The family nurse practitioner knows that an infant who is exclusively breast-fed is at risk for developing iron-deficiency anemia at age:

    1. 1 month.

    2. 2 months.

    3. 4 months.

    4. 6 months.

Urinary/Renal

22. Physical examination for a child reveals 2+ proteinuria. What would be the next step in the differential diagnosis?

    1. Quantify protein excretion.

    2. Evaluate for orthostatic proteinuria.

    3. Reassure parent and follow up in 6 months.

    4. Evaluate for nephritis.

23. In children, hypertension and history of a sore throat may indicate which disorder?

    1. Heart failure.

    2. Glomerulonephritis.

    3. Vasculitis.

    4. Cushing's syndrome.

24. When assessing a child with glomerulonephritis, what symptoms would the family nurse practitioner expect to be present?

    1. Fever >102°F (38.9°C) and bilateral flank pain.

    2. Periorbital edema and increased blood pressure.

    3. Anorexia and complaints of dysuria.

    4. Oliguria with strong concentrated urine.

25. When instructing the parents regarding the course of poststreptococcal glomerulonephritis in their child, the family nurse practitioner would tell them to expect bloody urine for how long after onset of diuresis?

    1. 1 week.

    2. 1–2 weeks.

    3. 2–3 weeks.

    4. 4–7 days.

26. A mother brings in her 3-year-old daughter to the clinic, stating that she noticed a swelling in the child's abdominal area just below the rib cage on the left side. The family nurse practitioner observes a bulging of the area, and the child does not want to be touched because of abdominal tenderness. What is the best action for the family nurse practitioner at this visit?

    1. Immediately contact a pediatrician for consultation.

    2. Schedule a referral with a pediatrician in the near future.

    3. Perform a UA and draw blood for creatinine and potassium.

    4. Explain to the child that it is necessary to examine the abdomen.

27. A mother brings her 6-year-old daughter to the clinic. The child is complaining of burning on urination, and the urine is cloudy. A dipstick test of the urine is positive for leukocyte esterase. The mother states the child had a fever with nausea and vomiting the last time she took sulfisoxazole (Gantrisin). An appropriate medication for this child is:

    1. Nitrofurantoin (Macrodantin) 50 mg PO qid × 7 days.

    2. Trimethoprim-sulfamethoxazole (Septra DS) 1 tab PO bid × 10 days.

    3. Ciprofloxacin (Cipro) 200 mg PO bid × 10 days.

    4. Clarithromycin (Biaxin) 250 mg PO bid × 10 days.

Cardiac

28. On examination of a child, the family nurse practitioner notes weak femoral pulses. This finding is associated with what condition?

    1. Patent ductus arteriosus.

    2. Coarctation of the aorta.

    3. Tetralogy of Fallot.

    4. Pulmonary stenosis.

29. In doing a cardiac assessment of a 4-month-old infant, the family nurse practitioner notes a continuous murmur. This finding is consistent with a diagnosis of:

    1. Coarctation of the aorta.

    2. Patent ductus arteriosus.

    3. Ventricular septal defect.

    4. Aortic stenosis.

30. Heart failure (HF) is a common clinical presentation occurring in a child with congenital heart disease (CHD). What is another common clinical presentation with CHD?

    1. Hypoglycemia.

    2. Hypertension.

    3. Peripheral edema.

    4. Cyanosis.

31. Clinical manifestations of heart failure (HF) in an infant are:

    1. Easily fatigued, central cyanosis, tachycardia, tachypnea, hepatomegaly.

    2. Coughing, diaphoresis, peripheral edema, hepatomegaly.

    3. Tachycardia, tachypnea, easily fatigued, pallor, hepatomegaly.

    4. Peripheral edema, coughing, splenomegaly, hepatomegaly, tachycardia.

32. A young child is scheduled for surgical repair of tetralogy of Fallot. What does the family nurse practitioner expect the child's hemoglobin (Hgb) values to show, and what kind of lesion does the child have?

    1. Hgb 18 g/dL, cyanotic.

    2. Hgb 3 g/dL, cyanotic.

    3. Hgb 10 g/dL, acyanotic.

    4. Hgb 18 g/dL, acyanotic.

33. The family nurse practitioner understands that the most likely cause of hypertension in a young child is:

    1. Glomerulonephritis.

    2. Pheochromocytoma.

    3. Rheumatic fever.

    4. Hyperthyroidism.

34. Which of the following would be pertinent in the past medical history of a child who is being evaluated for cardiovascular disease?

    1. Kawasaki disease.

    2. Hypothyroidism.

    3. Osteogenic sarcoma.

    4. Tourette's syndrome.

35. The family nurse practitioner would refer a child with the following findings to a pediatric cardiologist for workup and evaluation within 1–2 weeks:

    1. Signs of exercise intolerance, dyspnea, and elevated pulse.

    2. Poor feeding, increased cyanosis with crying, and dizziness.

    3. Nonfunctional heart murmur, respiratory crackles, and retarded growth and development.

    4. Systolic ejection murmur, grade II, which disappears on sitting.

36. Infective endocarditis prophylaxis may be required for children with congenital heart defects in which of the following procedures?

    1. Dental procedures such as simple adjustment of orthodontic appliances.

    2. Cardiac catheterization.

    3. Tonsillectomy and/or adenoidectomy.

    4. Insertion of tympanostomy tubes.

37. For the child with congenital heart disease (CHD) and a permanent pacemaker, electrical safety precautions include avoidance of:

    1. Cellular phones.

    2. Microwave ovens.

    3. Household electrical appliances.

    4. Metal detectors.

38. A child is having a workup for rheumatic fever. His physical findings are temperature of 103.6°F (39.8°C), migratory joint pain, and increased ESR. According to the Jones criteria, what is essential for the diagnosis of rheumatic fever?

    1. History of group A beta-hemolytic streptococcal throat infection.

    2. Carditis.

    3. Sydenham's chorea.

    4. History of erythema marginatum for the past 3 days.

Respiratory

39. Cystic fibrosis (CF) is the preliminary diagnosis for a young girl who was brought to the clinic for evaluation. The test that will be used to rule out CF is:

    1. Hemoccult test.

    2. Sweat chloride test.

    3. Sputum culture and sensitivity.

    4. Glucose tolerance test.

40. An 18-month-old infant brought to the emergency department (ED) is awake, lethargic, and in severe respiratory distress. His mother states that he has not been sick and was playing on the floor when he suddenly began coughing, choking, and gagging. He has expiratory wheezes with decreased breath sounds over the right lower lobes, respirations of 36 breaths/min, pulse of 130 beats/min, and temperature normal. Portable chest x-ray shows hyperinflation on expiratory views. The best treatment for the infant is:

    1. Bronchoscopy as soon as possible.

    2. Cool-mist therapy with racemic epinephrine.

    3. Antibiotics with chest physiotherapy.

    4. Immediate endotracheal intubation and ventilation.

41. A 4-month-old patient presents to the office with a history of several days of rhinorrhea, cough, low-grade fever, and increased respiratory rate. What is the most likely diagnosis?

    1. Croup.

    2. Epiglottitis.

    3. Tracheitis.

    4. Bronchiolitis.

42. During a physical examination of a 2-year-old diagnosed with possible cystic fibrosis, the child passes a stool. The family nurse practitioner would expect the stool's appearance to be:

    1. Yellow and loose.

    2. Small and constipated.

    3. Green and odorous.

    4. Large and bulky.

43. A 6-year-old patient with a history of asthma presents to the office for evaluation by the family nurse practitioner. The child has never used a peak flowmeter. What quick tool can the family nurse practitioner use to assess the severity of the child's distress?

    1. ABGs.

    2. Child's inability to complete a sentence.

    3. Chest x-ray.

    4. Presence of runny nose.

44. The family nurse practitioner understands the following about tuberculosis (TB):

    1. Infants are more likely than children to present with wheezing and rales.

    2. Older children develop disseminated disease and meningitis more often than infants.

    3. Affected infants and young children are more likely to have a PPD skin test ≥15 mm.

    4. Adults are rarely the source of the disease when a child develops TB.

45. During a triannual visit to the clinic for routine care, the mother reports that her infant diagnosed with bronchopulmonary dysplasia (BPD) has been vomiting after each gastrostomy feeding. The family nurse practitioner notes that the infant's weight gain is adequate and would recommend:

    1. Referral to the pediatrician for follow-up.

    2. Reduction in amount of formula for the gastrostomy feeding.

    3. Addition of 3 oz of Pedialyte for the next two feedings.

    4. Positioning of the infant in a prone position after feedings with head and trunk elevated.

46. A 3-year-old child with up-to-date immunizations is brought to the office by his mother with a fairly rapid onset of stridor and a high-pitched wheeze. In view of this information, what would be the least important condition to consider for the differential diagnosis?

    1. Croup.

    2. Foreign body aspiration.

    3. Epiglottitis.

    4. Bacterial tracheitis.

47. A 15-year-old girl comes to the emergency department (ED) with complaints of extreme shortness of breath. She is confused, and her past medical history is not available.

Her vital signs are pulse of 124 beats/min, respirations of 32 breaths/min, BP of 124/80 mm Hg, and temperature normal. Physical examination reveals diffuse expiratory wheezes, hyperresonance on percussion, and prolonged expiratory phase. The best treatment for this patient includes:

    1. Aminophylline by mouth.

    2. Beclomethasone (Beclovent) inhaler.

    3. Epinephrine by injection.

    4. Albuterol (Proventil) by MDI.

48. The family nurse practitioner understands that an appropriate medication regimen for a child with drug-susceptible pulmonary tuberculosis (TB) is:

    1. Montelukast (Singulair) therapy with rifampin (Rifadin).

    2. Streptomycin, pyrazinamide, and rimantadine (Flumadine).

    3. Isoniazid (INH), pyrazinamide, and rifampin.

    4. Montelukast therapy with pyrimethamine (Fansidar).

49. During a routine well-child examination of a 4-year-old, the family nurse practitioner learns that the paternal grandmother has just been diagnosed with active TB. The mother states that the grandmother had stayed in their home for a week during the summer. The child has no signs of TB and has a negative PPD. What action should the family nurse practitioner take?

    1. Prescribe no medications, but schedule a repeat PPD in 2 months.

    2. Administer 1 mL gamma globulin IM.

    3. Start combination therapy with isoniazid (INH) and rifampin (Rifadin) for 15 months.

    4. Start isoniazid (INH) therapy for 4 months and then reevaluate.

50. Indications for antibiotic use in a child with bronchiolitis would include:

    1. History of two episodes in 4 months.

    2. Rhinitis and a productive cough.

    3. High fever and rales.

    4. Low-grade fever and sibilant wheezes.

51. A 10-year-old taking isoniazid (INH) prophylactically for exposure to TB complains of headache, palpitations, rash, and diarrhea. Management would be based on:

    1. Avoidance of foods containing tyramine and histamine.

2. Addition of pyridoxine to the diet.

3. Change in therapy from INH to rifampin.

4. Evaluation for hepatic impairment.

52. What is the initial treatment of choice for children diagnosed with bronchiolitis?

    1. Increase fluids; antipyretics as needed.

    2. Prednisolone (Pediapred) immediately and continue over 3–5 days.

    3. Diphenhydramine HCl (Benadryl) as long as symptoms persist.

    4. Amoxicillin over 10–14 days; aerosol humidification.

53. A 10-year-old boy is experiencing problems with wheezing, coughing, and shortness of breath about 4 hours after basketball practice. He has normal respirations and only experiences the problems after exercise. He is experiencing no other respiratory problems, and the physical findings are within normal limits. What is the treatment of choice for this child?

    1. Albuterol (Ventolin) 2 puffs MDI 20–30 minutes before exercise.

    2. Cromolyn sodium (Intal) 2 puffs each morning.

    3. Theophylline (Theo-24; methylxanthine) 100 mg PO bid.

    4. Beclomethasone (Beclovent) 2 puffs 3–4 times daily.

Immune and Allergy

54. The family nurse practitioner is evaluating the tuberculosis (TB) skin test on an immunocompetent 6-year-old child who has no risk factors for TB. The PPD is considered positive for this patient when it measures:

    1. 5 mm.

    2. 10 mm.

    3. 15 mm.

    4. 20 mm.

55. Children who have chronic allergic rhinitis often present with clinical symptoms that include:

    1. Mouth breathing and nasal polyps.

    2. Allergic "shiners" and Dennie-Morgan lines.

    3. Thick nasal discharge and sneezing.

    4. Flushed face and fever.

56. What are common sites for adolescent atopic dermatitis?

    1. Cheeks, forehead, and scalp.

    2. Wrists, ankles, and antecubital fossae.

    3. Antecubital fossae, face, neck, and back.

    4. Palmar creases and extensor surface of legs.

57. The clinic is notified that a child is being brought in with a bee sting and that the child is having difficulty breathing. Which medication should the family nurse practitioner have available for the child's initial care?

    1. Lidocaine topical ointment.

    2. Epinephrine.

    3. Prednisone.

    4. Diphenhydramine (Benadryl) elixir.

58. What is an appropriate antihistamine to recommend for a child with allergic rhinitis?

    1. Diphenhydramine (Benadryl).

    2. Chlorpheniramine (Chlor-trimeton).

    3. Brompheniramine (Dimetane).

    4. Loratadine (Claritin).

59. A child who weighs 30 lb (13.6 kg) arrives in the office. The mother is concerned that the child is having an allergic reaction to peanuts. The child has hives on most of her body and is beginning to wheeze; she is in acute distress. The family nurse practitioner administers:

    1. Diphenhydramine (Benadryl) 50 mg PO.

    2. Diphenhydramine (Benadryl) 25 mg PO.

    3. Epinephrine (Adrenalin) 0.14 mL of a 1:1000 solution.

    4. Epinephrine (Adrenalin) 0.3 mL of a 1:1000 solution.

60. A 2-year-old presents with mother with symptoms of atopic dermatitis, rhinorrhea, and recurrent otitis media with effusion. The house is nonsmoking and there are no pets in the home. The family nurse practitioner recognizes that the most likely cause of these symptoms in this age group would be from:

    1. Dust mite exposure.

    2. Internal mold exposure.

    3. Milk ingestion.

    4. Wheat ingestion.

61. A mother of a 5-year-old patient is concerned that they have a significant reaction to poison ivy every spring with a rash that appears on the ventral surfaces of the arms in the antecubital fossa. The rash is flat and erythematous and comes on suddenly with exposure to grass. Which statement would best describe the trigger of this dermatologic symptom?

    1. Poison ivy is very common in the spring and exposure results in immediate onset of symptoms.

    2. Plants that flower in the spring are laden with pollen that most likely will cause this type of symptom.

    3. Type IV hypersensitivity reactions are common in the spring with direct exposure to the allergen.

    4. Type I hypersensitivity reactions result in immediate symptoms upon exposure to the allergen.

HEENT

62. In examining the mouth of a school-age child, the family nurse practitioner notes that the central and lateral permanent incisors have surface pitting and are stained brown. This condition is most suggestive of:

    1. The mother taking tetracycline during pregnancy.

    2. Poor dental hygiene.

    3. Dental fluorosis.

    4. Going to bed with a bottle during infancy.

63. The visual screening for a 4-year-old boy is recorded as 20/40 in both eyes. The family nurse practitioner should now:

    1. Have the child return in 1 month to have his vision rechecked.

    2. Refer the child to an ophthalmologist.

    3. Recheck his vision to make sure that it is accurate.

    4. Record the findings as normal for age.

64. During a preschool screening for visual acuity, the family nurse practitioner would also assess for:

    1. Pupils that are equal and reactive.

    2. Intraocular pressure by tonometry.

    3. Diplopia.

    4. Strabismus.

65. A 4-year-old child's pure-tone audiometry reveals 25 decibels (dB) in the left ear and 43 dB in the right ear.

The family nurse practitioner would interpret these findings as:

    1. Inconclusive; pure-tone audiometry is not accurate in children less than 5 years of age.

    2. Within normal limits for age.

    3. Normal hearing in the left ear and moderate hearing loss in the right ear.

    4. Mild hearing loss in the left ear and normal hearing in the right ear.

66. The family nurse practitioner knows that an infant with low or obliquely set ears also has an increased incidence of:

    1. Cataracts.

    2. Hyaline membrane disease.

    3. Genitourinary defects.

    4. Cardiovascular anomalies.

67. Which of the following statement is true regarding tonsils?

    1. Children with large tonsils are more prone to tonsillitis than those with small tonsils.

    2. Tonsils enlarge as the child grows older.

    3. Hypertrophied tonsils in children usually represent a normal finding.

    4. Most cases of tonsillitis are caused by a β-hemolytic streptococcal infection.

68. An adolescent arrives at the clinic with a complaint of low-grade fever, sore throat, slight headache, and fatigue for the past week. On physical examination, the family nurse practitioner finds exudative tonsils bilaterally, red pharynx with white patches, and enlarged posterior cervical neck nodes. The family nurse practitioner would expect which laboratory test result?

    1. Positive rapid strep test.

    2. Positive monospot test.

    3. Increased white blood cell (WBC) count.

    4. Positive viral throat cultures.

69. The family nurse practitioner taking a preschooler's history learns that the family does not have fluoridated drinking water. With consideration of the concerns about fluorosis, what is the most appropriate nursing intervention?

1. Prescribe 5 mL of 0.02% fluoride solution (Fluorinse) once daily.

2. Instruct patients to use a pea-size fluoridated dentifrice and to supervise toothbrushing.

3. Instruct parents to use bottled drinking water.

4. Refer to dentist for topical application of fluoride.

70. A mother reports that her toddler awoke this morning with eyelid redness and a swelling. The family nurse practitioner notes that the child is afebrile and the eyelid is nontender and uniformly swollen. The most likely diagnosis is:

    1. Blepharitis.

    2. Hordeolum.

    3. Insect bite.

    4. Dacryocystitis.

71. On examination, the family nurse practitioner notes that a 2-week-old infant's left eye is watering and crusted material is on the eyelids. No edema or erythema is noted. The family nurse practitioner would make the diagnosis of:

    1. Nasolacrimal duct obstruction.

    2. Conjunctivitis.

    3. Congenital dacrocystocele.

    4. Corneal abrasion.

72. A mother brings her 6-week-old infant to the clinic because she is concerned that the child's eyes are crossed. What is the family nurse practitioner's most appropriate response?

    1. Explain to the mother that this is normal; reevaluate the child at 3 months of age.

    2. Refer the infant to an ophthalmologist.

    3. Provide the mother with normal saline eye drops for the infant.

    4. Have the mother alternate patching one eye and then the other every 6 hours.

73. In assessing a child with bacterial conjunctivitis, the family nurse practitioner finds:

    1. Minimal tearing, moderate itching, and profuse exudate.

    2. Severe itching, moderate tearing, and minimal discharge.

    3. Minimal itching, moderate tearing, and mucoid exudate.

    4. Minimal itching, moderate tearing, and profuse exudate.

74. The family nurse practitioner makes the diagnosis of nasolacrimal obstruction in a 1-week-old infant who presents with "leaking" of the right eye and a yellow discharge in the inner canthus of both eyes. Which of the following interventions would be contraindicated?

    1. Neosporin ophthalmic drops.

    2. Massaging the lacrimal duct for 1 minute four times daily.

    3. Cleansing the eye with warm water four times daily.

    4. Dexamethasone (Decadron) ophthalmic drops.

75. A child is diagnosed by the family nurse practitioner with acute otitis media (AOM). During a pneumatic otoscopy, the family nurse practitioner expects the tympanic membrane (TM) to be:

    1. Immobile, painful, with absent or decreased landmarks.

    2. Mobile, painful, with absent or decreased landmarks.

    3. Immobile, not painful, with landmarks visualized.

    4. Mobile, not painful, full and bulging.

76. A 6-year-old child is seen by the family nurse practitioner for ear pain. The child is afebrile. The left ear canal is extremely edematous and moderately inflamed with thick yellowish drainage at the external meatus. The child denies putting anything in the ear canal, but the family nurse practitioner finds that the child swims frequently. The most likely diagnosis is:

    1. Acute otitis media.

    2. Serous otitis media.

    3. Sinusitis.

    4. Otitis externa.

77. Risk factors for acute otitis media (AOM) include:

    1. Second-hand smoke, attending daycare, American Indians, and Eskimos.

    2. Chinese race, previous otitis media, many siblings.

    3. Higher socioeconomic level, full-time daycare, allergies.

    4. Summer season, full-time daycare, premature at birth.

78. A 6-year-old child is examined by the family nurse practitioner because of fluctuating hearing problems. The child is afebrile and denies otalgia. The mobility of the tympanic membrane (TM) is decreased when the family nurse practitioner performs pneumatic otoscopy. The TM is opaque with no visible landmarks. The child denies putting anything in the ear, and the mother states the child does not swim frequently. The most likely diagnosis is:

    1. Acute otitis media (AOM).

    2. A foreign body.

    3. Otitis media with effusion (OME).

    4. Otitis externa.

79. The family nurse practitioner teaches the mother of a school-age child the following as the most effective preventive measure against the common cold:

    1. Judicious use of vitamin C during cold season.

    2. Ensuring adequate sleep and fluids.

    3. Meticulous handwashing, preferably with an antibacterial soap and warm water.

    4. Avoiding contact with children and adults who have a runny nose, cough, and sore throat.

80. Which antibiotic would be appropriate for the family nurse practitioner to prescribe for beta-lactamase production by strains of *Haemophilus influenzae* and *Moraxella catarrhalis* in a child with acute otitis media?

    1. Amoxicillin (Amoxil).

    2. Erythromycin-sulfisoxazole (Pediazole).

    3. Penicillin V potassium (Pen-Vee K).

    4. Amoxicillin with clavulanic acid (Augmentin).

81. A 4-year-old boy (weight 18 kg) is diagnosed with bilateral otitis media. His last ear infection was 6 months ago, and he has no known drug allergies. An appropriate medication to prescribe would be:

    1. Ampicillin 40–50 mg/kg/day tid × 7 days.

    2. Corticosteroid otic solution 3 gtt both ears × 10 days.

    3. Amoxicillin 75–90 mg/kg/day bid × 10 days.

    4. Doxycycline 250 mg 1 tsp PO tid × 10 days.

82. An adolescent patient has had yellowish-green nasal discharge and a frontal headache for a week. The adolescent's temperature has gone up to 101.2°F (38.4°C) on most afternoons, and she has a cough that worsens when she lies down. The physical exam is within normal limits except for the drainage and a slightly erythematous pharynx. She does not have any drug allergies and has not been taking any medications in the past few months. Which medication would be best to prescribe for her?

    1. Diphenhydramine (Benadryl).

    2. Erythromycin (E-Mycin).

    3. Pseudoephedrine (Sudafed).

    4. Amoxicillin/clavulanate (Augmentin).

Integumentary

83. The nurse is examining a 6-week-old infant of Latin-American descent. There are irregular areas of deep-blue pigmentation across the infant's buttocks. The nurse would identify this as characteristic of:

    1. Child abuse.

    2. Telangiectatic nevi.

    3. Cutis marmorata.

    4. Mongolian spots.

84. A mother brings her school-age child in for an examination. She reports that the child frequently scratches and that the itching seems to be worse at night. On examination, the family nurse practitioner notes lesions on the sides of the fingers and inner aspect of the elbows. These lesions are short, irregular "runs" that are approximately 2–3 mm long and the width of a hair. The family nurse practitioner tells the mother she suspects:

    1. Scabies.

    2. Hives.

    3. Fleas.

    4. Ticks.

85. When treating atopic dermatitis in children, which of the following instructions are applicable?

    1. Eliminate foods thought to induce flares, one food at a time.

    2. Encourage moisturizing bubble baths.

    3. Keep well dressed during winter.

    4. Encourage bathing two or three times a day.

86. A family nurse practitioner is teaching the mother of a child how to use permethrin 1% cream rinse (Nix)

for treatment of pediculosis capitis. What is the most important information the family nurse practitioner should give to the mother?

1. Shampoo the child's hair daily for 1 week, followed by permethrin rinse.

2. Shampoo and towel-dry hair, apply permethrin to scalp and hair, and wait 10 minutes before rinsing.

3. The shampoo should not be used again because it is toxic and may absorb systemically.

4. It is not necessary to launder bedding or clothing.

87. The family nurse practitioner understands that nonintentional scalding in young children usually occurs:

1. On the back of the body.

2. On the front of the body.

3. In a circular or glove pattern.

4. With no specific pattern.

88. An infant has pruritus caused by eczema. The family nurse practitioner teaches the mother the following regarding the infant's care:

1. Dress the infant in cotton shorts and short-sleeved shirts.

2. Dress the infant in wool-blend, long-sleeved jump suits.

3. Give the infant cornstarch or Aveeno baths.

4. Give the infant salt baths three times a day.

89. A new mother is concerned about the hemangioma on her infant's neck. What is the treatment of choice for the majority of infants with hemangioma?

1. Cryosurgery.

2. Intralesional injection of steroids.

3. Observation.

4. Injection of a sclerosing agent.

90. The family nurse practitioner is examining an infant with atopic dermatitis. What would the physical examination reveal?

1. Dry, scaly rash with pruritus.

2. Distribution of rash on face and extensor surfaces.

3. Erythematous raised areas on flexor surfaces.

4. Moist, crusting rash with no pruritus.

91. The family nurse practitioner is examining a 6-year-old child and identifies 8 to 10 patches of coffee-colored areas on the trunk. The areas are nontender, the border is irregular, and most of the areas are larger than 1.5 cm and nonpalpable. What is the best recommendation to the child's parents?

1. The child should be evaluated further by a pediatrician for possible referral to a neurologist.

2. These areas are normal pigmentation and will disappear.

3. A dermatologist should be consulted for removal of lesions.

4. Emollients should be applied to keep skin moist, and sunlight on the areas should be avoided.

92. An infant is noted at his well-child visit to have a yellowish, greasy scaly rash on his scalp, forehead, and ears. What is the most likely diagnosis?

1. Seborrheic dermatitis.

2. Atopic dermatitis.

3. Erythema toxicum.

4. Eczema.

93. A 1-month-old infant is being seen by the family nurse practitioner for a diaper rash. On examination, the practitioner notes moderate erythema and poorly marginated, dry patches of skin localized to the buttocks. The deep folds are not affected. There are no satellite lesions. What is the most likely diagnosis?

1. Infantile seborrheic dermatitis.

2. Allergy to disposable diapers.

3. Contact dermatitis.

4. Candidal diaper rash.

94. A mother brings her preschool child to see the family nurse practitioner because of sores on his arms and legs. On examination, the family nurse practitioner notes several honey-colored crusted lesions with an erythematous base on the arms and legs. There is a history of exposure to mosquitoes. The rest of the exam is essentially negative. What is the most likely diagnosis?

1. Scabies.

2. Impetigo.

3. Pityriasis rosea.

4. Varicella.

95. A mother returns to the clinic with her 6-month-old infant to have his ears rechecked after a 10-day course of antibiotics for an ear infection. During the visit, the mother states that the child is now eating better and appears to be recovering, but he now has a bad diaper rash. What is the most likely cause of this rash?

    1. Poor hygiene.

    2. Cellulitis.

    3. Seborrheic diaper dermatitis.

    4. *Candida albicans.*

96. A school-age child presents with erythematous, papular lesions and scaly plaques in the antecubital and popliteal fossae and on the neck, wrists, and ankles. The mother states that the child has been scratching the areas, especially at night. History reveals that the child also has been treated for asthma. The family nurse practitioner would make the diagnosis of:

    1. Scabies.

    2. Atopic dermatitis.

    3. Tinea corporis.

    4. Contact dermatitis.

97. While attending a rural public school, a 7-year-old child was bitten on the hand by a raccoon. At the rural clinic, the family nurse practitioner cleansed the wound. What would be the next action?

    1. Administer tetanus antitoxin.

    2. Contact local animal control authorities.

    3. Administer rabies immune globulin (RIG) and human diploid cell vaccine (HDCV).

    4. Teach the family how to do hourly soaks to the hand using normal saline and peroxide.

98. A toddler is brought to the clinic with a history of an insect bite last evening. What presenting symptom would be associated with the bite of a brown recluse spider?

    1. Paresthesias in all extremities.

    2. Edematous, erythematous area with coalescing macules.

    3. Tissue sloughing in the bite area within 8–10 hours.

    4. Development of a central black eschar of "sinking infarct" within 12–24 hours.

99. The family nurse practitioner understands that cat bites become infected more often than dog bites because:

    1. Dogs have a "cleaner mouth" than cats.

    2. Cat bites are often deep puncture wounds.

    3. Dog bites are usually on the face, which makes them less susceptible to infection.

    4. Cat bites are usually associated with clawing and spreading of microorganisms.

100. An adolescent was bitten by a neighbor's dog 3 days ago. He has developed an infection in a large wound on his lower leg. What would be an appropriate management for the patient?

    1. Prescribe amoxicillin-clavulanate (Augmentin).

    2. Approximate the edges of the wound together with suture.

    3. Prescribe cephalexin (Keflex).

    4. Have the adolescent return to the clinic for follow-up in 2 weeks.

101. A young adolescent has been bitten by a black widow spider while doing yard work. He is having a severe reaction; the family nurse practitioner expects:

    1. Hypotension and shock.

    2. Localized pain, erythema, and edema in the area.

    3. Black eschar of sloughing tissue within 4 hours of the bite.

    4. Abdominal cramping, nausea, and headache.

Childhood Diseases

102. Phone consultation with a mother reveals that her child has been taking TMP-SMX (Septra) for 3 days for a urinary tract infection. She has been treated with the drug previously with no problems. Currently, the child is experiencing blister-like sores in the skinfold areas (axilla and groin), oral ulceration, and a few genital sores. Her temperature is 104°F (40°C), and she is very weak. Differential diagnosis includes:

    1. Kawasaki disease.

    2. Erythema multiforme (major).

    3. Viral exanthem.

    4. Early scalded-skin syndrome.

103. A daycare center director calls to confirm when a child can return to the center after having fifth disease (erythema infectiosum). The family nurse practitioner's

response is based on the knowledge that the period of communicability lasts until:

1. The rash is gone.

2. The rash appears.

3. Upper respiratory symptoms are gone.

4. The transient joint pain disappears.

104. Examination of a nontoxic, but ill-appearing 6-year-old reveals vesicular and ulcerative oral lesions and a maculopapular rash on the hands and feet; temperature is 100.4°F (38°C) and the child has feelings of malaise. Differential diagnosis includes:

1. Hand-foot-and-mouth disease.

2. Roseola.

3. Drug rash.

4. Varicella.

105. The family nurse practitioner understands that the rash of roseola differs from that of rubella. Which statement is correct?

1. Rash of roseola starts on the trunk.

2. Rash of rubella is pruritic.

3. Rash of roseola fades in 3–5 days.

4. Rash of rubella clears on the extremities, when facial rash erupts.

106. What is an appropriate treatment for a child with roseola?

1. Antiviral medications, fluids, and rest.

2. Antipyretics, rest, and hydration.

3. Antibiotics, hydration, and rest.

4. Hospitalization, antipyretics, and IV fluid replacement.

107. In treatment of severe inflammatory acne for a female adolescent, the family nurse practitioner understands that:

1. Isotretinoin (Accutane) provides an effective first-line therapy.

2. The benefits of treatment will be noted in 5–7 days.

3. Counseling on stringent dietary changes is important.

4. Systemic antibiotics are effective treatment.

108. A young mother brings her infant to the family nurse practitioner with a complaint of diaper rash present

for about 1 week. The diaper area appears beefy red with sharply marginated dermatitis. Satellite lesions are also noted. The family nurse practitioner recommends:

1. Changing from disposable diapers to cloth diapers with plastic pants.

2. Nystatin cream (Mycostatin) after each diaper change.

3. Wet soaks three times daily.

4. Liberally applying oil after bathing.

109. The family nurse practitioner is examining lesions around a child's nose and mouth. His mother states that the lesions appeared several days ago and now seem worse. Some of the vesicular, edematous, red, and tender lesions have yellow crusts and an erythematous base. What is the recommended treatment for this child?

1. Mupirocin ointment (Bactroban) qid × 10 days.

2. Gently soaking the lesions with antibacterial soap and removing the crusts.

3. Amoxicillin-clavulanate (Augmentin).

4. Diphenhydramine (Benadryl) to decrease itching and spreading.

110. A mother brings her 1-year-old child to the clinic for problems with a "rash." She states the child has not been feeling well since the rash started 2 days ago. The family nurse practitioner observes numerous macules and vesicles in clusters over the child's trunk and mucous membranes; some are clear, some are crusting. The child is irritable but does not have a fever. What would be the diagnosis and treatment for the child?

1. Varicella; immunize with varicella-zoster vaccine to decrease symptoms, and begin acyclovir (Zovirax) therapy to prevent/decrease complications.

2. Impetigo; treat with amoxicillin-clavulanate (Augmentin) for 10 days, and return to clinic in 2 weeks.

3. Contact dermatitis; apply diphenhydramine (Benadryl) spray over rash, cut child's fingernails to decrease scratching, and thoroughly review any changes in care with the mother.

4. Varicella; treat first with diphenhydramine (Benadryl) in age-appropriate dose, apply hydroxyzine (Atarax) for itching, and give daily baths with colloidal oatmeal (Aveeno).

111. A 6-month-old infant is brought to the clinic for a rash on the face and diaper area that consists of linear erythematous burrows. An older sibling has a similar rash on his wrists and between his fingers. An appropriate intervention would be:

    1. Bacitracin ointment.

    2. Mycitracin ointment.

    3. Acitretin (Soriatane).

    4. Permethrin 5% cream (Elimite).

112. A mother brings her school-age child to the family nurse practitioner's office. She states that the child developed a blistering rash on his face 2 days ago that has since spread to his hands and forearms. Examination reveals multiple small vesicular lesions across the child's face, arms, and hands. Some of the lesions are covered with a honey-colored crust. The family nurse practitioner diagnoses impetigo and recommends:

    1. Frequent scrubbing of the lesions with a washrag and antibacterial soap.

    2. Isolation of the child from other children for 7 days and discarding the clothing the child has been wearing since the lesions appeared.

    3. Amoxicillin-clavulanate (Augmentin) for 10 days and gentle washing of the lesions.

    4. Referral to a dermatologist and that the mother practice better personal hygiene.

113. An adolescent female presents to the office with a long history of facial acne. She has been seen by several dermatologists and has been treated over the past 3 years with multiple therapies, including topical antibiotics, drying agents, intralesional injections of corticosteroids, and multiple systemic antibiotics, without success. After consulting with the collaborating physician, the family nurse practitioner prescribes isotretinoin (Accutane). Teaching/counseling related to the use of this medication includes:

    1. No dietary/alcohol restrictions are necessary.

    2. Exposure to sunlight without burning can be helpful in hastening the healing process.

    3. Eliminate all fat from the patient's diet.

    4. Emphasize the importance of effective contraception if the patient is sexually active.

114. A father brings in his 4-year-old son to the emergency department after the boy ingested a small bottle of aspirin approximately an hour or so ago. What is the family nurse practitioner's priority?

    1. Insert a nasogastric tube and attach to low suction.

    2. Give 16 oz of orange juice.

    3. Give 8 oz of milk.

    4. Give activated charcoal.

115. The family nurse practitioner is aware that the toxic symptoms of salicylate poisoning are:

    1. Tinnitus and nausea.

    2. Itching and blurred vision.

    3. Fruity odor to the breath.

    4. Fever and chills.

Musculoskeletal

116. The family nurse practitioner is assessing a preadolescent girl for scoliosis. How is this test conducted?

    1. Have the girl bend at the waist, and look for asymmetry in the back and hip area.

    2. Examine the child fully clothed, paying particular attention to the hips and back.

    3. Have the child walk heel-to-toe, and observe the gait and pelvis.

    4. Place the child on her back, and flex the knees and observe for misalignment.

117. In doing a physical assessment on a newborn, the family nurse practitioner notes a "hip click." What other findings are associated with this condition?

    1. Shortened quadriceps.

    2. Lateral deviation of patella.

    3. Limited abduction.

    4. Lax hamstrings.

118. An adolescent complains of right knee pain immediately after running in track practice. On examination, the knee is warm to touch, and a tender, swollen tibial tuberosity is noted. The family nurse practitioner suspects:

    1. Osgood-Schlatter disease.

    2. Rheumatoid arthritis.

    3. Acute tendinitis.

    4. Posttraumatic knee effusion.

119. Nighttime extremity pain in school-age children that is deep but not present in the joints and that may be caused by inflammation of the muscle bodies in tight fascial sheaths and by periods of high activity is:

    1. Osgood-Schlatter disease.

    2. Patellofemoral stress syndrome.

    3. Growing pains.

    4. Shin splints.

120. The family nurse practitioner is teaching crutch walking to an adolescent with a lower leg cast for a fractured tibia. Instructions for assisting the adolescent to walk up the stairs would include:

    1. Place both crutches on the upper step and step up with unaffected leg while balancing on crutches.

    2. Position the affected leg on the upper step and use the crutches to move up.

    3. Place the unaffected leg on the upper step and move affected leg and crutches up together.

    4. Position the affected leg and the crutch on the upper step and bring the unaffected leg up with the crutch.

121. An adolescent patient is being evaluated by the family nurse practitioner for knee pain. The patient is active in sports in his school but can recall no specific injury to the knee. On examination, the family nurse practitioner finds unilateral swelling of the anterior aspect of the tibial tubercle, which is tender. The most likely diagnosis is:

    1. Stress fracture.

    2. Patellar dislocation.

    3. Osgood-Schlatter disease.

    4. Neuman's syndrome.

122. Which of the following is the most accurate statement about juvenile rheumatoid arthritis (JRA)?

    1. Symptoms present in much greater severity than in adult RA.

    2. Complete remission occurs in three fourths of patients.

    3. More than 90% of cases progress to severe joint destruction.

    4. Cytotoxic drugs should be initiated as early as possible in the treatment regimen.

123. Children with juvenile rheumatoid arthritis (JRA) must be screened regularly for:

    1. Ulcerative colitis.

    2. Iridocyclitis.

    3. Diabetes mellitus.

    4. Adrenal insufficiency.

124. An adolescent who twisted his knee while skateboarding comes to the clinic complaining of knee pain. He also states that in the past few weeks his knee has "locked up a couple of times." On examination, a positive McMurray's test is elicited. This is consistent with a diagnosis of:

    1. Anterior cruciate ligament tear.

    2. Dislocated patella.

    3. Medial meniscus tear.

    4. Chondromalacia patella.

125. In young children, a complaint of hip pain without a history of trauma suggests several differential diagnoses. Which diagnosis is considered a true orthopedic emergency?

    1. Toxic synovitis of the hip.

    2. Legg-Calvé-Perthes disease.

    3. Increased femoral anteversion.

    4. Avascular necrosis of the femoral head.

126. Differentiation between structural and functional scoliosis can be done by placing the child in Adam's position. Which of the following occurs in this position?

    1. Structural scoliosis disappears, and functional scoliosis is enhanced.

    2. Persistent functional scoliosis is indicated.

    3. Functional scoliosis disappears, and structural scoliosis is enhanced.

    4. Curves greater than 10 degrees are indicated.

Neurology

127. In infants, especially preterm infants, seizures can present as:

    1. Coughing spells.

    2. Poor feeding.

    3. Awake apnea.

    4. Regurgitation.

128. The family nurse practitioner is caring for a 10-year-old child with meningitis. To assess for the presence of nuchal rigidity, the family nurse practitioner would:

    1. Have the child bend forward at the waist, and observe the line of the spine.

    2. Place hand on child's forehead and ask child to press nurse's hand with his head.

    3. With the child relaxed, attempt to move his head side to side.

    4. Place hand on back of child's head and assist him to put his chin on his chest.

129. An adolescent girl is accompanied to the clinic by her mother, who states the school reports that she "stares off into space a lot" and does not seem to pay attention during these brief periods, which typically last 1–3 minutes. The neurologic examination is within normal limits. What should the family nurse practitioner suspect in the patient?

    1. Grand mal seizure.

    2. Complex partial seizure.

    3. Absence seizure.

    4. Simple partial seizure.

130. A child is admitted to the rural clinic after a car accident in which she sustained a closed head injury and fractured femur. The child is lethargic and follows commands slowly, and her pupils are equal and reactive. The child is to be transferred to a hospital by air ambulance. In assessing the child, what would the family nurse practitioner consider as a significant change in her condition?

    1. Urine output is less than 500 mL in 24 hours.

    2. She complains of a headache in the frontal area.

    3. She is able to move her lower extremities to command.

    4. Vital signs are BP of 130/50 mm Hg and pulse of 70 beats/min.

131. A parent whose son was recently diagnosed with Tourette's syndrome asks the family nurse practitioner about the condition. The family nurse practitioner understands that:

    1. Tourette's syndrome is usually treated with antianxiety agents, such as diazepam (Valium).

    2. The tics may occur often throughout the day and may change over time.

    3. Children rarely have ADHD in conjunction with Tourette's syndrome.

    4. Tics are typically neuromuscular (e.g., facial grimacing, tongue protruding, neck twitching) and rarely vocal.

132. A 3-week-old infant has been diagnosed with bacterial meningitis. The family nurse practitioner is aware that the most common causative organism is:

    1. *Streptococcus pyogenes.*

    2. *Escherichia coli.*

    3. *Neisseria meningitidis.*

    4. Group B streptococcus.

133. The family nurse practitioner is seeing a 3-year-old child with a history of hospitalization at 18 months for bacterial meningitis and treatment with ampicillin and gentamicin. Which test should the family nurse practitioner make sure to include in the examination?

    1. Vision testing.

    2. Hearing testing.

    3. Lumbar puncture.

    4. ECG.

134. Which is considered a likely cause of seizures in adolescents and young adults?

    1. Congenital abnormalities and metabolic disturbances.

    2. Metabolic disorders, CNS infection, and fever.

    3. Idiopathic disease, trauma, and substance abuse.

    4. Trauma, malignant tumor, and cerebrovascular accident.

135. A child presents with a history of a purpuric rash with a centrifugal distribution and a fever. After the family nurse practitioner examines this child, what would be the most important condition to rule out at this time?

    1. Rubella.

    2. Lyme disease.

    3. Meningococcemia.

    4. Roseola.

136. A mother brings her 5-year-old son to the clinic with complaints that he is "acting funny." She states there are brief periods when he does not respond to her, and then he suddenly responds and acts as if nothing has happened. The nurse would initially evaluate the child further for the presence of:

    1. Petit mal or absence seizures.

2. Attention deficit disorder.

3. Horner's syndrome.

4. Avoidance disorder of childhood.

137. Which finding would lead the family nurse practitioner to consider shaken baby syndrome in an infant?

1. Visible head trauma.

2. Subconjunctival hemorrhages.

3. Anisocoria.

4. Retinal hemorrhages.

138. Which statement about autism is correct?

1. Autism has no gender preference.

2. There is no genetic predisposition.

3. Delay in motor development is an expected co-morbidity.

4. Language skills are delayed or underdeveloped.

139. Which of the following statements is true regarding cerebral palsy?

1. Cerebral palsy can be reversed.

2. It is more common in males than in females.

3. Cognitive impairment is the hallmark of the disorder.

4. Hypertonia is an expected finding in infancy.

140. During physical examination of a child diagnosed with chronic recurrent seizures who is currently receiving antiepileptic medication, the family nurse practitioner notes hyperplasia of the gums. The nurse understands that hyperplasia of the gums is:

1. An unusual side effect of phenobarbital.

2. A common side effect of phenytoin.

3. Common with chronic recurrent seizures.

4. Caused by poor oral hygiene.

Gastrointestinal

141. The viral gastroenteritis seen in older children and adults has a short incubation (18–72 hours) and short duration (24–48 hours), is characterized by abrupt onset of nausea and abdominal cramps, followed by vomiting and diarrhea, and is often accompanied by headache and myalgia. What causes this disorder?

1. Enteric adenovirus.

2. Enteric calicivirus (Norwalk).

3. Rotavirus.

4. Cytomegalovirus.

142. The family nurse practitioner is interpreting the notation of "string sign" on an upper GI series performed on an infant. This is associated with a diagnosis of:

1. Intussusception.

2. Hirschsprung's disease.

3. Pyloric stenosis.

4. Gastroesophageal reflux.

143. The family nurse practitioner identifies the following condition as most conducive to the development of metabolic alkalosis in a child:

1. Severe anxiety resulting in hyperventilation.

2. Excessive vomiting related to gastroenteritis.

3. Depressed respirations from excessive narcotic ingestion.

4. Decreased renal function with glomerular damage.

144. The family nurse practitioner in the emergency department examines a child with severe diarrhea and vomiting, which results in dehydration. One of the orders is to start an IV line of 500 mL normal saline with 10 mEq potassium to run at 23 mL/hr. The child is NPO. What would be a priority action before initiating the IV fluid with potassium?

1. Weigh the child.

2. Obtain serum electrolyte values.

3. Make sure the child is voiding adequately.

4. Determine amount of previous fluid loss.

145. An 18-month-old child is brought to the clinic by her mother and is complaining of abrupt onset of vomiting, followed by more than 10 liquid stools with mucus for the past 48 hours. The temperature is 100°F (37.8°C) orally. The stool smear obtained by the family nurse practitioner is negative for WBCs. What is the most likely etiologic pathogen for this young child's gastroenteritis?

1. Rotavirus.

2. *Shigella dysenteriae.*

3. *Campylobacter jejuni.*

4. *Salmonella.*

146. The symptoms of abdominal discomfort after meals, diarrhea or constipation, anorexia, weight loss, and failure to grow are most often associated with:

    1. Ulcerative colitis.

    2. Irritable bowel syndrome.

    3. Carcinoma of the colon.

    4. Crohn's disease.

147. What are the most consistent clinical findings in children with acute appendicitis?

    1. An elevated WBC count and pyuria.

    2. High fever and tenderness around the umbilicus.

    3. Low-grade fever and periumbilical abdominal pain.

    4. Nausea, vomiting, and diarrhea.

148. What question by the family nurse practitioner would be appropriate to ask the parents of an infant suspected of intussusception?

    1. "Does the infant have clay-colored stools?"

    2. "Does the infant have projectile vomiting?"

    3. "Does the infant have constant abdominal pain?"

    4. "Does the infant have red currant jelly stools?"

149. The major symptom of reflux in infants is:

    1. Vomiting or regurgitation, especially after feeding.

    2. Poor weight gain in infants.

    3. Hyperirritability and refusal of feeding.

    4. Fever and diarrhea.

150. Optimal medical therapy for young infants with vomiting or regurgitation of gastroesophageal reflux disease (GERD) consists of:

    1. Frequent small feedings and burping after each feeding.

    2. Placing the infant prone after frequent feedings.

    3. Placing the infant supine after feedings.

    4. Thickening the feedings and using proton pump inhibitors.

151. What is true regarding the management of an infant born to a HBsAg-positive mother?

    1. No prophylaxis against hepatitis B is required because the infant is not at risk for the development of hepatitis B based on exposure to mother.

    2. One dose of hepatitis B immunoglobulin should be administered by 36 hours after birth.

    3. The family nurse practitioner should administer one dose of hepatitis B vaccine.

    4. One dose of hepatitis B immunoglobulin should be administered within 12 hours of birth and a complete three-dose immunization of hepatitis B vaccine administered at the usual recommended intervals.

152. What physical findings would lead the family nurse practitioner to suspect Hirschsprung's disease in a 6-month-old infant?

    1. Rectal bleeding, diarrhea, and prolonged jaundice at birth.

    2. History of constipation and current abdominal distention.

    3. Irritability, vomiting, and dehydration.

    4. History of colic, bloody diarrhea, and nausea.

153. A common cause of acute abdominal pain in children under 5 years old is:

    1. Appendicitis.

    2. Intussusception.

    3. Incarcerated hernia.

    4. Gastroenteritis.

154. The family nurse practitioner understands that common causes of recurrent abdominal pain in children are:

    1. Intussusception, gastroenteritis, and right lower lobe pneumonia.

    2. Psychogenic pain, trauma, and urinary tract infection.

    3. Parasitic infestation, lactose intolerance, and chronic stool retention.

    4. Incarcerated hernia, appendicitis, and inflammatory bowel disease.

155. A mother brings her adolescent son to the family nurse practitioner for evaluation after a dirt-bike accident. The patient states that the bike flipped over and struck him on the abdomen. He has a hematoma just below the left anterior rib area. The family nurse practitioner must be particularly aware of which possibility?

    1. Ruptured bowel due to blunt trauma.

    2. Bladder trauma.

3. Hypovolemia due to ruptured spleen.

4. Arrhythmias.

156. A 2-year-old Asian American comes to the clinic with her parents and infant brother. The chief complaint is abdominal pain with flatulence and diarrhea after eating. Until 3 months ago, the patient had continued to be breast-fed twice a day. The family nurse practitioner would suspect:

   1. Irritable bowel syndrome.

   2. Hirschsprung's disease.

   3. Lactose intolerance.

   4. Food allergy.

157. A 10-year-old girl comes to the clinic with complaints of nausea, vomiting, and right upper quadrant pain during vigorous play. She is also more tired than usual. Serologic tests for IgM antibodies are ordered to rule out:

   1. Cholecystitis.

   2. Hepatitis A.

   3. Infectious mononucleosis.

   4. Hepatitis B.

158. A 5-year-old presents to the clinic with diffuse abdominal pain, irritability, and a low-grade fever. The mother states the child has not had a bowel movement since the previous morning. Physical examination reveals umbilical tenderness, guarding, and hypoactive bowel sounds. The family nurse practitioner's next step is to:

   1. Refer to physician/surgeon for further evaluation.

   2. Assess for rebound tenderness and do a rectal exam.

   3. Prescribe pediatric Fleet enemas.

   4. Assess dietary intake for past 24 hours.

159. A 2-year-old child is seen for a foreign body in the GI tract. The family nurse practitioner pays particular attention to the size of the object, knowing that passing the ligament of Treitz is difficult with objects larger than:

   1. 5 cm.

   2. 8 cm.

   3. 10 cm.

   4. 12 cm.

160. A 2-month-old infant presents with coughing, which results in emesis that occurs when laid supine after eating. The infant has lost 1.3 lb since birth with a birth weight of 7.5 lb. The family nurse practitioner focuses the assessment toward the possibility of:

   1. Suck-swallow incoordination.

   2. Gastroesophageal reflux.

   3. Tracheoesophageal fistula.

   4. Infantile colic.

161. Shigellosis is diagnosed in a young child with bloody diarrhea. The family nurse practitioner knows *Shigella* is a bacteria that is transmitted by the fecal–oral route or swimming in contaminated water and is treated by:

   1. Amoxicillin in weight-based dosing for 10 days.

   2. Symptomatic treatment and antidiarrheal agent loperamide (Imodium) as needed.

   3. Symptomatic treatment, including fluid replacement, such as Pedialyte, and avoid any antidiarrheals.

   4. TMP-SMX (Bactrim) dosed age appropriate for 7 days.

162. A 3-year-old child is seen in the clinic for chronic, relapsing diarrhea. A stool for ova and parasites is obtained and is positive for *Giardia*. What is the most appropriate pharmacologic intervention?

   1. Ampicillin (Omnipen).

   2. Erythromycin (E-Mycin).

   3. Metronidazole (Flagyl).

   4. Tetracycline (Achromycin).

Male Reproductive

163. Circumcision can prevent which of the following?

   1. Paraphimosis.

   2. Epididymitis.

   3. Sexually transmitted disease.

   4. Prostatitis.

164. A 15-year-old male presents with complaints of severe scrotal pain for the past 2 hours. The scrotum is swollen and extremely tender; palpation of the epididymis is not possible. What does the family nurse practitioner recognize as the immediate treatment?

   1. Narcotic analgesics and bed rest.

   2. Warm packs and scrotal support.

   3. Antibiotics, ice packs, and analgesics.

   4. Referral to a surgeon for exploration.

165. Cryptorchidism is defined as:

    1. Testicular underdevelopment.

    2. Imbalance of estrogen/androgen ratio.

    3. Undescended testicles.

    4. Absence of spermatogenesis.

166. A 14-year-old boy comes into the clinic from school with complaints of sudden, severe scrotal pain radiating inguinally. He has no difficulty voiding and has some nausea but no vomiting. Examination reveals scrotal edema and erythema. The scrotum on the affected side is slightly higher than on the unaffected side, and the cremasteric reflex is negative. What would the family nurse practitioner determine as the best treatment for the patient?

    1. Bed rest with ice pack and scrotal elevation.

    2. Warm scrotal pack and return to clinic the next day.

    3. Immediate referral to a urologist.

    4. Schedule for an ultrasound in the morning.

Female Reproductive

167. While assessing a 16-year-old girl, the family nurse practitioner was asked about douching. What information would be used in the family nurse practitioner's teaching plan?

    1. Douching during menstruation is safe.

    2. Daily douching is important because the patient has copious vaginal discharge.

    3. Hypoallergenic douches include flavored or perfumed types.

    4. Douching removes natural mucus and upsets normal vaginal flora.

168. A high school athlete presents to the clinic with concerns regarding her menstrual periods. She states she has not had a period in the past 2 months. She has been in training and running about 3 miles a day for the past 3 months. She has lost approximately 15 lb. Her height is about 63 inches, and she currently weighs 100 lb. What is the best response by the family nurse practitioner?

    1. Determine the patient's percentage of body fat and body mass.

    2. Obtain FSH serum levels.

    3. Determine serum levels of hCG.

    4. Order thyroid function tests.

169. During a gynecologic examination at the family planning clinic, an underweight 17-year-old presents with bruising around her upper torso and genitalia. She is minimally interactive and avoids eye contact as much as possible. Priority intervention should focus on:

    1. Lab work to rule out bleeding disorder.

    2. Nutritional assessment to determine possible anemia.

    3. Determination of possible physical abuse.

    4. Finding out if she has a support system.

Newborn

170. The family nurse practitioner is measuring a newborn's frontal-occipital circumference (FOC). Correct technique involves:

    1. Placing the paper tape measure at the maximal occipital prominence and just above the eyebrows.

    2. Placing the cloth tape measure at a level 2 inches above the ears.

    3. Using a cloth tape to prevent inaccuracy due to stretchable materials.

    4. Having another person hold the tape in the center of the forehead and repeating the measurement.

171. Which newborn screening tests are mandatory state requirements?

    1. CBC and urinalysis.

    2. Thyroid function test and PKU.

    3. PKU and alpha-fetoprotein.

    4. Glucose and thyroid function tests.

172. The family nurse practitioner notes an undescended testicle on a newborn. She understands that testicular function and the ability to produce healthy sperm as an adult may be impaired if the repair is not made by age:

    1. 6 years.

    2. 2 years.

    3. 1 year.

    4. 6 months.

173. The family nurse practitioner is examining a full-term infant who developed physiologic jaundice and is being treated with phototherapy. What is the mechanism of action of phototherapy in the treatment of this infant?

1. The light is absorbed by bilirubin and promotes the conversion of a toxic bilirubin to an unconjugated product that can be excreted in the bile.

2. It increases hemolysis of the excessive red blood cells that are received by the full-term infant during labor and delivery.

3. The ultraviolet light decreases sensitivity to the destruction of red blood cells secondary to the Rh incompatibility.

4. It increases enzymatic activity in breaking down the unconjugated bilirubin to a nontoxic form to be eliminated by the kidney.

174. A 4-day-old infant who is being breast-fed begins to develop jaundice. What is a common theory regarding the precipitating cause of this jaundice?

    1. Decreased intake in the first few days and the subsequent weight loss.

    2. Decreased tolerance and digestion of the breast milk.

    3. Increased destruction of red blood cells with release of bilirubin.

    4. Antigen–antibody reaction that increases destruction of fetal red blood cells.

175. Which infant is at an increased risk for development of "bronze baby syndrome"?

    1. Premature infant with ABO incompatibility.

    2. Asian infant who is bottle-fed.

    3. Caucasian infant who is breast-fed.

    4. Presence of obstructive liver disease.

176. A mother brings her 6-week-old infant to the office with concern over the child's "constant crying." She states she did not have this problem with her other two children. She is bottle-feeding the infant, and there is no problem with feeding. The infant has a bowel movement every day, and the stools are soft. The infant is afebrile with no evidence of ear, throat, lung, or abdominal problems. What is the best diagnosis for this infant?

    1. Infantile colic.

    2. Spastic colon.

    3. Infant stress syndrome.

    4. Lactose intolerance.

177. The family nurse practitioner suspects infantile colic in a 2-month-old infant. A complete physical examination reveals no abnormalities. What further study might the family nurse practitioner order?

    1. Chest radiograph.

    2. CBC and differential.

    3. Blood culture.

    4. None of the above.

178. The family nurse practitioner is discussing with the parents the care of their 1-month-old infant, who has been diagnosed with infantile colic. What is important to explain to the parents?

    1. The problem may be decreased by not feeding the infant more often than every 3 hours.

    2. No specific medication is indicated to treat the problem.

    3. The problem is often related to increased stress in the home; family therapy may be indicated.

    4. The formula should be changed from a milk-based to a soy-based formula.

179. The family nurse practitioner is assessing an infant who was delivered by cesarean section. What is a complication frequently associated with cesarean delivery?

    1. Increased levels of serum bilirubin.

    2. Respiratory distress.

    3. Meconium aspiration.

    4. Hypoglycemia.

180. The family nurse practitioner is assessing an infant's respiratory status immediately after birth. Breath sounds are normal, no retractions present, acrocyanosis present, respirations of 70 breaths/min and irregular with 5-second periods of apnea, pulse regular at 160 beats/min, and first and second heart sounds normal with no murmurs. What is the initial interpretation of these findings?

    1. Normal newborn findings for immediately after birth.

    2. Symptoms suggestive of respiratory distress syndrome.

    3. Increased probability of neonatal asphyxia.

    4. Presence of choanal atresia.

181. The family nurse practitioner is performing a new-born assessment on a full-term infant approximately 6 hours after birth. When evaluating the infant's head, the family nurse practitioner identifies an edematous area that crosses the cranial suture lines, is soft, and varies with size. The cranial suture lines have minimal space between them. What is the family nurse practitioner's interpretation of these findings?

    1. A cephalhematoma is present.

    2. The cranial suture lines indicate premature closing.

    3. Molding of the infant's head is present.

    4. A caput succedaneum is present.

182. The nurse is evaluating an infant 8 hours after delivery. The infant was full term, weighed 10 lb at birth, and is being breast-fed. The mother has a history of gestational diabetes during the pregnancy. What findings indicate the need for further evaluation?

    1. Blood glucose of 50 mg/dL with glucose screening strips.

    2. Respirations of 70 breaths/min, tremors, and jitteriness.

    3. Bilirubin level 3 mg/dL.

    4. No passage of meconium stool.

183. The family nurse practitioner is assessing a postpartum patient about 12 hours after delivery. On assessment of the uterus, at what position would the family nurse practitioner expect to palpate the uterus?

    1. At the level of the umbilicus.

    2. Two fingerbreadths below the umbilicus.

    3. About 2 cm above the umbilicus.

    4. Three fingerbreadths above the symphysis pubis.

Mental Health

184. A child is being evaluated for ADHD. Which test is helpful in evaluating the difference between ADHD and a learning disability?

    1. Standardized IQ achievement test.

    2. Denver Developmental Screening Test.

    3. Audiologic and visual testing.

    4. Complete neurologic examination.

185. While taking a history, the family nurse practitioner is aware that the following drug is most commonly first used by an adolescent:

    1. Nicotine.

    2. Alcohol.

    3. Marijuana.

    4. Crystal methamphetamine.

186. A mother brings her young child to the clinic, stating she fell off the porch swing. What assessment finding would cause the family nurse practitioner to consider the possibility of child abuse?

    1. Mother is very upset and stroking her daughter's hair.

    2. Child is crying and says her head and arm hurt.

    3. Child has red-, blue-, and green-colored bruised areas on her trunk.

    4. Child has a bruised, edematous area on forehead and shoulder.

187. In evaluating a 16-year-old female patient, which symptom would indicate anorexia nervosa?

    1. Refuses to discuss questions pertaining to food.

    2. Reflects a positive body image.

    3. States she is eating very well but has episodes of vomiting.

    4. The family states she refuses to stop her severe dieting.

188. A mother is concerned about her child having nightmares. The family nurse practitioner understands the difference between nightmares and night terrors is:

    1. Nightmares are vivid, frightening dreams recalled by the child.

    2. Nightmares rarely occur in children before age 4.

    3. Nightmares are accompanied by gross motor movements, labored breathing, and enuresis.

    4. Nightmares and night terrors are essentially the same and are unrelated to stressful events.

189. A 16-year-old adolescent boy is 54 inches in height. The family nurse practitioner identifies the following as a positive, effective coping behavior:

    1. Acts as the class clown.

    2. Has a rehearsed reply to teasing comments.

    3. Spends most of his free time watching television.

    4. Has predominantly friends who are short statured.

190. The family nurse practitioner is examining an older adolescent who has been a long-term intravenous cocaine user. What other findings would alert the family nurse practitioner to a frequent complication?

    1. Epistaxis and chronic rhinorrhea.

    2. Cardiac arrhythmias and hypertension.

    3. Chest congestion and wheezing.

    4. Hepatitis and cellulitis.

191. The family nurse practitioner is comparing the typical signs of depression in the adolescent with the adult patient. The depressed adolescent would present with:

    1. Lonely feelings.

    2. Sad, flat affect.

    3. Anger and acting-out behavior.

    4. Feelings of powerlessness and anxiety.

192. The effects of prenatal cocaine exposure on newborns include:

    1. Increased incidence of prematurity.

    2. Large for gestational age.

    3. Caput succedaneum.

    4. Hypotonia and lethargy.

193. While interviewing a teenager to determine her level of health, the family nurse practitioner recognizes symptoms of anorexia nervosa. Which characteristics of anorexia nervosa would be noted in the admission assessment interview?

    1. Below-to-average intelligence.

    2. Increased libido.

    3. Vigorous daily exercise.

    4. Tachycardia.

194. The family nurse practitioner expects a preschool child with ADHD to have:

    1. Delayed growth and development, especially language skills.

    2. Negativism, overactivity, and active curiosity.

    3. Diminished fine motor skills and frequent mood swings.

    4. Easy distractibility, impulsiveness, and fidgeting.

195. The family nurse practitioner is completing a history and physical exam on a child who she suspects may be autistic. Findings associated with autism include:

    1. Delay in language development.

    2. Delay in physical growth.

    3. Overprotective parents who provide minimal social interaction for the child.

    4. Warm, cuddling child with excessive need for interaction.

196. The mother of a preschooler is concerned because her child has begun to stutter. The family nurse practitioner should:

    1. Refer the child to a speech pathologist.

    2. Encourage the mother to correct the child when she stutters.

    3. Give the child verbal exercises to perform at home.

    4. Reassure the mother that stuttering is normal in a preschooler.

197. A teenage female patient is brought to the family nurse practitioner for evaluation by her grandmother with whom she lives. The teenager has been vomiting and her grandmother believes that she is becoming confused. The grandmother relates that the patient has been upset lately over a breakup with her boyfriend. What will the family nurse practitioner investigate as a possible cause for the teenager's symptoms?

    1. Appendicitis.

    2. Ectopic pregnancy.

    3. Drug overdose.

    4. Sexually transmitted disease.

198. A teenager comes to the office of the family nurse practitioner and states that she was raped several hours ago by her boyfriend. The immediate action taken by the family nurse practitioner is:

    1. Perform a pelvic examination to determine injuries to the patient.

    2. Accompany her to the emergency department for an exam.

    3. Send her immediately for counseling to help her deal with this situation.

    4. Call the patient's parents so they can be with her.

199. The parents of a 7-year-old boy ask advice regarding sugar intake, stating the teacher has said not to allow the child to have any sugar products, such as cookies at lunch, because of behavior problems. Advice would include:

    1. The child needs further assessment for ADHD.

    2. Moderate sugar consumption rarely produces inappropriate behavior.

    3. Increase the protein and fat in his diet to decrease nerve overstimulation.

    4. Research has shown increased sugar intake directly affects cognitive performance.

200. What condition of a child would the family nurse practitioner identify as most likely to be the result of abuse?

    1. Concussion in a 4-year-old.

    2. Fractured wrist in a 6-year-old.

    3. Femur fracture in a 6-month-old.

    4. Scald burn on the arm of a 1-year-old.

201. While interviewing an adolescent female presenting with her mother for birth control counseling and examination, you detect signs of family tension. During the physical exam, while the mother is out of the room, the daughter admits to frequent marijuana use and occasional drinking. What assessment information would most confirm the presence of active or potential violence in the home?

    1. Signs of general neglect.

    2. Injuries at different stages of healing.

    3. Patient's response to a direct question.

    4. Admitted fear of mother's boyfriend.

202. The family nurse practitioner's physical exam on an adolescent is as follows: disheveled appearance, 5-lb weight loss since the last visit 2 months ago, pulse strong and regular at 128, 4+ deep tendon reflexes (DTRs), nasal mucosa erythematous and ulcerated. His mother relates that he has been getting in trouble at school, avoids the family, has no appetite, and is not sleeping much at night. The family nurse practitioner suspects drug use of:

    1. Heroin.

    2. Marijuana.

    3. LSD.

    4. Cocaine.

Endocrine

1. Answer: 4

Rationale: All these contribute significantly to difficulty controlling diabetes in the teenage years. Hormonal changes and the desire to become independent increase emotional conflicts. Teens have a great desire to be like their peers and do not want to be regimented in following a specific diet and adhering to a treatment plan.

2. Answer: 3

Rationale: Thyroid replacement is lifelong maintenance therapy and should be given as one dose in the morning. Weight loss, diarrhea, and tachycardia are signs of overmedication.

3. Answer: 4

Rationale: No consensus exists on adapting glycemic goals in the pediatric population. The goals for glucose control must be individualized with each family based on the child's age and ability to recognize symptoms of hypoglycemia and a past history of hypoglycemia or seizures.

4. Answer: 1

Rationale: This is the best choice for the initial examination because the history may reveal normal variation in pattern of growth related to race, heredity, size of other family members, and psychosocial status. Skeletal maturation ("bone age") can be assessed through radiography if child is in the fifth-growth percentile or lower. Other choices are inappropriate without history and physical exam, and growth hormone would not be administered without lab evaluation.

5. Answer: 3

Rationale: Pubertal (physiologic) gynecomastia is a visible or palpable glandular enlargement of the male breast that can occur in healthy adolescents. Typically the breasts are unequal in size and may be tender; nipples are often irritated from rubbing against clothing; and Tanner stages II–IV of pubertal development are noted. The symptoms of lymphadenopathy, goiter, asymmetrical testes, and repaired hypospadias are associated with pathologic gynecomastia.

6. Answer: 2

Rationale: Hyperthyroidism in children most often affects girls and is an autoimmune disorder (Graves' disease) in which the body produces antibodies that stimulate TSH receptors, causing overproduction of thyroid hormones and goiter. Hypothyroidism is associated with iodine deficiency.

7. Answer: 4

Rationale: These findings are consistent with Turner's syndrome: short stature, gonadal dysgenesis, lymphedema (usually appearing in infancy), left-sided heart or aortic abnormalities, primary amenorrhea, and delayed onset of puberty. Fragile X syndrome is an inherited condition usually affecting males and characterized by a long, narrow face and prominent ears, mild to profound mental retardation, hyperactivity and poor attention span, and autistic-type behavior. Marfan's syndrome is a connective tissue disorder of tall and thin adolescents that is characterized by long limbs, narrow hands, long, slender fingers, and nearsightedness. Klinefelter's syndrome is characterized by small testes, sterility, gynecomastia, and long legs.

8. Answer: 4

Rationale: Hypogonadism, associated with delayed sexual development, sexual infantilism, and small testes, is most often the contributing factor to growth retardation after age 10 years for girls and 12 years for boys. Other causes of decelerated growth or short stature include hypothyroidism, diabetes, and hypopituitarism. Chromosomal abnormalities would be noted at an earlier age.

9. Answer: 3

Rationale: Most children have a target goal to maintain blood sugar at 80–140 mg/dL if they can recognize the symptoms of hypoglycemia. A blood glucose of 60–75 mg/dL is too low and may predispose the child to hypoglycemia. The other options are too high.

10. Answer: 1

Rationale: Type 1 diabetes usually (but not always) appears before age 30 and is heralded by the three "P's": polydipsia, polyuria, and polyphagia.

11. Answer: 4

Rationale: Tight glycemic control is contraindicated in infants <2 years of age and should be instituted with extreme caution in children <7 years of age to avoid injuring the developing brain.

12. Answer: 1

Rationale: Infants with hypothyroidism often have an abnormally pitched cry because of lethargy and delayed mental responsiveness. Hypertelorism does not produce an abnormal cry unless accompanied by microcephaly.

13. Answer: 3

Rationale: A low temperature and pulse, constipation, and fatigue are all signs of hypothyroidism; therefore, the dose of levothyroxine needs to be increased. Levothyroxine toxicity would manifest with signs of hyperthyroidism. Constipation is a symptom of hypothyroidism and is not related to the child's fluid intake. Congenital hypothyroidism requires lifelong drug therapy.

Hematology

14. Answer: 4

Rationale: This clinical presentation would make the family nurse practitioner consider the diagnosis of leukemia, necessitating a workup. CBC with differential, along with platelet count (indicators of bone marrow function), is the diagnostic approach for leukemia. Further testing may be necessary, but the workup should always include a CBC.

15. Answer: 1

Rationale: The findings associated with iron-deficiency anemia include low mean corpuscular volume (MCV), decreased hemoglobin/hematocrit, and low reticulocyte count. Elevated MCV is associated with macrocytic anemias (e.g., pernicious anemia).

16. Answer: 4

Rationale: Dolls and puppets are effective teaching tools for the preschool child. Using the doll reflects the child's understanding of the procedure. Children will often withdraw and appear calm when they have feelings of anxiety.

17. Answer: 3

Rationale: Early presenting symptoms of acute lymphocytic leukemia (ALL) include pallor, bleeding, pain, and fever associated with infiltration of the bone marrow of proliferative lymphocytic cells, which ultimately leads to bone marrow failure. The symptoms of splenomegaly, facial rash, cough, expiratory wheezing, bleeding, and hepatomegaly are often found in juvenile chronic myelogenous leukemia (CML). Bone pain, fever, and night sweats are often noted in CML.

18. Answer: 3

Rationale: With iron-deficiency anemia, the amount of oxygen-carrying hemoglobin is reduced. Long-term oxygen deprivation can lead to impaired cognitive and motor development.

Pernicious anemia is associated with lack of intrinsic factor. Crohn's disease has a familial incidence and leads to diarrhea-related problems. The liver and spleen are both involved in RBC production.

19. Answer: 4

Rationale: Sickle cell disease is an autosomal recessive inherited disease transmitted by both parents, who are carriers of the sickle cell trait. Each pregnancy carries a 25% chance of sickle cell disease, a 25% chance of an unaffected child, and a 50% chance of the child carrying the trait.

20. Answer: 3

Rationale: Iron-deficiency anemia is often found in this age group, especially in infants who do not eat a balanced diet that includes foods rich in iron (e.g., iron-fortified cereals). This is a microcytic, hypochromic anemia with a decrease in serum iron (ferritin). Mean corpuscular volume (MCV) would be decreased.

21. Answer: 4

Rationale: The normal, full-term infant is born with sufficient iron stores to prevent iron deficiency for the first 6 months of life.

Urinary/Renal

22. Answer: 2

Rationale: In children, 25%–60% of proteinuria is orthostatic in nature and must be evaluated first.

23. Answer: 2

Rationale: Acute hypertension in children and adolescents is usually caused by an identifiable secondary cause, such as glomerulonephritis, because of a streptococcal infection.

24. Answer: 2

Rationale: The facial edema and increased BP are common. Generally, the child does not have a high fever, and the urine is not concentrated, but it may be decreased in amount.

25. Answer: 2

Rationale: Gross hematuria may occur for 1–2 weeks after the diuresis and microscopic hematuria for up to 2 years. It is essential that parents be educated about poststreptococcal glomerulonephritis to ensure they know what to expect and to ensure that they know what is considered abnormal. Appropriate education will ensure that the parent will know when to notify a health care professional.

26. Answer: 1

Rationale: The family nurse practitioner should contact the pediatrician immediately; this is frequently the first sign of a Wilms' tumor, which can be malignant. Because Wilms' tumor is very fragile, the abdomen should not be examined. The family nurse practitioner should not wait for a referral because the child may not be seen immediately. The family nurse practitioner should contact the pediatrician by telephone to discuss the clinical findings and to arrange for an emergency appointment. A urinalysis (UA) and blood testing can be done, but often these tests are negative.

27. Answer: 1

Rationale: The clinical presentation indicates a urinary tract infection (UTI). The dipstick is positive for bacteria. The child may have had a reaction to sulfisoxazole, so it would be best to avoid sulfa drugs at this time. The other appropriate medication for UTI in children is amoxicillin. Ciprofloxacin is not recommended for children under 18 years old, and clarithromycin is not a first-line drug for UTI.

Cardiac

28. Answer: 2

Rationale: Weak or absent pulses are associated with coarctation of the aorta and are not indicative of the other cardiovascular diseases.

29. Answer: 2

Rationale: A continuous murmur is consistent with patent ductus arteriosus (PDA). The turbulent flow of blood from the aorta through the PDA to the pulmonary artery results in this characteristic murmur. Coarctation presents with upper extremity hypertension, systolic murmur, and weak or absent femoral pulses. Ventricular septal defect is characterized by a loud, harsh, pansystolic murmur heard best at the lower left sternal border. Aortic stenosis has a systolic murmur.

30. Answer: 4

Rationale: Most cases of heart failure (HF) in children result from congenital heart disease, and most occur during the first year of life. Although the clinical presentation of a child with CHD will vary with the specific defect, the clinical manifestations usually relate to the degree of HF or cyanosis.

31. Answer: 3

Rationale: Most cases of heart failure (HF) in infants result from congenital heart disease during the first 12 months of life.

Symptoms result from the decreased cardiac output and the infant's compensatory mechanisms. Symptoms include tachypnea, dyspnea, tachycardia, pallor, and easy fatigability. Additional symptoms include periorbital edema, hepatomegaly, difficult feeding, and persistent cough. Diaphoresis, central cyanosis, and peripheral edema are not necessarily associated with HF but may be manifestations of the underlying congenital heart defect.

32. Answer: 1

Rationale: Congenital heart disease is usually classified as acyanotic or cyanotic. Cyanotic heart defects (right-to-left shunts) include tetralogy of Fallot, severe pulmonary stenosis, pulmonary atresia, tricuspid atresia, and transposition of the great vessels. Children with cyanotic heart disease develop polycythemia to increase the oxygen-carrying capacity of the blood. Additionally, the child with a cyanotic heart defect should have hemoglobin of at least 16 g/dL.

33. Answer: 1

Rationale: Although all these conditions can lead to hypertension, the most common in infants and young children is secondary hypertension because of renal disease (e.g., glomerulonephritis; polycystic kidneys; nephrosis). Endocrine-induced hypertension is the second most common cause.

34. Answer: 1

Rationale: The two major conditions known to play a causative role in the development of cardiovascular disease in children are untreated streptococcal infections involving group A β-hemolytic streptococci (leads to cardiac valve problems) and Kawasaki disease (leads to coronary artery aneurysm).

35. Answer: 4

Rationale: Children with a murmur need to be evaluated further, but affected children are not considered emergencies as long as they are asymptomatic, have normal activity and exercise, and are growing normally. The other options are considered unstable and acute, and these children should be immediately referred to a pediatric cardiologist.

36. Answer: 3

Rationale: Procedures for which endocarditis prophylaxis is recommended include dental procedures known to induce gingival bleeding. It is also recommended for surgical procedures that involve the respiratory mucosa tonsillectomy/adenoidectomy. Endocarditis prophylaxis is not recommended for insertion of tympanostomy tubes, cardiac catheterization, simple dental procedures, or endotracheal intubation.

37. Answer: 4

Rationale: Metal detectors have an electromagnetic field that could alter the pacemaker's function temporarily. In addition, the alarm will be set off as a result of the metal in the pacemaker. For the child with a pacemaker, an electric shock may irreparably damage the pacemaker, and immediate surgical replacement would be necessary. There is no risk of electromagnetic interference between the permanent pacemaker and household items, such as electrical appliances, radios, electronic equipment, cellular phones, or microwave ovens. Ovens and pacemakers have filtering systems that prevent interference with the pacemaker's function.

38. Answer: 1

Rationale: According to the Jones criteria, in addition to two major manifestations (carditis, polyarthritis, Sydenham's chorea, erythema marginatum, and subcutaneous nodules) or one major and two minor manifestations (arthralgia, fever, elevated ESR, C-reactive protein, and prolonged PR interval), a diagnosis of rheumatic fever is highly likely if there is evidence of a previous group A beta-hemolytic streptococcal infection.

Respiratory

39. Answer: 2

Rationale: Sweat chloride test is positive for cystic fibrosis (CF) because of the abnormal amount of sodium chloride in the sweat. Hemoccult is a test for blood in the stool. Sputum culture and sensitivity help determine which medication is effective against an organism. Glucose tolerance test is performed to diagnose diabetes.

40. Answer: 1

Rationale: The child has the symptoms and history that are consistent with a partial airway obstruction from aspiration of a foreign body. Direct laryngoscopy or bronchoscopy is necessary to remove the foreign body. Chest physiotherapy may dislodge the object and force it farther into the airway. Antibiotics and epinephrine will not be effective. There is no need to intubate the infant if the foreign body can be removed.

41. Answer: 4

Rationale: Croup, epiglottitis, and tracheitis are all middle respiratory tract infections with a rapid onset. Bronchiolitis is a lower respiratory tract infection that has a more gradual onset and no "barking" sound to the cough.

42. Answer: 4

Rationale: In cystic fibrosis (CF), the stools are large, bulky, and foul smelling (steatorrhea). Yellow stools are indicative of liver or gallbladder problems. Green stools often indicate a rapid transit time and may be associated with an infection.

43. Answer: 2

Rationale: In children too young to use a peak flow meter properly, the inability to cry or complete a sentence may indicate an acute asthma attack. Obtaining an arterial blood gas (ABG) is usually not performed in office settings, and a chest x-ray will most likely agitate the child and take too long to process.

44. Answer: 1

Rationale: In addition to symptoms of wheezing and rales, infants with tuberculosis (TB) are more likely to develop disseminated disease, such as meningitis, and to have a negative purified protein derivative (PPD) skin test. Usually, the transmission of the disease can be traced to an affected adult living in the household.

45. Answer: 4

Rationale: Maintaining a high-caloric intake is important in the care of infants with bronchopulmonary dysplasia (BPD) to promote growth and nourishment of developing lung tissue. Infants may have gastroesophageal reflux (GER) after feedings. Initially, positioning should be tried, and then feedings may be thickened or given in smaller amounts more frequently. If the problem persists or weight gain is inadequate, referral to a pediatrician is indicated.

46. Answer: 3

Rationale: If the child is up-to-date on immunizations, he should have had his vaccine for *Haemophilus influenzae* type b (Hib), the most common cause of epiglottitis. A dramatic decline in the incidence of epiglottis and *H. influenzae* type b infections is associated closely with the history of Hib vaccines. Considering the age of this child and the suddenness of the onset, the most likely diagnosis is foreign body aspiration.

47. Answer: 4

Rationale: Beta-agonist (albuterol) by MDI is the first line of treatment to decrease airflow obstruction. Aminophylline by mouth would take too long to be effective. Epinephrine is used predominantly for anaphylactic reaction. Beclovent is a steroid inhaler that is most effective when used prophylactically rather than in acute episodes.

48. Answer: 3

Rationale: These are the common drugs used for combination therapy for the treatment of tuberculosis in children.

Rimantadine is an antiviral; pyrimethamine is an antimalarial. Montelukast therapy is not indicated because of the virulence of the tubercle bacillus.

49. Answer: 4

Rationale: Close contacts of patients with an active case of TB should be placed on isoniazid single-drug therapy, even if the tuberculin skin test is negative. This early treatment will destroy the tubercle bacilli before hypersensitivity develops. The isoniazid should be continued for 4 months for those whose skin test remains negative and who show no evidence of disease. If there is a positive skin test conversion, isoniazid (10–20 mg/kg) should be continued for 1 year. If the child develops TB symptoms, he should be given isoniazid and rifampin (10 mg/kg) for 1 year.

50. Answer: 3

Rationale: Rhinitis and a productive cough are common and are not cause for concern unless the mucus begins to change color and is accompanied by a high fever. The wheezes are also common, if the mucus is loose. A high fever and rales indicate further deterioration and possible bacterial infection.

51. Answer: 2

Rationale: Pyridoxine (vitamin B_6) is added to prevent peripheral neuropathy. Foods containing tyramine and histamine (e.g., tuna, aged cheese, yeast, vitamin supplements) cause interaction with monoamine oxidase (MAO) inhibitors. Anorexia, jaundice, malaise, and fatigue would be signs of hepatic involvement.

52. Answer: 1

Rationale: Bronchodilators are strongly discouraged in current evidence-based bronchiolitis guidelines. Antibiotics and antihistamines are not effective and should not be used. The condition is usually treated symptomatically. If the child does not improve, consult a physician.

53. Answer: 1

Rationale: Medications should be taken only when the child is planning to exercise and anticipates respiratory difficulty. Cromolyn and beclomethasone are steroids and do not provide immediate relief. Theophylline should be avoided unless symptoms progressively worsen and cannot be controlled with inhalation therapy.

Immune and Allergy

54. Answer: 3

Rationale: A positive purified protein derivative (PPD) for an immunocompetent child is 15 mm. A child who is HIV positive, immunocompromised, or exposed to an active case of TB is considered positive at 5 mm. The child (<4 years of age) who has chronic disease or has been exposed to HIV-positive individuals or persons born in a foreign country is considered positive at 10 mm.

55. Answer: 2

Rationale: The typical allergic facies consists of allergic "shiners" (black eyes), Dennie-Morgan lines (extra crease below the lower eyelids), and mouth breathing. Nasal polyps are uncommon in childhood allergic rhinitis. The nasal discharge with allergies is usually clear.

56. Answer: 3

Rationale: In adolescent and through adult atopic dermatitis, common sites are the popliteal and anticubital fossae, face, neck, upper arms and back, dorsa of the hand, feet, fingers, and toes.

57. Answer: 2

Rationale: Epinephrine would be the first-line drug to be injected for the treatment of the respiratory distress associated with an anaphylactic reaction. The dose for epinephrine (1:1000, SC) is 0.01 mL/kg for a child and 0.3–0.5 mL/kg for an adult. The onset of action of Benadryl is not fast enough. Lidocaine would only topically treat the pain and not the respiratory problem. Anti-inflammatory drugs would not be given initially but may be given later, if needed, for generalized discomfort or pain at the sting site.

58. Answer: 4

Rationale: Although both diphenhydramine, brompheniramine, and chlorpheniramine are antihistamines and could be prescribed, loratadine would have less central nervous system (CNS)-sedating effects.

59. Answer: 3

Rationale: Although diphenhydramine could be administered for itching after the child's distress is relieved, the immediate concern is to prevent respiratory arrest from swelling of the throat's mucosa. The usual epinephrine dose for children is 0.01 mL/kg of the 1:1000 solution.

60. Answer: 3

Rationale: The most common food allergy worldwide is cow's milk, with egg and peanut as second and third most common, respectively. Wheat allergy is in the top eight of food allergens, but milk must be ruled out first through an elimination diet. Dust mite and internal mold allergy as an inhalant trigger is unlikely in this age group and may be present by 4 or 5 years of age.

61. Answer: 4

Rationale: Type IV hypersensitivity reactions are delayed hypersensitivity disorders with symptoms that start after 1 day of exposure, such as with poison ivy contact; symptoms are not immediate. Flowering plants are nonallergenic because their pollen is heavy and spread by insects, not the wind as in grass and tree and weed pollen. Tree and grass pollen results in a type I hypersensitivity reaction that is immediate on exposure, resulting in atopic dermatitis, allergic rhinitis, asthma, or urticaria.

HEENT

62. Answer: 3

Rationale: Dental fluorosis causes surface pitting and staining, especially to the central and lateral permanent incisors. Tetracycline would have caused staining of all the teeth. Dental caries would be more indicative of poor dental hygiene. "Baby teeth," not the permanent teeth, would be affected by going to bed with a bottle.

63. Answer: 4

Rationale: A 4-year-old's normal acuity is 20/40; therefore, none of the other answers are appropriate.

64. Answer: 4

Rationale: Strabismus (malaligned eyes) can be a precursor for amblyopia (decreased visual acuity). It is important to detect strabismus as early as possible in preschool children. Checking pupils and assessing for double vision (diplopia) are components of a neurologic assessment. Tonometry exams are performed to assess for glaucoma.

65. Answer: 3

Rationale: Pure-tone audiometry is appropriate after age 3 years; 0–25 dB = normal, 26–40 dB = mild hearing loss, and 41–55 dB = moderate hearing loss.

66. Answer: 3

Rationale: Low-set or obliquely set ears occur more frequently in children who also have genitourinary defects. None of the other defects is associated with low-set ears.

67. Answer: 3

Rationale: Enlarged tonsils are common in young children. As the child grows older, the tonsils recede in size. Only about 25%–30% of tonsillitis is caused by the β-hemolytic streptococcus. Having large tonsils does not make a child more prone to tonsillitis.

68. Answer: 2

Rationale: The patient in this situation had risk factors (age) and symptoms of mononucleosis, so the monospot or heterophile antibody test should be conducted. The classic triad of mononucleosis symptoms includes sore throat, fever, and posterior cervical lymphadenopathy with or without mild tenderness. Rapid screening for streptococcal infection can be done from throat swab with antigen agglutination kits and would be obtained first, but it would probably be negative. WBC count would be ordered for bacterial pharyngitis; an increased WBC is found with bacterial infection and a decreased WBC with viral agents.

69. Answer: 2

Rationale: A fluoridated dentifrice should be used in a small amount (pea size), and children under 6 should be supervised so that they do not swallow too much toothpaste, which would put them at risk for fluorosis. The dose of fluoride rinse is too high, and it is inappropriate to prescribe to a preschooler. Bottled water does not contain fluoride. Topical application, although appropriate, is not the best answer.

70. Answer: 3

Rationale: Generalized, diffuse swelling and erythema of the eyelid are associated with an insect bite. Blepharitis is a chronic inflammatory condition characterized by erythema and scaling of the lid margins. Hordeolum, or stye, is an acute, purulent inflammation of the sebaceous glands (usually the glands of Zeis or meibomian glands) of the eyelids and usually does not involve the entire eyelid. It may be painful, especially over the gland. Dacryocystitis is an inflammation of the lacrimal sac that is characterized by erythema and swelling over the lacrimal duct.

71. Answer: 1

Rationale: Nasolacrimal obstruction occurs in up to 6% of infants. Signs and symptoms include a wet eye with mucoid discharge. Irritated skin and conjunctivitis also may be associated with this condition. There is no redness, which would suggest conjunctivitis. Congenital dacryocystocele presents at birth as a bluish subcutaneous mass. There would be more signs of irritation and pain with a corneal abrasion.

72. Answer: 1

Rationale: Strabismus is not an uncommon or abnormal occurrence in infants up until 3 months of age.

73. Answer: 4

Rationale: Classic signs of bacterial conjunctivitis include those symptoms listed along with complaints of eyelids being "glued shut" on awakening. Severe itching, moderate tearing, and minimal discharge symptoms are indicative of allergic conjunctivitis. Minimal itching, moderate tearing, and mucoid exudate symptoms are indicative of viral conjunctivitis.

74. Answer: 4

Rationale: Steroid (dexamethasone) medications are not used to treat nasolacrimal obstruction in infancy. Because of the yellow discharge in the eye, it would be appropriate to prescribe an antibiotic to prevent or treat conjunctivitis. Cleansing the eye with warm water and massaging the lacrimal duct are both appropriate interventions.

75. Answer: 1

Rationale: The diagnosis of acute otitis media (AOM) is clinical, made by otoscopy based on the appearance of the tympanic membrane (TM). The bony landmarks are absent or decreased. The TM may be full, bulging, or retracted, with pus, and the light reflex is distorted. A pneumatic otoscopy reveals decreased or absent TM mobility. Erythema is an inconclusive finding, especially in children, because the redness may be caused by crying rather than infection.

76. Answer: 4

Rationale: The patient has the clinical findings of otitis externa, an inflammation and infection of the external ear canal predisposed by excessive wetness, such as swimming. Common organisms responsible for otitis externa include *Pseudomonas aeruginosa, Proteus mirabilis,* and *Enterobacter aerogenes* or fungal organisms of the *Aspergillus or Candida* species. Sinusitis clinical findings focus on sinus tenderness and a purulent nasal discharge. Clinical findings of otitis media include ear pain, full or bulging tympanic membrane, decreased or negative mobility, and possible erythema. Findings associated with serous otitis media include opaque or translucent tympanic membrane with air bubbles; landmarks may be absent, and the light reflex may be diffuse or absent.

77. Answer: 1

Rationale: Acute otitis media (AOM) occurs more during the fall, winter, and spring than summer. American Indians and Eskimos have more repetitive and severe otitis media than members of other races. Children who attend daycare centers have more frequent infections than those who do not. Members of lower socioeconomic levels are more at risk than those at higher levels. Other risk factors are children who live with many siblings or in homes with smokers, children who have developmental abnormalities, and male gender.

78. Answer: 3

Rationale: The patient with otitis externa, "swimmer's ear," or inflammation of the external auditory canal presents with ear pain. The most common clinical findings include redness and swelling of the external ear canal, pain with manipulation of movement of auricle, no swelling or pain over mastoid, and usually no involvement of the tympanic membrane (TM). The TM is involved in acute otitis media (AOM). No evidence indicated that the child placed a foreign body in the ear. The most significant distinction between otitis media with effusion (OME) and AOM is that clinical findings of acute infection (e.g., fever, otalgia) are lacking in OME. Clinical findings of OME, the most common cause of hearing loss in children, include relatively asymptomatic, decreased mobility, and bulging, opaque TM with no visible landmarks.

79. Answer: 3

Rationale: Transmission of cold viruses is indirect (e.g., self-inoculation from virus on surfaces of inanimate objects to mucous membranes of nose and mouth). Virus is less likely to be spread by the aerosol route. Thus, the patient should avoid touching the nose and mouth unless the hands have been thoroughly washed. It is impractical to avoid contact because cold viruses are found everywhere. Although many individuals believe vitamin C prevents colds, research to support this claim is minimal.

80. Answer: 4

Rationale: Amoxicillin with clavulanic acid is effective against beta-lactamase production. Cephalexin, cefuroxime, or cefixime can be used as alternatives. Erythromycin-sulfisoxazole has recently been reported as less effective. Cephalosporins are effective against beta-lactamase production by *Haemophilus influenzae* and *Moraxella catarrhalis.* Amoxicillin is ineffective against beta-lactamase production, as is penicillin V.

81. Answer: 3

Rationale: The recommended treatment for otitis media in a child is amoxicillin 75–90 mg/kg/day, or, for this child (18 kg), 250 mg/5 mL, 2.75 tsp bid × 10 days. The other drugs and doses listed are not appropriate treatment for acute otitis media (AOM).

82. Answer: 4

Rationale: The patient is experiencing symptoms of moderately severe acute sinusitis based on the symptoms of facial pressure, headache, and postnasal discharge. The first-line antibiotic to prescribe is amoxicillin/clavulanate for its safety and efficacy. Oral antihistamines, such as diphenhydramine, should not be used unless the patient has allergies. Oral decongestants (pseudoephedrine) are not as effective in patients with sinusitis as are topical agents. Erythromycin is not a first-line antibiotic for sinusitis.

Integumentary

83. Answer: 4

Rationale: This best describes Mongolian spots, which are characteristic in newborns of African, Asian, or Latin descent. When closely evaluated, these spots do not resemble the ecchymoses that occur with trauma. Telangiectatic nevi are commonly known as "stork bites" and are deep-pink lesions most often found on the back of the neck. Cutis marmorata is the transient mottling that occurs when an infant is cold.

84. Answer: 1

Rationale: The location and appearance of the lesions are typical of scabies: short, irregular "runs" that are approximately 2–3 mm long and the width of a hair.

85. Answer: 1

Rationale: Food allergies and other causative triggers should be identified and avoided. Excessive bathing dries the skin, which irritates the atopic dermatitis. Bubble baths can irritate skin, as can sweating.

86. Answer: 2

Rationale: This is the correct procedure for the permethrin cream rinse. After rinsing, remove nits with a nit comb. Repeat shampoo treatment after 7 days if living lice are still observed. Clothing and bedding should be washed or dry-cleaned.

87. Answer: 2

Rationale: Nonintentional scalding is usually splash-related and occurs on the front of the body. The family nurse practitioner should be suspicious of any burns on the back of the body or any well-defined, uniform burn areas on the buttocks or extremities, which may indicate physical abuse. Immersion burns on the buttocks may be seen as punishment for toileting or wetting "accidents."

88. Answer: 3

Rationale: The cornstarch or Aveeno baths will temporarily help relieve the itching, followed by application of a heavy cream emollient (the thicker and greasier the emollient, the more effective). The shorts and short-sleeved shirt would expose too much skin, which would be scratched by the infant. Wool irritates the skin. Salt would also be an irritant.

89. Answer: 3

Rationale: The most common treatment is observation because most hemangiomas resolve over time, usually beginning about 18 months of age. The other treatments may be performed, especially for hemangiomas proliferating rapidly.

90. Answer: 2

Rationale: Infantile atopic dermatitis, as contrasted to atopic dermatitis in older children and adolescents, is a moist, oozing, crusting pruritic rash found mainly on the extensor surfaces of the body and the face. It usually begins about 2 months of age, often with a family history of atopy.

91. Answer: 1

Rationale: In prepubertal children, café-au-lait spots larger than 1 cm and present in more than 5 areas are a concern and may be associated with neurofibromatosis. The child should be referred to a pediatrician for further evaluation.

92. Answer: 1

Rationale: Seborrheic dermatitis is usually salmon in color and has a yellowish, greasy appearance. It occurs in infants under 6 months of age. It does not itch. The distribution is mainly to the face, postauricular scalp, axillae, and groin. Rashes in atopic dermatitis and eczema are pink, or red if inflamed, and have a whiter, nongreasy appearance. Rash may begin at 2–12 months and continues through childhood and is associated with a family history of allergy. Itching may be severe. The distribution is to the cheeks, trunk, and extensors of extremities. Erythema toxicum consists of yellow or white papules on the face. It occurs in 30%–50% of term infants and disappears in 2 weeks.

93. Answer: 3

Rationale: Given the distribution of the rash, the most likely cause is a contact dermatitis, such as that caused by the use of baby wipes. Allergy to disposable diapers would involve the entire diaper area. Seborrheic dermatitis presents as large, confluent, sharply marginated bright plaque on the anterior surface of the groin. Candidal rashes are bright red with satellite lesions that involve the deep folds and may spread to the entire diaper area.

94. Answer: 2

Rationale: Impetigo presents with honey-colored crusted lesions with an erythematous base. Staphylococci and group A beta-hemolytic streptococci are important pathogens in this disease. Scabies presents with linear burrows about the wrists, ankles, finger webs, anterior axillary folds, genitals, or face (in infants). Pityriasis rosea presents as erythematous papules that coalesce to form oval plaques preceded by a large oval plaque with central clearing and a scaly border (the herald patch). Varicella (chickenpox) presents as crops of red macules that rapidly become tiny vesicles with surrounding erythema that form pustules. The pustules become crusted, and then scabs form. The rash appears predominantly on the trunk and face.

95. Answer: 4

Rationale: After a course of antibiotics, the normal flora is destroyed, making the child a prime target for *Candida albicans*. The classic signs of a yeast infection include a beefy red, sharply marginated, maculopapular rash with satellite lesions. Poor hygiene and a contact dermatitis would present as erythema and thickening of the skin in the perianal area. Seborrheic dermatitis consists of an erythematous, scaly dermatitis, accompanied by overproduction of sebum in areas rich in sebaceous glands (face, scalp, and perineum).

96. Answer: 2

Rationale: Atopic dermatitis typically presents in the flexural areas of children. The lesions are characteristically erythematous and papular, with scales and pruritus often noted. A personal or family history of atopy is noted in about 70% of patients with atopic dermatitis. Scabies lesions appear as gray or skin-colored ridges, vesicles, and papules. Tinea corporis lesions are generally distributed over the body and face, with an area of clearing in the center of the lesion. Contact dermatitis usually produces vesicular lesions in the shape of the object causing the reaction.

97. Answer: 3

Rationale: Any bite potentially associated with an animal that may harbor rabies (skunks, bats, raccoons, foxes, coyotes, and rats) should be treated with both active and passive rabies immunization. Tetanus antitoxin would be indicated if the patient was not current on the immunization. Animal authorities would be called after the initial treatment to locate the animal and sacrifice it, so that the brain could be examined for rabies.

98. Answer: 4

Rationale: Brown recluse spiders produce sharp pain at the instant of the bite, with subsequent minor swelling and erythema. Tissue necrosis may occur within the next few hours. A blue-gray to black macular halo may surround the bite, with eventual widening and sinking of the center of the lesion, leading to a "sinking infarct." This leaves a deep ulcer that requires weeks or months to heal.

99. Answer: 2

Rationale: Deep puncture wounds are more likely to become infected with anaerobic organisms. The narrow, sharp feline incisors deeply puncture tissue and may easily penetrate a bone or joint. Bites on the hand have the highest infection rate, whereas bites on the face have the lowest rate.

100. Answer: 1

Rationale: Amoxicillin-clavulanate is an excellent choice for the empiric treatment of animal bites. Cephalexin is not indicated because of resistant strains of *Pasteurella multocida,* an organism present in 25% of dog bites and 50% of cat bites. An infected bite should be followed up daily until the infection clears. Open wound management is indicated, not suturing.

101. Answer: 4

Rationale: In addition to these symptoms, bronchospasm, hypertension, seizures, and altered mental status may occur. Black eschar is associated with a brown recluse spider bite.

Childhood Diseases

102. Answer: 2

Rationale: Erythema multiforme is a major side effect of sulfa drug use that presents with a sudden onset of high fever, weakness, blisters, bulla, and ulcerations of the mucous membranes. Kawasaki disease presents with a more diffuse erythematous rash. Viral exanthems are centrally located and do not resemble blisters. Scalded-skin syndrome is staphylococcal in origin and causes the skin to peel off and turn bright red.

103. Answer: 2

Rationale: The incubation period for erythema infectiosum is 4–14 days, with communicability until the rash appears.

104. Answer: 1

Rationale: The symptoms are indicative of coxsackievirus 5 or 16 group A (usually A16), called hand-foot-and-mouth disease. The lesions may appear in one or all three areas. Children are usually uncomfortable, but not seriously ill, and may refuse fluids with severe oral lesions. Varicella lesions begin on the trunk with classic "teardrop" vesicles.

105. Answer: 1

Rationale: In roseola, an erythematous, maculopapular rash appears on the trunk after abrupt onset of fever and spreads to the extremities, neck, and face. It fades within 24 hours. The pink maculopapular rash of rubella begins on the face and spreads down the trunk. Often the facial rash will disappear as the rash erupts on the extremities, clearing in 3–5 days.

106. Answer: 2

Rationale: The primary treatment for roseola is supportive, including control of fever, adequate rest, and hydration. No preventive measure or immunization is available.

107. Answer: 4

Rationale: Systemic antibiotics (e.g., tetracycline) offer the most effective treatment in inflammatory acne. Isotretinoin is also very effective, but, because of serious teratogenic side effects, it is not first-line treatment. Improvement in acne will not be noted for 4–8 weeks, and dietary changes have not been demonstrated to have any beneficial effect.

108. Answer: 2

Rationale: The appearance is indicative of *Candida albicans,* which is best treated with nystatin. The other choices would aggravate the diaper rash by promoting overhydration.

109. Answer: 3

Rationale: The child's lesions are characteristic of impetigo and should be treated with an antibiotic if present on the face; amoxicillin-clavulanate (Augmentin) is considered the first-line medication. The ointment, soaking, and Benadryl will not stop the spread of the infection, which could lead to post-streptococcal glomerulonephritis.

110. Answer: 4

Rationale: Varicella (chickenpox) should be treated symptomatically unless the child is at high risk secondary to other medical problems. Acyclovir is not recommended for routine treatment of uncomplicated varicella. The current bathing therapy is with colloidal oatmeal products, taking preference over the traditional baking soda baths. Impetigo usually occurs on the face and neck with no diffuse lesions over the trunk. Contact dermatitis is characterized by erythema and scaling, possibly with weeping vesicles. The area of distribution of rash offers clues to diagnosis.

111. Answer: 4

Rationale: Permethrin 5% cream is used in infants but is not recommended in those under 2 months of age. Bacitracin could be used to treat secondary infections but would not help eradicate the scabies. Mycitracin is also not effective for the treatment of scabies. Acitretin is used for the treatment of psoriasis.

112. Answer: 3

Rationale: Impetigo is communicable until the patient has been on antibiotic therapy for 48 hours. Washing clothing and linens separately with hot water is recommended, along with

surveillance of close contacts for the appearance of lesions. Isolation is not necessary, except to keep the child home from school until 48 hours of antibiotic therapy has been completed. Amoxicillin-clavulanate (Augmentin) is the most effective antibiotic. Gentle washing is recommended to keep the lesions clean and to prevent scarring (potentially caused by vigorous scrubbing).

113. Answer: 4

Rationale: Because isotretinoin is extremely teratogenic, sexual assessment and pregnancy testing (as appropriate) and contraceptive counseling should be done for all patients. The combination of alcohol and isotretinoin can cause a disulfuram-like reaction, so alcohol should be avoided. Isotretinoin can cause photosensitivity, so the family nurse practitioner should counsel the patient to avoid sunlight, wear protective clothing and sunglasses, and apply sunscreen to all sun-exposed areas that are without acne. No conclusive relationship between diet and acne has been established.

114. Answer: 4

Rationale: An age-appropriate dose of activated charcoal (1 g/kg of body weight) would be indicated. Gastric lavage may be of little benefit if used later than 1 hour after ingestion.

115. Answer: 1

Rationale: Tinnitus and nausea are toxic symptoms of salicylate poisoning. Fruity odor to the breath is usually associated with diabetic ketoacidosis.

Musculoskeletal

116. Answer: 1

Rationale: The child should remove her shirt (leave on bra or swimsuit top) and bend at the waist. The family nurse practitioner should examine for uneven hips and shoulders.

117. Answer: 3

Rationale: Typical findings include Ortolani's (hip click) sign, limited abduction, shortening of the extremity on the affected side, and asymmetric gluteal folds. The lax hamstrings allow for full extension of the hip when the knee is fully flexed.

118. Answer: 1

Rationale: Osgood-Schlatter disease (tibial tubercle apophysitis) is characterized by a painful, self-limiting tibial tubercle swelling that leads to knee pain, especially during periods of rapid growth. Extension of the knee against resistance or application of pressure over the tibial tubercle aggravates the pain. Pain worsens with activity and subsides with rest.

119. Answer: 3

Rationale: Growing pains usually occur at night and resolve by morning. The pain is deep and does not involve the joints. Osgood-Schlatter disease results from degeneration of the tibial tubercle because of overuse and a rapid growth spurt. Pain and swelling occur over the tibial tubercle. Symptoms are exacerbated by activities that involve the quadriceps muscle. Another form of overuse syndrome is patellofemoral stress syndrome. Pain of a dull, aching quality is present in the knee, sometimes with clicking. Long periods of sitting or activities that involve knee flexion as well as compression of the patella in the groove cause increased pain. In shin splints, inflammation of muscles along the medial shaft of the tibia results from overuse and causes aching pain. Rest improves the pain. Improper warm-up exercises or extended exercise by an unconditioned person, especially in unsuitable shoes, can lead to this pain.

120. Answer: 3

Rationale: The unaffected leg goes up the step first, and then the crutches, followed by the affected leg. This allows for stability and weight bearing on the unaffected leg, with the crutches supporting the affected leg.

121. Answer: 3

Rationale: Osgood-Schlatter disease is common in late childhood and adolescence. The risk for disease increases in patients who are involved in strenuous activity, especially involving the quadriceps muscle. The usual treatment is NSAIDs and rest.

122. Answer: 2

Rationale: Most do not have disease persistent into adulthood. Juvenile rheumatoid arthritis (JRA) symptoms present very similarly to adult arthritis. Most disease activity diminishes with age; although some do have some residual joint damage, the percentage is not this high. Aspirin is the treatment of choice, and cytotoxic drugs are reserved for patients in whom other therapies have failed.

123. Answer: 2

Rationale: Development of iridocyclitis may be insidious and asymptomatic and, if untreated, may cause blindness. Although children may develop any of the other listed diseases, there is no correlation with juvenile rheumatoid arthritis (JRA).

124. Answer: 3

Rationale: A positive McMurray's test (palpable click and pain when rotating the foot laterally and extending the leg) along with the symptoms is indicative of a medial meniscus tear. The drawer test evaluates for anterior cruciate ligament tears (knee flexed with foot on table; sit on foot and grasp both sides of tibia at knee; pull tibia forward; abnormal if movement of tibia away from the joint).

125. Answer: 4

Rationale: Avascular necrosis results in death of the femoral head with revascularization. Toxic synovitis and increased femoral anteversion, while causing pain, are not bone threatening. Legg-Calvé-Perthes disease results in necrosis of the proximal femoral epiphysis; however, there is later revascularization.

126. Answer: 3

Rationale: In Adam's position (forward bending, arms loose at side, and thumbs hooked together), true scoliosis (structural) is demonstrated (by an elevated rib hump), whereas the functional type related to other conditions is not apparent. Persistent functional scoliosis can eventually become structural.

Neurology

127. Answer: 3

Rationale: Although it is important to investigate all episodes of apnea in infants, premature infants may not exhibit the typical tonic–clonic type-seizures but may have awake apnea.

128. Answer: 4

Rationale: Nuchal rigidity is a stiff neck; the child cannot move his head forward and cannot bring his chin in contact with his chest. Movement of the head from side to side does not elicit nuchal rigidity.

129. Answer: 3

Rationale: This accurately fits the description of a petit mal or absence seizure, which is a type of generalized seizure that begins in childhood and usually ends in early adulthood (30s). There is usually impairment of consciousness, automatic symptoms, and mild tonic–clonic symptoms. Classically, "staring off into space" is the reporting symptom.

130. Answer: 4

Rationale: An increase in the pulse pressure and decrease in pulse rate are indications of increasing cerebral edema and intracranial pressure, which would necessitate immediate intervention. A child's urine output should be 20–30 mL/hr.

131. Answer: 2

Rationale: Tourette's syndrome is a hereditary, chronic neuromuscular disorder consisting of various motor and vocal tics. Tics are sudden, involuntary, brief, repetitive, motor movements that often begin in childhood and change over time. Attention deficit/hyperactivity disorder (ADHD) frequently occurs concomitantly with Tourette's syndrome.

132. Answer: 4

Rationale: The most common cause of bacterial meningitis in the first month of life is the group B streptococci. *Streptococcus pneumoniae* and *Neisseria meningitides* are usually associated with meningitis after age 1 month in areas where the conjugate *Haemophilus influenzae* type b (Hib) vaccines are used.

133. Answer: 2

Rationale: A formal hearing acuity test is most important in a child with a history of bacterial meningitis because of the ototoxic medications used to treat the disease. A vision test should be done on all children but is not specific for a child with a history of meningitis. A lumbar puncture or ECG would not be appropriate.

134. Answer: 3

Rationale: The most likely causes of seizures in adolescents and young adults are idiopathic disease, trauma, and substance abuse. Congenital abnormalities are the likely cause of seizures in newborns. In children under 6 years old, metabolic causes, CNS infection, and fever can cause seizures. Trauma, malignant tumor, and stroke are likely causes for seizures in elderly patients.

135. Answer: 3

Rationale: The most common finding in children with meningococcemia (71%) is fever and a purpuric rash. The rash of rubella, Lyme disease, and roseola is finer, and none of these problems is life-threatening, unlike with meningococcemia, which makes it a "do not miss" diagnosis.

136. Answer: 1

Rationale: The description is that of a petit mal or absence seizure. Although the etiology of the majority of seizures is unclear, the patient should be referred for neurologic evaluation to determine whether an underlying abnormality is present.

137. Answer: 4

Rationale: Retinal hemorrhages may be evident on fundoscopic assessment. This finding should lead the family nurse practitioner to suspect shaken baby syndrome or hypertension. Visible head trauma would typically be absent in shaken baby syndrome. Subconjunctival hemorrhages are not an associated finding. Anisocoria is a common finding in up to 20% of the population and not associated with increased intracranial pressure.

138. Answer: 4

Rationale: Delayed language development is an early sign of autism, along with impaired social interactions. Males are diagnosed more commonly than females, and there is a genetic influence with the genome responsible for early brain development. Motor skills are not affected in autism.

139. Answer: 2

Rationale: Cerebral palsy (CP) affects males more often than females. It is not a reversible condition, and movement and posture disturbances are the hallmark of the condition. Cognitive impairment is not always present in CP. Hypotonia is a cardinal finding of CP in infancy.

140. Answer: 2

Rationale: Hyperplasia of the gums is a common side effect of phenytoin (Dilantin). The child should have regular dental prophylactic hygiene to deal with the problem.

Gastrointestinal

141. Answer: 2

Rationale: Gastroenteritis is a common cause of abdominal pain in children. Symptoms vary depending on the type of viral infection. Rotavirus mainly affects infants 3–15 months of age in the winter months, causing voluminous watery diarrhea without leukocytes. Enteric adenoviruses are the second most common viral infection in infants, with symptoms similar to rotavirus except the duration of the illness may be longer. Enteric calicivirus (Norwalk) mainly causes vomiting but also diarrhea in older children and adults. Duration of symptoms is short, usually 24–48 hours. Cytomegalovirus rarely causes diarrhea and is common after bone marrow transplants and in late stages of HIV infection.

142. Answer: 3

Rationale: The string sign is indicative of a narrow pyloric channel and is associated with pyloric stenosis. Intussusception would be evaluated by a barium enema. Hirschsprung's disease (congenital aganglionic megacolon) can be diagnosed with a Wagenstein-Rice series (air rises in the inflated colon). Gastroesophageal reflux is usually diagnosed by clinical findings in infants. Barium swallow will reveal free regurgitation of barium from stomach to esophagus. An upper GI series would be performed to rule out causes of vomiting.

143. Answer: 2

Rationale: Excessive vomiting with loss of acid and gastric juice is the most common cause of metabolic alkalosis. Respiratory problems do not precipitate primary metabolic acid–base imbalance, and renal disease most often causes metabolic acidosis. Severe anxiety resulting in hyperventilation results in respiratory alkalosis. Hyperventilation results in an increase in pH.

144. Answer: 3

Rationale: It is critical that a child is voiding before starting an intravenous (IV) solution with potassium. The problem with renal compromise is always a possibility, and adequate output should be established before initiating fluid therapy. The other three options are important but not the priority in this situation. Clinical evaluation of the child patient with dehydration should be prioritized as the volume of fluid intake, urine output, fever, and underlying medical conditions. Weight is also important in estimating dehydration but needs to be compared with prior weights. Important laboratory values include urine specific gravity, blood urea nitrogen (BUN), creatinine, hematocrit, and serum albumin.

145. Answer: 1

Rationale: Rotavirus is the most frequent cause of gastroenteritis in children 6 months to 2 years of age. The Norwalk virus is more predominant in school-age children. Up to 58% of diarrhea in children results from viral infections, causing vomiting and then diarrhea. The stool smear is negative for WBCs in viral causes and positive in bacterial causes. In viral diarrhea, the fever is mild, and diarrhea is watery and non-bloody.

146. Answer: 4

Rationale: Clinical features of Crohn's disease include severe weight loss, abdominal pain, growth failure, and weight loss. In irritable bowel syndrome (IBS), abdominal pain predominates. Altered bowel habits with either diarrhea or constipation are also seen. Clinical findings associated with carcinoma of the colon include mild occult blood loss with intermittent episodes of acute bleeding. Ulcerative colitis clinical features include diarrhea, rectal bleeding, and moderate weight loss.

147. Answer: 3

Rationale: Appendicitis usually begins as periumbilical abdominal pain accompanied by anorexia and nausea, but not necessarily vomiting or diarrhea. Within hours the patient may develop a low-grade fever. Most laboratory tests are normal. A WBC count >15,000/mm³ is often noted but neither confirms nor excludes the diagnosis of appendicitis. Pyuria is not indicative of appendicitis and suggests renal disease.

148. Answer: 4

Rationale: Red currant jelly stools are seen in intussusception and are caused by a mixture of stool, mucus, and blood. Clay-colored stools are seen with hepatitis. Projectile vomiting is associated with pyloric stenosis. Infants with intussusception usually have periods of severe pain, followed by intervals in which they appear comfortable. Constant or recurrent abdominal pain is experienced by about 10% of healthy children 5–15 years of age. School phobia may be associated with the etiology of the pain. An organic etiology is found in less than 10% of patients.

149. Answer: 1

Rationale: The major symptom of reflux is vomiting or regurgitation. It may occur during sleep, and frequently after feeding. Poor weight gain, hyperirritability, and refusal of feeding may be signs in some infants but are not the major symptoms. Fever or diarrhea may be present in patients with acute otitis media, gastroenteritis, or urinary tract infections.

150. Answer: 1

Rationale: The optimal therapy for gastroesophageal reflux disease (GERD) should include small, frequent feedings, burping after each feeding, and placing the baby on an inclined surface at 30 degrees. The prone position is not advocated because it allows gravity to promote reflux and sudden infant death syndrome (SIDS). The supine position leads to more reflux compared with the prone position. The effectiveness of thickened feedings has not been demonstrated because it is believed to delay gastric emptying and thus promotes reflux. Proton pump inhibitors are useful in controlling esophagitis, but long-term effects in infants are not defined. Pharmacologic therapy in young infants has received scant justification in research literature.

151. Answer: 4

Rationale: The recommendations for an infant born to a hepatitis B surface antigen (HBsAg)-positive mother are that the baby should have one dose of hepatitis B immunoglobulin (by 12 hours after birth) and a complete three-dose immunization of hepatitis B vaccine. The vaccine will stimulate the newborn's active immunity.

152. Answer: 2

Rationale: Classic signs and symptoms of Hirschsprung's disease in later infancy include alternating diarrhea and constipation and abdominal distention. The stools are offensive and ribbon-like, the abdomen is enlarged, and the veins are prominent. The other listed physical findings are not usually found in Hirschsprung's disease but are prevalent in other gastrointestinal (GI) disorders.

153. Answer: 4

Rationale: Gastroenteritis is the most common cause of abdominal pain in all age groups. The incidence of appendicitis increases after age 5 and peaks between ages 15 and 30. Intussusception and incarcerated hernia are uncommon and certainly occur less often than gastroenteritis in children.

154. Answer: 3

Rationale: Parasitic infestations cause recurrent episodes of abdominal pain, often with diarrhea, nausea, and vomiting, depending on the type of infestation. Lactose intolerance can cause recurrent abdominal pain in the lower abdomen with cramping and distention. Chronic stool retention occurs in a child with a history of ineffective toilet training. There is often a family history of constipation. All other conditions present with acute symptoms, except for psychogenic pain, which is recurrent and is a diagnosis of exclusion.

155. Answer: 3

Rationale: The location of the injury suggests a ruptured spleen. Although bowel and bladder problems are possible with blunt trauma to the abdomen, the upper abdominal location makes a spleen injury more likely. Older children may complain of dizziness, fatigue, chest pain, and palpitations because of arrhythmias, but hematomas are not usually present.

156. Answer: 3

Rationale: Lactose intolerance is common among Asian patients. The primary symptoms are bloating, flatulence, abdominal cramps, and diarrhea 2 hours after eating food containing lactose. Symptoms of irritable bowel syndrome (IBS) include abdominal pain and diarrhea, alternating with constipation. IBS is more common during late adolescence. Hirschsprung's disease is four times more common in boys than girls; 10%–15% of patients have Down syndrome. Food allergies are common in children under age 3 years. Clinical findings occur minutes to 2 hours after ingestion of the food. Clinical findings include hives, facial angioedema, flushing, and throat itching.

157. Answer: 2

Rationale: Right upper quadrant pain during exercise, malaise, nausea, and vomiting are early signs of hepatitis A. Elevated IgM antibodies indicate a recent or current infection. Clinical findings of cholecystitis include colicky pain in the right upper quadrant with radiation to the flanks after a large meal. Mononucleosis, common in college-age adults and young children, has the classic triad of fever, exudative pharyngitis, and adenopathy (particularly posterior cervical).

Hepatitis B causes symptoms ranging from asymptomatic seroconversion to acute illness with malaise, anorexia, and nausea to fatal hepatitis.

158. Answer: 2

Rationale: To rule out appendicitis (although rare, it can occur in young children), further physical examination is necessary, as well as diagnostic testing and assessment for lactose intolerance, urinary tract infection, or extra-abdominal causes. Assessment of dietary intake and prescribing pediatric Fleet enemas would not be appropriate if surgery is indicated.

159. Answer: 1

Rationale: Objects 5 cm or larger have difficulty passing the ligament of Treitz and other points of narrowing, such as the gastroesophageal junction. Ingested foreign bodies tend to lodge in areas of natural constriction.

160. Answer: 2

Rationale: When the infant is in a supine position, increased abdominal pressure after eating can result in passage of gastric contents into the esophagus, which often would be aspirated during sleep, and result in the forceful coughing, resultant emesis, and esophageal reflux. Suck-swallow incoordination can cause the same problems regardless of position, as can tracheoesophageal fistula. Colic is characterized by severe crying in healthy, well-fed infants for more than 3 hours a day.

161. Answer: 3

Rationale: Shigellosis usually is self-limited, lasting 5–7 days. Prevention of hydration is key, and fluid replacement should be diligent. For children, the most common age is 2–4 years for *Shigella* infection. A mild case can be managed with fluids, such as Pedialyte and good handwashing. Antidiarrheals should not be used because the course could worsen. Treatment with TMP-SMX (Bactrim) shortens the course and prevents further spread of the organism but is not required in mild cases. Prevention of dehydration also includes a clear liquid diet for 24–48 hours, no dairy products, electrolyte-rich sports drinks, and advance to a bland diet as tolerated.

162. Answer: 3

Rationale: The drug of choice for treating *Giardia* is metronidazole 5 mg/kg (up to 250 mg) tid × 5 days (80%–95% effective). This drug is well tolerated in children. Metronidazole has a disulfiram-like effect and should not be used in children or adolescents receiving ethanol-containing medications. All other drugs are ineffective for *Giardia*.

Tetracycline should not be prescribed to children under age 8 for any reason.

Male Reproductive

163. Answer: 1

Rationale: Paraphimosis is a retraction disorder related to a constricted prepuce that can be relieved through circumcision.

164. Answer: 4

Rationale: This involves the differential diagnosis between epididymitis and testicular torsion. Irreversible damage will be done to the testicles if torsion is not released in 3–4 hours. Time should not be wasted with other treatments if torsion is strongly suspected.

165. Answer: 3

Rationale: Cryptorchidism is the result of undescended testes, either bilateral or, more often, affecting the right testis. Normally, descent is in the seventh to eighth month of gestation.

166. Answer: 3

Rationale: The symptoms described are consistent with testicular torsion. This is an emergent surgical problem, and the patient should be referred immediately.

Female Reproductive

167. Answer: 4

Rationale: Douching is never necessary. It changes the normal pH and upsets the normal vaginal flora. Douching during menstruation could cause "retrograde menstruation," a potential precursor to endometriosis. Copious vaginal discharge can be a symptom of infection and warrants workup.

168. Answer: 3

Rationale: Pregnancy is the most common cause of amenorrhea in young women. It is important to rule out pregnancy by obtaining a serum human chorionic gonadotropin (hCG) level in patient with a problem of amenorrhea, even if she is very athletic. Interviewing the patient regarding her sexual practices is unreliable. The presence or absence of pregnancy should be determined before other diagnostic studies.

169. Answer: 3

Rationale: The presence of bruising, particularly on genitalia, should raise suspicion of abuse. Combined with her nonver-

bal behavior, the bruising should prompt the family nurse practitioner to explore the possibility of abuse.

Newborn

170. Answer: 1

Rationale: Using a paper or a plastic tape, rather than cloth, prevents error because of the stretching of the fabric. Measurements should be repeated to confirm accuracy. The tape should not lie over the ears.

171. Answer: 2

Rationale: Neonatal screening for PKU and congenital hypothyroidism is done in all states. Other tests are up to the primary care provider. Alpha-fetoprotein is usually a maternal blood test done during the prenatal period to screen for genetic defects, primarily neural tube anomalies.

172. Answer: 3

Rationale: Normal morphology and testes tissue development will be impaired if the testes are not descended by age 1 year. These children are at higher risk for development of testicular cancer in the young adult male (20–30 years old).

173. Answer: 1

Rationale: Phototherapy is effective secondary to the absorption of the light by bilirubin across the infant's skin. The light energy is absorbed by bilirubin and promotes the conversion of bilirubin to a nontoxic form that can be excreted in the bile without the need for conjugation. The increase in hemolysis will increase the bilirubin level, and this is physiologic jaundice that is not associated with an Rh-incompatibility problem.

174. Answer: 1

Rationale: Neonatal jaundice is more common in breast-fed infants and is thought to result from the decreased intake in the first few days. It usually begins between 4 and 7 days after birth, and the bilirubin levels range from 10 to 30 mg/dL. Increasing the infant's intake of water does not improve the condition. Breast-feeding may be temporarily interrupted, but phototherapy is usually unnecessary.

175. Answer: 4

Rationale: Bronze baby syndrome describes a grayish-brown pigmentation that occurs in neonates. It may occur in infants undergoing phototherapy but is usually associated with infants who have obstructive liver problems. The pigmentation is not permanent but may last for several months.

176. Answer: 1

Rationale: Infantile colic is unexplained crying and restlessness that lasts longer than 3 hours per day, 3 days a week. Most often it stops spontaneously at about 3 months. Other causes, particularly infections, should be ruled out. Spastic colon and lactose intolerance are unlikely and would include problems with diarrhea and constipation. Infant stress syndrome is not a valid problem.

177. Answer: 4

Rationale: With a normal physical exam, in the absence of fever or sepsis, the listed lab tests are not necessary to diagnose colic. If there were positive findings or fever, the complete laboratory workup should be obtained, with the addition of urinalysis and lumbar puncture.

178. Answer: 2

Rationale: After the infant has been carefully evaluated and there is no evidence of other problems, it is important to explain to the parents that no medication is available to treat the condition. The condition is not resolved by changing the feeding schedule of the infant nor is it related to stress within the home, and a change to soy formula will not solve the problem. The parents must be informed that the colic most often resolves with no residual problems by age 3 months.

179. Answer: 2

Rationale: The physiology of normal vaginal delivery causes pressure against the infant's thorax and helps remove amniotic fluid. If the cesarean section was done as an emergency before term, the infant may have inadequate surfactant for good pulmonary function. Increased levels of bilirubin, meconium aspiration, and hypoglycemia are not associated with an increase in cesarean delivery.

180. Answer: 1

Rationale: These are normal newborn findings. The respiratory rate is increased but is usually increased immediately after birth (transient tachypnea) and during the second period of reactivity. Continued tachypnea is abnormal. The respiratory rate should be counted for a full minute because of the irregularity of the infant's breathing. Periodic pauses may occur for up to 10 seconds, but apnea lasting longer than 20 seconds is abnormal. Acrocyanosis is normal immediately after birth. Choanal atresia occurs when one or both of the nasal passages are blocked by an abnormality of the septum. In respiratory distress syndrome, the infant exhibits other symptoms that are consistent with hypoxia.

181. Answer: 4

Rationale: Caput succedaneum results from pressure against the mother's cervix during labor. The edematous area crosses the suture lines and will resolve within hours to days after birth. There is normally a space between the cranial suture lines; if there is no space or an overriding suture line, it may be caused by molding. Widening of the suture line may indicate increased intracranial pressure. Cephalhematoma is characterized by bleeding between the bone and the periosteum, and it does not cross the suture line.

182. Answer: 2

Rationale: Early signs of hypoglycemia are jitteriness, poor muscle tone, tremors, and symptoms of respiratory difficulty. The blood sugar of 50 mg/dL is within normal limits at this time (40–60 mg/dL the first 24 hours). If blood sugar levels are less than 45 mg/dL on the screening strip, a follow-up serum glucose should be done. The meconium stool should be passed within the first 24 hours, and the bilirubin level is normal.

183. Answer: 1

Rationale: Within a few hours after birth, the fundus rises to the level of the umbilicus and remains there for about 24 hours. After 24 hours, the fundus begins to descend by about 1 cm or one fingerbreadth per day. It often is not palpable by day 10.

Mental Health

184. Answer: 1

Rationale: Children with learning disabilities and attention deficit/hyperactivity disorder (ADHD) are often impulsive, inattentive, and overactive. Usually, children with ADHD do not have lower IQ achievement scores; however, children with a learning disability usually demonstrate a level of educational achievement substantially below that of the IQ.

185. Answer: 1

Rationale: Nicotine is commonly the first drug used by adolescents.

186. Answer: 3

Rationale: The family nurse practitioner must determine whether the bruised areas match the type of trauma the parent describes. Bruises in various stages of healing turn different colors and are indicative that the injuries did not occur at the same time, which could be indicative of child abuse.

187. Answer: 4

Rationale: Adolescents with anorexia nervosa will severely reduce their nutritional intake by dieting constantly on high fiber and low calories. They usually have an inappropriate body image and may admit to occasional episodes of vomiting.

188. Answer: 1

Rationale: Nightmares peak in incidence around ages 3–4 years and are often associated with abandonment issues and posttraumatic stress disorder (following gun shootings, fires, and abuse). Night terrors are typically accompanied by gross motor movements (sleepwalking and enuresis), tachypnea, labored breathing, and tachycardia.

189. Answer: 2

Rationale: Role playing and planning a rehearsed reply to teasing comments about short stature are helpful tools to deal with this issue. Although humor can be effective, constantly clowning around for attention is not positive coping behavior. Withdrawal (i.e., watching television or reading) is not effective coping and may indicate depression. Spending time and associating only with younger adolescents who are his height is not a positive coping behavior and may hinder normal maturation.

190. Answer: 4

Rationale: More than 50% of intravenous cocaine users develop hepatitis, phlebitis, endocarditis, and acquired immunodeficiency syndrome (AIDS). Epistaxis, rhinorrhea, and nasal congestion are seen most often in intranasal users of cocaine. Chest congestion, wheezing, and eventual emphysema occur with chronic free-base (crack) smokers. Although cardiac arrhythmias, hypertension, and respiratory arrest can occur, they are not the common complications.

191. Answer: 3

Rationale: Adolescents often act out to protect themselves from feelings of vulnerability and dependency. It is important to evaluate signs of anger and frustration in the adolescent because the significance of the behavior may indicate symptoms of depression. Adults who are depressed typically display findings noted in the other three options.

192. Answer: 1

Rationale: The newborn exposed to cocaine is often premature, small for gestational age, has low birth weight, and has a low Apgar score. Intrauterine growth retardation occurs along with symptoms of hypertonia, irritability, tremulousness, irregular sleeping patterns, and frequent gaze aversion.

193. Answer: 3

Rationale: People with anorexia nervosa will exercise up to 4 hours a day. They are above average intelligence in most cases, suffer from bradycardia, and have decreased libido.

194. Answer: 4

Rationale: In a preschool child, it may be difficult to distinguish attention-deficit/hyperactivity disorder (ADHD) because problems of overactivity, inattention, and negativism are common. Problems with language-skill development, along with fine motor skills, are more likely found with learning disabilities. Active curiosity and negativism are normal behaviors for preschoolers.

195. Answer: 1

Rationale: Autism is a developmental disorder that starts early in a child's life and is characterized by avoidance of eye contact, indifference to caregivers, language and communication delays, failure to develop a social smile, repetitive movements, and an excessive need for routine.

196. Answer: 4

Rationale: Repetition of whole words and phrases is normal for preschoolers; therefore, it would be inappropriate to refer to a speech pathologist at this time. Parents should not correct or criticize the child because it could contribute to low self-esteem. Verbal exercises are unnecessary and could be very stressful to the child and contribute to low self-esteem.

197. Answer: 3

Rationale: The grandmother's concern is warranted. In teenage girls, the most common form of suicide attempt is by drug overdose. The combination of vomiting and confusion suggests a drug overdose, and the family nurse practitioner should run a toxicology screen.

198. Answer: 2

Rationale: This patient should be examined by emergency department personnel, many of whom are specially trained to collect the evidence needed to testify in court about rape. The exam should not be done in the office unless the family nurse practitioner has been trained in evidence collection and has a rape evidence collection kit. The exam must be done quickly, before evidence is destroyed. The patient decides who should be called for support. Although she is encouraged to call her parents, she is also offered the support of rape crisis and other resources.

199. Answer: 2

Rationale: Woraich's 1994 study failed to demonstrate a link between sugar and behavior or cognitive performance. Further assessment is indicated before labeling as attention-deficit/hyperactivity disorder (ADHD).

200. Answer: 3

Rationale: Based on developmental levels, a 6-month-old is not walking or pulling up, so a femur fracture is unlikely. A 4-year-old is beginning to run and jump, a 6-year-old is playing outside and riding a bicycle, and a 1-year-old is beginning to pull up and cruise around cabinets and tables.

201. Answer: 4

Rationale: Although all answers may contribute to a family nurse practitioner's suspicion of family violence, the admission of genuine fear of a household member is considered an excellent indicator of actual or potential violence and the level of danger in a home. The family nurse practitioner should involve Social Services to assist the adolescent female in this situation.

202. Answer: 4

Rationale: Often, the first indication of drug use in adolescents is a sudden change in behavior or school performance. Symptoms of heroin use are constricted pupils, respiratory depression, needle tracks, and poor nutrition. Symptoms of marijuana use are slow reflexes, tachycardia, conjunctival injection, nasal congestion, and increased appetite. Symptoms of LSD use are dilated pupils, reddened eyes, hypertension, increased appetite, and hallucinations. The use of central nervous system stimulants, like crack cocaine, leads to hypertension, weight loss, anorexia, insomnia, hyperreflexia, and a perforated or ulcerated nasal septum.

19

Mental Health

Psychosocial Exam & Diagnostic Tests

1. The mental status exam enables the family nurse practitioner to identify:
   1. Intelligence quotient (IQ) and reasoning.
   2. Abstract thinking and memory functioning.
   3. Reasoning and coordination.
   4. Memory functioning and IQ.

2. A patient with a history of psychiatric problems arrives at the clinic shouting that he is a messenger of God and knows the meaning of the prophecies in Revelations. This behavior is assessed as:
   1. A delusion.
   2. A hallucination.
   3. Magical thinking.
   4. An illusion.

3. An assessment of a patient experiencing auditory hallucinations would most likely reveal:
   1. Patient mumbling to self, tilted head, eyes darting back and forth.
   2. Performance of obsessive-compulsive rituals of turning off and on a radio, talking to self.
   3. Hyperactivity, expansive mood, easy distractibility.
   4. Cool, aloof, unapproachable, avoiding enclosed areas.

4. CAGE is a screening instrument for which disease process?
   1. Glaucoma.
   2. Depression.
   3. Alcoholism.
   4. Diabetes.

5. When receiving records from another agency, the family nurse practitioner notes on the summary sheet that the patient has a dual diagnosis. This means the patient has:
   1. Both manic and depressive symptoms of bipolar affective disorder.
   2. Two closely related psychiatric disorders (e.g., panic disorder and bulimia nervosa).
   3. Coexistence of both a psychiatric disorder (e.g., depression) and a substance abuse disorder (e.g., alcohol dependence).
   4. Coexistence of a personality disorder (e.g., borderline personality) and a psychiatric disorder (e.g., panic disorder).

6. While completing the history on an older adult, the family nurse practitioner understands that when a patient "makes up stories or answers" to questions, it is known as:
   1. Perseveration.
   2. Confabulation.
   3. Echolalia.
   4. Alcoholic encephalopathy.

7. **QSEN** In taking a history from a patient with depression, which is the most important question for the family nurse practitioner to ask?
   1. Have you ever experienced hallucinations, delusions, or illusions?
   2. Have you ever been hospitalized in a psychiatric facility?
   3. Do you regularly take antidepressants or other medications?
   4. Have you thought about or attempted suicide?

8. A common laboratory finding associated with bulimia nervosa is:

   1. Hyperkalemia.

   2. Hypochloremia.

   3. Elevated liver enzymes.

   4. Platelet abnormalities.

9. An 85-year-old woman comes in with her daughter with the primary complaint of worsening confusion over 6 months. The family nurse practitioner has already ordered a urine analysis and it was negative. The basal metabolic panel was unremarkable. Complete blood count showed a mild anemia. What other tests might the family nurse practitioner consider ordering for this patient?

   1. A1C, folic acid, TSH.

   2. TSH, lipid panel, vitamin B$_{12}$, vitamin D.

   3. Folic acid, vitamin B$_{12}$, TSH.

   4. Lipid panel, A1C, vitamin D.

10. The family nurse practitioner knows drug tolerance is suggested when a patient gives a history of:

    1. Reduced effects with the same dose of the drug.

    2. Less of the medication produces the desired effects.

    3. No withdrawal symptoms when the drug is stopped.

    4. Increasing side effects with an increase in the dose of the drug.

11. When doing a mental status exam, which questions would be helpful to assess the patient for the ability to think abstractly?

    1. Can you repeat the following numbers: 1, 3, 5, 7, 9?

    2. What is today's date?

    3. How are a carpet and a hardwood floor alike?

    4. Can you tell me the names of three past U.S. presidents?

Psychiatric Disorders

12. An older adult patient is experiencing a recent onset of confusion. The family nurse practitioner is trying to determine whether the confusion is related to depression or dementia. In evaluating the patient, what specific assessment finding would be helpful in making this distinction?

    1. Determining whether confusion worsens in the evening.

    2. Assessing early morning agitation, hyperactivity, and insomnia.

    3. Noting signs of anger, hostility, and loss of control.

    4. Assessing reality distortions and preoccupation with family matters.

13. **QSEN** A patient calls the clinic and asks to speak to the family nurse practitioner. When the family nurse practitioner answers the telephone, the patient states that he is going to commit suicide. The priority goal is to:

    1. Refer the patient to an appropriate treatment facility.

    2. Encourage ventilation of angry and depressed feelings.

    3. Assess the lethality of the suicide plan.

    4. Establish rapport with the patient.

14. During an intake interview with a 26-year-old man diagnosed with generalized anxiety disorder, the family nurse practitioner might observe what type of behavior?

    1. An inflated sense of self.

    2. Constant relation to future events.

    3. Inability to concentrate and irritability when questioned.

    4. Nervousness and fear of the family nurse practitioner during the interview.

15. An older adult woman answers the family nurse practitioner's questions by mumbling in low tones with answers that seem inappropriate. What would be initial findings associated with a diagnosis of dementia?

    1. Sees people floating across the ceiling of her room.

    2. Has problems with cognition and confusion.

    3. Hears voices at night telling her to change her clothes.

    4. Shows fear when the nurse makes any movements toward her.

16. An older patient comes to the office with the complaint of confusion. The daughter is concerned that her mother is developing Alzheimer's disease. Which of these assessments would indicate the patient is experiencing delirium versus dementia?

    1. The confusion has been slowly developing.

    2. The confusion started after the patient started taking cimetidine (Tagamet).

    3. The patient's attention span has been affected.

    4. The patient's memory has been impaired.

17. When the family nurse practitioner talks with a patient about his chemical dependency, the patient states, "I wish I would have never used cocaine. It has ruined my life!" What would be the most appropriate response by the family nurse practitioner?

    1. "You should think before you do something."

    2. "Things will work out, don't worry."

    3. "It sounds like you've thought a lot about your cocaine use."

    4. "You shouldn't be so hard on yourself. You can change."

18. The family nurse practitioner would expect which symptoms in a patient with a diagnosis of schizophrenia?

    1. High energy with varying sleep patterns and nonstop conversation.

    2. Extreme and frequent mood swings with hyperactivity and difficulty concentrating.

    3. Paranoia, delusions, hallucinations, and diminished self-care.

    4. Antisocial behavior, manipulative, charismatic, and ability to lie convincingly.

19. Dementia can be distinguished from delirium because:

    1. Dementia lasts days to weeks compared to delirium, which lasts months to years.

    2. Dementia is often associated with medications or systemic illness.

    3. Dementia exhibits a disturbance in attention that is not present in delirium.

    4. Dementia is a chronic medical condition and delirium is an acute illness.

20. An older adult patient is brought to the family nurse practitioner by his family for evaluation of increasing confusion over the past few days. The patient has a history of dementia; however, the family states that there is a definite change. What course of action would the family nurse practitioner consider?

    1. Help the family look for a nursing home.

    2. Order an MRI scan.

    3. Order a non-contrast head CT.

    4. Order a UA.

21. **QSEN** A middle-aged, upper-middle-class married woman presents to your clinic for the third time in 2 months with a complaint of headache, gastrointestinal upset with abdominal pain, and difficulty sleeping. Past exams have been essentially negative. You suspect the patient suffers from depression, but she has been reluctant to complete even the briefest of screenings for this. Today, the patient requests "something for sleep" again stating that she "doesn't have time to take a bunch of tests." Which tentative diagnosis seems most likely?

    1. Hypochondriasis.

    2. Domestic violence.

    3. Addiction.

    4. Irritable bowel syndrome.

22. An older adult patient was taken to the clinic in a confused state that began suddenly 24 hours ago. She fails to be oriented to person, time, or place. She was incontinent of urine because of her confusion. She looks apathetic and is drowsy. The family nurse practitioner would suspect:

    1. Delirium.

    2. Dementia.

    3. Depression.

    4. A psychotic disorder.

23. **QSEN** Which of the following groups of patients fall under mandatory reporting laws for abuse and neglect in a majority of states in the United States?

    1. Children, adult women, dependent older adults.

    2. Children, disabled individuals, adult women.

    3. Disabled individuals, adult women, dependent older adults.

    4. Children, disabled individuals, dependent older adults.

24. Physical findings of cocaine abuse include:

    1. Bradycardia, miosis, hypertension.

    2. Hypertension, tachycardia, tremor.

    3. Hypotension, bradycardia, abdominal cramps.

    4. Decreased level of consciousness, tachycardia, excessive salivation.

25. What three behaviors meet the criteria for alcohol use disorder in the *Diagnostic and Statistical Manual of Mental Disorders, Fifth Edition (DSM-V)?*

    1. Repeated arrests for drunk driving.

    2. Multiple absences from work due to substance use.

    3. Chronic anxiety attacks.

    4. Recurrent arguments with spouse about his/her drinking behavior.

    5. Obsessively washing hands.

26. An older adult patient's wife is concerned about her husband's increasing confusion and agitation. Not only has he exhibited symptoms of increased confusion, but he also is unable to care for his physical needs. He has been incontinent of urine and feces and sometimes is totally unaware of other people. What would be an assessment priority for the patient?

    1. Evaluate changes in social habits.

    2. Assess for hallucinations and impaired reality testing.

    3. Evaluate his orientation to person, place, and time.

    4. Determine if he is experiencing a problem with impaired judgment.

27. **QSEN** A 42-year-old male comes in to the office with his friend. The friend states that he found the patient confused with some shaking and seeing things that are not there. The patient typically drinks two six packs of beer every day. The patient decided to stop drinking 2 days ago. Vital signs show elevated blood pressure, fever, and tachycardia. The family nurse practitioner transfers the patient to the hospital as he:

    1. Is overdosing on heroin.

    2. Has thyroid storm.

    3. Is septic from pneumonia.

    4. Has delirium tremens.

28. What four items are risk factors for a major depressive disorder in an adult?

    1. Female gender.

    2. Male gender.

    3. Lack of social support.

    4. Married women.

    5. Married men.

    6. Family history of depression.

29. A patient is transferred to the alcohol treatment unit from the emergency room. What is important to include in the therapeutic milieu during detoxification?

    1. Keep the environment adequately lit to diminish hallucinations.

    2. Keep a radio or television on in the room to assist in maintaining orientation.

    3. Speak quietly when in the room to avoid overstimulation.

    4. Keep the suction equipment available in case of seizures.

Pharmacology

30. **QSEN** A patient has been receiving fluphenazine (Prolixin) for the past 3 weeks. The family nurse practitioner's assessment notes the following: temperature elevated 105.8°F (41°C), marked muscle rigidity, agitation, and confusion. The family nurse practitioner understands these findings are often associated with the diagnosis of:

    1. Acute dystonia.

    2. Tardive dyskinesia.

    3. Neuroleptic malignant syndrome.

    4. Extrapyramidal disorder.

31. The preferred antidepressant for an older adult patient is:

    1. Amitriptyline (Elavil).

    2. Citalopram (Celexa).

    3. Trazodone (Desyrel).

    4. Haloperidol (Haldol).

32. A patient has been referred to the family nurse practitioner. The patient's medical history reveals long-term use of benzodiazepines, which the patient considers harmless. The family nurse practitioner understands that benzodiazepines can:

    1. Cause drug dependency.

    2. Produce nephrotoxicity.

    3. Lead to functional damage of the cardiopulmonary system.

    4. Cause profound dissociative personality problems.

33. An older female has a diagnosis of dementia and is taking haloperidol (Haldol) 2 mg every evening. The family nurse practitioner observes her engaging in a restless, repetitive movement with her legs. She states that, not only does she have ongoing movement, but she also feels jittery. The family nurse practitioner would interpret this activity to be:

1. Ataxia.

2. Akathisia.

3. Agitation.

4. Dyskinesia.

34. What is the best initial treatment plan for a sleep disorder in the older adult patient?

    1. Medicate with amitriptyline (Elavil).

    2. Medicate with trazodone (Desyrel).

    3. Discuss the importance of naps daily.

    4. Decrease noise and light in the environment.

35. An older adult patient presents with a new symptom of acute confusion over the past 24 hours. Which assessment would be a priority for the family nurse practitioner to evaluate during the exam?

    1. Drug history.

    2. Electrocardiogram.

    3. Mini-Mental status exam.

    4. Thyroid profile.

36. The family nurse practitioner is aware that the following class of drugs is most likely to precipitate a hypertensive crisis in the older adult:

    1. Narcotic analgesics.

    2. MAO inhibitors.

    3. Barbiturates.

    4. Phenothiazines.

37. The family nurse practitioner knows that the following class of drugs would have the greatest effect on memory in the older adult patient:

    1. Phenothiazines.

    2. Tricyclic antidepressants.

    3. Benzodiazepines.

    4. MAO inhibitors.

38. The family nurse practitioner understands that adolescents who use LSD:

    1. Experience withdrawal symptoms within 24 hours.

    2. Will quickly become addicted.

    3. Experience flashbacks and depression.

    4. Experience disorientation and delusional feelings.

39. Of the following antidepressants, which one has the most sedating side effects, making it a good sleeping agent?

    1. Fluoxetine (Prozac).

    2. Doxepin (Sinequan).

    3. Trazodone (Desyrel).

    4. Paroxetine (Paxil).

40. In the management of acute alcohol withdrawal delirium, which three drugs would the family nurse practitioner consider using?

    1. Bupropion (Wellbutrin).

    2. Chlordiazepoxide (Librium).

    3. Lorazepam (Ativan).

    4. Citalopram (Celexa).

    5. Thiamine.

    6. Chlorpromazine (Thorazine).

41. Which three laboratory results would be important to assess before placing a patient on lithium?

    1. TSH, T_4, T_3.

    2. Fasting lipids.

    3. BUN, creatinine.

    4. Electrolytes.

    5. ESR.

    6. ALT, AST, LDH.

42. **QSEN** A patient comes to the rural clinic having taken an undetermined amount of heroin. Before transferring the patient to a psychiatric treatment facility, the family nurse practitioner anticipates the drug of choice for an opioid overdose is:

    1. Clonidine (Catapres).

    2. Methadone (Dolophine).

    3. Naloxone (Narcan).

    4. Naltrexone HCl (Revia).

43. Benzodiazepines are useful in the treatment in which of the three following disorders:

    1. Alcohol withdrawal.

    2. Schizophrenia.

    3. Anxiety.

    4. Obsessive-compulsive disorder.

    5. Seizures.

    6. Bipolar affective disorder.

44. When starting a psychotropic medication in the older adult, a good rule of thumb is:

    1. Start low, go slow.

    2. Higher doses are almost always needed.

    3. Side effects of psychotropic medications will usually not impact other medications.

    4. The same adult dosages can be used initially without any problems.

45. A patient is a 20-year, 2-pack-a-day smoker with a history of chronic bronchitis. What is the prescription to give the patient who wishes to stop smoking?

    1. Nicotine polacrilex (Nicorette) gum 2-mg piece, chew for 30 minutes, q1–2h × 6 weeks, then q2–4h × 3 weeks, then q4–8h × 3 weeks, and then discontinue.

    2. Nicotine patch (Nicoderm) 21 mg/24 hr qd × 6 weeks, then 14 mg/24 hr qd × 2 weeks, then 7 mg/24 hr qd × 2 weeks, and then discontinue.

    3. Bupropion HCl (Zyban) 150 mg qd × 3 days, then 150 mg bid for 7–12 weeks, and to stop smoking when medication is started.

    4. Nicotine patch (Nicoderm) 14 mg/24 hr qd × 6 weeks, then 7 mg/24 hr qd × 6 weeks, and then discontinue.

46. A young woman tells the family nurse practitioner that she no longer wants to be on sertraline (Zoloft). She had a traumatic event a few years ago but has been doing much better and has a strong support structure from family and friends. The family nurse practitioner advises her to:

    1. Stop taking the medication.

    2. Taper the dose slowly.

    3. Keep taking the medication.

    4. Switch to citalopram (Celexa).

47. A patient with bipolar disorder is on divalproex sodium (Depakote) for mania. What test(s) would the family nurse practitioner monitor?

    1. Liver function test and CBC.

    2. Pulmonary function test.

    3. ECG.

    4. UA and C&S.

48. An 82-year-old male, who is on a stable dose of furosemide (Lasix) for heart failure, comes in with complaints of feeling down for the past year after losing his wife. After assessing the patient, the family nurse practitioner diagnoses the patient with depression and starts him on citalopram (Celexa). The family nurse practitioner knows that by starting citalopram the patient is at risk for:

    1. Hypernatremia.

    2. Hyponatremia.

    3. Hyperkalemia.

    4. Hypokalemia.

49. A 75-year-old female comes to see the family nurse practitioner to follow up on an upper respiratory infection that she has had for 1 week. She has been taking diphenhydramine (Benadryl). The family nurse practitioner knows this is a poor medication for older adult patients because diphenhydramine (Benadryl) can cause:

    1. Sedation.

    2. Prolonged QT.

    3. Bradycardia.

    4. Hypertension.

50. **QSEN** What is the maximum dose of citalopram (Celexa) for a patient over 60 years old?

    1. 40 mg once daily by mouth.

    2. 20 mg twice daily by mouth.

    3. 20 mg once daily by mouth.

    4. 10 mg once daily by mouth.

51. The family nurse practitioner understands the following about the use of benzodiazepines in the older adult:

    1. Withdrawal symptoms may occur within 24 hours of abruptly stopping the medication.

    2. Adverse side effects are minimal and tend to minimize the incidence of falls and other injuries.

    3. Long-acting medications (i.e., chlordiazepoxide [Librium]) are preferred over the shorter-acting medications (i.e., lorazepam [Ativan]).

    4. Larger doses are needed to maintain therapeutic levels for the anxious or agitated patient.

19 Mental Health Answers and Rationales

Psychosocial Exam & Diagnostic Tests

1. Answer: 2

Rationale: The mental status exam provides a basic assessment of the patient's intellectual functioning (reasoning, abstract thinking, and memory). The intelligence quotient (IQ) is determined by neuropsychological evaluation. Coordination is part of a neurologic exam and can be tested by rapid alternating movements and heel-to-shin or finger-to-nose tests.

2. Answer: 1

Rationale: Delusions are false, fixed beliefs that can be of a persecutory or grandiose nature. In this instance the patient is experiencing a delusion of grandeur. Often older adults with a diagnosis of dementia will have delusions, which worsen with acute illnesses. A person may have delusions as a symptom of a disorder, such as schizophrenia. They may also occur as part of a delusional disorder, such as grandiose, jealousy, persecutory, somatic, or mixed. A hallucination is a false sensory experience. An illusion is a misinterpretation of reality. Magical thinking is when the patient feels that his or her thoughts or wishes can control other people.

3. Answer: 1

Rationale: The patient experiencing the auditory hallucination will often look out into space and act as if he or she is listening to someone talking. This is associated with behaviors such as tilting the head, mumbling, and eye movement.

4. Answer: 3

Rationale: CAGE (Cut down, Annoyed, Guilty, Eye opener) is a screening instrument used to alert providers to possibility of alcoholism.

5. Answer: 3

Rationale: Dual diagnosis involves both a psychiatric diagnosis and a substance abuse diagnosis.

6. Answer: 2

Rationale: Patients who experience confabulation are fabricating events or situations to fill in gaps in their memory, usually in a plausible way. Confabulation is a common symptom of alcohol amnesic disorder, or Korsakoff's syndrome. Echolalia is the parroting or automatic, meaningless repeating of another's words. Perseveration is the involuntary persistent repetition of an idea or response (e.g., patient keeps repeating the same phrase over and over).

7. Answer: 4

Rationale: Although it is important to know whether the patient has ever experienced hallucinations, delusions, or illusions and had ever been hospitalized in a psychiatric facility, the single most important factor to ascertain is whether or not the patient has contemplated suicide. In addition, determination of a specific plan and the means to do it are also involved in the questioning about suicidal ideation. Asking a patient whether or not he or she is suicidal does not increase the risk of the patient committing suicide. It is also important for the family nurse practitioner to determine whether the patient regularly takes antidepressants or other medications. Patients may have stopped taking their antidepressant, causing an acute exacerbation of their depression, or another medication that may be causing an increase in their depression.

8. Answer: 2

Rationale: The other abnormalities are not usually associated with bulimia. The hypochloremia is associated with the purging (self-induced vomiting). Other fluid and electrolyte imbalances that may be seen include hyponatremia, hypokalemia, and metabolic alkalosis and acidosis.

9. Answer: 3

Rationale: It is appropriate to check for other conditions that cause confusion, such as hypothyroidism and folic acid and vitamin B_{12} deficiency. The other tests listed are important for patient health but will not help determine the cause of confusion.

10. Answer: 1

Rationale: Drug tolerance exists when the same dose of the drug produces reduced effects and is usually seen with the development of physical dependence on any medication. Addiction occurs when there is a deep-seated psychological need for the drug/medication.

11. Answer: 3

Rationale: Abstract thinking requires the patient to compare and tell how two things are alike or different, involving the thought process that is oriented toward the development of an idea without application to a particular object; it is independent of space and time. Today's date assists to determine orientation, the names of past presidents assists to demonstrate long-term memory, and repetition of numbers assists to demonstrate short-term memory.

Psychiatric Disorders

12. Answer: 1

Rationale: Confusion can occur in both dementia and depression. However, with dementia, symptoms worsen at night and are commonly referred to as sundowning. Additionally, the family nurse practitioner must also ensure that the increased confusion is not a result of an acute illness. Often the only sign or symptom the demented older adult may present with is confusion. Usually the culprit is a urinary tract infection. The family nurse practitioner should order a urine analysis (UA) to ensure that the confusion is not the result of an acute illness and is reversible.

13. Answer: 4

Rationale: The family nurse practitioner must first establish trust and rapport with the caller before an assessment can be made. If rapport is not established, the patient will hang up the phone. The family nurse practitioner understands that, by keeping the patient talking, he or she is prevented from acting out the suicidal threat.

14. Answer: 3

Rationale: Impaired concentration and irritability are major characteristics of generalized anxiety disorder. Other symptoms of generalized anxiety disorder include excessive anxiety and worry; inability to control the worry and restlessness; easily fatigued; difficulty concentrating; muscle tension; and sleep disturbance. Patients often pace the exam room because of their irritability; they are more focused on the here and now and have low self-esteem.

15. Answer: 2

Rationale: Confusion and cognitive function problems (i.e., short-term memory loss) are initial signs of dementia. Other signs of early-stage Alzheimer's dementia include time and spatial disorientation, poor judgment, personality changes, depression or withdrawal, and perceptual disturbances. The severity of the symptoms depends on what stage of cognitive degeneration the patient is manifesting. The other options are characteristic of hallucinatory experiences and may occur later. This patient may also be exhibiting signs and symptoms of an acute illness. The culprit is commonly a urinary tract infection (UTI), and the family nurse practitioner should order a urinalysis (UA) to ensure that the cause of the confusion is not related to a reversible cause.

16. Answer: 2

Rationale: Cimetidine (Tagamet) is not tolerated well in the older adult patient, and one of the major side effects is confusion. Any time a new medication is added to an older adult patient's medication regimen, an abrupt onset of confusion must be reviewed closely, because it may be attributed to the new medication or a –drug interaction with an existing medication. Another possibility is the onset of an acute illness, which often manifests as acute confusion in the older adult patient. Most often the culprit is a UTI; therefore, in addition to a careful medication review, obtaining a UA could also rule out a UTI. When a patient has true dementia, the onset of confusion develops slowly, over a longer period of time, and not acutely, which would indicate that there is another underlying problem causing the acute confusion. Attention span and memory may be affected in each diagnosis.

17. Answer: 3

Rationale: The family nurse practitioner's statement acknowledges the patient's feelings and is open ended, which promotes open discussion and helps the patient clarify feelings and thoughts. Telling the patient to think before doing something is condescending and punitive. Telling the patient to not worry and things will work out offers false reassurance. When the family nurse practitioner tells the patient to not be so hard on himself or herself, it tends to discount the patient's feelings.

18. Answer: 3

Rationale: The characteristics of schizophrenia are paranoia, delusions, tangential thought, suspiciousness, disorganized behavior, and hallucinations.

19. Answer: 4

Rationale: Dementia lasts for months to years and the patient never recovers. Delirium is an acute process that is often associated with medications or a systemic illness and is reversible once the acute problem is addressed and resolved.

20. Answer: 4

Rationale: One of the most common reasons for an acute change in mental status in the demented older adult patient is an acute infection. This is usually a urinary tract infection (UTI). Usually the demented older adult patient is incontinent and because of the changes of aging, does not recognize the normal signs or symptoms of a UTI (burning, urgency, frequency, and suprapubic tenderness). Older adults also do not typically run elevated temperatures. The family nurse practitioner should order a UA to ensure that an acute infectious process is not the cause of the acute confusion. The family nurse practitioner should also conduct a medication review to ensure that no new medications have been added or that no new over-the-counter or herbal medications have been added because this is the second major reason for acute confusion in the older adult patient.

21. Answer: 2

Rationale: The indicators to domestic violence in this case are the multiple vague physical complaints without supporting objective data, the suspected depression, and the reluctance to wait around in the clinic for extended periods of time. This patient is on the verge of disclosing if a provider would only ask her about domestic violence.

22. Answer: 1

Rationale: Based on the state of acute confusion and the incontinence, she is experiencing delirium. This is most likely secondary to sepsis, with the source of infection being a UTI. The fact that she has mental status changes (disoriented to person, place, or time, in addition to the acute confusion, delirium, and incontinence) gives you the clues to sepsis. Dementia is more insidious versus acute. Depression and psychosis are not consistent with the assessments. The major symptoms in depression would include loss of interest, sleep disorder, decreased appetite, loss of concentration, inactivity, guilt, lack of energy, and potential suicidal thoughts. Psychotic disorders include thoughts and behavior indicating the patient is not in touch with reality.

23. Answer: 4

Rationale: The laws in most states require the reporting of suspected or actual abuse and neglect of any person considered to be dependent or with a reduced ability to make life choices. Children, disabled individuals, and dependent older adults fall into these categories. Very few states require reporting for adult women unless a weapon is involved; this is a different situation, requiring a report.

24. Answer: 2

Rationale: Bradycardia and excessive salivation are not found with cocaine abuse. There are no drug antagonists that can be used for cocaine overdose, although benzodiazepines are used to treat cocaine toxicity such as seizures, tachycardia, and hypertension. Naloxone is given to reduce the concurrent toxic effects of other narcotic drugs that may be in the patient's body system but is not effective against cocaine toxicity.

25. Answer: 1, 2, 4

Rationale: Chronic anxiety attacks and obsessive-compulsive disorder (OCD) behaviors are not part of the *Diagnostic and Statistical Manual of Mental Disorders, Fifth Edition (DSM-V)* criteria for alcohol use disorder.

26. Answer: 4

Rationale: Although all of the items listed are appropriate to assess in the patient, it is most important to determine

judgment. If he cannot make safe judgments, he is at high risk for unsafe behaviors, such as driving, walking along the sidewalk, running the bath water, etc.

27. Answer: 4

Rationale: Delirium tremens is severe alcohol withdrawal that typically develops 24–72 hours after the last drink. The patient may be confused and disoriented and have hallucinations, tremors, elevated blood pressure, tachycardia, a rise in body temperature, and tonic–clonic seizures. A patient with heroin overdose may also be confused, but he or she would have hypotension, slowed respirations, and a decreased pulse. A patient septic from pneumonia may present with cough, chills, low oxygen saturation, fever, hypotension, and tachycardia. Thyroid storm is severe hyperthyroidism that presents with elevated temperature, weakness, sweating, confusion, tachycardia, and gastrointestinal symptoms.

28. Answer: 1, 3, 4, 6

Rationale: The risk factors for depression include the following: female gender, history of depression, unmarried men, married women, within 6 months of having a baby, pain, lack of social support, medical illness, substance abuse, and a negative or traumatic event.

29. Answer: 1

Rationale: The patient needs to be able to easily interpret his surroundings. Shadows or areas of poor lighting will increase the hallucinations. When in the room, it is important to speak in clear tones and make sure to include the patient in the conversations to decrease the paranoia and feelings that people are talking about him or her. Radio and television may provide too much stimulation and may not be of any assistance in maintaining orientation. Suction equipment is for physical safety, not therapeutic milieu.

Pharmacology

30. Answer: 3

Rationale: The patient is experiencing a rare problem called neuroleptic malignant syndrome. The patient would require immediate referral and hospitalization. This can also occur with the medication prochlorperazine. Acute dystonia, parkinsonism, and akathisia are associated with extrapyramidal disorder or acute movement disorder. Tardive dyskinesia occurs late in therapy and is often irreversible. Slow, wormlike movements of the tongue are the earliest symptom, followed by grimacing, lip smacking, and involuntary limb movements.

31. Answer: 2

Rationale: The favorable side effect profile of citalopram (Celexa) makes it a useful antidepressant in the older adult because it has a short half-life. Amitriptyline (Elavil) has the most anticholinergic and sedating side effects of the antidepressants. There may be pronounced effects on the cardiovascular system (hypotension). Geropsychiatrists agree it is best to avoid amitriptyline (Elavil) in the older adult; however, low dose (10 mg, PO every evening) is low cost and can be effective at controlling neuropathic pain. Trazodone (Desyrel) is very sedating for the older adult patient but can be used for insomnia and for behavioral issues with dementia patients. Haloperidol (Haldol) is an antipsychotic medication and is not to be used at all in long-term care facilities.

32. Answer: 1

Rationale: Physical dependence can occur, even with low doses of benzodiazepines. This is a particular problem in the older adult, who is sensitive to low-dose ranges. If possible, it is better to slowly taper the patient from benzodiazepines; often they can be tapered to a much lower dose.

33. Answer: 2

Rationale: Akathisia is a feeling of restlessness and can be challenging to distinguish from anxiety. The family nurse practitioner should slowly taper the patient from the haloperidol (Haldol) 2 mg.

It is possible that she may not need the medication or that one of the newer atypical antipsychotics would be more effective with a lesser side effect profile. Patients may complain of a feeling of muscular quivering. Ataxia is a disorder wherein muscular incoordination occurs with voluntary muscular movements. Agitation is a general assessment that may be part of the psychotic behavior. Dyskinesia is a defect in voluntary movement.

34. Answer: 4

Rationale: Correction of environmental factors and treatment of underlying iatrogenic and medical problems should be addressed initially. Amitriptyline (Elavil) can cause excessive somnolence. Trazodone (Desyrel) may be of particular use when sleep disturbance is prominent; however, it does not address the best initial plan. The goal is to begin with good sleep hygiene before pharmacologic therapy. Eliminating naps during the day may be useful in facilitating sleep.

35. Answer: 1

Rationale: Drug-drug interactions are a common cause of acute confusion in the older adult patient. This assessment can minimize the need to do further costly interventions if the patient only needs medication adjustment. The other options should be included in the plan after the drug history is completed and has been ruled out as a potential problem. The family nurse practitioner must always consider that an acute illness, such as a UTI, may be the cause of acute confusion. A UA should also be obtained because the patient can quickly progress to sepsis.

36. Answer: 2

Rationale: In combination with tyramine-rich foods that have undergone an aging process such as cheese, wine, beer, salami, and yogurt, catecholamines are released from the nerve endings, causing a hypertensive crisis. The other drugs listed cause hypotension.

37. Answer: 3

Rationale: The benzodiazepines cause sedation and decreased attention, which, in turn, affect the memory. Although phenothiazines and antidepressants may also cause sedation, they do not affect memory.

38. Answer: 3

Rationale: Flashbacks, depression, and psychotic behavior can occur with lysergic acid diethylamide (LSD) use. There are no withdrawal symptoms or physical dependence associated with use; however, tolerance develops quickly. Commonly, the adolescent remains oriented but experiences hallucinations and altered bodily sensations.

39. Answer: 3

Rationale: Trazodone (Desyrel) has sedation as a side effect, which has made it less popular as an antidepressant; however, it is commonly prescribed for insomnia.

40. Answer: 2, 3, 5

Rationale: Lorazepam (Ativan) is a short-acting benzodiazepine and may be used in acute alcohol withdrawal delirium. Chlordiazepoxide (Librium) is also a benzodiazepine and can be used for acute alcohol withdrawal. Thiamine (B_1) deficiency is often seen with alcoholism and should be given as a supplement. Citalopram (Celexa) and bupropion (Wellbutrin) are antidepressants and are not used in acute alcohol withdrawal. Chlorpromazine (Thorazine), which is an antipsychotic, would not be used in the management plan.

41. Answer: 1, 3, 4

Rationale: Lithium has adverse side effects on renal, cardiac, and thyroid function. Baseline electrolytes are also important to obtain. It is not important to evaluate liver function, fasting lipids, and ESR before initiating treatment with lithium.

42. Answer: 3

Rationale: Naloxone (Narcan) is a narcotic antagonist and is used for the reversal of narcotic depression, including respiratory depression. Clonidine (Catapres) is a central-acting α_2-agonist and is indicated for treatment of hypertension. Methadone is used in the treatment of opioid addiction. The Food and Drug Administration (FDA) has placed methadone in a special drug category that allows medically supervised administration of the drug to addicts with chronic, intractable addiction to heroin. In addition, methadone can be used for pain management. The therapeutic classification of naltrexone (Revia) is as a narcotic detoxification adjunct.

43. Answer: 1, 3, 5

Rationale: Seizures, alcohol withdrawal, and anxiety are commonly treated with benzodiazepines. They are not the first drug of choice for obsessive-compulsive disorder; selective serotonin reuptake inhibitors are usually used. Schizophrenia and bipolar affective disorder are treated with antipsychotics.

44. Answer: 1

Rationale: The rule of thumb for starting medications in the older adult patient is to start low and go slow; therefore, doses should be reduced by 30%–50% to start therapy and gradually increased as necessary. Adverse effects are likely to occur because of slowed drug metabolism, which occurs with aging. These include hypotension, arrhythmias, and sedative and anticholinergic effects.

45. Answer: 2

Rationale: A highly nicotine-dependent patient benefits from intense counseling and prescription of alternative nicotine delivery during the smoking cessation process. The nicotine patch is usually the preferred form of replacement because the gum is noncontinuous and withdrawal symptoms may occur during nonchewing times. The nicotine patch delivers a fixed dose of nicotine on a continual basis, is applied once daily, and eliminates the gastrointestinal upset that often occurs with the gum. If this patient insisted on using the gum, the dose should be 4 mg, not 2 mg. A nicotine patch with 14 mg is too low a dose to start on this patient and is not the correct dosing schedule. Underdosing can cause patients to start smoking again. Bupropion HCl (Zyban) would be used in conjunction with the nicotine patch, and patients are to quit smoking 1–2 weeks after starting the bupropion HCl (Zyban), not immediately.

46. Answer: 2

Rationale: When stopping a selective serotonin reuptake inhibitor (SSRI), such as sertraline (Zoloft), it is important to taper the dose over at least 2 weeks. Stopping the medication abruptly can lead to flulike symptoms. There is no need to continue the medication or switch to a different antidepressant because the patient was assessed for safety and it is reasonable to stop the medication. The family nurse practitioner should make a follow-up appointment to assess how the patient is doing off the medication.

47. Answer: 1

Rationale: Divalproex sodium (Depakote) is an antiepileptic used to treat seizures and mania in bipolar disorder and prevent migraine headaches and is used for agitation in dementia patients. Divalproex sodium (Depakote) can cause hepatotoxicity, especially in the first 6 months of starting the medication. It can also cause thrombocytopenia and pancreatitis in some incidences.

48. Answer: 2

Rationale: Selective serotonin reuptake inhibitors (SSRIs), such as citalopram (Celexa), can lead to hyponatremia from syndrome of inappropriate antidiuretic hormone (SIADH). The patient is at particular risk because he is an older adult and is on furosemide (Lasix). The patient may be at risk for hypokalemia secondary to furosemide (Lasix), but it is not aggravated with the addition of citalopram (Celexa).

49. Answer: 1

Rationale: Diphenhydramine (Benadryl) is an antihistamine with anticholinergic properties. Anticholinergic drugs may cause confusion, urinary retention, orthostatic hypotension, tachycardia, dry mouth, constipation, sedation, and blurred vision. Anticholinergic drugs are particularly dangerous in the older adult because they can lead to falls and confusion.

50. Answer: 3

Rationale: The maximum dose of citalopram (Celexa) for a patient older than age 60 is 20 mg once a day. Citalopram (Celexa) has a risk of prolonged QT interval, which can lead to torsades de pointes. Torsades de pointes is a ventricular dysrhythmia that can lead to sudden death.

51. Answer: 1

Rationale: Benzodiazepines should be tapered in all patients but especially in the older adult. Withdrawal symptoms may include sweating, vomiting, muscle cramps, tremors and/or seizures. Rebound or withdrawal symptoms occur within 24 hours in patients taking the shorter-acting medications and may not occur for several days in patients taking long-acting medications. The adverse effects of oversedation—dizziness, confusion, and orthostatic hypotension—contribute to falls and other injuries in the older adult. Short-acting medications are preferred. Typically, larger doses are not needed but rather small initial doses with gradual increases.

Research & Theory

Research

1. When designing a research study that will involve patients, what is the most important point to be included in the written consent to participate?

   1. Role of the primary research investigator.

   2. Anticipated date for publication of the completed research report.

   3. Assurance of patient privacy and confidentiality.

   4. Number of previously published research studies about this topic.

2. When determining whether to incorporate a new procedure into a clinical practice based on the findings of a recent quantitative research study, which of the following should be considered? Select two responses.

   1. Statistical significance of the findings.

   2. Statistical relevance of the findings.

   3. Statistical software program used.

   4. Statistical background of the researcher.

   5. Methodological limitations of the study.

3. The research process is similar to the processes that family nurse practitioners use to provide patient care. What steps are involved in the research process and process of family nurse practitioners in providing direct patient care?

   1. Assessing, teaching, evaluating, and discussing.

   2. Defining, planning, implementing, and charting.

   3. Questioning, evaluating, diagnosing, and teaching.

   4. Assessing, planning, implementing, and evaluating.

4. Both descriptive and inferential statistics are used in research. However, their purposes are different in that: (Select two responses.)

   1. Inferential statistics are used for assigning participant code numbers.

   2. Descriptive statistics are used for assigning participant code numbers.

   3. Descriptive statistics are used to provide information about the study variables.

   4. Inferential statistics are used for hypothesis testing.

   5. Descriptive statistics are used for hypothesis testing.

5. In an ambulatory care setting run exclusively by family nurse practitioners, the family nurse practitioner might find it difficult to conduct collaborative research because:

   1. Health care professionals outside of nursing are needed for conducting collaborative research, and this would be difficult in a family nurse practitioner–only care setting.

   2. Procedures for conducting collaborative research have not been well defined in the literature.

   3. Studies involving collaborative research published in professional journals are too difficult to access by clinicians.

   4. Ambulatory care settings have little in common with the settings used for most types of research.

6. The scientific method for conducting research uses the null hypothesis, which is statistically based. What is the correct format for stating the null hypothesis?

   1. There is no significant difference between two groups.

   2. Group "A" is greater than group "B."

   3. Group "A" is less than group "B."

   4. There is a 95% probability that group "A" is different from group "B."

7. When evaluating claims made on advertisements, such as "Drug X has been used for 5 years with over 1 million doses administered in the United States, Canada, and Great Britain. Drug X stops heartburn, aids in digestion, and prevents esophageal reflux and is the 'treatment of choice' to relieve GERD," the family nurse practitioner realizes that the claim is:

   1. Invalid; there is no control or comparison group, and no statistics are stated.

   2. Valid; there are sufficient numbers of users who have had success.

   3. Invalid; the level of significance is not mentioned to be at the 0.05 level or higher.

   4. Valid; the cohort and Hawthorne effects are operating.

8. Reviewing labor and delivery in the practice, the family nurse practitioner notes that pregnant patients who are still in their teens generally seem to go into labor before their due date (as determined by ultrasound), whereas women in their mid-20s usually go into labor at or after their due date. Which statistical analysis would answer the research question, "Among pregnant women in a family nurse practitioner practice, what are the differences between the length of gestation for women ages 16–19 compared with women ages 23–26?"

   1. Multiple regression.

   2. Cronbach's alpha.

   3. Two-tailed *t*-test.

   4. Pearson's product-moment correlation.

9. The Stetler model of research utilization in nursing practice can be equated with:

   1. Nursing theory.

   2. Change theory.

   3. Discharge planning.

   4. Patient education.

10. The family nurse practitioner is compiling monthly statistics for the practice, and one of the elements of the analysis is the ethnicity of patients. What level of measurement data can be used to analyze the variable of ethnicity?

    1. Nominal level.

    2. Ordinal level.

    3. Interval level.

    4. Ratio level.

11. A family nurse practitioner working with a physician in short-term rehabilitation is compiling end-of-month statistics. The patients who received care are 55 years of age and over. Which of the following data from the monthly report is most likely to be normally distributed?

    1. Laboratory tests scheduled for the patients.

    2. Gender of the patients.

    3. Primary diagnosis of the patients.

    4. Height of the patients.

12. A family nurse practitioner is compiling statistics at the end of the month for an older adult patient population with coronary artery disease. The family nurse practitioner and physician in the general practice want to know the average total cholesterol levels of their patients. Which would be the most appropriate statistical measure of the average cholesterol level for the patient population?

    1. The mean.

    2. The median.

    3. The mode.

    4. The range.

13. A family nurse practitioner is evaluating research articles for a research utilization project. The majority of the articles report that either random selection or random assignment was used. Because certain procedures in research are used across disciplines, what can be assumed for studies where randomization has been used?

    1. The ages of the research subjects in these studies will be negatively skewed.

    2. The researchers were attempting to select research subjects who fit certain demographic criteria.

    3. The ages of the research subjects in these studies will be positively skewed.

    4. The researchers were attempting to obtain the most representative sample by randomly assigning research subjects to either a control or treatment group.

14. The ability to predict outcomes of care is desirable both in research and in practice. If a family nurse practitioner wanted to determine whether there was a relationship among providing annual physical exams and immunizations to predict patient outcomes, which statistical analysis method would be used to analyze the clinical data?

    1. Descriptive statistics.

    2. Paired *t*-test.

    3. Multiple regression.

    4. Chi-square (χ^2) test.

15. Quantitative research articles are being evaluated by a family nurse practitioner for a utilization project. What three steps are essential in providing a critical appraisal of quantitative research? (Select three responses.)

    1. Read the discussion findings section.

    2. Determine the strengths and limitations of the study.

    3. Verify the educational background of the research author(s).

    4. Identify the steps of the research process.

    5. Evaluate the credibility and meaning of the study to nursing practice.

16. The family nurse practitioner has determined that the current policy and procedures for diagnosing and stabilizing new diabetic patients need to be evaluated and possibly updated. Which would be the best choice for the first phase of the evaluation?

    1. Design and conduct a double-blind clinical trial.

    2. Design and conduct a research utilization project.

    3. Design and conduct a research project comparing men and women.

    4. Design and conduct a study to test Callista Roy's theoretic model.

17. A family nurse practitioner has read a nursing research article in which there were no statistically significant findings. What would be the family nurse practitioner's most appropriate response?

    1. "Reading this article was a waste of my time."

    2. "Because of this article, there is no reason to conduct similar studies."

    3. "Reading this article raises new questions for my practice."

    4. "Because of this article, I will immediately change my practice."

18. In a recent study, the researcher reports that "the statistical analysis used was Pearson's product-moment correlation." Based on this information, when is it appropriate to use Pearson's product-moment correlation as the statistical analysis for analyzing data in research? Select two responses.

    1. Pearson's product-moment correlation can be used for comparing interval or ratio levels of measurement among one or more variables.

    2. Pearson's product-moment correlation actually determines if a causal relationship exists between one or more variables.

    3. Pearson's product-moment correlation can be used only when there is a single variable.

    4. Pearson's product-moment correlation is used to identify the relationship between one or more variables.

19. When might a qualitative research design be employed over a quantitative or mixed methods research design?

    1. Qualitative research is the preferred methodology for exploring and understanding a particular phenomenon of interest.

    2. With qualitative methods, there are no concerns about the rights of research subjects.

    3. Qualitative research will provide precise measures for statistical analysis.

    4. Qualitative research ensures tight control during data collection and data analysis.

20. The normal ranges of blood chemistry values are most similar to which statistical concept?

    1. The standard error.

    2. The mean.

    3. The standard deviation.

    4. The median.

21. Variance is a key statistical concept. How would current research methods change if there were no variance?

    1. Nurse researchers would need to increase the sample size in all research studies to 100 research subjects or greater.

    2. Since current research methods do not depend on the presence of variance, researchers would not need to change the current methods.

    3. Nurse researchers would need to decrease the sample size of all research studies to 15 research subjects.

    4. Since current research methods are based on the presence of variance, researchers would not be able to use current methods.

22. A family nurse practitioner understands that an incidence rate is: (Select two responses.)

    1. Often a percentage and describes the characteristics of a population.

    2. A sensitive indicator of the changing health of a community.

    3. The number of new cases of a disease in those exposed to a disease.

    4. The number of cases of a specific disease or condition in a population at a specified point in time relative to the population at the same point in time.

    5. The occurrence of new cases of a disease or condition in a population over a period of time relative to the size of the population at risk for the disease or condition in the same time period.

23. A community screening for hypertension revealed 15 patients previously diagnosed with hypertension and 22 new cases for a total of 37 cases. What is this called?

    1. Morbidity.

    2. Incidence.

    3. Attack.

    4. Prevalence.

24. A state public health region reported 21 cases of measles in children 7 years of age and younger to date this year with 2 children who died. The total population for this geographic region is 11,533, of whom 4420 are children age 7 years and younger. What is the prevalence rate of measles in the region thus far in the current year?

    1. 1.8/1000

    2. 2/1000

    3. 21/1000

    4. 4.7/1000

25. The four major sequential steps of evidence-based practice are:

    1. Establish a patient relationship, perform a health assessment, make a diagnosis, devise a plan of care, perform prescribed treatments, and evaluate efficacy of the treatments.

    2. Identify the problem and generate a clinical question, conduct a literature review of scholarly research articles, critically appraise published research, implement useful findings in practice and clinical decision making, and disseminate findings.

    3. Review the popular literature, review the institution's policy and procedures, summarize the findings from the literature review, policies and procedures, and evaluate applicability of the study findings to practice setting.

    4. Review the patient's lab reports, complete a thorough health assessment, diagnose, collaborate with the health care provider in developing a treatment plan, implement the treatment, and evaluate the efficacy of the treatment.

26. A family nurse practitioner is planning to conduct a study to examine the efficacy of a high-protein, high-fiber diet in weight reduction of obese patients. The family nurse practitioner develops the following research question to guide the study: *What is the effect on obese patients' weight who follow a high-protein, high-fiber diet compared with obese patients' weight who do not follow a high-protein, high-fiber diet over a 12-week period?*

    What is the independent variable and dependent variable in the research question?

    1. The independent variable is the 12-week time frame, and the dependent variable is the high-protein, high-fiber diet.

    2. The independent variable is the high-protein, high-fiber diet, and the dependent variable is the patients' weight.

    3. The independent variable is the patients' weight, and the dependent variable is the high-protein, high-fiber diet.

    4. The independent variable is the high-protein, high-fiber diet, and the dependent variable is the 12-week time frame.

27. The family nurse practitioner is a member of a research team conducting a study to evaluate the efficacy of yoga as a treatment in children with attention-deficit hyperactivity disorder (ADHD). When reviewing the literature, which type of research study does the nurse practitioner recognize as the highest level of evidence?

    1. A qualitative research study using a grounded theory approach.

    2. A quantitative research study using a correlational research design.

    3. A quantitative research study using a randomized-controlled trial design.

    4. A qualitative research study using a phenomenological approach.

28. When the family nurse practitioner determines whether or not being exposed to second-hand smoke leads to lung cancer in a group of residential home patients with another group of residential patients who have not been exposed to second-hand smoke, the family nurse practitioner is determining the:

    1. Prevalence rate.

    2. Incidence rate.

    3. Confidence interval.

    4. Relative risk.

29. The family nurse practitioner explains to a group of nursing students that 6 babies out of 1000 live births die during their first year of life. This type of statistic is called:

    1. Prevalence rate.

    2. Infant mortality rate.

    3. Infant morbidity rate.

    4. Incidence rate.

30. The family nurse practitioner is conducting a meta-analysis on the effectiveness of patient teaching on how to use an MDI in the treatment of asthma patients. Which three statements are accurate concerning a meta-analysis?

    1. Assesses clinical effectiveness of health care interventions.

    2. Provides a precise estimate of the treatment effect.

    3. Focuses on a few targeted studies with homogeneity.

    4. Can add bias to the review of specific research studies.

    5. Provides a qualitative review of pertinent research literature.

    6. Provides highest level of evidence due to statistical analysis and integration of many studies.

Theory

31. Martha Rogers' theory of principles of homeodynamics focuses on several principles that explain how individuals interact with the environment. Which of the following three principles are included in Rogers' theory of principles of homeodynamics? (Select three responses.)

    1. Carative factors.

    2. Resonancy.

    3. Primary prevention.

    4. Integrality.

    5. Helicy.

32. A family nurse practitioner is providing a wellness screening to a 4-month-old infant. The mother expresses concern that her infant cannot roll over in either direction without assistance and that there is a developmental delay with his gross motor development. The mother indicates that her toddler's lack of movement is her fault because she works full-time and has to keep her son in daycare full-time. Based on the patient case scenario, what type of nursing theory could be applied here?

    1. Neuman's Systems Model.

    2. Watson's Theory of Caring.

    3. King's Theory of Goal Attainment.

    4. Mercer's Theory of Becoming a Mother.

33. King's Theory of Goal Attainment specifically focuses on:

    1. Effective communication among patient, family, and health care provider.

    2. Reducing stressors that may contribute to illness and disease.

    3. Interaction, transactions, and mutually shared outcomes between the nurse and patient.

    4. The nurse assisting the patient with improving and meeting self-care needs.

34. The theoretical basis for nursing practice is:

    1. A recent development in nursing practice.

    2. Developed from the medical model.

    3. Traced back to Florence Nightingale.

    4. Unrelated to the practice of nursing.

35. The verification of the more abstract nursing theories (e.g., of Martha Rogers) is often hampered by:

    1. Lack of adequate instrumentation for the theoretical concepts.

    2. Prior studies that did not support the theory.

    3. Lack of adequate settings for conducting experiments.

    4. Prior studies that were conducted in other countries.

36. Basing nursing practice on nursing theory contributes to the professionalization of nursing practice by:

    1. Adapting the medical model to nursing care.

    2. Limiting the choice of treatments for patients.

    3. Determining what types of patients will be seen by the nurse.

    4. Providing a consistent perspective for providing care to patients.

37. A family nurse practitioner has decided to incorporate a theoretical nursing model into the ambulatory care practice, which emphasizes patients doing as much as possible to maintain their own health. Which nursing model is most applicable to this setting?

    1. Orem's Self-Care Deficit Theory of Nursing.

    2. Roy's Adaptation Model.

    3. Roger's Science of Unitary Human Beings.

    4. King's Theory of Goal Attainment.

38. Which of the following nursing theorists is considered to have general systems theory as the philosophical orientation to her model?

    1. Callista Roy.

    2. Martha Rogers.

    3. Rosemarie Parse.

    4. Betty Neuman.

39. Which nursing theory addresses nursing outcomes in terms of primary, secondary, and tertiary prevention?

    1. Roy's Adaptation Model.

    2. Neuman's Systems Model.

    3. King's Theory of Goal Attainment.

    4. Watson's Human Caring Theory.

40. Which nursing model includes a concept that explores the individual's desire to improve health and well-being?

    1. Watson's Theory of Caring.

    2. Neuman's Systems Model.

    3. Pender's Health Promotion Model.

    4. Roy's Adaptation Model.

41. The family nurse practitioner is planning to conduct an educational program to encourage smoking cessation in a group of adult smokers. The family nurse practitioner knows that they must employ interventions that facilitate the participant's recognition of the health risk associated with continued smoking to facilitate the participant's desire to utilize the proposed interventions to improve overall health. Based on the goals and desired outcomes of the educational program, the family nurse practitioner knows that the most appropriate theoretical model to guide the development of the program would be:

    1. Roy's Adaptation Model.

    2. The Health Belief Model.

    3. The Conservation Model.

    4. The Intersystem Model.

42. The family nurse practitioner is reviewing nursing theories that utilize the nursing metaparadigm. The family nurse practitioner knows that the nursing metaparadigm is composed of which four concepts? (Select four responses.)

    1. Human being.

    2. Research.

    3. Environment.

    4. Nursing.

    5. Health.

    6. Education.

43. The family nurse practitioner is discussing methods to facilitate independence with a recent stroke patient, who is experiencing residual hemiplegia. The family nurse practitioner is using which concept of Orem's Self-Care Deficit Theory during this interaction?

    1. Universal self-care requisites.

    2. Developmental self-care requisites.

    3. Health deviation self-care deficits.

    4. Nursing system.

44. The family nurse practitioner is working in a culturally diverse medical clinic and plans to develop an educational program to facilitate improvement in health in the patient population. Based on the patient population and the purpose of the program, which of the following nursing theorists would be most appropriate to review to use as a theoretical framework for the educational program?

    1. Calista Roy.

    2. Dorothea Orem.

    3. Margaret Newman.

    4. Madeleine Leininger.

45. The family nurse practitioner is working with a group of colleagues to develop a research study that will use Roy's Adaptation Model as the theoretical framework to develop the study. Which three theoretical concepts will the team be sure to include in the study? (Select three responses.)

    1. Adaptation.

    2. Cognator subsystem.

    3. Exploitation phase.

    4. Contextual stimuli.

    5. Culture care re-patterning.

    6. Orientation phase.

20 Research & Theory Answers and Rationales

Research

1. Answer: 3

Rationale: By federal law, the rights of human research subjects must be protected. Patients must be assured of their privacy and confidentiality through informed consent. The other information is interesting and may be included but is not required by federal law.

2. Answer: 1, 5

Rationale: In published research reports, of the options listed, statistical significance of the findings and methodological limitations of the study are consistently reported by researchers. The statistical significance of a study's findings provides consumers of research with information about the likelihood that the results may have occurred by chance. It is also equally important to have knowledge of a study's limitations to determine whether the findings could be applicable in a different population or setting. The clinical relevance is considered, not the statistical relevance. The specific statistical software program used does not make a difference because all are based on the same statistical formulas. Researchers frequently work with statistical consultants, so a researcher's background is not a limitation to a published study.

3. Answer: 4

Rationale: The elements common to both processes are assessing, planning, implementing, and evaluating.

4. Answer: 3, 4

Rationale: Neither type of statistics is used to assign participant code numbers. Descriptive statistics are used to describe the independent and dependent variables used in the study. Inferential statistics conducts hypothesis testing to analyze data from a sample to determine whether the findings could be generalized to an entire population.

5. Answer: 1

Rationale: Limited interaction with medical and health care professionals can be a barrier to conducting collaborative research in any setting. The process of collaborative research is well delineated by researchers. With the ever-increasing availability of professional journals offered online and via mobile devices, access is rarely a problem. A considerable body of research has been conducted in ambulatory care settings.

6. Answer: 1

Rationale: The correct format for the null hypothesis is, "There is no significant difference between two groups." The alternate or research hypothesis may take the other forms. Probability theory uses percentages or decimal values to evaluate the likelihood that an outcome will occur in a particular situation.

7. Answer: 1

Rationale: Even though the claims detail extensive use of "Drug X," there must be statistical evidence reported. Additionally, randomization, as demonstrated through the use of control or comparison groups, should be implemented that will render a level of significance. The Hawthorne effect is a limitation and threat to a study's validity, as the study participants' behaviors and responses are changed because of being in the study, not necessarily from the intervention or treatment performed.

8. Answer: 3

Rationale: Only the two-tailed t-test compares two independent groups on a variable to determine whether the means of the two independent groups differ. Multiple regression analyzes the relationships between two or more independent variables on a dependent variable. Cronbach's alpha is used for reporting the reliability of an instrument used in a study. Pearson's product-moment correlation is used to analyze the relationship between two variables.

9. Answer: 2

Rationale: Incorporating evidence-based research findings into practice often results in a change in practice. Nursing theory uses concepts to explain phenomena. Discharge planning and patient education are responsibilities carried out by family nurse practitioners and do not necessarily relate to research utilization.

10. Answer: 1

Rationale: The variable of ethnicity is categorical data or nominal-level data. Ordinal-level measurements are also categorized, but the categories can be ranked. Interval-level measurements of data are categorized, ranked, and have equal interval scales where the distance between intervals is always the same. Ratio-level measurement has all of the criteria as interval-level data but also has an absolute zero point.

11. Answer: 4

Rationale: The gender and primary diagnosis are nominal-level data. The laboratory tests would be skewed and are considered a ratio level of measurement data, whereas the height would have a symmetric bell-shaped curve for patients 55 years of age and over.

12. Answer: 2

Rationale: The median cholesterol level would be most representative of the average because the cholesterol level of 50% of the patients is above and 50% is below the median. The mean could be influenced by one patient with a very high or very low cholesterol level. The mode identifies only the cholesterol level that is reported most often. The range identifies only the lowest and the highest cholesterol levels and does not represent an average.

13. Answer: 4

Rationale: Randomization is a research technique used to increase the amount of control and reduce potential threats of internal validity in any research design. The other three options are false; they do not occur because of randomization.

14. Answer: 3

Rationale: Of the options, only multiple regression examines the relationship between two or more independent variables in a way that permits prediction on an outcome or dependent variable. Descriptive statistics provides information about the study variables and sample. A paired *t*-test is used to determine differences between two groups (e.g., control and experimental group) on an outcome. Chi-square (χ^2) test compares percentages in one category to another category.

15. Answer: 2, 4, 5

Rationale: In conducting a critical appraisal of quantitative research, it is necessary to identify the steps of the research process, determine the strengths and limitations of the study, and evaluate the overall credibility of the study to nursing practice. Reading the discussion of findings section and verifying the educational background of the researchers are actions completed under the three comprehensive steps for critically appraising quantitative research.

16. Answer: 2

Rationale: As a first step, a research utilization project would provide a thorough review of the published literature on which to make a change based on evidence. A full study may not be needed, and testing a theoretic nursing model is not appropriate for this situation.

17. Answer: 3

Rationale: The lack of significant findings is an important piece of information about the topic of the research and definitely is not a waste of time. Particularly when findings are not statistically significant, additional studies need to be conducted about this topic. Ideally, changes in practice are based on the findings of more than one study.

18. Answer: 1, 4

Rationale: Pearson's product-moment correlation is the preferred statistical analysis to use for variables that consist of ratio or interval levels of measurement, whereas Spearman's correlation would be an appropriate statistical test to use when the research variables are ranked. Pearson's product-moment correlation also identifies the relationships among variables, not causal relationships among variables. Two or more variables may be used for Pearson's product-moment correlation.

19. Answer: 1

Rationale: The purpose of qualitative research designs is to learn more about a particular phenomenon of interest by exploring the beliefs, values, and experiences of individuals. Qualitative designs do not yield precise measures, are usually not analyzed statistically, and carry the same concerns about the rights of subjects as all other research designs. Quantitative research designs ensure tight control over data collection and analysis.

20. Answer: 3

Rationale: The normal ranges of blood chemistry values are based on studies that identified the standard deviation for each blood chemical value, e.g., normal serum sodium value range 135–145 mEq/L. The mean is an average of the blood chemistry values, the median is the middle blood chemistry value, and the standard error is not applicable to this situation.

21. Answer: 4

Rationale: All current research and statistical analysis methods rely on the presence of variance or variation; if variance is no longer present, current methods could no longer be used. If there is no variance, a sample of one would be adequate.

22. Answer: 2, 5

Rationale: The incidence rate is the occurrence of new cases of a disease or condition in a population over a period of time relative to the size of the population at risk for the disease of condition in the same time period. Incidence rates are helpful for monitoring short-term changes in a disease (influenza, chickenpox, measles, etc.) and are a sensitive indicator of the changing health of a community because the rate captures the fluctuations of a disease. A prevalence rate is the number of cases of a specific disease or condition in a population at a specified point in time relative to the population at the same point in time. An attack rate is the number of new cases of a disease in those exposed to the disease.

23. Answer: 4

Rationale: Prevalence is a measure of disease that allows family nurse practitioners to determine a person's likelihood of having a disease. A prevalence rate is the total number of cases of a disease existing in a population divided by the total population. The incidence is a measure of the frequency with which a disease occurs in a population over a period of time. Morbidity is another term for illness, injury, or disability. Attack rate often refers to the risk of getting a disease during a specified period, such as during an outbreak of measles.

24. Answer: 4

Rationale: A prevalence rate is the total number of cases of a disease existing in a population divided by the total population. The formula to calculate is:

$$\frac{number\ of\ existing\ cases}{total\ population} \times 1000$$

The number of existing cases is 21 and the total pediatric population is 4420.

25. Answer: 2

Rationale: Identify the problem and generate a clinical question, conduct a literature review of scholarly research articles, critically appraise published research, implement useful findings in practice and clinical decision making, and disseminate findings contained in the published steps of evidence-based practice. All other options are nursing actions taken on behalf of the patient (in no particular order).

26. Answer: 2

Rationale: The independent variable is the measure that can be manipulated in a study; the high-protein, high-fiber diet. The dependent variable is the response from the independent variable and is measurable, i.e., the obese patients' weight. The population of interest is the obese patients and the length of the study is 12 weeks.

27. Answer: 3

Rationale: A randomized, controlled trial is one of the highest levels of evidence in determining if a cause and effect relationship exists between an experimental intervention (treatment) and dependent variable (outcome). By randomizing participants into either a control or treatment group, rigor is

increased. A quantitative correlational research design examines the relationship between one or more variables; correlational research does not predict causality. Qualitative research designs are lower on the hierarchal level of evidence pyramid as they do not attempt to predict causality or determine the effectiveness of an intervention.

28. Answer: 4

Rationale: The relative risk or risk ratio (RR) is a measure of the risk of a certain event (getting lung cancer) happening in one group exposed to a factor (second-hand smoke) compared to the risk of the same event happening in another group not exposed to a factor. A prevalence rate is the total number of cases of a disease existing in a population divided by the total population. The incidence is a measure of the frequency with which a disease occurs in a population over a period of time. The confidence interval describes the amount of uncertainty associated with a sample estimate of a population parameter, e.g., usually at 95% level, and assists in representing how good an estimate is.

29. Answer: 2

Rationale: Infant mortality is the death of an infant less than one year of age and is measured as the infant mortality rate (IMR), which is the number of deaths of infants under one year of age per 1000 live births. Infant morbidity is a measure of disease, illness, or injury within a population. A prevalence rate is the total number of cases of a disease existing in a population divided by the total population. The incidence rate is the new (or newly diagnosed) cases of a disease and is generally reported as the number of new cases occurring within a period of time (e.g., per month, per year).

30. Answer: 1, 2, 6

Rationale: A meta-analysis is a summary of a number of independent studies focused on one question or topic, and uses a specific statistical methodology to synthesize the findings in order to draw conclusions about the area of focus that ultimately seeks new knowledge, as well as confirming knowledge, from existing research data. It is used to assess clinical effectiveness of health care interventions and is helpful in providing a precise estimate of a treatment or intervention outcome. Meta-analysis provides Level I evidence, which is considered the highest level of evidence, as it statistically analyzes and integrates the results of many independent studies. An effective, robust meta-analysis aims for complete coverage of all relevant studies, examines for the presence of heterogeneity in the studies, and explores the studies' main findings using sensitivity analysis. Meta-analysis, when carried out as a rigorous systematic review, can overcome inherent bias by offering an unbiased synthesis of the empirical data. Meta-analyses offer a systematic and quantitative (not qualitative) approach to synthesizing research evidence to analyze clinical interventions.

Theory

31. Answer: 2, 4, 5

Rationale: Resonacy, integrality, and helicy are principles of homeodynamics that Rogers developed and defined to explain how individuals interact with their environment. Carative factors refer to Jean Watson's 10-carative factors under the Theory of Human Caring, and primary prevention relates to Neuman's Systems Model.

32. Answer: 4

Rationale: Mercer's Theory of Becoming a Mother is applicable to this case scenario because it involves a mother's emotional response to her infant's development. Maternal role identification and infant/child outcomes are two characteristics associated with Mercer's Theory. Neuman's Systems Model focuses on health promotion and prevention. Watson's Theory of Caring and King's Theory of Goal Attainment are not as applicable to the patient's case scenario.

33. Answer: 3

Rationale: King's Theory of Goal Attainments focuses on human interaction between the nurse and patient. During this interaction, information sharing and mutual patient goal-setting occurs between the nurse and patient. Although King's Theory focuses on communication, additional factors make up King's Theory. Minimizing stressors in the patient's environment refers to Neuman's Systems Model. Orem's Self-Care Theory focuses on assisting the patient with meeting self-care needs.

34. Answer: 3

Rationale: The theoretic basis for nursing practice began with Florence Nightingale and has been used in practice and research for more than a century. Nursing theories are specifically developed for nursing.

35. Answer: 1

Rationale: The lack of adequate tools and instruments for theoretical concepts is a major roadblock in many areas of research, and particularly so with the more abstract theories. Prior studies always provide information about the theory, even when conducted in other countries. The setting of the study plays no role in testing the theory.

36. Answer: 4

Rationale: Theory-based practice contributes the consistent perspective that permits the comparison of care across settings. This practice does not necessarily limit treatments or determine patient types. Theory-based practice specifically eliminates reliance on the medical model and provides nurs-

ing with a method to explain and explore the relationships between phenomena specific to nursing.

37. Answer: 1

Rationale: Orem's theory focuses on the patient participating in their own health care. Roy's model focuses on adaptation. Rogers' theory focuses on the synchronicity between the patient and the environment. King's theory is focused on the patient and nurse working together to achieve health-related goals.

38. Answer: 4

Rationale: Neuman's Systems Model is based on general systems theory. Roy's Adaptation Model is based on stress and adaptation as the framework. Martha Rogers' and Rosemarie Parse's theories are based on a humanistic developmental framework.

39. Answer: 2

Rationale: Betty Neuman identified the need to implement nursing interventions through the use of one or more of three modalities: primary, secondary, and tertiary prevention. Watson, Roy, and King's theories do not employ these concepts in their theories.

40. Answer: 3

Rationale: Pender's Health Promotion Model explores the concept of health promotion in which the individual seeks to improve health. Watson, Neuman, and Roy do not focus on the concept of health promotion.

41. Answer: 2

Rationale: The Health Belief Model purports that an individual's desire to employ health-promoting interventions is directly related to their perceived risk of developing a negative outcome if the intervention is not employed. The Intersystem Model, the Conservation Model, and Roy's Adaptation Model do not employ the risk and benefit concepts to facilitate participation in improving health or participating in health promotion activities.

42. Answer: 1, 3, 4, 5

Rationale: The nursing metaparadigm is comprised of four concepts: human being, environment, health, and nursing. Research and education are not concepts within the nursing metaparadigm.

43. Answer: 3

Rationale: Health deviation self-care deficits relate to facilitating self-care when a health care deficit exists. Universal self-care requisites relate to general human needs. Developmental self-care deficits refer to necessary developmental processes that occur throughout life. Nursing systems, according to Orem's Self-Care Deficit Theory, refer to the relationship between the nurse and the patient.

44. Answer: 4

Rationale: Madeleine Leininger's Theory of Transcultural Nursing explores cultural diversity and aims to recognize similarities and differences with various cultures and the role of nursing in working with these cultures in the health care setting. Calista Roy's Adaptation Model, Dorothea Orem's Self-Care Deficit Theory, and Margaret Newman's Health as Expanding Consciousness Theory all explore the interrelationship of nursing and the patient, but only Leininger's Theory of Transcultural Nursing explores the aspect of cultural diversity in addition to these concepts.

45. Answer: 1, 2, 4

Rationale: Adaptation, cognator subsystem, and contextual stimuli are all theoretical concepts of Roy's Adaptation Model and should be addressed in a study in which the model serves as the theoretical framework. The exploitation phase and orientation phase are theoretical concepts associated with Peplau's Art and Science of Nursing theory and would not be addressed in the study. Culture care re-patterning is a construct of Leininger's Culture Care Theory and would not be applicable as a theoretical framework for the study.

21

Professional Issues

Legal and Ethical

1. An occurrence-form professional liability insurance policy is preferred because:

   1. The amount of insurance money available to pay a claim increases with each renewal of the policy.

   2. The policy proceeds are available to pay claims regardless of when the claim is reported to the carrier.

   3. The carrier will be notified of a potential claim during the policy period.

   4. The coverage is broader than that provided by a claims-made policy form.

2. Early reporting of a potential professional liability claim is advantageous because:

   1. Insurance carriers have a 10-day reporting window, after which the coverage is canceled.

   2. Documents and witnesses needed to defend the claim are more likely to be available at the time of the event.

   3. Insurance premiums will be reduced with a good-faith showing of cooperation with the carrier.

   4. Risk management personnel require such reporting in order to comply with Joint Commission on the Accreditation of Healthcare Organizations (JCAHO) mandates.

3. A family nursing practitioner's nursing license may be in jeopardy if:

   1. The family nurse practitioner appropriately delegates medication administration to a trusted registered nurse (RN) employee, who administers a fatal dose.

   2. The family nurse practitioner delegates patient assessment tasks to a licensed practical nurse (LPN), who has been "floated" to the outpatient clinic for the day.

   3. The family nurse practitioner provides nursing care services consistent with established standards of practice in the jurisdiction.

   4. The medical assistant in the supervising physician's office exceeds the scope of her authority, but the family nurse practitioner takes prompt action to correct the problem.

4. A 46-year-old mentally challenged man has been diagnosed with colon cancer. Consent for his corrective surgery should be obtained from:

   1. The patient himself.

   2. The patient's 84-year-old mother, who is his closest relative.

   3. The patient's court-appointed guardian.

   4. The administrator of the group home where the patient lives.

5. A family nurse practitioner has a 75-year-old female patient with metastatic cancer. Her affairs are in order; she has arranged all her finances and her own funeral rites. She has systematically secured enough barbiturates to successfully end her life. The patient asks the family nurse practitioner to mix the drugs for her in some pudding to make them palatable for ingestion. What would be the family nurse practitioner's best course of action?

   1. Mix the medications as requested and stay with her while she consumes the preparation.

   2. Consult with family and attending physician to warn them about the patient's proposed course of action.

   3. Seek an immediate order for an antidepressant.

   4. Sit down with the patient and conduct a physical and psychological assessment.

6. The Patient Self-Determination Act (PSDA), passed by the U.S. Congress in 1990, resulted in which of the following policy changes?

   1. Hospitals are mandated to assist every patient to create a "living will."

   2. Federally funded managed care organizations (MCOs) are required to inform subscribers about their rights under state law to create "advance directives."

   3. Home health agencies are required to have "do not resuscitate" (DNR) orders on file for all terminally ill patients.

   4. Hospitalized patients are obligated to select a surrogate decision maker to make health care decisions for them if they become incapacitated.

7. Both the U.S. Food and Drug Administration (FDA) and Department of Health and Human Services (DHHS) have regulations governing research activities on human subjects. The principal investigator is responsible for:

   1. Securing a signed special research consent form.

   2. Reporting back to the Institutional Review Board if a subject is injured during the course of the study.

   3. Appearing before the Institutional Review Board to present the study and secure approval to proceed with subject recruitment at the facility.

   4. All the above.

8. If served with a summons and complaint (lawsuit documents), the family nurse practitioner should take which of the following actions as the first step?

   1. Call the patient to determine the basis for the action and nature of the alleged wrongdoing.

   2. Call the patient's lawyer (listed on first page of lawsuit) to obtain more information.

   3. Call the insurance company for instructions on how to proceed.

   4. Confer with colleagues and review the chart to determine if notes need to be clarified.

9. A family nurse practitioner in an impoverished rural area frequently encounters a female patient in a situation of domestic violence with few community options for referral. To address the situation, the family nurse practitioner participates in community education forums and fundraising for a safe house. The family nurse practitioner's participation is an example of applying what ethical principle?

   1. Autonomy.

   2. Nonmaleficence.

   3. Justice.

   4. Veracity.

10. Nurses practicing in expanded roles should carry professional liability insurance for which of the following reasons?

    1. Premiums are often modest and are a tax-deductible business expense.

    2. Even if the employer insures the family nurse practitioner, situations of conflict between employer and nurse may necessitate separate legal counsel.

    3. As roles expand, so does the liability potential.

    4. All the above.

11. The confidentiality of medical records is always a valid concern, especially with widespread computerization and fax machines. Release of medical information to third parties is:

    1. A "creature of state law," meaning that state statutes control the processing of such requests.

    2. Prohibited without the informed consent of the patient.

    3. Automatic when the requesting party is a third-party payer or insurer.

    4. Disallowed if the records contain proof of a diagnosis of acquired immunodeficiency syndrome (AIDS).

12. Which population is not included in the definition of disability under the Americans with Disabilities Act (ADA)?

    1. Profoundly deaf employees.

    2. Persons who are wheelchair bound.

    3. Current users of illegal drugs.

    4. Persons with mental retardation.

13. If a patient is having a problem with a managed care plan, the family nurse practitioner can offer to assist in which of the following ways?

    1. Suggest that the patient contact the customer service department (or "member services") for the care plan to resolve the issue; a formal grievance filing may be necessary.

    2. Remind the patient, who is a member of the "senior" plan for Medicare recipients that the patient may complain to the federal Office of Personnel Management (OPM).

    3. Remind the patient that the state's insurance department also investigates complaints against health plans.

    4. All the above.

14. If a piece of equipment malfunctions while being used on a hospitalized patient, the risk manager would probably recommend which of the following courses of action?

    1. Return the item to the manufacturer with a description of the problem and a request for analysis.

    2. Tag and sequester the item at the facility and defer analysis pending risk management review of the litigation potential.

    3. Send the item to the biomedical engineering department with a request for immediate equipment breakdown and troubleshooting.

    4. Repair the item, either in house or by an outside contracted firm, and return it to service as soon as possible.

15. Nurse expert witnesses are essential in the adjudication of most professional negligence claims against nurses. Which of the following criteria do attorneys use in selecting family nurse practitioner experts?

    1. Appropriate professional education, preferably at the technical level.

    2. Relevant and recent professional work experience.

    3. Ability to understand and articulate the legal issues involved in the claim.

    4. Published authors of medical texts in the clinical subject areas.

16. Which federal law mandates the tracking of implantable medical devices?

    1. Administrative Procedures Act (APA).

    2. Patient Self-Determination Act (PSDA).

    3. Safe Medical Devices Act (SMDA).

    4. Omnibus Budget Reconciliation Act (OBRA) of 1987.

17. Which of the following are elements of a broad-based risk management program?

    1. Hazardous materials compliance program as part of a comprehensive safety and security system.

    2. Early-warning/incident reporting program to identify elements of risk.

    3. System of contract review to avoid assuming liabilities that should be borne by others.

    4. All the above.

18. What the type of insurance coverage is purchased (or self-insured) by an organization to address employee job-related injuries?

    1. Professional liability insurance.

    2. Business interruption insurance.

    3. Directors and officers insurance.

    4. Workers' compensation insurance.

19. While driving your personal vehicle on a job-related errand, you are struck by a semitrailer on the interstate. The car is totaled and you are severely injured. Which insurance policies will respond to these losses?

    1. Your personal auto policy and your employer's workers' compensation policy.

    2. The employer's business auto policy and workers' compensation policy.

    3. Your homeowner's policy.

    4. The semitrailer driver's personal auto policy.

20. Family nurse practitioners with hospital privileges may be impacted by the part of the Health Care Quality Improvement Act known as the National Practitioner Data Bank (NPDB). Which of the following statements about the Data Bank is not true?

    1. Professional liability insurance claims payments made on behalf of family nurse practitioners are reported to the NPDB.

    2. The facility granting medical staff privileges must query the NPDB before approving a practitioner's privileges.

    3. The purpose of the NPDB is a nationwide flagging system that provides information about malpractice claims, licensure actions, and restrictions on privileges so that practitioners may not easily move from one jurisdiction to another to escape quality review.

    4. Insurance companies report all malpractice payments made on behalf of affected family nurse practitioners within 30 days of the date the payment was made, if the amount of the claim is in excess of $11,000 and no matter how it was settled.

21. In 1985, the U.S. Congress took action against a phenomenon known as "patient dumping" by enacting what was known at the time as the COBRA law, now referred to the Emergency Medical Treatment and Active Labor Act (EMTALA). Which three statements about EMTALA are true?

    1. The original purpose of the statute was to prohibit the transfer of uninsured and untreated patients from the emergency department of one hospital to another (usually the county hospital).

    2. Subsequent rules and case law have expanded the statute so that almost any unauthorized transfer of a patient from one facility to another is potentially problematic.

    3. To effect a proper transfer, the forwarding facility need not notify or secure the acquiescence of the receiving facility.

    4. The transferring facility must utilize appropriate transport methods and send copies of patients' medical records.

    5. The patient can be transferred by family members to another facility awaiting the patient's arrival.

22. A family nurse practitioner who wants to effect change in the state's laws regarding the dispensing of prescription medications by family nurse practitioners would take this case to the:

    1. State legislature.

    2. State board of nursing.

    3. State board of pharmacy.

    4. Nursing specialty organization.

23. What is the common meaning of "gag clauses" or "gag orders" in managed care?

    1. The managed care organization (MCO) declines to publish, in its subscriber contracts, the treatments that are excluded from coverage under the plan.

    2. The MCO refuses to allow its member services personnel to answer certain subscriber questions about covered benefits.

    3. The MCO contracts with providers to disallow providers from offering treatment alternatives that the providers know are not covered by patient plans.

    4. Providers are prohibited from offering experimental treatment to patients.

24. Under the Safe Medical Devices Act of 1990, which of the following health care providers or organizations are required to report the death of a patient to the Food and Drug Administration (FDA) if the death is related to the use of a medical device?

    1. Physician office staff.

    2. Hospitals, home health agencies, and ambulance companies.

    3. Nurse family members treating patients without compensation.

    4. Physicians making home visits.

25. A patient receives a medication that was intended for another person. Which is an appropriate way for the family nurse practitioner to document this event in the medical record?

    1. "Patient was given X mg of Y drug in error."

    2. "X mg of Y drug administered to patient. No adverse effects noted. Physician notified."

    3. "Patient received wrong medication. Incident report filed. Practitioner disciplined."

    4. "Practitioner inadvertently administered Y drug to wrong patient. Supervisor notified. Family threatening litigation."

26. What is the primary reason that patients give for suing family nurse practitioners for medical negligence?

    1. The care they received was substandard.

    2. The provider made an honest mistake.

    3. The patient was not "heard" when attempting to communicate with the provider.

    4. The patient participated fully in all aspects of medical decision making, but the results were disappointing.

27. Informed consent is based on the ethical principle of:

    1. Beneficence.

    2. Respect for persons.

    3. Nonmaleficence.

    4. Autonomy.

28. The four elements of a professional negligence claim are:

    1. Duty, fulfillment of duty, professional relationship, and wrongful act.

    2. Professional responsibility, fault, harm to patient, and wrongful act.

    3. Duty, breach of duty, causal connection between act and harm, and harm to patient.

    4. Professional relationship, intentional wrongful act, proximate cause, and damage to patient.

29. A family nurse practitioner is making an initial home health care visit to an older adult woman. Her spouse states that she is often confused; he answers all the questions and dominates the discussion. On the initial assessment, the patient does seem to be oriented to time, place, and person. Who is the proper party to sign the written form to request consent for services?

    1. Spouse.

    2. Patient.

    3. Attending physician.

    4. Home health aide who will be providing continuing care.

30. Why is an expert witness usually required in a nursing negligence case?

    1. Knowledge of medical or nursing facts is not considered intuitive to a lay jury.

    2. Jurors are allowed to use their "sixth sense" regarding the facts presented to them.

    3. Fact witnesses are not able to present an unbiased account of the circumstances in dispute.

    4. Appropriately credentialed experts have more credibility in the eyes of lay jurors.

31. The standard of care for a family nurse practitioner will be established by an expert witness(es) in a trial. The expert opinion will be based on which three items:

    1. National norms for the specialty.

    2. Facility policies and procedures.

    3. Professional literature.

    4. Opinions of other nurse practitioners.

    5. Current events.

32. Alternative dispute resolution (ADR) is a process in which the parties to a dispute resolve their differences outside of a court trial. Advantages to this system of problem solving include three of the following:

    1. The parties usually prefer the process because they have their opportunity to be heard in a less formal and less intimidating environment.

    2. The process is often less time-consuming and less costly than traditional litigation.

    3. Damage awards are less likely to include nonfinancial compensation.

    4. Insurers are amenable to working with mediators with a track record of fairness and successful case resolution.

    5. The losing party may appeal the ADR decision to the court system.

33. The statute of limitations is:

    1. The state law that prescribes the time frames within which a nursing negligence action may be filed.

    2. The law that states that minors have no legal authority to sue nurses for malpractice.

    3. The law that limits the right of patients to sue family nurse practitioners for negligent acts.

    4. The federal law that limits a family nurse practitioner's right to countersue a patient for malicious prosecution.

34. A family nurse practitioner is driving to a nursing seminar on an interstate highway. The family nurse practitioner observes a head-on collision and decides to stop to render aid. Which three statements are accurate with respect to the family nurse practitioner's potential liability for malpractice?

    1. There is no legal obligation to stop to render assistance; if the family nurse practitioner had driven by the accident, there would be no liability on the nurse's part.

    2. If appropriate nursing care is provided, gratuitously, the family nurse practitioner will be protected from liability under that state's Good Samaritan Law.

    3. Even if the family nurse practitioner acts in a grossly negligent manner, the Good Samaritan Law will shield the nurse from liability.

    4. The protections afforded by the Good Samaritan Law may differ from state to state; the family nurse practitioner should research the state's law on the subject.

    5. The family nurse practitioner must stop and render aid.

35. If a family nurse practitioner is subpoenaed to appear for a deposition in a nursing negligence case, appropriate preparation is prudent. Which advice from the attorney is appropriate? Select three responses.

    1. "Discreetly chew gum to calm your nerves, and dress for dinner because depositions usually take all day and you won't have time to change."

    2. "Review the patient's medical record and other pertinent material before appearing for questioning."

    3. "Take as much time as needed to think about your responses before answering; don't let the other lawyer put words in your mouth."

    4. "Be straightforward and truthful; remember that 'I don't know' and 'I don't remember' are acceptable responses."

    5. "Try to confuse the other attorney by displaying sophisticated medical knowledge and information."

36. Which of the following four suggestions for documentation is recommended?

    1. "Carefully document your criticism of a fellow provider's clinical decision in the patient's medical record. This will protect you if your treatment decisions need to be defended later."

    2. "Use standard abbreviations in the medical record so that subsequent readers will have no doubt as to your meaning and intent."

    3. "Document telephone conversations with the patient and family in the medical record. Be particularly vigilant about recording changes in the patient's medications."

    4. "Document noncompliant patient behaviors in the medical record; be thorough, yet factual."

    5. "Always make notation of errors in the medical record according to agency policy."

37. If a patient is under the "age of majority" for the state, what three factors would be considered to determine whether the patient is "emancipated" and able to consent to medical treatment?

    1. The patient is married.

    2. The patient is in the military.

    3. The patient is living outside the "care, custody, and control" of a parent or guardian.

    4. A personal friend of the patient's tells you that the patient has been emancipated by an order of the court.

38. In 1987 and 1994, the U.S. Congress updated many of the regulations that govern the provision of long-term care services. What is important for an employer or family nurse practitioner working in the long-term care environment to know?

    1. Nursing assistants working in long-term care facilities must be formally trained and certified.

    2. Patients or residents have specific rights, such as information about their physical condition, medical benefits, and associated costs.

    3. New and swifter sanctions are available to reviewers to impose on facilities with deficiencies.

    4. All the above.

39. A family nurse practitioner is employed in a private medical office. There is constant activity at the front desk, with patients checking in for appointments, staff scheduling tests, and telephone advice triage in progress. To preserve patient confidentiality, what changes should be implemented?

    1. Orient the computer monitor and printer, so that persons other than staff cannot read incoming reports and other data.

    2. Do all telephone scheduling from a more secure location, such as a conference room in the back office.

    3. Create a more private space to confer with patients who need follow-up information or explanations of tests or treatments.

    4. All the above.

40. Which activity could be considered grounds for a sexual harassment claim?

    1. A male employee tells an off-color joke to another man. The joke is overheard by a female co-worker who seems to appreciate the humor in it. The joke telling is an isolated incident.

    2. A nurse supervisor conducts an employee performance review. The supervisor does not mention a prior social relationship with the employee. The ratings are appropriate for the level of performance, and the employee receives a salary increase.

    3. A co-ed locker room is decorated with multiple centerfold photos from a popular men's magazine. The female employees find this offensive and have filed several complaints.

    4. A nurse is complimented on her appearance and asked on a date by her boss. She informs the boss that she is married and not seeking another relationship. The incident is forgotten.

41. A comatose female patient requires a feeding tube inserted for long-term nutritional needs. Her husband presents the family nurse practitioner with a document that he says is his wife's living will. It is signed by him, and he says that it sets out the wishes of his wife with respect to the feeding tube. Why is this living will not a legally binding document?

    1. The wife did not sign the document.

    2. The husband is not authorized to execute a living will on behalf of his wife.

    3. This type of advance directive must be signed by the individual (wife/patient) while this person is legally competent to execute the documents.

    4. All the above.

42. A family nurse practitioner is helping out at a clinic for homeless women. A diabetic patient in her third trimester of pregnancy has been reasonably compliant with respect to insulin therapy. Now, however, she has announced her intent to abandon her insulin regimen because she has heard "on the streets" that some drugs are harmful to fetuses. Which option is **not** legally appropriate for the family nurse practitioner, as this patient's health care provider, to consider?

    1. Seek the support of the clinic's attorney to file a petition for court-ordered treatment for the patient.

    2. Attempt to engage the patient in dialogue to provide her with accurate medical information.

    3. Detain the patient in the homeless shelter and administer the insulin, with or without her consent.

    4. Confer with social services to find an appropriate interim placement for the patient until her medical and legal issues can be addressed.

43. What is the purpose of the Americans with Disabilities Act (ADA)?

    1. "Level the playing field" with respect to employment and other opportunities for disabled persons.

    2. Create a federal entitlement program for AIDS patients.

    3. Guarantee wheelchair access to every residential and commercial building.

    4. Authorize interpreters for deaf employees at all private businesses.

44. As a result of the U.S. Supreme Court's ruling on assisted suicide, which of the following is the current state of the law on this topic?

    1. Assisted suicide is still a criminal offense in most jurisdictions.

    2. A physician may prescribe a fatal dose of medication with the concurrence of the ethics committee.

    3. A family nurse practitioner may prescribe a fatal dose of medication with the concurrence of the supervising physician.

    4. A pharmacist may instruct a patient on how to mix and ingest a fatal dose of prescription medication.

45. A professional negligence or medical malpractice case is a civil action. What is the difference between a civil lawsuit and a criminal lawsuit?

    1. The damages sought in a civil suit are monetary; one private party sues another for money.

    2. If convicted in a criminal case, you are still covered by your professional liability insurer.

    3. In a criminal case, your state sues you for money; other penalties do not apply.

    4. In a civil suit, if you do not prevail, you could be incarcerated.

46. Which of the following are forms of alternative dispute resolution (ADR)? Select three responses.

    1. Court or bench trial (judge's decision).

    2. Binding and nonbinding arbitration.

    3. Settlement conference.

    4. Jury trial.

    5. Mediation.

47. Why is it especially important for family nurse practitioners caring for children to have adequate professional liability insurance coverage?

    1. Damages are always higher when a child is the injured party.

    2. Juries tend to award fewer dollars to injured children because the children are eligible for a variety of social programs that cover their medical expenses.

    3. The statute of limitations is often tolled (put on hold) until the minor reaches majority, so the time frame within which the child can file a lawsuit is extended.

    4. Insurers are sensitive to the increased risk posed by minor claimants, so the coverage is difficult to obtain.

48. A health care provider has a duty to disclose certain information to the patient as part of the informed consent process. Exceptions to this duty would include all the following **except**:

    1. The patient has waived the right to receive the data.

    2. It is a bona fide emergency situation.

    3. The provider believes that the information would be harmful to the patient and invokes the therapeutic privilege.

    4. The patient is 80 years old, and older adult persons are unable to comprehend complex medical facts.

49. Before deciding to provide a detailed reference on a former employee, it would be important for the family nurse practitioner to consider which of the following?

    1. The requirements of the human resources department should be determined.

    2. If the comments are perceived as negative and the former employee becomes aware of them, the family nurse practitioner could be subjected to suit for defamation.

    3. If the employee exhibits unsafe patient care practices, it may be wiser to risk legal action from the employee than to subject future patients to this unsafe employee.

    4. All the above.

50. What is the primary purpose of a preemployment physical exam?

    1. Identify existing health problems that might adversely affect the company's insurance rates.

    2. Determine the mental status of the applicant.

    3. Determine if the applicant is physically capable of doing the job.

    4. Document any existing disabilities and recommend accommodations.

51. A family nurse practitioner involved in work-related surveillance knows all employers must report, according to Occupational Safety and Health Administration (OSHA), the following: (Select two responses.)

    1. Keep all OSHA records for 5 years.

    2. Report all work-related fatalities within 8 hours.

    3. Report all work-related inpatient hospitalizations, amputations, and losses of an eye within 24 hours.

    4. Report hospital–employee fatalities occurring 90 days following a work-related incident.

52. When treating a work-related injury, what is the family nurse practitioner required to do?

    1. Document thoroughly because of the high probability of legal action.

    2. Communicate directly with the patient's employer.

    3. File a report with the industrial commission documenting the injury and treatment.

    4. Notify the Occupational Safety and Health Administration (OSHA).

53. Which of the following situations would be considered reportable under the Occupational Safety and Health Administration (OSHA)?

    1. 3-cm abrasion of forearm.

    2. Warehouse worker with back strain reassigned to office work for a week.

    3. Twisted ankle that responded to ice and Ace wrap.

    4. Minor closed-head injury with no loss of consciousness.

54. The purpose of an Occupational Health and Safety Administration (OSHA) 300 log (form) is to record:

    1. Occupational injuries and illnesses.

    2. Only work-related deaths.

    3. Dangerous workplace situations.

    4. Lost work days.

55. The Americans with Disabilities Act (ADA) regulates how employers treat disabled persons. Under the ADA, disability is defined as a physical or mental impairment that substantially limits one or more major life activities of an individual, or a record of a situation in which an individual is regarded as having such an impairment. What would be included under this definition?

    1. History of addiction.

    2. Paralysis.

    3. Bipolar disorder.

    4. All the above.

56. Bioethical practice dilemmas are best described as situations in which proposed treatment alternatives are:

    1. Ranked from most acceptable to least acceptable.

    2. Not appealing to involved parties.

    3. Lacking acceptance by anyone.

    4. Less-than-perfect approaches to the situation.

Issues and Trends

57. The family nurse practitioner understands which of the following about the Health Insurance Portability and Accountability Act (HIPAA) of 1996?

    1. The HIPAA allows health insurance providers to deny insurance to patients because of preexisting medical conditions.

    2. The HIPAA provides easier access to all providers to obtain secure and private health information.

    3. A National Provider Identifier and Employer Identifier facilitates enrollment, eligibility, and claims processing and provides a mechanism to identify a specific provider, insurer, or patient.

    4. Health care organizations, insurers, and payers using electronic storage of patient data and performing claims submission must comply with the Final Rule for National Standards for Electronic Transactions.

58. Considering the four advanced practice roles of the clinical nurse specialist, family nurse practitioner, certified nurse midwife, and nurse anesthetist, which role became accepted by and included into the practice arena without significant controversy?

    1. Clinical nurse specialist.

    2. Family nurse practitioner.

    3. Certified nurse midwife.

    4. Nurse anesthetist.

59. Historically, who was one of the most outspoken opponents of the family nurse practitioner role?

    1. Loretta Ford.

    2. Hildegard Peplau.

    3. Martha Rogers.

    4. Dorothea Orem.

60. Who started the first family nurse practitioner program?

    1. Hildegard Peplau.

    2. Mary Breckenridge.

    3. Agnes McGee.

    4. Loretta Ford.

61. Which is the most important action in developing health policy skills in the family nurse practitioner?

    1. Develop political allies in the U.S. Congress.

    2. Work on a campaign.

    3. Support causes (e.g., teen pregnancy, AIDS).

    4. Write letters and editorials.

62. Which is the least important barrier to collaborative advanced nursing practice?

    1. Prescriptive authority.

    2. Reimbursement privileges.

    3. Legal scope of practice.

    4. Political activism.

63. To obtain reimbursement, the family nurse practitioner must understand which of the following?

    1. MNDS.

    2. ICD-10, CPT, and HCPC codes.

    3. HCPC codes and NANDA diagnoses.

    4. Medicare and Medicaid numbers.

64. According to Kurt Lewin, steps in the change process are as follows:

    1. Unsolving, mobilizing, recruiting, and finalizing.

    2. Building relationships, acquiring resources, choosing solution, and stabilizing.

    3. Unfreezing, moving, and refreezing.

    4. Forming, storming, and norming.

65. What was the major impetus for family nurse practitioner development?

    1. Need for an expert nurse clinician.

    2. Shortage of primary care physicians.

    3. Trend for specialized nurses to diagnose and manage unstable acute and chronic patients.

    4. Movement of graduate nursing education to diagnosis and treatment of major illness.

66. The family nurse practitioner understands that Medicare B provides:

    1. Hospitalization costs for insured patients.

    2. Health insurance benefits for low-income families.

    3. Benefits that cover physicians, family nurse practitioners, medical equipment, and outpatient services.

    4. Outpatient laboratory services, radiography services, and skilled nursing care in appropriate facilities.

67. What was the impact of the Balanced Budget Act of 1997 on family nurse practitioner practice?

    1. Authorized all states to provide family nurse practitioners prescriptive authority.

    2. Provided for only well visits and primary care services.

    3. Prevented a physician from billing 100% for a family nurse practitioner's services.

    4. Allowed direct Medicare payments to family nurse practitioners in both rural and urban settings.

68. In the clinic, the family nurse practitioner must resolve a conflict between two medical assistants. The family nurse practitioner has observed that one assistant is usually pleasant and helpful and the other is often abrasive and angry. What is the most important guideline that the family nurse practitioner must observe in resolving such a conflict?

    1. Require the medical assistants to reach a compromise.

    2. Weigh the consequences of each possible solution.

    3. Encourage ventilation of anger and use humor to minimize the conflict.

    4. Deal with issues, not personalities.

69. A family nurse practitioner approaches his friend, another family nurse practitioner, and tells him that a female physician at the clinic often follows him into the supplies room and tells him how "good looking" he is. Yesterday she patted his hand and said, "I wish we would get to know each other better. I would make it worth your while—better benefits at the clinic, more money." The family nurse practitioner asks his friend, "What do I do? I don't want to date her, but I don't want to lose my job. I just want her to leave me alone." What would be the friend's best reply?

    1. "Tell her that her behavior makes you feel uncomfortable and that you want her to stop."

    2. "Go for it; date her and see if you get what she promises."

    3. "Go to the human relations office at the agency right away and relate to them the entire situation."

    4. "Contact your lawyer and get advice as soon as possible, in case she decides to turn the tables and accuse you of advances."

70. The family nurse practitioner understands that "incident to" services are reimbursed at which percentage?

    1. 75%.

    2. 80%.

    3. 85%.

    4. 100%.

71. What is the purpose of the Agency for Healthcare Research and Quality (AHRQ)?

    1. Develop cost-cutting strategies for health care.

    2. Provide assessment and treatment protocols and algorithms.

    3. Promote health care policy by lobbying efforts.

    4. Produce evidence to make a safer health care that is equitable and affordable.

21 | Professional Issues Answers and Rationales

Legal and Ethical

1. Answer: 2

Rationale: The most important advantage of an occurrence policy is that the coverage is available regardless of how long it takes to become aware of a claim (the long "tail" of a medical malpractice claim). The limits do not automatically increase. The carrier need not be notified during the policy period as is required with claims-made coverage. The coverage under each policy may be as broad as the carrier allows.

2. Answer: 2

Rationale: Fact witnesses and necessary paperwork are always easier to discover the sooner they are sought after a medical misadventure. Memories are fresh, and documents are less likely to be misplaced or destroyed. No rigid reporting window is required by insurance carriers, although they do want to be notified in a timely manner. Insurance premiums may be reduced if the insured's track record is clean (i.e., no claims), but not by mere compliance with policy requirements. Risk management employees prefer early notification so that damage-control efforts may be implemented promptly, not for regulatory reasons.

3. Answer: 2

Rationale: Assessment skills are presumed to be within the purview of the professional nurse, not those with fewer years of nursing education. Also, in this option, the LPN is an unknown entity to the delegator. Delegating to the LPN should be done cautiously after determining that person's skill level. The family nurse practitioner's license is not in jeopardy as they delegated appropriately to the RN, but an error was made and is attributed to the delegatee (RN). Activities such as providing nursing services and intervening when medical assistant personnel exceed their authority are appropriate for the role.

4. Answer: 3

Rationale: The patient's capacity to consent is questionable, so alternatives must be sought. If the patient has a court-appointed guardian, that person is the decision maker. The court has already made a determination of the patient's legal incapacity and appointed the person to whom the nurse will look for consent. If there were no guardian, the family nurse practitioner would analyze whether the patient himself may be able to consent or whether to look to his mother as the most appropriate surrogate decision maker. The group home employee has no automatic legal authority to consent to treatment for any resident.

5. Answer: 4

Rationale: Assisted suicide is still a criminal activity in most states (and in legal limbo in others). Circumventing the patient may seem to be an appealing option, but it substitutes paternalism for the autonomy we all claim as our due. A diagnosis of depression cannot be made with inadequate data; the necessary information can be determined only by conferring with the patient herself.

6. Answer: 2

Rationale: Managed care organizations (MCOs) are one group of health care organizations impacted by this law. All subscribers must be provided with the stated information at the time of enrollment. Advance directive documents, although extremely helpful in the health care setting, are never mandatory.

7. Answer: 4

Rationale: These are the basic requirements for conducting research at health care facilities.

8. Answer: 3

Rationale: Insurance carriers are thoroughly familiar with the processes of handling a claim. They will assist with every step, first by meeting their obligation to put the family nurse practitioner in contact with a lawyer. Conferring with the patient or the patient's lawyer is never a wise move. Colleagues can only offer moral support at this stage; the lawyer is the professional of choice at this time. The family nurse practitioner must never consider altering a record; it can turn a defensible case into a nondefensible one.

9. Answer: 3

Rationale: Lobbying for underserved patients is an example of justice, which is the duty to treat all patients fairly, without regard to age, socioeconomic status, or other variables. Autonomy is the patient's right to self-determination without outside control. Nonmaleficence is the duty to prevent or avoid doing harm, whether intentional or unintentional. Veracity is the duty to tell the truth.

10. Answer: 4

Rationale: These are all valid reasons to protect assets in the event of litigation. In an opposing view regarding the need for professional liability insurance, some professionals think that, if there are few assets to protect, insurance is an unnecessary expense. Family nurse practitioners with professional liability coverage ("deep pockets") could be retained as defendants in a case for a longer time.

11. Answer: 1

Rationale: State law must be examined to define the circumstances under which confidential medical information may be disclosed. There may be additional requirements imposed by federal regulations (e.g., the handling of certain psychiatric records), but the bulk of the rule making on this issue is accomplished at the state level. Exceptions to the requirement of patient consent include communicable disease reporting to public health authorities and court-ordered record production. Third-party payers, although powerful with their fiscal controls, must produce some proof of patient consent to acquire records. An AIDS diagnosis does not shield a record from production, although many states have enacted extra levels of protection for this information. Again, knowledge of state laws is crucial.

12. Answer: 3

Rationale: The Americans with Disabilities Act (ADA) does not protect this population. In fact, employers may test for illegal drug use; this is not considered a medical exam, which ordinarily is subject to specific requirements under the law.

13. Answer: 4

Rationale: These are all ways to achieve satisfaction from a health plan. The family nurse practitioner could also offer to help explain clinical issues to personnel who may not be clinically oriented.

14. Answer: 2

Rationale: The best immediate solution is to identify the item and remove it from service to avoid further patient injury. Then the risk manager, in consultation with the facility's attorneys and insurers, will determine how to proceed with equipment analysis. Returning the item to the manufacturer removes it from the nurse's control and diminishes the opportunity to defend against a charge of user error. Immediate repair may fail to uncover the real cause of the patient injury and impair a successful defense of a claim. If the litigation potential is high, the parties may want to pool their efforts (and costs) to conduct a third-party review of the equipment. If litigation is likely, it is also likely that the manufacturer and others in the distribution chain will be codefendants with the facility and staff.

15. Answer: 2

Rationale: The level of education preferred is that of a master's or doctoral of nursing practice (DNP) degree with family nurse practitioner specialization, not an associate's degree conferred on the technical nurse. The legal issues are the province of the attorneys and the judge; the nurse is expected to be the expert in the clinical issues. Published authorship on nursing issues do add an aura of credibility; specific work experience coupled with the educational credentials are more desirable.

16. Answer: 3

Rationale: The Safe Medical Devices Act (SMDA) of 1990 mandates the regulation and tracking of medical devices. The Administrative Procedures Act (APA) describes the workings of federal agencies. The Patient Self-Determination Act (PSDA) deals with advance directives, and the Omnibus Budget Reconciliation Act (OBRA) of 1987 changed the rule dealing with long-term care.

17. Answer: 4

Rationale: These and other elements combine to produce a program of systematic risk identification, analysis, treatment, and evaluation, with the overall goal of loss prevention.

18. Answer: 4

Rationale: Liability insurance is acquired to protect the organization from suits by patients arising from negligent acts of employees. Business interruption coverage is usually purchased in tandem with fire insurance. It reimburses an organization for losses sustained while the business is partially or completely shut down after a catastrophic event. The organization's management team (CEO and senior staff) is insured against losses based on business judgment errors through directors and officers (D&O) coverage. Workers' compensation is the line of coverage that protects employees after on-the-job injuries. It is a no-fault system (negligence is not a factor) that covers employee medical bills and pays a percentage of wages while an employee is unable to work.

19. Answer: 1

Rationale: You were driving your personal vehicle, so your own auto insurer is "primary" (i.e., responds first to a loss). Because you were on company business, your injuries were sustained "within the course and scope of your employment," so there is coverage under the employer's workers' compensation policy for your medical bills and wage replacement. Depending on the circumstances and policy definitions, there could be some "excess" or additional coverage available under the employer's auto policy, but in no event would that carrier be primarily responsible for your losses. This is not the type of incident that homeowner's insurance is intended to cover. The semitrailer, presumably in use as a business vehicle, would not be insured under a driver's personal auto policy.

20. Answer: 4

Rationale: The intent of the National Practitioner Data Bank (NPDB) is to improve the quality of health care by encouraging state licensing boards, hospitals, and other health care entities and professional societies to identify and discipline those who engage in unprofessional behavior and to restrict the ability of incompetent physicians, dentists, and other health care practitioners to move from state to state without disclosure or discovery of previous medical malpractice payment and adverse action history. Adverse actions can involve licensure, clinical privileges, professional society membership, and exclusions from Medicare and Medicaid.

21. Answer: 1, 2, 4

Rationale: The forwarding facility needs to know whether the receiving facility has space for the new arrival and, more important, the ability to treat the particular illness for which the patient needs therapy. The receiving agency needs to be contacted and agrees on the transfer. The transferring agency must send the patient's medical records. The transfer must be with qualified personnel and transportation equipment. A familiar example of a patient transfer is that of the burn victim, for whom specialty care is mandatory, and the locations of that specialty care are usually limited.

22. Answer: 1

Rationale: Health care policy within the states is codified or enacted into law by the respective state legislature. The state boards of nursing and pharmacy should have significant input in the process, providing the research data and expert "testimony" that the legislature needs to make informed decisions. Nursing organizations should also be willing to provide background information and nurse experts to educate the lawmakers.

23. Answer: 3

Rationale: The managed care organization's (MCO) cost-containment strategy is enhanced if providers practice within the treatment guidelines suggested by the plans. Providers who inform patients that a certain treatment regimen is the preferred alternative create difficulties if that alternative is excluded from coverage. MCOs usually clearly set out the exclusions in the plan documents, and member services personnel are expected to be able to explain the coverage to subscribers. Experimental treatment, if excluded, would be listed as such in the plan documents.

24. Answer: 2

Rationale: These are three of the agencies required to report. Events occurring in the other settings are exempt from reporting requirements under this federal law.

25. Answer: 2

Rationale: This is the most factual note; the writer does not apportion blame or assume liability. The other notes would be "red flags" for a chart reviewer. The mention of an incident report makes it virtually impossible to protect these documents from disclosure, especially in those jurisdictions still affording protection to these internal early warning documents that seek to alert risk management personnel to a potential claim.

26. Answer: 3

Rationale: Patients are often unable to evaluate the quality of the care they receive, but they do react to the way in which the care is delivered. Patient perceptions of rudeness or "uncaring" actions by the provider often spur patients to pursue legal action. Patients tend to be more forgiving of less-than-optimal outcomes if they have been involved in the process and are treated with respect.

27. Answer: 4

Rationale: Making one's own decisions is the basis for informed consent and the ethical underpinning of the Patient Self-Determination Act. "Doing good" (beneficence) and its corollary, "avoiding harm" (nonmaleficence), are ethical principles that are usually cited as the basis for other health care activities, such as maintaining professional competency. Respect for persons is a more global ethical principle supporting much of a nurse's personal philosophy of caring.

28. Answer: 3

Rationale: Usually phrased as duty, breach, proximate cause, and damages, these are the four elements of proof required to prevail in a medical negligence action. Intentional acts are not synonymous with negligent acts. Duty presumes a professional relationship and obligation to provide services. The breach is the error or mistake ascribed to the provider that results in the harm to the patient.

29. Answer: 2

Rationale: A competent adult patient is the person to whom the family nurse practitioner looks for consent to treat. A surrogate decision maker is sought only when the patient is unable to consent. Individual state laws must be checked for selection and priority of surrogate decision makers.

30. Answer: 1

Rationale: Lay jurors are not expected to know the clinical facts and circumstances involved in a professional negligence claim. The expert witness is necessary to educate the jurors about the medical facts and to testify to the standard of care to be applied. Witnesses with direct involvement in the case are no less credible because of their involvement; their testimony and personal bias, if any, will be evaluated by the jurors in the context of their roles.

31. Answer: 1, 2, 3

Rationale: With respect to nursing specialties, the standard of care is usually a national one. Facility policies, books, and journals are important to review, and physician input may be sought. In some cases, physicians may even be allowed to testify about the standard of care. Opinions of other nurse practitioners and current events are not considered a component of expert opinion.

32. Answer: 1, 2, 4

Rationale: One particular advantage of alternative dispute resolution (ADR) is the flexibility of the system. In mediation, for example, the mediator can assist with crafting a solution package that meets all the needs of a party, including such an apology from the health care provider. Money is not always the only answer. Insurers' goals, however, usually do focus on cash, avoiding huge damage awards to plaintiffs. If a mediator is successful in facilitating case settlements, the costs are usually significantly lower than the costs of a court trial. Insurers focusing on the bottom line are not averse to these advantages. Damage awards in the ADR process are generally financial awards. The parties may invest substantial time and money in the ADR process. The arbiter's decision can then be appealed to the district court, which is a disadvantage.

33. Answer: 1

Rationale: Statutes of limitations set out each state's rules for the timing of the filing of lawsuits, including malpractice actions. These statutes are procedural laws in that they describe the "how-to" parameters within which legal rights may be exercised. Minority is considered a legal disability; other state laws usually define it and describe its effects. Rights to sue are not governed by statutes of limitations.

34. Answer: 1, 2, 4

Rationale: Statutes may indeed differ from state to state with respect to the breadth of the protection, but most will protect a family nurse practitioner who renders aid, without expectation of compensation and in a competent manner. Gross negligence will usually void the statutory protections. The family nurse practitioner is not required to stop and render aid.

35. Answer: 2, 3, 4

Rationale: A professional appearance boosts credibility as a witness. Inappropriate attire and gum chewing detract from the family nurse practitioner's professional demeanor. Preparation is critical because the family nurse practitioner's words are recorded and transcribed as part of the official litigation transcript. The family nurse practitioner should review documents but should refrain from bringing any materials to the deposition without the attorney's approval. The nurse should always ask for clarification of ambiguous questions. Speculation is not appropriate, as is trying to use sophisticated language and knowledge to confuse the other attorney. Questions about professional work history are always asked, so a copy of the family nurse practitioner's curriculum vitae (CV) is a useful tool to bring to a deposition.

36. Answer: 2, 3, 4, 5

Rationale: Jousting in the patient's medical record is never a good approach; it provides fodder for plaintiffs' lawyers and does not contribute to quality nursing care. The family nurse practitioner who has a conflict with another provider should deal with the provider directly, preferably in person. Another arena for resolving such disputes is the quality review process. The remaining options are good practice for documentation.

37. Answer: 1, 2, 3

Rationale: All these factors enter into an analysis of whether it is appropriate to accept a minor's consent to treatment. Another factor to consider is the type of treatment sought. Some states have statutes allowing minors to consent to specific therapies, such as treatment for venereal disease. A statement from a third party without supporting documentation to show that the patient is emancipated is not a factor.

38. Answer: 4

Rationale: Long-term care is a specialized area with layers of regulatory requirements, most stemming from the federal government. Nurses who work in this environment need to be vigilant about learning the rules and maintaining compliance. Ongoing, effective communication with regulators is essential.

39. Answer: 4

Rationale: Family nurse practitioners tend to become careless with information management and the way they interact with patients and their personal data. The often wide-open and frantic front desk atmosphere of an office does little to calm patient fears that their information will be too easily accessible to those without a need to know.

40. Answer: 3

Rationale: The co-ed locker room with centerfold photos seems to fit the criteria for a hostile environment, a form of sexual harassment. The harassment seems to be pervasive and longstanding; the women have complained, and apparently no action has been taken. The isolated incident and single date request do not rise to the level of harassment. The participants did not find the actions objectionable, and job performance was not affected. Although the potential was there for the nurse to use the prior relationship either to downgrade the employee or to deny a benefit during the employee performance review, this result did not occur.

41. Answer: 4

Rationale: Advance directives are documents crafted by individuals who personally decide how they wish their future health care decisions are to be handled. The documents must be prepared while the signer is fully capable of understanding their content and importance. Because the wife in this scenario is already comatose, she has missed her opportunity to prepare advance directives. This does not mean that the spouse is unable to decide on her medical treatment, only that a different consent process needs to be employed.

42. Answer: 3

Rationale: The option of detaining the patient would create liability potential for the family nurse practitioner under at least two legal theories, battery and false imprisonment. Talking with the patient would be the first prong of a planned approach to convince this patient that she needs the prescribed medical therapy. Conferring with social services would be the next choice. Court-ordered treatment is a consideration with a viable fetus.

43. Answer: 1

Rationale: This is the overall goal of Americans with Disabilities Act (ADA). It is not another entitlement program, and it cannot impose wheelchair ramp requirements on every building owner in America. Access ramps and interpreters may be required as a "reasonable accommodation" to qualified people in certain defined circumstances. No across-the-board mandate exists for these types of aids to the handicapped population.

44. Answer: 1

Rationale: The U.S. Supreme Court essentially deferred to the states to legislate on this topic. In most states, the activity is not permitted. In one of the states involved in the high court's case, a statute permitting assisted suicide is being challenged. Family nurse practitioners need to look at their state laws on this topic for guidance. The providers referenced in the other options would act at their peril if their state laws followed the current majority view.

45. Answer: 1

Rationale: The purpose of a medical malpractice action is to make the claimant whole by the awarding of money damages. The award compensates the claimant or plaintiff for the wrong (or tort) he or she has suffered at the hands of the defendant.

On the criminal side, the state sues on behalf of society for violations of society's criminal laws. The punishment is fines, imprisonment, or both. Professional liability insurance usually excludes criminal and intentional acts, so coverage for these types of activities is unlikely.

46. Answer: 2, 3, 5

Rationale: The full-blown jury trial and a bench or court trial are what alternative dispute resolution (ADR) seeks to avoid. Mediation and arbitration are the most well-known forms of ADR. Some jurisdictions use the settlement conference as a technique to attempt settlement after a lawsuit has been filed but before a trial begins. ADR hybrids include "med-arb," in which a proceeding starts out as a mediation, but if the case does not settle, it is referred to an arbitrator for resolution.

47. Answer: 3

Rationale: This is the so-called long tail of professional liability; there is always a time lag from the date of injury to the date a claimant files a malpractice action. In the case of an infant, the time lag may be many years because of the statute of limitations. This extends the period of potential risk to the nurse who cares for children. Although a sympathy factor may be involved when jurors decide damage awards, the judgment is usually proportional to the injury and not the age of the claimant. Insurance coverage for pediatric providers is no less available than for other specialties; insurers adjust premiums to account for the level of risk.

48. Answer: 4

Rationale: All patients are entitled to medical information to make an informed decision about treatment. Age, in and of itself, is not an exclusionary criterion. Providers may treat in the other circumstances.

49. Answer: 4

Rationale: If the human resources department has established guidelines for the handling of references, it would be wise to follow them. It is also an effective mechanism to deflect potentially problematic queries by passing requests to the department most equipped to handle them. Most employers will be very circumspect about the information released, often limiting the data to dates of employment only. Without protective state legislation, employers should be prudent about sharing comments on former employees' work histories.

50. Answer: 3

Rationale: The purpose is to determine the appropriateness of the applicant for the job. Identifying health problems to prevent hiring an individual is discriminatory. The mental status and disabilities may also be a part of the pre-employment physical but are not the primary purpose.

51. Answer: 2, 3

Rationale: As of January 1, 2015, the Occupational Safety and Health Administration (OSHA) requires that all employers must report all work-related fatalities within 8 hours and all work-related inpatient hospitalizations, all amputations, and all losses of an eye within 24 hours. Fatalities occurring within 30 days of a work-related incident must be reported to OSHA.

52. Answer: 3

Rationale: It is required by law that a report of any work-related injury be filed with the industrial commission of the state in which the injury occurred.

53. Answer: 2

Rationale: The Occupational Safety and Health Administration (OSHA) requires the report of any injury or illness that requires more than first-aid treatment and/or involves loss of work time, limited work status, loss of consciousness, or death.

54. Answer: 1

Rationale: The purpose of form 300 is to record or log occupational injuries and illnesses, including mortality reports and lost workdays, which could also reveal dangerous working conditions.

55. Answer: 4

Rationale: All the conditions listed would qualify under the Americans with Disabilities Act (ADA) and may require accommodation in the workplace.

56. Answer: 4

Rationale: The crux of a bioethical dilemma is that the proposed solutions are not perfect and, therefore, create some aspect of moral conflict.

Issues and Trends

57. Answer: 4

Rationale: The four major goals of the Health Insurance Portability and Accountability Act (HIPAA) of 1996 are to ensure health insurance portability by eliminating "job-lock" because of preexisting medical conditions, reduce health care fraud and abuse, enforce standards for health information, and guarantee security and privacy of health information. Because of protests from civil libertarians and others concerned about privacy issues, the National Individual Identifier has been put on hold until some compromise can ensure that no abuses of such an identifier system will occur. The first compliance HIPPA rule relates to national standards for electronic transactions.

58. Answer: 1

Rationale: According to the National Commission on Nursing (1983) and the Task Force on Nursing Practice in Hospitals (1983), the clinical nurse specialist (CNS) role was accepted quite rapidly. The psychiatric CNS role is considered the oldest and most highly developed of the CNS specialties and helped initiate the growth of other CNS specialties.

59. Answer: 3

Rationale: Martha Rogers argued that the development of the family nurse practitioner role was a ploy to lure nurses out of nursing and into medicine, thus weakening and undermining nursing's unique role in health care. This led to a major division within nursing, hindering the establishment of family nurse practitioner educational programs within the mainstream of graduate nursing education.

60. Answer: 4

Rationale: Loretta Ford, RN, PhD, and Henry Silver, MD, established the first pediatric nurse practitioner program at the University of Colorado. Hildegard Peplau started the first psychiatric clinical nurse specialist (CNS) program at Rutgers University. Mary Breckenridge established the Frontier Nursing Service in the depressed, rural mountain area of Kentucky, which led to training nurse midwives. Agnes McGee is credited with offering the first postgraduate program for the nurse anesthetist role at St. Vincent's Hospital in Portland, Oregon.

61. Answer: 1

Rationale: Although all these answers are important for the family nurse practitioner in developing policy skills, the most important is developing political allies. Having political allies in decision-making places (legislature) will enable the family nurse practitioner to be active and informed regarding issues of regulation, limitations on admitting privileges and prescriptive authority, and managed care.

62. Answer: 4

Rationale: Three major issues are central to the expansion of the family nurse practitioner role: prescriptive authority, reimbursement privileges, and legal scope of practice. Although political activism is important, it is not specific to collaborative practice.

63. Answer: 2

Rationale: The International Classification of Diseases (ICD-10) diagnostic codes identify the condition, illness, or injury to be treated and are used for billing insurance carriers. Physicians' Current Procedural Terminology (CPT) codes specify the procedure or medical service given. Medicare and state Medicaid carriers are required by law to use CPT codes. The Health Care Financing Administration Common Procedure Coding System (HCPC) is used for reporting supplies and medical equipment. Minimum Nursing Data Set (MNDS) is a classification system of a set of items of essential nursing data with specific definitions and categories related to nursing and nursing care. Having a Medicare and Medicaid number is important, but additional information is required for reimbursement.

64. Answer: 3

Rationale: Lewin described three processes of change. Unfreezing involves "breaking the habit" or "disturbing the equilibrium." Moving involves the development of new responses based on new information, with a change in attitudes, feelings, behaviors, or values. Refreezing involves reaching a new status quo by stabilizing and integrating new behaviors, with appropriate support to maintain the change. Forming, storming, and norming refer to the stages of group process development. Building relationships, acquiring resources, choosing a solution, and stabilizing list steps in Havelock's change theory.

65. Answer: 2

Rationale: According to most sources, the family nurse practitioner role developed as a result of a shortage of primary care physicians in the 1960s and 1970s, when medical specialization was the trend.

66. Answer: 3

Rationale: Medicare B is regulated by the federal government and includes the services described, plus outpatient laboratory and radiography. Hospitalization costs are covered under Medicare A.

67. Answer: 4

Rationale: The Balanced Budget Act is a crucial piece of legislation that allows direct payments to family nurse practitioners at "80% of the lesser of either the actual charge or 85% of the fee schedule amount of the same service if provided by a physician." This does not change the "incident to" rule, which allows a physician to bill for 100% of a family nurse practitioner's services, provided the physician is in the suite at the time of the service and readily available to provide assistance.

68. Answer: 4

Rationale: Conflict must be addressed directly by the family nurse practitioner. The personal characteristics of the medical assistants must not enter into the conflict resolution process. The family nurse practitioner should determine the issue of conflict and then work on possible solutions to resolve the issue. Compromise, in which both parties must be willing to give up something, is only one method of conflict resolution.

69. Answer: 1

Rationale: There are two ways to deal with sexual harassment at work: informally and formally through a grievance procedure. The harassed person should always start with the direct approach and ask the person to **stop.** The male family nurse practitioner should tell the female physician in clear terms that her behavior makes him uncomfortable and that he wants it to stop immediately.

70. Answer: 4

Rationale: The family nurse practitioner is reimbursed at 100% of "incident to" services. Medicare services provided entirely by the family nurse practitioner are reimbursed at 80% of the lesser of the actual charge or 85% of the fee schedule amount of physicians.

71. Answer: 4

Rationale: The Agency for Healthcare Research and Quality's (AHRQ) purpose or mission statement is to produce evidence-based practice and research to make health care safer for all individuals that is of higher quality, more accessible, equitable, and affordable. The AHRQ works within the U.S. Department of Health and Human Services (USDHHS) and with other agencies to make sure that the evidence-based research is understood and used.

Bibliography

Adams, M., Holland, N., & Urban, C. (2014). *Pharmacology for nurses: A pathophysiologic approach* (4th ed.). Boston, MA: Pearson.

Academy of Nurse Practitioners Certification Program (AAN-PCP). (2016). *Candidate handbook and renewal of certification handbook.* Retrieved from http://www.aanpcert.org/ptistore/resource/documents/2016%20Certificant_Candidate_Handbook%20(Final)%2001%2004%2016.pdf.

AGS Beers Criteria for Potentially Inappropriate Medication Use in Older Adult. (2012). *American Geriatrics Society.* Retrieved from http://www.americangeriatrics.org/files/documents/beers/2012AGSBeersCriteriaCitations.pdf.

Allen, P. J., Vessey, J., & Schapiro, N. (2010). *Primary care of the child with a chronic condition* (5th ed.). St. Louis, MO: Mosby.

Alligood, M. R. (2014). *Nursing theory: Utilization and application* (5th ed.). St. Louis, MO: Elsevier.

American Academy of Orthopedic Surgeons. (2015). How to use crutches, canes, and walkers. Retrieved from http://orthoinfo.aaos.org/topic.cfm?topic=a00181.

American Academy of Pediatrics, Report of the Committee on Infectious Diseases. (2015). *Red book* (30th ed.). Elk Grove, IL: American Academy of Pediatrics.

American Academy of Pediatrics. (2015). Car seats: Information for families for 2015. Retrieved from https://www.healthychildren.org/English/safety-prevention/on-the-go/Pages/Car-Safety-Seats-Information-for-Families.aspx?nfstatus=401&nftoken=00000000-0000-0000-0000-000000000000&nfstatusdescription=ERROR:+No+local+token.

American Cancer Society. (2015). What are the risk factors for oral cavity and oropharyngeal cancers? Retrieved from http://www.cancer.org/cancer/oralcavityandoropharyngealcancer/detailedguide/oral-cavity-and-oropharyngeal-cancer-risk-factors.

American Psychiatric Association. (2013). *Diagnostic and statistical manual of mental disorders* (5th ed., text rev.). Arlington, VA: American Psychiatric Association.

American Nurses Credentialing Center (ANCC). (2013). *Certification: General testing and renewal handbook.* Retrieved from http://nursecredentialing.org/GeneralTestingRenewalHandbook.

American Nurses Credentialing Center (ANCC). (2016). *Test content outline.*

American Society of Clinical Oncology. (2015). Head and neck cancer: Risk factors and prevention. Retrieved from http://www.cancer.net/cancer-types/head-and-neck-cancer/risk-factors-and-prevention.

American Society for Colposcopy and Cervical Pathology (ASCCP). (2013). Management guidelines. Retrieved from http://www.asccp.org/Guidelines-2/Management-Guidelines-2.

Anderson, B. (2014). General evaluation of the adult with knee pain. In T. W. Post (Ed.), *UpToDate.* Waltham, MA.

Arabi, Z., Aziz, N. A., Abdul Aziz, A. F., Razali, R., & Wan Puteh, S. E. (2013). Early dementia questionnaire (EDQ): A new screening instrument for early dementia in primary care practice. *BMC Family Practice, 14*(49). http://dx.doi.org/10.1186/1471-2296-14-49.

Askgaard, G., Grønbæk, M., Mette, S., et al. (2015). Alcohol drinking pattern and risk of alcoholic liver cirrhosis: A prospective cohort study. *Journal of Hepatology, 62*(5), 991–1220.

Augenbraun, M. H., & McCormack, W. M. (2015). Urethritis., In J. Mandell., E. Bennett., R. Dolin., & M. J. Blaser (Eds.), *Mandell, Douglas, and Bennett's principles and practice of infectious disease* (8th ed.). (pp. 1349–1357). Philadelphia, PA: Elsevier.

Ball, J., Dains, J., Flynn, J., Solomon, B., & Stewart, R. (2015). *Seidel's guide to physical examination* (8th ed.). St. Louis, MO: Elsevier. Retrieved from http://online.vitalsource.com/#/books/9780323112406/pages/115630823.

Bartlett, J. (2014). Diagnostic approach to community-acquired pneumonia in adults. *UpToDate.* Waltham, MA.

Beitz, J. (1997). Unleashing the power of memory: The mighty mnemonic. *Nurse Educator 22*(2), 25–28.

Bickley, L. S., & Szilagyi, P. G. (2007). *Bates' guide to physical examination* (9th ed.). New York, NY: Lippincott Williams & Wilkins.

Bloomingfield, R. (1982). *Mnemonics, rhetorics, and poetics for medics.* Salem, NC: Harbinger Medical Press.

Burns, C. (2013). *Pediatric primary care* (5th ed.). St. Louis, MO: Elsevier/Saunders.

Buttaro, T., Trybulski, J., Bailey, P., & Sandberg-Cook, J. (2013). *Primary care: A collaborative practice* (4th ed.). St. Louis, MO: Mosby.

Centers for Disease Control and Prevention. (2015). Hepatitis B FAQ's for health professionals. Retrieved from www.cdc.gov/hepatitis/hbv/hbvfaq.htm.

Centers for Disease Control and Prevention. (2016). *Immunization schedules.* Retrieved from http://www.cdc.gov/vaccines/schedules/index.html.

Centers for Disease Control and Prevention. (2015). *Meningococcal vaccination.* Retrieved from http://www.cdc.gov/vaccines/vpd-vac/mening/default.htm.

Centers for Disease Control and Prevention. (2015). *Pneumococcal vaccination.* Retrieved from http://www.cdc.gov/vaccines/vpd-vac/pneumo/default.htm.

Centers for Disease Control and Prevention. (2015). *Shingles (Herpes zoster).* Retrieved from http://www.cdc.gov/shingles/about/transmission.html.

Centers for Disease Control and Prevention. (2014). *Latent tuberculosis infection: A guide for primary health care providers.* Retrieved from http://www.cdc.gov/tb/publications/ltbi/diagnosis.htm#3.

Centers for Disease Control and Prevention. (2012). *Tuberculosis fact sheet.* Retrieved from http://www.cdc.gov/tb/publications/factsheets/testing/skintesting.htm.

Centers for Disease Control and Prevention. (2013). *Varicella vaccination: Information for health care providers.* Retrieved from http://www.cdc.gov/vaccines/vpd-vac/varicella/default-hcp.htm.

Centers for Disease Control and Prevention. (n.d.). *Improving the nation's vision health: A coordinated public health approach.* Retrieved from http://www.cdc.gov/visionhealth/pdf/improving_nations_vision_health.pdf.

Centers for Disease Control and Prevention. (n.d.). *Preventing lead poisoning in young children: Chapter 6.* Retrieved from http://www.cdc.gov/nceh/lead/publications/books/plpyc/chapter6.htm.

Chernecky, C., & Berger, B. (2013). *Laboratory tests and diagnostic procedures* (6th ed.). St. Louis, MO: Saunders.

Chinn, P. L., & Kramer, M. K. (2011). *Integrated theory and knowledge development in nursing* (8th ed.). St. Louis, MO: Mosby.

Chow, A. W., & Doron, S. (2015). Evaluation of acute pharyngitis in adults. In M. D. Aronson (Ed.), *UpToDate.* Waltham, MA.

Creanga, A. A., Shapiro-Mendoza, C. K., Bish, C. L., Zane, S., Berg, C. J., & Callaghan, W. M. (2011). Trends in ectopic pregnancy mortality in the United States: 1980-2007. *Obstetrics & Gynecology, 117*(4), 837–843. http://dx.doi.org/10.1097/AOG.0b013e3182113c10.

Diekema, D. S. (April 29, 2013). (2005). Responding to parental refusals of immunization of children. *Pediatrics, 115*(5), 1428–1431. http://dx.doi.org/10.1542/peds.2013-0430 American Academy of Pediatrics. (2013). Reaffirmed: Responding to parental refusals of immunization of children. *Pediatrics, 131*(5), e1696; originally published online. Retrieved from http://pediatrics.aappublications.org/content/pediatrics/131/5/e1696.full.pdf.

Domino, F. J., Baldor, R. A., Golding, J., & Stephens, M. B. (2015). *The 5 Minute Clinical Consult Standard 2015.* Philadelphia, PA: Wolters Kluwer Health.

Drug Facts. (2014). Hallucinogens – LSD, Peyote, Psilocybin, and PCP. National Institute on Drug Abuse. Retrieved from http://www.drugabuse.gov/publications/drugfacts/hallucinogens-lsd-peyote-psilocybin-pcp.

Dunphy, L. M., Winland-Brown, J. E., Porter, B. O., & Thomas, D. J. (2011). *Primary care: The art and science of advanced practice nursing* (3rd ed.). Philadelphia, PA: F.A. Davis.

Edmunds, M., & Mayhew, M. (2014). *Pharmacology for the primary care provider* (4th ed.). Retrieved from. http://online.vitalsource.com/#/books/9780323087902/pages/232443p963.

El-Ghar, M., Refaie, H., Sharaf, D., & El-Diasty, T. (2014). Diagnosing urinary tract abnormalities: Intravenous urography or CT urography? *Reports in Medical Imaging, 7,* 55–63. http://dx.doi.org/10.2147/RMI.S35592.

Estes, M. (2010). *Health assessment & physical examination* (4th ed.). Independence, KY: Delmar Cengage Learning. 20150728201413179951787.

Faes, M. C., Spigt, M. G., & Rikkert, O. (2007). Dehydration ingeriatrics. *Geriatrics and aging, 10*(9), 590–596.

Ferri, F. (2013). *Ferri's clinical advisor.* St. Louis, MO: Mosby.

Fischer, B. L., Gleason, C. E., Gangnon, R. E., Janczewski, J., Shea, T., & Mahoney, J. E. (2014). Declining cognition and falls: Role of risky performance of everyday mobility activities. *Physical Therapy, 94*(3), 355–362.

Freda, M. C. (2004). Issues in patient education. *Journal of Midwifery & Women's Health, 49,* 203–209. http://dx.doi.org/10.1016/S1526-9523(04)00004-2.

Fuller, K. (2014). Diagnosis of testicular cancer. *Journal for Nurse Practitioners, 10*(6).

Garcia-Tsao, G., Sanyal, A. J., Grace, N. D., et al. (2007). Prevention and management of gastroesophageal varices and variceal hemorrhage in cirrhosis. *Hepatology, 46*(3), 922–938.

Garneau, A. M. (2015). Nursing theory. In J. Zerwekh & A. M. Garneau (Eds.), *Nursing today: Transition and trends* (pp. 170–187). St. Louis, MO: Elsevier.

Gilbert, D. N., Chambers, H. F., Eilopoulos, G. M., & Saag, M. S. (2015). *The Sanford guide to antimicrobial therapy 2015* (45th ed.). Sperryville, VA: Antimicrobial Therapy, Inc.

Global Initiative for Asthma. (2015). *Pocket guide for asthma management and prevention.* Retrieved from http://www.ginasthma.org/.

Global Initiative for Chronic Obstructive Lung Disease. (2015). *Global strategy for the diagnosis, management, and prevention of chronic obstructive pulmonary disease.* Retrieved from http://goldcopd.com/guidelines-global-strategy-for-diagnosis-management.html.

Gomella, L. G. (2010). *The 5 minute urology consult* (2nd ed.). Philadelphia, PA: Lippincott Williams & Wilkins.

Grove, S. K., Gray, J. R., & Burns, N. (2015). *Understanding nursing research: Building an evidence-based practice* (6th ed.). St. Louis, MO: Elsevier.

Grove, S. K., Burns, N., & Gray, J. R. (2013). *The practice of nursing research: Appraisal, synthesis, and generation of evidence* (7th ed.). St. Louis, MO: Elsevier.

Hall, M. A. (2013). Sinusitis. In T. M. Buttaro, J. Trybulski, P. P. Bailey, & J. Sandberg-Cook (Eds.), *Primary care: A collaborative practice* (pp. 376–379). St. Louis, MO: Elsevier.

Halter, J. G., Ouslander, J. G., Tinetti, M. E., Studenski, S., High, K. P., & Asthana, S. (2009). *Hazzard's geriatric medicine and gerontology* (6th ed.). New York, NY: McGraw-Hill.

Hamric, A. B., Hanson, C. M., Tracy, M. F., & O'Grady, E. T. (2014). *Advanced practice nursing: An integrative approach* (5th ed.). St. Louis, MO: Elsevier.

Hartig, M. T. (2013). Otitis media. In T. M. Buttaro, J. Trybulski, P. P. Bailey, & J. Sandberg-Cook (Eds.), *Primary care: A collaborative practice* (pp. 359–363). St. Louis, MO: Elsevier.

Heller, J. (2013). Heroin overdose. *U.S. National Library of Medicine: Medline Plus.* Retrieved from http://www.nlm.nih.gov/medlineplus/ency/article/002861.htm.

Hill, D. L. (2015). Infant constipation. Retrieved from https://healthychildren.org/English/ages-stages/baby/diapers-clothing/Pages/Infant-Constipation.aspx.

Hsu, S., Le, E., & Khoshevis, M. (2001). Differential diagnosis of annular lesions. *American Family Physicians, 64*(2), 289–297.

Hwang, P. H., & Patel, Z. M. (2015). Acute sinusitis and rhinosinusitis in adults: Treatment. In D. G. Deschler & S. B. Calderwood (Eds.), *UpToDate.* Waltham, MA.

Institute of Medicine. (2009). *Weight gain during pregnancy: Reexamining the guidelines.* Retrieved from http://iom.nationalacademies.org/~/media/Files/Report%20Files/2009/Weight-Gain-During-Pregnancy-Reexamining-the-Guidelines/Report%20Brief%20-%20Weight%20Gain%20During%20Pregnancy.pdf.

Isaac, A. (2015). Treatment of neck pain. In T. W. Post (Ed.), *UpToDate*. Waltham, MA.

Jacobs, D. S. (2015). Cataract in adults. In J. Trobe (Ed.), *UpToDate*. Waltham, MA.

Jacobs, D. S. (2015). Open-angle glaucoma. In J. Trobe (Ed.), *UpToDate*. Waltham, MA.

Jacobs, D. S. (2015). Photokeratitis. In J. Trobe (Ed.), *UpToDate*. Waltham, MA.

James, P. A., Oparil, S., Carter, B. L., et al. (2014). Evidence-based guideline for the management of high blood pressure in adults: Report from the panel members appointed to the Eighth Joint National Committee (JNC8). *JAMA, 311*(5), 507–520. http://dx.doi.org/10.1001/jama.2013.284427.

Jarvis, C. (2016). *Physical examination & health assessment* (7th ed.). St. Louis, MO: Elsevier.

Kaji, A., & Hockberger, R. (2015). Evaluation of thoracic and lumbar spinal column injury. In T. W. Post (Ed.), *UpToDate*. Waltham, MA.

Keltner, N., & Steele, D. (2015). *Psychiatric nursing* (7th ed.). (pp. 401–417). St. Louis: Elsevier/Mosby Retrieved from http://online.vitalsource.com/#/books/9780323185790/pages/226796402.

Kern, B., & Rosh, A. J. (2014). Hyperventilation syndrome treatment & management. Retrieved from http://emedicine.medscape.com/article/807277-treatment#d10 .

Kossler, A. L., & Banta, J. T. (2013). Blepharitis, hordeolum, and chalazion. In T. M. Buttaro, J. Trybulski, P. P. Bailey, & J. Sandberg-Cook (Eds.), *Primary care: A collaborative practice* (pp. 324–326). St. Louis, MO: Elsevier.

Kozy, M., & Halter, M. (2014). Depressive disorders. In M. Halter (Ed.), *Varcarolis' foundations of psychiatric mental health nursing: A clinical approach* (7th ed.). (pp. 249–276). Retrieved from http://online.vitalsource.com/#/books/978-1-4557-5358-1/pages/163134622.

Lemaine, V., Cayci, C., Simmons, P., & Petty, P. (2013). Gynecomastia in adolescent males. *Seminars in Plastic Surgery, 27*(1), 56–61.

LoBiondo-Wood, G., & Haber, J. (2014). *Nursing research: Methods and critical appraisal for evidence-based practice* (8th ed.). St. Louis, MO: Mosby.

Logical Images (2013). *Psoriasis*. Retrieved from http://www.skinsight.com/adult/psoriasis.htm.

Lowdermilk, D. L., Perry, S. E., Cashion, K., & Alden, K. R. (2016). *Maternity & women's health care* (11th ed.). St. Louis, MO: Elsevier.

Mandell, L. A., Wunderink, R. G., Anzueto, A., Bartlett, J. G., Campbell, G. D., Dean, N. C., & Whitney, C. G. (2007). Infectious Diseases Society of America/American Thoracic Society consensus guidelines on the management of community-acquired pneumonia in adults. *Clinical Infectious Diseases, 1* (44) (Suppl 2), S27–S72.

Marcdante, K. J., & Kliegman, R. M. (2015). *Nelson essentials of pediatrics* (7th ed.). St. Louis, MO: Saunders.

Margulis, V., & Sagalowsky, A. I. (2011). Assessment of hematuria. *Medical Clinics of North America, 95*, 153–159.

Mast, E. E., Margolis, H. S., Fiore, A. E., et al. (2005). A comprehensive immunization strategy to eliminate transmission of hepatitis B virus infection in the United States. Recommendations of the Advisory Committee on Immunization Practices. National Center of Infectious Diseases, Division of Viral Hepatitis. *MMWR, 54*(RR-16), 1–37.

Maughan, K. (2015). Ankle sprain. In T. W. Post (Ed.), *UpToDate*. Waltham, MA.

McCaffrey, R., & Youngkin, E. Q. (2014). *NP notes* (2nd ed.). Philadelphia, PA: F.A. Davis.

McCance, K., & Huether, S. (2015). *Pathophysiology: The biological basis for disease in adults and children* (7th ed.). St. Louis, MO: Elsevier.

McDonagh, A. F. (2011). Bilirubin, copper-porphyrins and bronze baby syndrome. *Journal of Pediatrics, 158*(1), 160–164.

Merriam-Webster Medical Dictionary. (2015). *Erythroplasia*. Retrieved from http://www.merriam-webster.com/medical/erythroplasia.

Michaelson, M. D., & Oh, W. K. (2015). Epidemiology of and risk factors for testicular germ cell tumors. In P. W. Kantoff & M. E. Ross (Eds.), *UpToDate*. Waltham, MA.

Mitchell, L. (2012). Long QT syndrome and torsades de pointes ventricular tachycardia. *Merck Manuals*. Retrieved from http://www.merckmanuals.com/professional/cardiovascular-disorders/arrhythmias-and-conduction-disorders/long-qt-syndrome-and-torsades-de-pointes-ventricular-tachycardia.

Mohan, R., & Schellhammer, P. F. (2011). Treatment options for localized prostate cancer. *American Family Physician, 84*(4), 414–420.

Munsell, D. S. (2013). Pharyngitis and tonsillitis. In T. M. Buttaro, J. Trybulski, P. P. Bailey, & J. Sandberg-Cook (Eds.), *Primary care: A collaborative practice* (pp. 399–403). St. Louis, MO: Elsevier.

Murphree, D. D., & Thelen, S. M. (2010). Chronic kidney disease in primary care. *Journal of the American Board of Family Medicine, 22*(4), 542-440. Retrieved from http://www.jabfm.org/content/23/4/542.long.

National Cancer Institute. (2013). Head and neck cancers. Retrieved from http://www.cancer.gov/types/head-and-neck/head-neck-fact-sheet#q1.

National Institutes of Health, National Cholesterol Education Program Expert Panel. (2001). *Detection, evaluation and treatment of high blood cholesterol in adults (Adult Treatment Panel III)*. Retrieved from http://www.nhlbi.nih.gov/files/docs/guidelines/atp3xsum.pdf.

National Institute of Neurological Disorders and Stroke. (n.d.). *Febrile seizures fact sheet*. Retrieved from http://www.ninds.nih.gov/disorders/febrile_seizures/detail_febrile_seizures.htm.

Niederhuber, J. E. (2014). *Abeloff's clinical oncology* (5th ed.). Philadelphia, PA: Elsevier.

Nopper, A., Markus, R., & Esterly, N. (1998). When it's not ringworm: Annular lesions of childhood. *Pediatrics Annuals, 27*(3), 136–148.

O'Connor, P. (2008). Cocaine. *Merck manual*. Retrieved from http://www.merckmanuals.com/professional/special-subjects/drug-use-and-dependence/cocaine.

Pezaro, C., Woo, H. H., & Davis, I. D. (2014). Prostate cancer: Measuring PSA. *Internal Medicine Journal, 44*(5), 433–440.

Rayner, A., O'Brien, J., & Schoenbachler, B. (2006). Behavior disorders of dementia: Recognition and treatment. *American Family Physician, 73*(4), 647–652. Retrieved from http://www.aafp.org/afp/2006/0215/p647.html.

Remedy Health Media. (2015). Allergy testing overview, types of allergy tests. Retrieved from http://www.healthcommunities.com/allergy-testing/overview-types-of-allergy-tests.shtml.

Rich, P., & Jefferson, J. (2015). Overview of nail disorder. In T. W. Post (Ed.), *UpToDate*. Waltham, MA.

Ross, D. S. (2015). Overview of the clinical manifestations of hyperthyroidism in adults. In D. S. Cooper (Ed.), *UpToDate*. Waltham, MA.

Schrier, S., & Camaschella, C. (2015). Anemia of chronic disease. In T. W. Post (Ed.), *UpToDate*. Waltham, MA.

Seidel, H. M., Ball, J. W., Dains, J. E., Flynn, J. A., Solomon, B. S., & Stewart, R. W. (2011). *Mosby's guide to physical exam* (7th ed.). St. Louis, MO: Elsevier.

Silberberg, C. (2013). Nephrotic syndrome. *MedlinePlus Encyclopedia*. Retrieved from http://www.nlm.nih.gov/medlineplus/ency/article/000490.htm.

Simon, R. S., Baker, C., Barden, G. A., III. Brown, O. W., Hardin, A., Lessin, H. R., Meade, K., Moore, S., & Rodgers, C. T. (2014). 2014 Recommendations for pediatric preventive health care. *Pediatrics*, *133*(3), 568. Retrieved from http://pediatrics.aappublications.org/content/pediatrics/133/3/568.full.pdf.

Simpson, K. R., & Creehan, P. A. (2014). *Perinatal nursing* (4th ed.). Philadelphia, PA: Wolters Kluwer/Lippincott Williams & Wilkins.

Smith, R. J. H., & Gooi, A. (2015). Hearing impairment in children: Evaluation. In G. C. Isaacson (Ed.), *UpToDate*. Waltham, MA.

Stanford School of Medicine. (2015). *Fundoscopic exam*. Retrieved from http://stanfordmedicine25.stanford.edu/th25/fundoscopic.html.

Swantz, M. H. (2014). *Textbook of physical diagnosis* (7th ed.). Philadelphia, PA: Elsevier.

Taketomo, C. K., Hodding, J. H., & Kraus, D. M. (2014). *Pediatric & neonatal dosage handbook*. Hudson, OH: Lexi-Comp, Inc.

U.S. Department of Health & Human Services. (2015). Office for Human Research Protections (OHRP). Retrieved from http://www.hhs.gov/ohrp/policy/consentckls.html.

U.S. Department of Health & Human Services, National Institutes of Health, National Kidney and Urologic Diseases Information Clearinghouse. (2007). Urinary incontinence in men (NIH Publication No. 07-5280). Retrieved from http://www.niddk.nih.gov/health-information/health-topics/urologic-disease/urinary-incontinence-in-men/Documents/uimen_508.pdf.

U.S. Preventive Services Task Force. (2013). Final recommendation statement lung cancer screening. Retrieved from Published Recommendations. http://www.uspreventiveservicestaskforce.org/Page/Document/RecommendationStatementFinal/lung-cancer-screening.

U.S. Preventive Services Task Force. (2012). Final recommendation statement prostate cancer: Screening, May 2012. U.S. Preventive Services Task Force. (2012). Retrieved from http://www.uspreventiveservicestaskforce.org/Page/Document/RecommendationStatementFinal/prostate-cancer-screening.

U.S. Preventive Services Task Force. (2011). Final Recommendation Statement Testicular Cancer: Screening, April 2011. Retrieved from http://www.uspreventiveservicestaskforce.org/Page/Document/RecommendationStatementFinal/testicular-cancer-screening.

Varcarolis, E. (2014). Communication and the clinical interview. In M. Halter (Ed.), *Varcarolis' foundations of psychiatric mental health nursing: A clinical approach* (7th ed.) (pp. 147–165). Retrieved from http://online.vitalsource.com/#/books/978-1-4557-5358-1/pages/163133636.

Vasavada, S. P. (2014). Urinary incontinence: Practice essentials, background, anatomy. *Medscape reference: Drugs, diseases & procedures*. Retrieved from http://emedicine.medscape.com/article/452289-overview.

Wallace, M., & Fulmer, T. (2008). Fulmer SPICES: An overall assessment tool for older adults. *Annals of Long Term Care*, *15*(3). Retrieved from http://www.annalsoflongtermcare.com/article/6911.

Weber, P. C. (2000). Noise-induced hearing loss. *American Family Physician*, *61*(9), 2749–2756.

Wein, A. J., Kavoussi, L. R., Novick, A. C., Partin, A. W., & Peters, C. A. (2012). *Campbell-Walsh urology* (10th ed.). Philadelphia, PA: Elsevier.

Weizer, J. S. (2015). Angle-closure glaucoma. In J. Trobe (Ed.), *UpToDate*. Waltham, MA.

Williams, M. E. (2007). Examining the ears, nose and oral cavity in the older patient. Retrieved from http://www.medscape.org/viewarticle/556144_2.

Wolf, J. S. (2014). Nephrolithiasis treatment & management. *Medscape: Drugs and diseases*. Retrieved from http://emedicine.medscape.com/article/437096-overview.

Woo, T., & Robinson, M. (2015). *Pharmacotherapeutics for advanced practice nurse prescribers* (4th ed.). Philadelphia, PA: F.A. Davis.

World Health Organization. (2014). Children: Reducing mortality. Retrieved from http://www.who.int/mediacentre/factsheets/fs178/en/.

Youngkin, E. Q., Davis, M. S., Schadewald, D. M., & Juve, C. (Eds.). (2013). *Women's health: A primary care clinical guide* (4th ed.) Upper Saddle River, NJ: Pearson/Prentice Hall.

Zerwekh, J. (2016). Test-taking strategies. In *NCLEX-RN®: A comprehensive study guide* (9th ed.). St. Louis, MO: Elsevier.

Zerwekh, J., Garneau, A. M., & Miller, C. J. (2016). *Memory notebook of nursing*, CD. Chandler, AZ: Nursing Education Consultants, Inc.